Physiological Chemistry
of
Domestic Animals

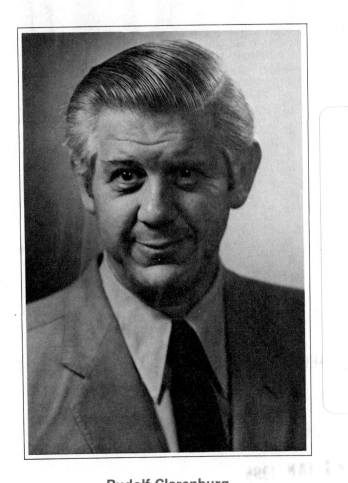

Rudolf Clarenburg

(1931-1991)

Physiological Chemistry
of
DOMESTIC ANIMALS

Rudolf Clarenburg, Ph.D.

Professor of Physiological Chemistry
Department of Anatomy and Physiology
Kansas State University
College of Veterinary Medicine
Manhattan, Kansas

with 317 illustrations

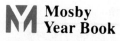
**Mosby
Year Book**

St. Louis   Baltimore   Boston   Chicago   London   Philadelphia   Sydney   Toronto

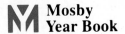
Mosby
Year Book

Dedicated to Publishing Excellence

Editor: Robert W. Reinhardt
Assistant editor: Melba Steube
Project supervisor: Barbara Bowes Merritt
Cover design: Susan Lane

Editing and production: The Bookmakers, Incorporated

Cover photo montage: *Cat* © Geoffrey Gove,
The National Audubon Society Collection/Photo Researchers, Inc.
Electron orbitals of hydrogen, carbon and iron atoms © Dave Parker,
SPL/Photo Researchers, Inc.

Printed in the United States of America.

Mosby-Year Book, Inc.
11830 Westline Industrial Drive
St. Louis, Missouri 63146

Library of Congress Cataloging in Publication Data

Clarenburg, Rudolf.
    Physiological chemistry of domestic animals/Rudolf Clarenburg.
        p.   cm.
    Includes index.
    ISBN 0-8016-6953-7
    1. Veterinary physiology.   2. Biochemistry.   I. Title.
SF768.C55   1992
636.089'2015—dc20   92-1334
                                                              CIP

92 93 94 95 96 GW/MV 9 8 7 6 5 4 3 2 1

RUDOLF CLARENBURG
(1931-1991)

Rudolf (Rudy) Clarenburg was born on May 3, 1931, in Utrecht, The Netherlands. He graduated from the State University of Utrecht in both Pharmacy and Chemistry, and went on to earn a Ph.D. with specializations in Physiological Chemisty and Radiochemistry (the latter at the Institute for Nuclear Research in Amsterdam). After immigrating to the United States in 1959, he became a research associate in the Department of Physiology, University of California at Berkeley, collaborating with Professor I.L. Chaikoff in the area of lipid metabolism and its disorders. Following seven years at the University of California, he became a U.S. citizen and accepted a professorial appointment in the Department of Anatomy and Physiology at Kansas State University's College of Veterinary Medicine, where he remained until his death in 1991.

Professor Clarenburg designed and taught courses in physiological chemistry, intermediary metabolism, research methods involving radioisotopes, and veterinary physiology for both graduate and veterinary students for more than twenty years. He wrote many publications in several areas of research, including metabolism of cholesterol and plant sterols, pharmacokinetics and metabolism of chloramphenicol, differences between embolic occlusion and mechanical ligation of blood circulation with regard to paralytic effects, transport of organic anions (e.g., bilirubin) across the liver cell plasma membrane and into bile, and hepatic and bacterial glycoprotein receptors.

Recognized by both colleagues and students as an outstanding and dedicated academician and teacher, Professor Clarenburg received the Norden Distinguished Teacher Award "for distinguished teaching in the field of veterinary medicine" in 1983. He could often be found in his office until the wee hours of the morning preparing for a lecture on intermediary metabolism, and his door was always open to any student wanting help. Professor Clarenburg's affinity for teaching stemmed from his love for learning, and he delighted in mastering all he could about the science of education. Classical guitar playing, comparative religious studies, and running were other favorite pursuits. Possessing a keen sense of humor and an extraordinary capacity for scholarly work, he was continually supported in this regard by two gracious and intelligent people, his wife Margalith and his son Nathan, both of whom deserve much credit for seeing this text through to its completion following his death.

Professor Rudy Clarenburg, a man who will be missed by his family, students, colleagues, and friends all over the world, has left us this text as his scientific legacy, so that memory of him and his teaching will survive.

Foreword

Physiological Chemistry of Domestic Animals is a practically oriented, concisely written, richly illustrated text designed to serve students of veterinary medicine, animal science, biochemistry, nutrition and mammalian physiology. Self-test questions of varying depths appear at the end of each chapter, with answers in the back of the book for questions that require information beyond the scope of this text.

Professor Clarenburg's text is organized to discuss general homeostatic control mechanisms over the animal's internal environment first at the cellular level, then at the organismic level. Throughout the text, topics are taken from the "global" picture of the whole animal, dissected, then put back into context before other topics are introduced. Because of this, a student who loses a few trees on the way still does not lose sight of the more global forest.

Although there is considerable overlap in two of the basic biomedical disciplines, physiology and biochemistry, Professor Clarenburg rightfully recognized long ago that most physiology texts fail to cover the field of physiological chemistry adequately and that biochemistry texts, in general, are not physiologically oriented:

Biochemistry texts tend to emphasize mechanistic aspects of reactions and pathways for their own sake in an attempt to prepare students for subsequent research in the field. However, few attempts are successfully made to integrate material into a picture of the whole animal; consequently, veterinary students most often leave their first year biochemistry and physiology courses with only fragmented bits of biochemical information which they are ill-equipped to apply to real-life situations.

He therefore directed his attention to the task of creating a text that would integrate relevant principles in both physiology and biochemistry, while at the same time retaining a practical focus on the whole animal:

My book on physiological chemistry is whole-animal oriented, and the material is presented in a form which is relevant and applicable to the intact organism. I believe that there is no comparable text (in the English language) available today.

Textbooks in physiology, biochemistry, or any other basic medical-science discipline cannot possibly be kept up to the minute, for they will inevitably run a losing race with the research reported in periodical literature. Nevertheless, Professor Clarenburg has clearly expended every effort to supplement established knowledge with current facts, theories, and hypotheses, insofar as this is possible, with full awareness I am sure that in some respects, obsolescence commences with the date of publication (if not before). This may be of more concern to the researcher, however, than to the student; and for that reason the former should take recourse to the original articles that augment basic concepts presented in this text.

Professor Clarenburg's sudden death in 1991 took away a dedicated teacher and scholar who will be missed by those of us who were fortunate enough to have benefited from his friendship and teaching. This work, his important contribution to veterinary science education, is in itself a fitting memorial. I have been privileged to work closely with the Clarenburg family, and Mosby–Year Book, Inc. during the final editorial stages of this book's development. While I have found the superb writings of Professor Clarenburg to be a renewed biochemical education for myself, I am also convinced that students who use this text will find their way through the maze of biochemical pathways a little easier because of his unique and effective organizational approach to the teaching of physiological chemistry.

Larry R. Engelking
Director of Contract Research;
Associate Professor of Medicine and Physiology
Tufts Veterinary School

Preface

The days of simply dispensing information to students are coming to an end. We cannot cope with the ongoing information explosion. It has been shown that students forget over 80% of factual information within one year; moreover, such information is available to students on computer disk. Traditional methods of teaching fail to train our students to synthesize ideas and solve problems. Clearly the focus of science education must be redirected. The best an instructor can hope to do is instill in students the desire to learn, a desire that derives from a sense of relevance, and then equip them with the tools for self-education.

This textbook offers a practical, functional approach to the live organism. In approaching each new process, it first seeks to answer the physiological questions. What is its function? Why do we need it? Then it looks into some of the biochemical background. How does it work? The combination of those questions, physiological chemistry, encourages learning about control. What factors (neuroendocrine, nutritional) are needed for control? How does lack of control manifest itself in a patient (diagnostics)? What can be done to regain control (therapy)?

Students enter veterinary or graduate school with a substantial knowledge-base and learning experience from their previous education. My objective in this book is to broaden that undergraduate knowledge-base to the point where students who have completed a year of graduate or professional training in veterinary and animal-health sciences, can read their professional literature and continue educating themselves. I aim to prepare theses students for a lifelong habit of self-education and to get them started in applying their information to clinical and research situations — a process that continues during the final years of formal education.

This is no all-inclusive tome into which the author packs everything he thinks we know today and through which the student is left to wade, sifting the debris in an effort to find what he or she is after. Since freshman students in either professional or graduate curricula spend so much time in classrooms and laboratories, they need a text in which relevant principles are succinctly explained and applied. This text provides a common denominator of applied medical science, addressing primarily the needs of students in veterinary medicine, mammalian physiology, animal sciences, and biology. For more elementary materials, the student is referred to textbooks used in prerequisite undergraduate courses. Instructors may add specialty areas such as pregnancy, lactation, neonatal metabolism, exercise, hibernation, aging, and nutrition. Those can be studied independently once the student has a good understanding of basics. For example, I have introduced in my course student-led journal laboratories in which a current publication of a clinical case with solid physiological underpinnings is discussed. This lays a bridge between clinics and preclinical sciences; it also gives students an active role in their/our learning.

I have compiled appropriate topics and abstracted the pertinent current literature. But where this text leaves off, students must find their own ways to keep up with the literature. For that purpose, I have listed at the end of the text some key journals that follow recent developments in biological and animal health–related sciences. A listing of databases is meant to encourage the use of computers for literature searching and updating.

The text has evolved from syllabi for 90-hour physiological chemistry courses in professional veterinary and graduate programs. It was written with the idea in mind that students taking several courses concurrently may be too pressed for time to look up referred texts. For that reason, short paragraphs are sometimes repeated; repetition of a topic in a different context may be beneficial for reinforcement. The text is intended to be read consecutively from cover to cover.

Study questions following each chapter are meant for group discussion. Answers that cannot readily be found in the text, even using the index, are given at the end of the book. Students are encouraged to use the general metabolism charts to trace their lines of reasoning in answering study questions.

I have included ruminant metabolism because I believe that learning comparative metabolism strengthens students' understanding of meatbolism in general (much as learning a foreign language enhances appreciation of one's native tongue). Besides, the ruminant is of interest in its own right for students in veterinary medicine and animal sciences.

It is with a sense of humility that I am releasing this text. I am well aware that my position as author prevents me from being perceived as the student I feel I really am. I owe a debt of gratitude to three decades of fellow-students who have taught me most of what they think I know about teaching. I shall be indebted to all who will take the time to make corrections or suggestions for improvement so that my text may meet the expectations of students interested in the health and science of domestic animals.

Rudolf Clarenburg

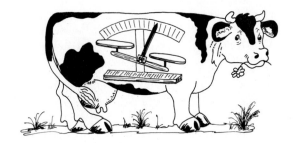

Contents

6 Cell surface phenomena, 92

7 Blood: composition and function, 125

8 Body fluids: volume, electrolytes, and acid-base homeostasis, 154

9   Gastrointestinal functions, 203

10   Introduction to metabolism, 218

11   Biological oxidation and energy metabolism, 223

12   Carbohydrate metabolism, 239

13 Lipid metabolism, 292

14 Nitrogen metabolism, 334

15 Whole body metabolism, 349

16 Nutritional energy requirements, 373

17 Comparative ruminant metabolism, 381

APPENDIXES

1 Introduction

DIRECTIVES AND OBJECTIVES

Physiology is a practical, functional approach to the understanding of the workings of nature. Therefore, when dealing with a subject in physiology, the first questions asked are, Why is it needed? What is its function? What controls it? What is needed to make it function normally? Then follows an exploration into the actual workings, into the How does it work? Unlike biochemistry, which emphasizes singular mechanistic answers to the "how" question, physiological chemistry concerns itself more with integrated, functional applications.

The following general outline of the field will be used. For proper orientation, the concept of homeostasis in the intact organism will be stressed. This text shows how animals are subject to the familiar laws of chemistry and physics but are able to adapt to their environment by means of their neuroendocrine system, which senses signals and transmits stimuli for adaptive actions to target tissues. The response of tissue cells to neuroendocrine stimuli, via cell surface phenomena, second messengers, and the activation of key enzyme activities is discussed in the context of cell physiology. Protein synthesis and the medical applications of genetic manipulations are also discussed. Turning then to the homeostatic maintenance of the composition of blood and other body fluids, the text focuses on erythrocytes' oxygen carrying capacity and metabolic properties, Na^+, K^+, Ca^{++}, HCO_3^-, Cl^-, water, phosphate, and acid-base balance in the context of which the functioning of

the kidneys is considered. After reviewing the metabolic functions of the gastrointestinal tract, there are discussions of intermediary metabolism with emphases on physiologic control, the metabolic functions of liver, fat cells, muscles, and other tissues and glands, nutritionally essential cofactors, and medical applications. Finally, intermediary metabolism in ruminants and monogastrics is compared.

The reader should focus on the following three objectives:

- Ability to read professional literature. Meeting this objective will allow for self-education and staying current with recent developments.
- Ability to condense a topic into a few words (or pictures) that can be remembered and used.
- Ability to apply physiological chemistry to neighboring areas such as pharmacology, nutrition, and clinical pathology.

To meet those objectives, the reader should do the following:

- Learn technical terms with their defined meanings and spellings.
- Reduce concepts to one-word or one-sentence abstracts where possible.
- Attach examples or applications to every new concept.
- Work through the study questions.

This text follows the mainstream of physiological chemistry. Prerequisite background information for the insufficiently prepared reader should be obtained from specialized textbooks. The student wanting more specialized, advanced material should consult the instructor. Literature recommended in conjunction with this text includes recent editions of (i) *Harper's Review of Biochemistry*: Martin, Mayes, and Rodwell, Lange; (ii) *Human Physiology: foundations and frontiers*: Schauf, Moffett, and Moffett, Mosby–Year Book, Inc.; and (iii) *Principles of Biochemistry, Mammalian Biochemistry*: Smith et al., McGraw-Hill.

THE GLOBAL PICTURE

The place and function of mammalian life within the framework of the biological universe (Figure 1-1) are best summarized by the ancient Greek maxim, "Everything flows; nothing stands still." Oxygen, food, and nitrogenous compounds needed to sustain mammalian life are obtained from plants, which, in turn, utilize the waste products of mammalian metabolism (CO_2, H_2O, and nitrogenous wastes) in a perpetual cycle. Thus mammalian life is in a state of flux: there is a continuous turnover of chemical and anatomical structures within the body. The same carbon, oxygen, hydrogen, and nitrogen atoms that once were created are still cycling around, since chemistry does not change the nuclei of atoms. Mammalian body chemistry simply borrows electrons from nutrients (via metabolic pathways), and sends that electrical current over the electron transport chain (maintained within mitochondria of cells) in order to generate energy. The electrons are then recycled by oxygen in the form of CO_2 and H_2O.

Solar energy, harvested at the sites of photosynthesis, drives mammalian life processes and is dissipated as metabolic heat loss and as continuous demise of the products of physical activity (see Figure 1-1). From this energy flowing through the body, enough is harvested to fuel the energy-consuming, or uphill, processes of life. However, it should be realized that for each uphill process there must be an energy-releasing, or downhill, process to drive it. Putting that more technically: an uphill process is never found without a corresponding downhill process, except in **isolated systems** where they are taken out of their biological context. Fat synthesis from acetate (uphill) is energetically driven by glucose conversion to acetate (downhill). While looking at the ascending limb of a water siphon, one only sees water going uphill; therefore, one is studying an isolated system.

This dynamic picture of mammalian life as a state of flux must never be forgotten. It shows the need for a constant supply of nutrient energy to keep life's

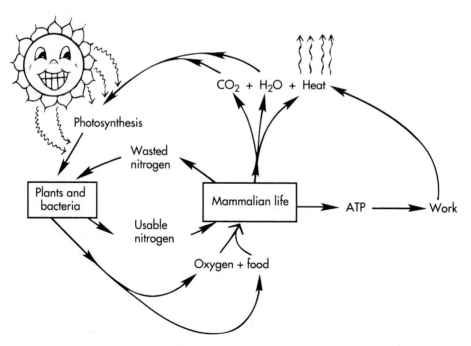

Figure 1-1. The place of mammalian life in the biological universe.

processes going. It makes one realize that all sorts of processes are going on while the body is in the seemingly uneventful state of homeostasis.

Homeostasis: maintaining the status quo in the body

The term homeostasis connotes that the body is able to cope with, and to compensate for, fluctuating outside conditions without undergoing permanent change. During a period of 40 years of adulthood, the human body remains in a steady state, both in weight and in composition, while processing approximately six tons of solid food and 10,000 gallons of water. This means that during all of those years the body is able to keep up structural integrity and maintain balances of temperature, calories, water, minerals, nitrogen, etc. In the process digestible food is continuously metabolized into CO_2, water, waste products, and heat. In short, there is dynamic equilibrium between the breakdown, or **catabolism,** and the (re)synthesis, or **anabolism**, of anatomical and chemical structures. For example: cells of the intestinal mucosa are constantly sloughed off while new ones are generated; fat and carbohydrate stores in the body

are constantly being used for various purposes, but over the period of a day the rates of synthesis of those energy stores equal their rates of expenditure.

What is the nature of this dynamic equilibrium? Why does a living being need food to maintain physical integrity, while inanimate objects such as automobiles do not? A car standing on a level street is in true equilibrium (Figure 1-2), but when positioned without brakes on a downslope, it is no longer in equilibrium and must be held in place by someone pushing from below, expending large amounts of energy. This apparently static situation belies the fact that in the surroundings of the automobile there are stormish activities that are ultimately keeping the car from rolling down the hill: the sun provides energy, plants harvest that energy to produce starches, animals eat the plants, and the person pushing the car feeds from the plants and animals. Here is the parallel with the living organism: as long as food is "pushed" into the organism, structural integrity and balances in temperature, water, minerals, calories, etc., are maintained; a steady state (homeostasis) exists. Without energy input, the body goes rapidly "downhill" and finally disintegrates. Not only do these considerations

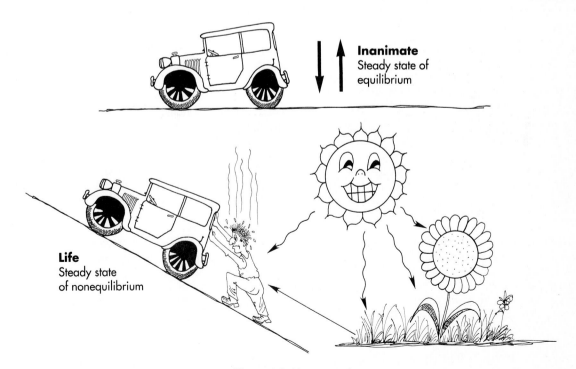

Inanimate
Steady state of equilibrium

Life
Steady state of nonequilibrium

Figure 1-2. Homeostasis.

apply to an intact organism in its surroundings, they are equally true for a cell culture in vitro, or any other form of life. Hence, life is defined functionally by the statement that food is needed to support a permanent steady state of **non-equilibrium**.

Maintaining the steady state of non-equilibrium (homeostasis) is the primary topic. This text discusses how physical, chemical, anatomical, and physiological properties are interwoven, organized, and controlled at the cellular level, organ level, and in the intact organism, and how one animal species differs from another.

Homeostatic control over body composition does not preclude transient variations in individual parameters that bring about ranges around average, or "normal" values. For example, in comparing blood glucose levels in different animal species, some factors that are responsible for the observed normal ranges can be recognized (Table 1-1).

Clearly, normal ranges of values are important criteria by which to interpret variations around normal values: for example, a body at a temperature of around 37° C has a blood glucose level at around 100 mg/dl. The science of statistics is used to determine the probability of an observed value being outside of the normal range so that it may be declared abnormal and a possible disease symptom. Eventually the causes and detection of failing homeostasis (disorder) and the methods by which to help nature correct the situation (therapy) must be considered.

Homeostatic control mechanisms

Maintaining homeostasis is a process in which all organ systems of the body are involved (Figure 1-3). Normal values are maintained by a system of checks and balances: small deviations from normalcy are monitored and signaled, via the nervous and endocrine systems, to organs that are instructed by those control systems to take corrective action. Therefore, an upset in just one parameter (e.g., osmolarity; pH; temperature) usually leads to a response in which various organ systems of the body interact; that is to say a **global response** occurs. This important idea is illustrated by considering the body's multifaceted (global) response to a lowered blood volume; numerous organs and homeostatic control systems are involved (Figure 1-4).

Students should not be overwhelmed by this description of physiological control; it will be discussed later in more detail. Rather, they should begin to appreciate the system of checks and balances at work

Table 1-1	Range of normal glucose levels in blood
Species	**Concentration (mg/dl)**
Human	70-110
Cat	65-130
Dog	70-125
Pig	80-120
Horse	60-130
Cow	40-80
Goat	40-75
Sheep	40-80

Various causes for the range in glucose concentration among the species listed here include time of day, gender, nutritional status, stress, and breed.

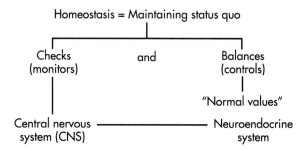

Figure 1-3. Homeostatic control mechanisms.

and to become thoroughly aware, right from the start, that the body, though consisting of a multitude of organs, is in fact one integrated organism that concertizes under the direction of the neuroendocrine system.

It is of fundamental importance to consider the integrated organism when studying one of its isolated parts. In the relative scheme, herein entitled "The Global Picture," the central nervous and endocrine systems exert corrective control over the main organs that influence whole-body homeostasis (Figure 1-5). This global picture will be the starting point for detailed discussion on each topic covered. For instance, when dealing with glycolysis in the liver, first the questions are asked, Why does the body need glycolysis? What is its function? Then the dietary sugars are traced through the scheme from the gut to the liver, where there is limited capacity to store carbohydrate in the form of glycogen. This necessitates storage of the sugars' energy as fat in adipose tissue.

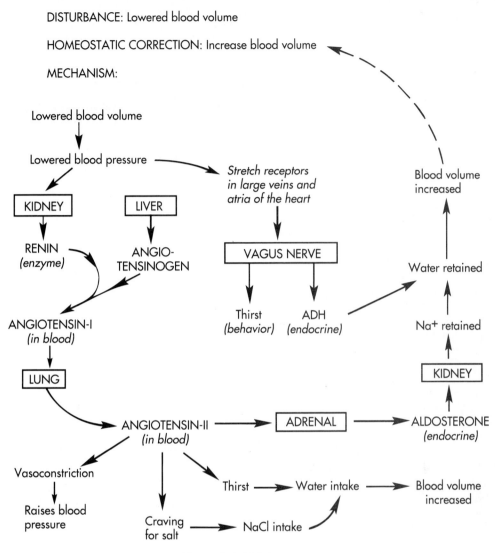

DISTURBANCE: Lowered blood volume

HOMEOSTATIC CORRECTION: Increase blood volume

MECHANISM:

Figure 1-4. Global response.

To that end, the liver converts the excess sugars into fat (here is where glycolysis comes in) and then exports that fat in the form of lipoproteins to fat cells. This process can be readily traced in the global scheme. Any new topic presented should first be placed in the global picture, where its function in the intact animal can be ascertained. Then the topic can be isolated, dissected into all of its details, studied closely, and finally put back into the global scheme before another topic is begun.

Blood is the common medium through which materials are transported into and out of cells, and its movement throughout the body also allows neuroendocrine monitoring to occur. Abnormal waste products in the blood are a readily available diagnostic source of deranged homeostasis (disease). The bloodstream is important for administering drugs or nutrients. Reasons for injecting materials intravenously, instead of giving them orally, include bypassing digestive actions of the gut and not having to wait for the

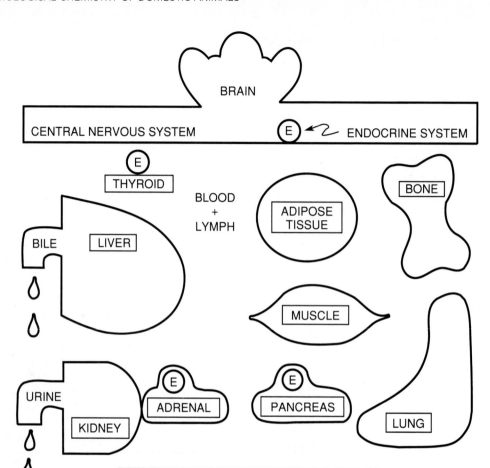

Figure 1-5. The global picture.

time-consuming process of intestinal absorption. Other modes of parenteral administration of materials include intraperitoneal, intramuscular, and subcutaneous injections.

Ideally studies could be limited to the intact animal; then there would be no possibility of losing sight of the "forest" when faced with the many "trees" of detailed information. Unfortunately this cannot be done. Out of necessity to understand the functioning of an organ, an in-depth study of the anatomical details of the organ's innervation, blood circulation, and individual cells must be made. And to understand cell functioning, it is necessary to take that cell apart into its constituent subcellular organelles (plasma membranes, mitochondria) and study the properties of those structures in terms of single molecules (DNA, enzymes, receptors).

The discussion starts with smaller, more detailed, fragments of the body in terms of their practical function in the body's homeostasis, and builds up to the functioning of the integrated organism. At all times, though, the global picture must be kept in mind!

METHODS EMPLOYED IN PHYSIOLOGICAL CHEMISTRY

Physiology is an experimental science. Hence, all published papers, be they research reports or textbooks, are based on interpretation of experimental data. It is important to realize that obtaining experimental data and interpreting them are subject to uncertainty; so printed texts should be open to challenge. This section describes some of the methods used to study physiological chemistry; at the same time, it reviews names and functions of subcellular structures.

Ideally, one would not have to disturb life in order to investigate it. However, since this is not always possible, a researcher often has to violate nature (e.g., killing an animal, isolating a system, etc.), and the experimental observations may or may not reflect the natural condition. Therefore, conclusions drawn from a study must be expressed in well-guarded terms as they may be one or more of the following:

- Valid only under the experimental conditions used and not applicable to the intact animal while living in its natural environment.
- Contaminated by artifacts resulting from the methods used.
- Influenced by sampling error: is the conclusion statistically significant; that is, does it have a probability of over 95% of being correct (or less than 5% of being just a freak, chance observation)?

In physiological sciences, the animal of study must be intentionally disturbed in order to learn something about it. Present knowledge and theories of metabolism are based on experiments in which the imposition upon nature ranges from observation of isolated intact animals, through parenteral administration of radioactively labeled compounds, to trials in which animals are killed, tissues taken, and subcellular fractions studied.

Although it may be possible, after extensive studies at various degrees of imposition, to extrapolate information gained from animal experiments to an undisturbed subject, it is extremely hazardous to do so from one animal species to another. The Food and Drug Administration (FDA), therefore, enforces strict rules requiring extensive testing of pharmaceuticals on a variety of animal species before granting permission to market a drug for human usage. And even then pitfalls occur; for example, dinitrophenol, causing rapid weight loss (by uncoupling oxidative phosphorylation) and having been found free of undesirable side effects in animal testing, was marketed as an aid in human weight control. Soon it had to be removed from the market as it caused blindness in people. Back at the drawing board, the pharmaceutical industry discovered that the only animal species that duplicated this side effect was the duck.

Experimental approaches to physiology will now be discussed in an order of increasing impositions upon nature.

Intact animals in their natural environment

This experimentation, seldom used in physiology, yields information on environmental adaptations, breeding seasons, life span, food preferences, and feeding patterns.

Isolated intact animals

Isolating and confining an animal is a severe imposition that alters mental and physical activities, as well as food intake. Examples are calf cutting as a rodeo event and wild animals failing to reproduce or even dying when isolated as pets or in laboratories. The following data were obtained in experiments performed on intact animals.

Circadian rhythm; entrainment

Circadian (from the Latin *circa* [about] and *dies* [day]) rhythm is a periodicity of about 24 hours in an animal's wake/sleep cycle, physical activity, feeding, body temperature, hormone levels, metabolic enzyme activities, urinary water and mineral excretions, etc. (Figure 1-6). In fact, so pervasive are the effects of circadian rhythm that this factor must be considered in any interpretation of animal experimentation. Those who have traversed time zones during east-west travel have experienced jet lag and its major upsets of sleeping, eating, and mental and physical activity levels. In the morning when tissue glycogen levels were high, rats' endurance to physical exercise was 60% higher than in the evening when glycogen levels were low.

The body has a **biological clock,** also referred to as the internal timekeeper, pacemaker, or primary circadian oscillator. In birds this clock is housed in the pineal gland, whose secretions and metabolic (enzyme) activities follow a seesaw rhythmicity, which can be demonstrated in vitro in pineal gland preparations. In mammals, the source of the wake/sleep cycle is associated with the suprachiasmatic nuclei of the hypothalamus—bilateral clusters of some 10,000 neurons that sit astride the optic chiasm. A special nervous tract (the retinohypothalamic tract), distinct from the optic tract, connects the retina of the eye with the suprachiasmatic nuclei and thus causes light-sensitivity of the circadian effects. The inborn circadian rhythm, which in man amounts to about 25 hours, is thereby synchronized to the 24-hour external

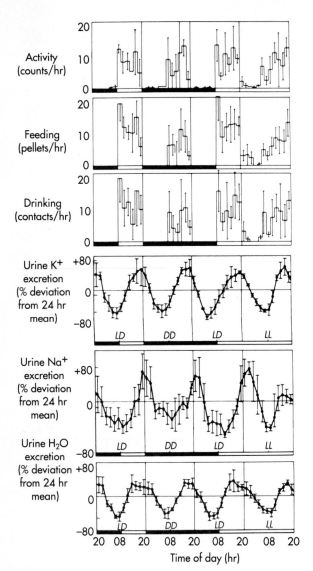

Figure 1-6. Circadian rhythms (mean ± SEM) of activity, feeding, drinking, and urinary potassium, sodium, and water excretion in four squirrel monkeys. After two equilibration days (not shown on the graph) with lights on from 08:00-20:00 hr daily, the animals were studied for a control day on the same light-dark cycle followed by a 36-hour period of constant darkness and then a 36-hour period of constant light. Despite the manipulations of the light-dark cycle each monitored circadian rhythm persisted with a period of approximately 24 hours. *Reproduced with permission from Moore-Ede MC and Sulzman FM: The physiological basis of circadian timekeeping in primates, Physiologist 20:17-25, 1977.*

rhythm of the light-dark cycle. That coupling of inborn rhythmicity to external rhythmicity is called **entrainment**; it gives rise to the diurnal oscillations in behavioral and metabolic characteristics. Placing a subject for extended periods in total darkness, uninterrupted light, or under an abnormal light-dark alternation (e.g., in space, fall-out shelters, improperly illuminated animal quarters) has profound effects on that subject's performance and well-being.

Feeding studies

In **balance** studies, the amount of a substance ingested is compared to the amount excreted. One use of this method is to check whether the potassium balance of an animal is normal.

Inferences as to the nature of a metabolic pathway can be made based on the identities of materials fed and excreted. For example, radiolabeled dietary cholesterol is recovered, in part, in fecal bile salts. The turnover time of drugs, and metabolic products formed from them, can be established by feeding studies.

Deletion or excessive addition of a given substance may affect growth rate, fertility, or other parameters. This method has been one of the mainstays of early experimentation on vitamins and minerals.

Parenteral administration of compounds

By infusion or injection, the digestive processes and influences of the intestines are bypassed. This approach is often used with compounds that, when fed, are too digestible or too large to be absorbed across the gut intact (e.g., polypeptide hormones, proteins, ^{14}C-sucrose).

In situ organ perfusion

The method of measuring arteriovenous concentration differences allows the study of the metabolic activity of a particular organ. For example, by determining that the glucose concentration in the hepatic vein is higher than in the portal vein in a starving animal, but in a fed animal this is reversed, the liver can be implicated in the regulation of blood glucose concentrations.

Animal after organ removal
Organ removal

Excision of an organ facilitates isolated study and experimentation, but may render the subject devoid of certain bodily functions. Examples would include the following: after surgical removal of the liver (hepatectomy) a rat cannot utilize dietary fructose to maintain an adequate blood sugar level; after surgical removal of the testes (castration) an animal can no longer reproduce.

Organ rendered nonfunctional but left in place

The great physiologist, Claude Bernard, ca. 1850, set out to settle once and for all the then controversial topic of pancreatic involvement in the regulation of the blood sugar level. To that end, he ligated the pancreatic duct of a dog. Thus, he blocked the exocrine secretions of the pancreas, such as digestive enzymes and bicarbonate secretion. Observing atrophy of the pancreas but no elevated level of blood glucose (hyperglycemia) or glucose in the urine (glucosuria), he concluded that the pancreas was not involved in blood sugar regulation. In 1869, Paul Langerhans, a senior medical student in Berlin, proved the great master wrong. He published a short paper on the histology of the pancreas in which he showed that the islets of Langerhans (as they are called today) produce insulin and release that hormone directly into the bloodstream via the endocrine (ductless) route (Figure 1-7).

While on the topic of secretions, a **paracrine** substance is defined as being elaborated by one cell and affecting neighboring cells; for example, in the pancreatic islets, somatostatin, elaborated by D cells, inhibits the secretions of glucagon and insulin by adjacent alpha and beta cells, respectively. The term **autocrine** is used for a cell secreting a substance that affects its own metabolism; for example, for the formation of lysosomes, a portion of the newly synthesized lysosomal enzyme precursors is secreted by the cell and then taken up again and directed to a prelysosomal compartment.

Organ extracts fed or injected into an animal

Roosters exhibit several changes after caponization: regression of comb and wattles, decreased red blood cell volume, cessation of crowing, and failure to reproduce. Testicular extracts (containing testosterone) injected into the capons can reverse all of the changes except for the failure to reproduce. In humans, injection of insulin compensates for pancreatic insufficiency caused by diabetes.

Isolated perfused organ

With this technique, endocrine and nervous controls are removed, and media that perfuse the organ of study can be controlled. Organ functions and drug metabolism are among items that can be studied this way; for example, the liver's removal of wastes from the circulation; factors in the perfusate that stimulate the pancreas to secrete insulin (secretagogues).

Tissue slices

Incubating freshly prepared tissue slices in a life-sustaining ("physiological") buffer solution is a great tool to establish metabolic pathways; for example, cholesterol synthesis from labeled intermediates, such as acetate, mevalonate, or squalene.

Isolated cells

Isolated cells are prepared by perfusing the organ, or incubating tissue slices, with a solution that contains collagenase, an enzyme that digests collagen and thereby disrupts cell adhesion. The cells are then sorted and propagated by incubation in cell culture flasks, often obviating the need to euthanize additional animals. Isolated cells are used to study metabolism in a pure cell type, or for cell recognition phenomena (e.g., receptors, hormone action, immunology), or for scanning suspected carcinogens.

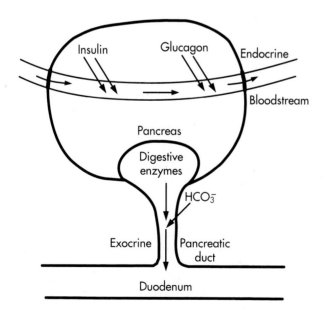

Figure 1-7. Endocrine and exocrine pancreas.

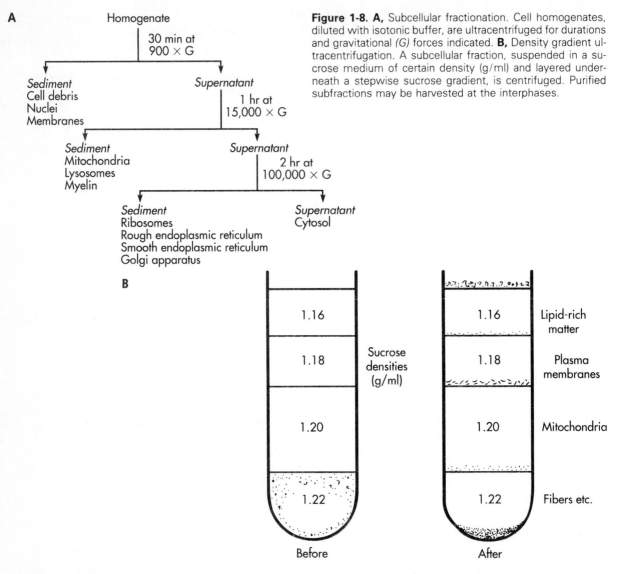

A

Homogenate
↓ 30 min at 900 × G

Sediment
Cell debris
Nuclei
Membranes

Supernatant
↓ 1 hr at 15,000 × G

Sediment
Mitochondria
Lysosomes
Myelin

Supernatant
↓ 2 hr at 100,000 × G

Sediment
Ribosomes
Rough endoplasmic reticulum
Smooth endoplasmic reticulum
Golgi apparatus

Supernatant
Cytosol

B

Sucrose densities (g/ml)

Before	After	
1.16	1.16	Lipid-rich matter
1.18	1.18	Plasma membranes
1.20	1.20	Mitochondria
1.22	1.22	Fibers etc.

Before

After

Figure 1-8. A, Subcellular fractionation. Cell homogenates, diluted with isotonic buffer, are ultracentrifuged for durations and gravitational (G) forces indicated. **B,** Density gradient ultracentrifugation. A subcellular fraction, suspended in a sucrose medium of certain density (g/ml) and layered underneath a stepwise sucrose gradient, is centrifuged. Purified subfractions may be harvested at the interphases.

Tissue homogenates

With a tissue homogenizer, cell membranes are ruptured, but subcellular organelles, (such as mitochondria, nuclei, and lysosomes), may remain intact if homogenization is done in an isotonic medium. The homogenate is used to assay for cellular constituents, such as proteins, glycogen, DNA, enzyme activities, etc., or as a starting material from which subcellular organelles may be isolated.

Subcellular fractions

Subcellular fractions may be obtained ultracentrifugally as diagrammed (Figure 1-8, A). Each of these fractions contains a mixture of subcellular entities, and may be further purified by density gradient ultracentrifugation in gradients established, for instance, of sucrose (Figure 1-8, B). Progress toward purification of organelles is monitored by electron microscopic inspection and by assaying for marker enzymes (e.g., cytochrome oxidase in mitochondria, or 5′-nucleotidase in plasma membranes) or marker constituents (e.g., DNA in nuclei or mitochondria).

Down to the smallest components

Ultimately, subcellular organelles may be dissected into their constituent parts; for example, from intact mitochondria the inner membranes may be isolated, and subsequently, **oligomolecular units** may be obtained from those inner membranes, which contain the essential features of oxidative phosphorylation. It should be realized that in physiology usually the smallest meaningful (i.e., functional) units are complexes made up of different molecules; for example, a unit membrane; a lipoprotein; an enzyme complex (metabolic pathway) attached to structures present in the cytoplasm. It is more in the realm of biochemistry to study individual molecules.

CELL MODEL AND FUNCTIONS OF SUBCELLULAR FRACTIONS

The cell model depicted in Figure 1-9 should serve to reacquaint the reader with cellular organization of the various subcellular structures shown in more detail in electromicrographs (Figures 1-10 through 1-14; see also Chapter 6). Some activities of purified subcellular fractions are listed in Table 1-2.

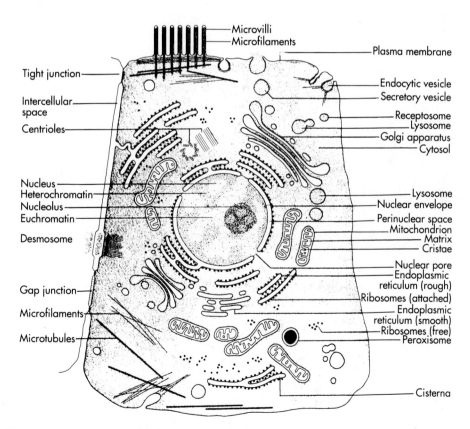

Figure 1-9. A cell model. *Reproduced with permission from Sheeler P and Bianchi DE: Cell and molecular biology, ed 3, p 27, New York, 1987, Wiley.*

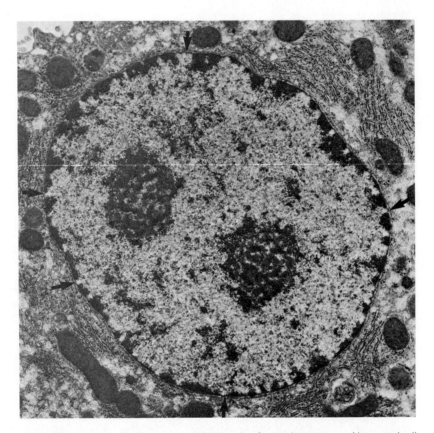

Figure 1-10. Cell nucleus. Electron photomicrograph of a rat hepatocyte. Note nucleoli, pores traversing the two nuclear membranes *(arrows)* for passage of nuclear macromolecules, rough endoplasmic reticulum, and mitochondria. *Courtesy Dr. Rick A. Rogers, Harvard School of Public Health.*

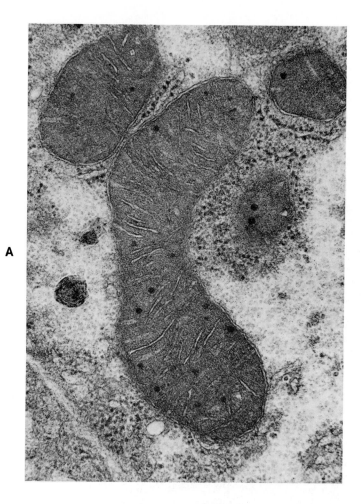

A

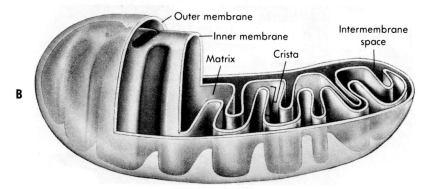

B

Figure 1-11. A mitochondrion. **A,** Electron photomicrograph of a rat hepatocyte. **B,** Schematic interpretation of the mitochondrial structure. **A** *Courtesy Dr. Rick A. Rogers, Harvard School of Public Health.* **B** *Reproduced with permission, from Schauf CL, Moffett DF, and Moffett SB: Human physiology: foundations and frontiers, St. Louis, 1990, Mosby–Year Book.*

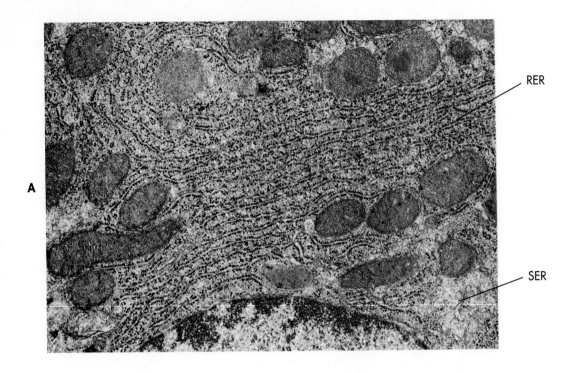

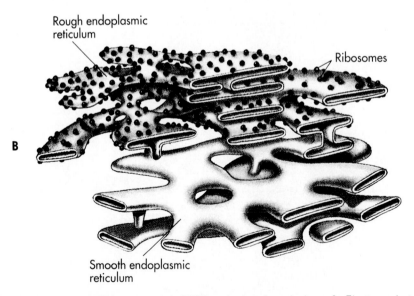

Figure 1-12. Rough (RER) and smooth (SER) endoplasmic reticulum. **A,** Electron photomicrograph of a cytoplasmic area in a rat hepatocyte. **B,** Diagram of the association between rough and smooth endoplasmic reticulum. *A Courtesy Dr. Rick A. Rogers, Harvard School of Public Health. B Reproduced with permission from Martini F: Fundamentals of anatomy and physiology, p 57, Englewood Cliffs, NJ, 1989, Prentice-Hall.*

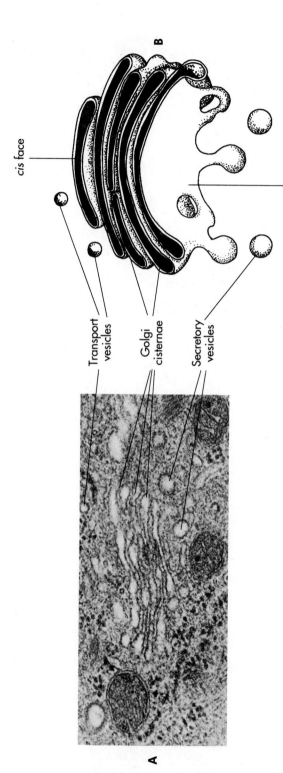

cis face

trans face

B

A

Transport
vesicles

Golgi
cisternae

Secretory
vesicles

Figure 1-13. The Golgi apparatus. **A,** Electron photomicrograph of an endothelial cell in rat liver. **B,** Interpretative drawing showing transport vesicles, that originate from the endoplasmic reticulum, fusing with the *cis* face of the Golgi apparatus, and the finished product leaving at the *trans* face in the form of secretory vesicles. **A** *Courtesy Dr. Rick A. Rogers, Harvard School of Public Health.*

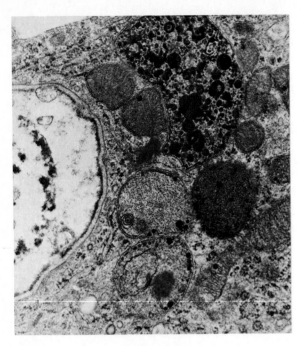

Figure 1-14. Lysosomes. The electron photomicrograph shows a Kupffer cell phagolysosomal compartment. A portion of a large phagolysosome, located on the left margin, contains enzymically degraded cellular material. The smaller vacuoles exhibit the typical lysosomal "halo" and are secondary lysosomes that have just formed by fusion of small primary lysosomes with endocytosed cellular material. *Courtesy Dr. Rick A. Rogers, Harvard School of Public Health.*

Table 1-2	Subcellular fractions and their activities

Fraction	Activities
Nuclei	DNA replication; mRNA synthesis
Nucleoli	rRNA synthesis
Mitochondria	Energy generators; β-oxidation
Ribosomes (rough ER)	Protein synthesis
Smooth ER	Steroid synthesis
Golgi apparatus	Macromolecular complexes
Peroxisomes	Detoxification; lipid synthesis
Cell membranes	Monitor import and export; transmit signals in ↔ out; protection; recognition
Cytoskeleton	Intracellular transport; support
Cytoplasm	Carbohydrate synthesis; fatty acid synthesis

STUDY QUESTIONS

1. List the most important course objective.
2. *a.* List technical term for maintaining normal balances and values in the face of impositions from outside the body.
   b. List factor that distinguishes steady state (life) from an inanimate equilibrium.
   c. Given that all natural processes go in the direction of lowering free energy, how then is life maintained?
   d. Exemplify an energy input required to maintain the body's steady state.
3. Name the chemical element that accepts metabolic electrons.
4. *a.* Define anabolism in terms of free energy, and list one specific example of anabolism.
   b. Name the opposite of anabolism, and list one specific example.
5. *a.* Voltage is a measure of electrical current, electrical potential, or electrical energy. (Choose one.)
   b. Name a unit in which energy of nutrients is expressed.
6. Taking homeostatic control into account, explain why a normal blood K^+ level does not guarantee that an animal is in proper K^+ balance.
7. *a.* Give one reason why blood glucose values in cows are lower than those in cats.
   b. Indicate, in the customary units, what the blood glucose level is in an animal that has .04 g of glucose in 50 ml blood.
8. List the two generalized controls over all of the body's physiology.
9. Give one example each of a hormone that is: proteinaceous; derived from one amino acid; derived from cholesterol.
10. What differentiates an endocrine gland from an exocrine gland?
11. Complete the following endocrine chain of events that corrects hypoglycemia:
    a. List the hypothalamic peptide released upon sensing hypoglycemia.
    b. List the pituitary hormone secreted under the influence of that peptide.
    c. List the adrenal cortical hormone class secreted under the influence of that factor.
    d. List the target organ of those adrenal hormones, and list corrective measures taken by that organ.
12. About global control of total osmotic pressure of blood, work through the following:
    a. Exemplify nervous control (monitoring).
    b. Exemplify hormonal regulation.

c. Exemplify behavioral adaptation to increase total osmotic pressure.

d. List four anatomical sites (organs) that contribute to the homeostatic response by which the body corrects hyperosmolality of blood.

e. Putting all of these controls together, explain decreased urination after salt intake.

13. *a.* If an osmoreceptor would sense a drop of 2% in the salt concentration of plasma, it would signal for the release of ADH. (True/False)

b. List the site of origin of antidiuretic hormone (ADH).

14. Name the body's drainage system that is under direct control by the liver.

15. What statistical probability (list the percentage) must be assured before one may state that a biological value is different from the norm?

16. *a.* What is basically incorrect when, in some literature, circadian rhythm is equated with the light-dark cycle?

b. List an observation that is influenced by circadian rhythm.

c. Give the technical term for adjustment of circadian rhythm to an environmentally imposed rhythmicity. List an example.

17. List the organ whose metabolic role is indicated by the finding that parenterally administered table sugar is excreted undigested.

18. *a.* Why does ligation of the pancreatic duct not affect the blood glucose level?

b. List an exocrine pancreatic contribution to the intestinal digestion of food.

c. Name the paracrine substance inhibiting glucagon release in the pancreas.

19. Hyperglycemia leads to glucagon release. (True/False)

20. Reason as to why it is ineffective to administer insulin via the diet if one wants to study the metabolic effects of insulin in an intact animal.

21. Name the breakdown product of hemoglobin the liver fails to remove from blood in cases of jaundice.

22. *a.* List two major control mechanisms that are lost in experiments with isolated perfused organs.

b. Why must red blood cells be included in the medium with which one perfuses an isolated liver when studying liver function?

23. The following four questions pertain to isolated fat cells incubated in a medium that allows them to combust glucose as a nutrient:

a. List the metabolic end products of glucose combustion.

b. How is glucose labeled to facilitate measurements?

c. List a hormone that must be added to the incubation medium.

d. Upon finding that a fat cell homogenate does not require that hormone for glucose combustion, what then would follow as the most likely subcellular site of action for that hormone?

24. *a.* After ultracentrifugation in a density gradient from 1.16 to 1.22 g/ml, where in the tube would one find myelin?

b. List the subcellular fraction, obtained by density gradient ultracentrifugation, that contains a high level of enzymes involved in phospholipid synthesis.

25. If density gradient centrifugation has yielded a subcellular fraction needed to test for the presence of plasma membranes, which of the following should be picked as the marker enzyme: Adenylate cyclase, Cytochrome oxidase, or Phosphorylase?

26. Based on what is known about the composition of nucleoli, which of these two tissues would contain the more visible nucleoli: the skeletal muscle or an oviduct cell of a laying hen?

27. *a.* Name the subcellular organelle largely responsible for a cell's ATP production.

b. List a metabolic function of the Golgi apparatus.

28. Definitions and terminology:

a. Define the following in one word: presence of glucose in urine.

b. Define the following in one word: abnormally low blood glucose level.

c. List the meaning of hepatectomy and gastrectomy.

d. After blood has been collected in the presence of an anticoagulant (e.g., heparin) and then centrifuged, what is the clear supernatant called?

e. Define hypocalcemia.

f. Define hypernatremia.

g. Define the following in one word: an injection given into a vein.

h. List the anatomical site where an intraperitoneal injection is given.

i. Define ischemia.

Some key principles

WATER: OUR LIFE-SUPPORTING MEDIUM

Dual function

Over half of the body weight of animals consists of water; therefore, it must be considered the medium in which life's processes occur. In addition, water is a chemical reactant; for example, in the following equation for hydrolysis (saponification) of an ester:

$$R-O-\underset{\underset{O}{\|}}{C}-R' + H_2O \leftrightarrow ROH + HO\underset{\underset{O}{\|}}{C}-R'$$

Water sources

Drinking is the primary method of water intake for most animals. Also, water contained in food must be considered, especially in carnivores. An appreciable water source is metabolic water generated by the oxidation of food in the body. Carbohydrates can be portrayed as $(C \cdot H_2O)_n$, and thus, their combustion with O_2 yields CO_2 and H_2O; likewise, lipids, mainly consisting of CH_2 chains, yield metabolic water when combusted as follows:

$$CH_2 + 1.5\ O_2 \rightarrow CO_2 + H_2O$$

Metabolic water is especially important to camels and birds.

Some physical characteristics

Physical constants based on water properties

The temperature scale of Celsius assigns a zero value (0° C) to the freezing point and a 100° C value to the boiling point of water at an atmospheric pressure of 1. As the scale has 100 divisions, values on that scale are expressed in centigrade. The Fahrenheit scale (with 32° F at freezing and 212° F at boiling) has 180 divisions.

The calorie (cal), a unit of energy, is defined as the amount of heat required to raise the temperature of 1 g of water from 14.5° C to 15.5° C. One thousand calories constitute 1 kilocalorie (Kcal, or Cal). Unfortunately, the difference between cal and Cal is totally obscured when the entire word CALORIE is capitalized, as is done on food product labels; in that case, Kcal is meant. One million calories, or 1000 Kcal, form one megacalorie (Mcal, or therm).

Water attains its maximal density at 4° C. The unit of mass has been defined so that 1 cm^3 of water at 4° C weighs exactly 1 g. The warmer water of summer and the cooler water (0-4° C) of winter, especially ice (with a density of about 0.9 g/cm^3), layer themselves above the denser water of 4° C to the benefit of aquatic life in deep water.

Heat capacity

Water has a high heat capacity: for example, it takes a large amount of heat to raise the temperature of water (1 cal per 1° C). This feature of water aids in temperature regulation, or thermoregulation, of the body. If the human body were made of copper, which has a low heat capacity, it would start to glow the minute it hit the beach!

Hydrogen bonding

In a solution, hydrogen atoms belonging to one molecule may be shared by oxygen and/or nitrogen

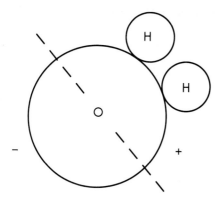

Figure 2-1. Dipolar nature of water.

site "pole" negatively charged, as the total water molecule is electrically neutral. Thus, water has a plus (+) and a minus (−) pole: it is dipolar (Figure 2-1).

Hydration of ions

The dipolar nature of water contributes to the solubilization of salts. Water dipoles orient themselves around ions (Figure 2-2), reducing the charge density on the surfaces of the hydrated ions and hence the attractive forces between them. The water coats also hinder the regrouping of ions in crystalline form.

A consequence of the hydration of salt ions is that in a concentrated salt solution there may be a paucity of uncommitted water molecules. Such a shortage leads to competition among ions for free water. In a salt solution, the charged (ionic) groups of protein molecules may not be hydrated such that protein molecules aggregate and precipitate. As one protein is more susceptible to this "salting out" than is another, individual proteins may be isolated from a mixture by a stepwise increase in the salt concentration of the solution and centrifuging after each addition of salt.

Polarity

As discussed, hydration of charged groups, or ions, facilitates solubilization in water. Organic compounds may contain ionic groups, both anionic (e.g., carboxyl group — $COOH$ which dissociate into — COO^- and H^+) and cationic (e.g., protonated amino groups — NH_3^+). Those ionized groups interact with water and lend water solubility to the compounds carrying those groups (e.g., acetic acid; or amino acids). In addition to ionized groups, there are electrically neutral groups with an uneven charge dis-

atoms belonging to different molecules. This sharing, or bonding between properly aligned adjacent molecules is called hydrogen bonding. If it were not for hydrogen bonding among adjacent oxygen atoms, water would not be a liquid at room temperature, for H_2S (S being under O in the 16th column of the periodic table of elements and about twice as heavy) is a gas. Hydrogen bonding is also a major stabilizing factor in the structures of proteins (helix, pleated sheath) and nucleic acids, which link the two strands of DNA.

Solubility of compounds in water
Dipolar nature of water

The two hydrogen atoms of a water molecule are attached to one side of the oxygen atom, rendering that side somewhat positively charged and the oppo-

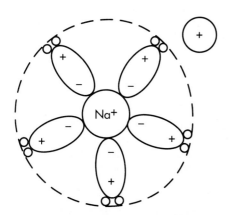

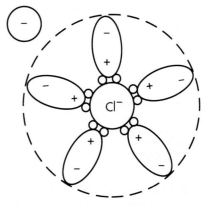

Figure 2-2. Hydration of ions.

tribution; like water, those groups are polarized, thus, their presence adds water solubility to the compound carrying those polar groups. Examples of polar groups are alcohol [$=CH(OH)$], ketone ($=CO$), aldehyde [$-CO(H)$], or nitro groups [$=CH(NO_2)$]. Just as increasing polarity adds to water solubility, a compound's water solubility is diminished by either the absence or the shielding of polar groups. For example, methane (CH_4) is not soluble in water, whereas methanol (CH_3OH) is; the solubility of an organic acid [$R_1-C(O)O^-$] is much diminished when the polar carboxyl group is shielded by making the corresponding ester [$R_1-C(O)O-R_2$].

Hydrophobic interactions

Compounds interacting with water are called **hydrophilic** (water-loving), and apolar compounds are **hydrophobic** (water-fearing). Weak forces attract apolar regions to each other and cause interaction between hydrophobic compounds. For example, fat droplets, being hydrophobic, float on the surface of a soup and coalesce due to the attraction of those weak forces (Figure 2-3, A). This attraction makes hydrophobic compounds soluble in oil; they are **lipophilic**, or fat-loving. An example of an oily medium in biology is the interior of cell membranes (Figure 2-3, B) in which lipids facing the interior of the cell interact with those on the outside. Lipophilic substances can traverse a lipid bilayer more easily than hydrophilic substances, so the degree of hydrophobicity (or lipophilicity) is a determining factor in the process of cellular uptake of compounds (e.g., nutrients, drugs). This is covered more fully in later chapters on cell physiology and lipid metabolism.

Amphoteric interactions

Amphoteric compounds have both hydrophilic and hydrophobic regions and, thus, are able to interact simultaneously with lipophilic substances and water (Figure 2-3, C).

Detergents

Amphoteric compounds can bind a lipid and then transport that lipid in an aqueous medium; they are detergents. The body's most important detergents are bile salts, which derive from apolar cholesterol by the addition of a number of polar (alcoholic and carboxyl) groups. The mode of action of bile salts, the formation of lipid micelles, and the stabilization of fat emulsion droplets by other amphoteric compounds (e.g., lecithin) is discussed later in this text.

Protein binding

Proteins are an important class of amphoteric compounds. They contain hydrophobic pockets, consisting of apolar amino acids (e.g., leucine, isoleucine, valine, phenylalanine) as well as hydrophilic pockets containing polar amino acids (e.g., aspartate, glutamate, serine, lysine, arginine). Apolar substances (e.g., lipids) may bind to the hydrophobic pockets while hydration of the numerous polar groups renders the complex water-soluble.

The physiological importance of this protein binding cannot be overstated. Some examples (to be discussed later in greater detail) are as follows:

- Transport of bilirubin (apolar breakdown product of hemoglobin) bound to albumin in the bloodstream.
- Protein binding protects small vital molecules (e.g., hormones) from being filtered by the kidney into the urine. The protein complex is too large to be filtered out of the bloodstream.
- A reversible dissociation equilibrium between protein-bound (inactive) and unbound (active) hormones in serum helps to regulate hormonal activities.
- Special transport proteins exist for various classes of compounds, including hormones (transcortin for cortisol), lipids (albumin for fatty acids, apoproteins for cholesterol and triglyceride), minerals (transferrin for iron, ceruloplasmin for copper), and vitamins (transcobalamin for vitamin B_{12}). Via receptors that are specific for these transport proteins, protein binding also aids in targeting compounds to the proper tissues.
- Proteins containing enzyme activities are often embedded in membranes, therefore they can use apolar compounds as their substrates.

pH AND BUFFERING
Definitions

$$pH = -\log[H^+]$$

The log scale is practical, since it covers a wide range of H^+ concentration values, but is also deceiving, because it makes curves out of straight lines; for example, at pH 7.1 the $[H^+]$ is twice that of pH 7.4. Also, the H^+ concentration in the viable pH range of serum (7.1-7.8) is on the order of 10^{-8} to 10^{-7} molar, which is less than one millionth the plasma $[Na^+]$.

An **H^+ donor** acts as an acid: $HA \leftrightarrow H^+ + A^-$; an **$H^+$ acceptor** acts as a base: $A^- + H^+ \leftrightarrow HA$. A

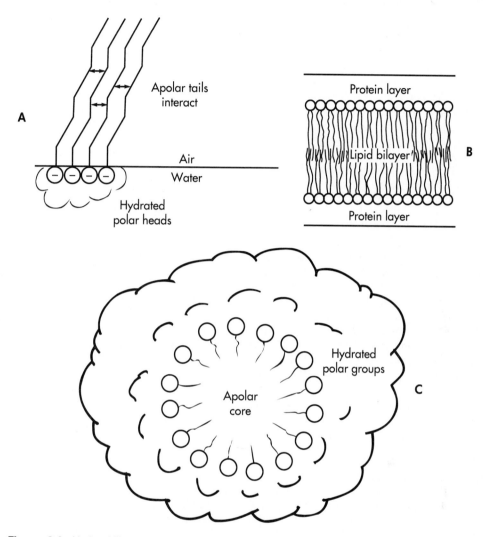

Figure 2-3. Hydrophilic and hydrophobic interactions. **A,** Fatty acids on a water surface. **B,** Simplified model of a cell membrane. **C,** Amphoteric compound.

compound such as $H_2PO_4^-$ can act as an acid or as a base by either donating or accepting a proton.

Strong electrolytes are completely dissociated, whereas **weak electrolytes** are partly dissociated. Hydrochloric acid is strong, whereas acetic acid is a weak acid, and proteins are weak electrolytes.

Buffering

In a solution of a weak acid (H^+ donor) the equilibrium is given by the equation $K = ([H^+] \cdot [A^-])/[HA]$. This equation, written in logarithmic form, $pH = pK + \log ([H^+ \text{ acceptor}]/[H^+ \text{ donor}])$, is known as the Henderson-Hasselbalch (H-H) equation, and is valid for all buffer systems. One can swamp the amount of H^+ acceptor that spontaneously dissociates from an acid by adding the conjugated salt of that acid (e.g., adding sodium acetate to acetic acid). In the latter case one can rewrite the H-H equation as follows, substituting the salt concentration for H^+ acceptor and the acid concentration for H^+ donor:

$$pH = pK + \log ([\text{salt}]/[\text{acid}])$$

pK is a nature-given constant (negative logarithm

of the dissociation constant). The value of pK equals the pH when concentrations of A^- (salt) and HA (acid) are equal, such that the log term in the H-H equation becomes zero.

Titration curve

Use of the illustrated titration curve of a buffer (Figure 2-4) aids in the review of the following features:
- Universal for all buffers
- Symmetric around pK
- Steepest slope (best buffering) around the pK
- Reversible over pH range
- Buffering capacity towards acids and bases

Chemical buffering in serum

As the physiologic pH of serum is about 7.4 under normal conditions, buffers in blood that have a pK in the vicinity of 7.4 have optimal buffering capacity at that pH. Although the following buffer systems may not possess the optimal pK for buffering at pH 7.4, they are nevertheless the three most important quantitative buffer systems in body fluids:
- Bicarbonate/carbonic acid; pK 6.1: H^+ + HCO_3^- ↔ H_2CO_3 ↔ CO_2 + H_2O). Though the pK of this buffer is far removed from the physiologic pH, this buffering system is important, since organ systems of the body homeostatically control the ratio of its H^+ acceptor/donor components.
- Phosphate system; pK 6.8: H^+ + $HPO_4^=$ ↔ $H_2PO_4^-$. Though the pK of this system is closer to the serum pH, this buffer is of little physiologic importance extracellularly owing to the low phosphate concentration in serum. The phosphate buffer system, however, is a quantitatively important intracellular buffer system.

- Proteins; ranging pK values: H^+ + Protein$^-$ ↔ HProtein. Proteins buffer best at pH values beyond the limits of viability. (Further explanation appears below.)

The concentrations of these buffers in human serum are small: Bicarbonate/CO_2 24-29 mmol/L; phosphates 1-1.5 mmol/L; and proteins 50-80 g/L. Moreover, judged by their pK values alone, none of these buffers would be expected to have a good buffering capacity at pH 7.4. The Henderson-Hasselbalch equation shows the following:
- Bicarbonate: $7.4 = 6.1 + \log ([HCO_3^-]/[H_2CO_3])$; ratio = 20:1;
- Phosphates: $7.4 = 6.8 + \log ([HPO_4^=]/[H_2PO_4^-])$; ratio = 4:1.

Stewart's concept of buffering

The following treatise of acid-base chemistry, proposed by Peter A. Stewart (Modern Quantitative Acid-Base Chemistry: Can J Physiol Pharmacol 61:1444, 1983), approaches serum as a composite of water, strong electrolytes, weak acids (including proteins), and the CO_2/bicarbonate system.

In water, $[H^+] \cdot [OH^-] = K_w \cdot [H_2O]$. As water has a molecular weight of 18, the $[H_2O]$ is about 55 molar. Water's dissociation constant, K_w, amounts to about 10^{-16} molar. The value of K_w, though influenced by temperature, osmolarity, and ionic composition, may be considered constant in homeostatically controlled body fluids, and so the product of K_w times $[H_2O]$ is written as a constant, K_w', called the ion product of pure water and having a numerical value of approximately 10^{-14} molar in plasma at 37° C. Since K_w' equals $[H^+]$ times $[OH^-]$, at neutrality (when $[H^+]$ and $[OH^-]$ are equal) both $[H^+]$ and $[OH^-]$ are the square root of K_w', about 10^{-7} molar.

Mixing HCl and NaOH (strong electrolytes) with water establishes a hydrogen ion concentration that must obey the following two equations:

$$[H^+] \cdot [OH^-] = K_w'$$
(ion product of water dissociation)
$$[Na^+] - [Cl^-] + [H^+] - [OH^-] = 0$$
(electroneutrality in a solution is required)

The difference between concentrations of strong cations and anions ($[Na^+] - [Cl^-]$) is termed **strong ion difference (SID)**. Substituting SID in the latter equation, and replacing $[OH^-]$ by $K_w'/[H^+]$ yields SID + $[H^+]$ + $K_w'/[H^+]$ = 0. This equation shows that the $[H^+]$ is controlled by the independent variable SID.

The next approach to serum composition is adding

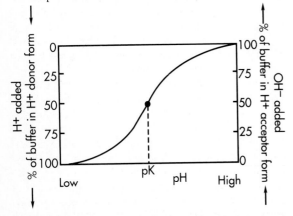

Figure 2-4. Titration curve of a buffer.

a weak acid (e.g., a protein) to the above NaCl solution. Now the $[H^+]$ must obey the following four equations:

$$[H^+] \cdot [OH^-] = K_w'$$
(ion product of water dissociation)

$$[H^+] \cdot [A^-] = K_A \cdot [HA]$$
(dissociation of weak acid)

$$[A^-] + [HA] = A_T$$
(total weak acid equals sum of dissociated and undissociated acid, or protein)

$$SID + [H^+] - [OH^-] - [A^-] = 0$$
(electroneutrality)

Solving these four simultaneous equations for $[H^+]$ yields the following cubic polynomial expression:

$$[H^+]^3 + (K_A + SID) \cdot [H^+]^2 +$$
$$\{K_A \cdot (SID - [A_T]) - K_w'\} \cdot [H^+]$$
$$- K_A \cdot K_w' = 0.$$

This expression shows how $[H^+]$ is a dependent variable whose numerical value is determined by the independent parameters SID and A_T (values over which there is direct control), and by the dissociation constants. In theory, estimating with the aid of a computer, the H^+ from this expression is the correct way to look at this solution of a weak acid in saline. One may ask, Does this mean that the Henderson-Hasselbalch equation is wrong? Maybe it is wrong in principle, but not in its practical way of estimating the pH in this solution. For if the numerically negligible entities are removed from the polynomial expression [i.e., eliminate $[H^+]^3$, K_A in the second term, K_w' in the third term, and the entire fourth term, $K_A \cdot K_w'$], we end up with the dissociation equilibrium equation of the weak acid, from which the H-H equation was derived.

To complete the serum composition, carbon dioxide is added to the aforementioned mixture of strong electrolytes and protein in water. Carbon dioxide dissolved in water forms carbonic acid (H_2CO_3), which equilibrates with bicarbonate (HCO_3^-); the latter, in turn, is in equilibrium with carbonate ($CO_3^=$). Thus, the $[H^+]$ must now obey the following six simultaneous equations:

$$[H^+] \cdot [OH^+] = K_w'$$
(water dissociation)

$$[H^+] \cdot [A^-] = K_A \cdot [HA]$$
(weak acid or protein dissociation)

$$[HA] + [A^-] = A_T$$
(accounting for all A)

$$[H^+] \cdot [HCO_3^-] = K_c \cdot pCO_2$$
(first dissociation)

$$[H^+] \cdot [CO_3^=] = K_3 \cdot [HCO_3^-]$$
(second dissociation)

$$SID + [H^+] - [A^-] - [HCO_3^-] - [CO_3^=] - [OH^-] = 0$$
(electroneutrality)

When these six equations are solved for $[H^+]$, the $[H^+]$ is found, with the aid of a computer, from the following fourth-power polynomial expression:

$$[H^+]^4 + [H^+]^3 \cdot (SID + K_A) + [H^+]^2 \cdot \{K_A \cdot (SID - A_T) - K_w' - K_c \cdot pCO_2\} - [H^+] \cdot \{K_A \cdot (K_w' + K_c \cdot pCO_2) - K_3 \cdot K_c \cdot pCo_2\} - K_A \cdot K_3 \cdot K_c \cdot pCO_2 = 0$$

This treatise shows that there are three independent variables (SID, A_T, and pCO_2), which, together with four nature-given constants, determine the pH of serum. Similarly, from the aforementioned six equations, it can be derived that, in addition to $[H^+]$, the values of $[HCO_3^-]$, $[CO_3^=]$, $[HA]$, $[A^-]$, and $[OH^-]$ are all dependent variables, whose values follow from the three independent variables, (SID, A_T, and pCO_2).

According to Stewart's concept, only changes in independent variables can affect pH. Whole-body acid-base balance can be understood in quantitative terms of the three independent variables and their physiologic regulation by the lungs, kidneys, gut, and liver. In contrast, the effects of strong ion differences and protein levels on the plasma pH cannot readily be understood on the basis of the traditional Henderson-Hasselbalch treatise.

Physiological buffering

Blood pH must be homeostatically regulated within the narrow limits of 7.1-7.8 that are compatible with life (Figure 2-5). A serum pH below the physiological value of 7.4 reflects a state of acidemia, which may indicate a general state of acidosis in the animal. Elevated serum pH, alkalemia, may reflect the general state of alkalosis in the animal.

Upsets in acid-base balance are very pervasive as the H^+ concentration influences nearly all vital processes, including: (i) enzyme activities and thus metabolism; (ii) transmembrane potentials and thus transport of compounds in and out of cells, and neuromuscular characteristics; (iii) breathing; (iv) oxygen-carrying capacity of hemoglobin; (v) regional blood flow; and many more. It is therefore of vital importance that the H^+ concentration is well monitored and buffered.

When the weak buffering capacity of the body's

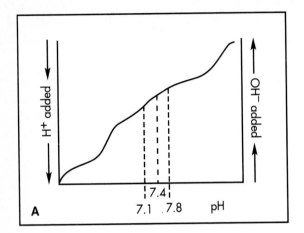

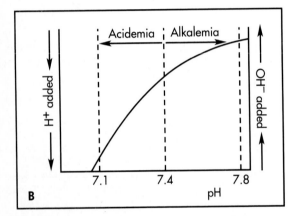

Figure 2-5. Titration curve of serum. Note that in the small pH range compatible with life chemical buffering is weak compared to regions beyond the viable pH range. **A,** Titration curve of serum. **B,** Viable range of serum pH.

chemical buffering systems in serum is considered, it is clear that organismic, physiological buffering systems must come to the rescue to maintain serum pH within the narrow limits of viability. Later, in a separate chapter on maintaining the body's acid-base balance, the following physiological control systems are discussed: the lungs' potential to eliminate or conserve acid (CO_2) by hyperventilating or hypoventilating; the kidneys' adaptive roles in acidosis and alkalosis, conserving or eliminating Na^+, Cl^-, K^+, NH_4^+, HCO_3^-, and other ions or compounds; the exchange of H^+ and other ions between tissues and blood; and the functions of liver, gut, and other organs in pH homeostasis.

ACID-BASE AND ELECTRICAL PROPERTIES OF PROTEINS
Acid-base properties
Amino acids

Amino acids have an α-carbon atom to which are attached the α-amino and α-carboxyl groups. Depending on the positioning of the four groups around the α-carbon, two stereoisomers can be distinguished: L- and D-amino acids. Only L-amino acids occur in proteins. D-amino acids are not metabolized; they are excreted in urine.

The amino and carboxyl groups are both protonated at low pH (Figure 2-6); the carboxyl group then loses its charge, whereas the amino group becomes cationic. Consequently, the net charge on the molecule at low pH is positive. Similarly, at high pH the net charge of the amino acid is negative, since the carboxyl group is fully dissociated and, thus, anionic, while the amino acid group loses an H^+ ion and, thus, its positive charge. Midway between the pK values of the α-amino and α-carboxyl groups, the number of positive and negative charges balance; at this **isoelectric point (IEP),** the amino acid has no net charge.

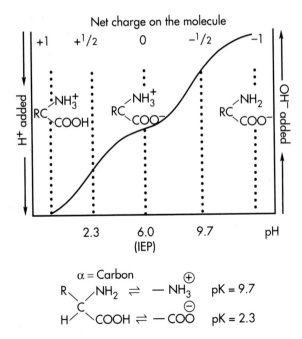

Figure 2-6. Electrical charge of an amino acide in relation to pH.

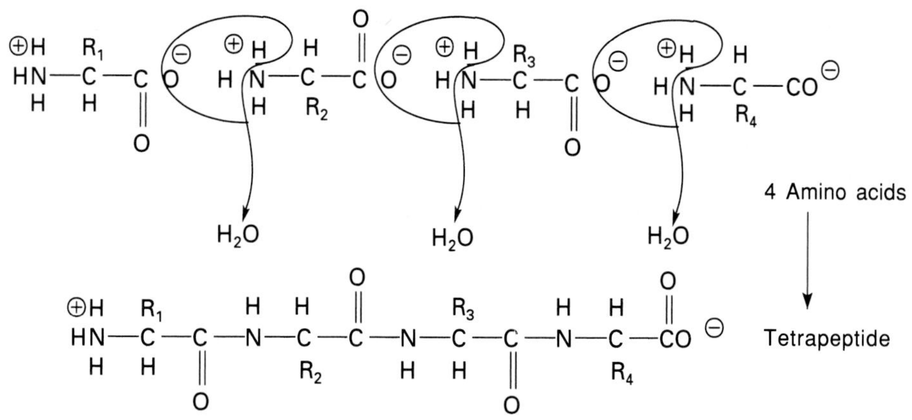

Figure 2-7. Peptide bond formation.

Peptides

The formation of peptide bonds is a condensation reaction as water is formed (Figure 2-7). Since the electrical charges on the $-NH_3^+$ and $-COO^-$ groups attached to the α-carbons are lost, a peptide chain is formed with one amino terminal ($-NH_3^+$) and one **carboxyl terminal** ($-COO^-$); in between are a variable number of amino acids with their specialty groups (R_x) branching off of the chain. It is common to define di-, tri-, tetra-, penta-, hexa-, hepta-, octa-, nona-, and deca-peptides according to their exact number (2-10), respectively, of constituent amino acids. Beyond 10, they are referred to as polypeptides. When the molecular weight of a polypeptide approaches 10,000 (approximately 50 amino acids in length), it is listed as a protein. Proteins consist mostly of several polypeptide chains to which non—amino-acid matter may be attached (e.g., heme; carbohydrates; lipids).

The peptide chain has no hydrophilic properties. Solubility of peptides (proteins) in water is, therefore, derived from charged specialty groups on the R portions of the constituent amino acids. As most of the amino acids in a peptide chain have no charges on R, they do not contribute to water solubility or to acid-base buffering. This explains why the body contains many insoluble proteins that function, for example, as structural elements (cytoskeleton; collagen; hair), contractile proteins in muscles (actin; myosin); and blood-clotting elements (fibrin). Many proteins are amphoteric; with their apolar regions they can interact with lipids, while their polar regions bring about water solubility (discussed earlier in the section entitled, "Amphoteric interactions").

Proteins

Two amino acids (aspartic acid and glutamic acid) contribute anionic charges, and three amino acids (lysine, histidine, and arginine) contribute cationic charges to a peptide chain. Judged by pK values (Figure 2-8), at the physiological pH of serum, the two acidic amino acids are totally dissociated (i.e., negatively charged), and the specialty groups of lysine and arginine are fully protonated (positively charged). Therefore, the only buffering group of any consequence is histidine's imidazole group (pK 6.0) that, at pH 7.4, is only partly protonated. Proteins, thus, have their best buffering capacities in nonphysiological pH ranges.

Electrical charges of proteins (Figure 2-9)
Influence of pH

β-lactoglobulin contains these charged amino acids: 3 carboxyl terminal groups, 60 aspartate/glutamate carboxyl groups, 3 amino terminal groups, 33 lysine, 7 arginine, and 4 histidine. Judged by the terminal groups, lactoglobulin has 3 peptide chains. It is a typical protein insofar as it contains more potential negative charges (63) than positive ones (47). Hence, at pH 7.4, the protein carries a net negative charge. At more alkaline pH, more cationic groups deprotonate (lose their positive charge), thus, the net

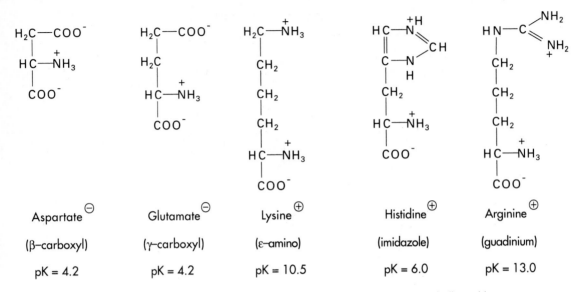

Figure 2-8. Anionic and cationic amino acids. Names of specialty groups are indicated in parentheses.

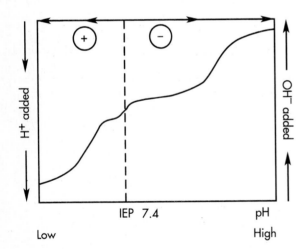

Figure 2-9. Net electrical charge of a protein depends on pH.

isoelectric point, or **isoelectric pH (IEP),** is specific for a given protein. Most proteins contain more aspartate and glutamate than basic amino acids, and, thus, have their IEP under pH 6.0. Hence, at physiologic pH, they carry a net negative charge. Notable exceptions are histones, proteins found in the nuclei of cells in close association with DNA. Because of excess lysine and arginine, histones have their IEP well above 7.0, thus, they are cationic at physiological pH.

Methods

- Electrophoresis: When a protein mixture is spotted on a solid support (e.g., gel or paper) that is saturated with buffer solution and an electrical field is applied to that support, the proteins move in proportion to their charge/mass ratio and, thus, are separated. They can then be fixed, stained, and quantified densitometrically (Figure 2-10).
- Electrofocussing: When a protein mixture is applied to a gel column that contains a continuous pH gradient and an electrical voltage difference is applied over the length of that column, each protein moves to its individual IEP and forms a band at that pH in the column.

negative charge of the protein increases. Similarly, by acidifying the medium, negative charges are lost by protonation. When 16 of the 63 negative charges of lactoglobin have been protonated, the remaining 47 anionic charges equal the 47 cationic charges. At this pH, the net charge of the protein is zero. The

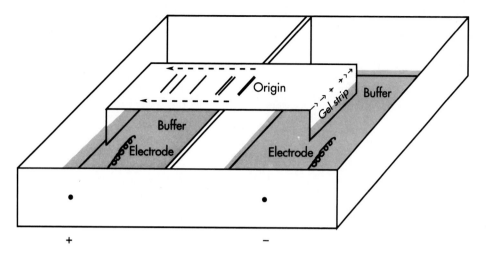

Figure 2-10. Electrophoresis. In the illustrated case, an alkaline buffer was used, giving the proteins a net negative charge so that they moved towards the anode.

STUDY QUESTIONS

1. *a.* What is meant when it is said that fat is a source of metabolic water in animals?
   b. Reason as to why protein is a poor source of metabolic water, and why fats yield more metabolic water than do carbohydrates.

2. *a.* List the subcellular structure held together largely by hydrophobic interactions within a lipid bilayer.
   b. List the kind of bonding that keeps water fluid (instead of gaseous) and helps stabilize DNA and protein structures.

3. The transport of apolar compounds in the body (which is aqueous) poses a solubility problem.
   a. In what form are these substances transported in the bloodstream?
   b. In what form are they transported in bile?

4. *a.* Why does protein binding of a compound prevent its loss through urination?
   b. List the organ with a special excretory route for waste products that are protein bound in the bloodstream.

5. *a.* A hormone's binding to a specific plasma protein increases that hormone's half-life in the circulation. (True/False)
   b. How is it possible that blood glucose, which isn't bound to plasma proteins, is not lost in the urine under physiologic conditions?

6. Homeostatic control of the body's pH is important for:
   a. Maintaining the H-bonding that holds DNA strands together. (True/False)
   b. Maintaining the disulfide bridges that provide tertiary structure to a protein. (True/False)
   c. Maintaining the proper balance of enzyme activities in cells. (True/False)
   d. Maintaining muscle cells' responsiveness to nervous stimulation. (True/False)

7. *a.* List the inorganic chemical buffer systems in serum.
   b. In arterial blood, the bicarbonate/carbonic acid ratio is higher than 20:1. (True/False)

8. In the condition of alkalemia:
   a. What are the kidneys' adaptive responses?
   b. What are the lungs' adaptive responses?

9. Two functions of the lungs have already been encountered
   a. List the overall purpose of converting angiotensin I to angiotensin II.
   b. List the overall purpose of hyperventilation during acidosis.

10. *a.* Most of the body's proteins have an isoelectric point above 7.4. (True/False)
   b. Adding acid would move an anionic protein closer to its isoelectric point. (True/False)

11. Why are aspartic acid and lysine in proteins unable to contribute to the acid-base buffering capacity of plasma in vivo?

12. *a.* List an amino acid that is abundantly present in the structure of histones, causing those proteins to have an isoelectric pH in the alkaline range.
    b. Would histones move toward the positive or the negative electrode when electrophoresed at physiologic pH?

13. *a.* Explain why lowering the body's pH decreases the net charge of a protein with an IEP of 5-6 (albumin).
    b. Reason as to why this effect causes the release of K^+ from cells (dangerous hyperkalemia).

14. Definitions and terminology:
    a. Exemplify a polar group of a protein.
    b. List the value of the physiological pH of serum.

c. List the general clinical term for a condition of low blood pH.
d. List a blood pH in the viable range of alkalemia.
e. List one chemical property, other than concentration, that determines whether a compound is a good buffer at physiologic pH.
f. List the independent variables that, according to Stewart, control pH in the body.
g. Name the hydrophilic group on glutamic acid in a peptide.
h. Name an "essential" amino acid.
i. List one anionic and one cationic amino acid that give charges to proteins.

Proteins: structure, function, and biosynthesis

PROTEIN STRUCTURE AND FUNCTION
Amino acids contained in proteins

Proteins consist of polypeptide chains in which twenty different amino acids may be included (Figure 3-1). Those amino acids can be divided into the following categories:

- Nonpolar amino acids: glycine, alanine, valine, leucine, and isoleucine. A preponderance of apolar amino acids is found where a protein interfaces with a lipid environment; for example, embedded in the lipid bilayer of a cell membrane.
- Amino acids with OH—groups: serine and threonine. In glycoproteins, carbohydrate chains are attached to the protein via OH groups (threonine) or amide groups (asparagine).
- Sulphur-containing amino acids: cysteine and methionine. The formation of cystine, linking two cysteine molecules by means of a disulfide (—S—S—) bridge, is a major determinant of tertiary protein structure. The —S—CH$_3$ group of methionine is vitally important in biological methylations.
- Anionic (acidic) amino acids: aspartate and glutamate. In addition to their α-carboxyl group, these amino acids have a second carboxyl group. Amide [—C(O)OH → −C(O)NH$_2$] formation from that second carboxyl group produces asparagine (from aspartate) and glutamine (from glutamate).
- Cationic (basic) amino acids: lysine, arginine, and histidine. In addition to their α-amino

group, these amino acids contain a second group that may be protonated.
- Aromatic amino acids: tryptophan, tyrosine, and phenylalanine. These amino acids are responsible for absorption of ultraviolet light at 280 nm by which protein concentrations in solutions can be quantified.
- Imino acids: proline and its posttranslational derivative, hydroxyproline.

Nutritionally, one distinguishes between essential and nonessential amino acids. An essential compound is one the body needs but cannot synthesize in adequate amounts; hence it must be provided by the diet. In most animal species, histidine, leucine, isoleucine, valine, methionine, lysine, threonine, phenylalanine, and tryptophan are essential. Nonessential amino acids are synthesized in the body when needed.

Physiologically active peptides

Between amino acids and proteins there exists a vast array of peptides that have vital physiological importance. Four examples are cited here.

Glutathione

This tripeptide consists of glutamic acid, cysteine, and glycine (Figure 3-2). Because of the —SH group of cysteine, glutathione is sensitive to the reduction/oxidation (redox) environment in a cell. By giving off electrons, two glutathione molecules are linked by a disulfide (—S—S—) bridge: 2 GSH ↔ GS—SG

Name	Abbreviation		Structural Formula	Chemical Nature of Side Chain
	Three-Letter	One-Letter		
Glycine	Gly	G	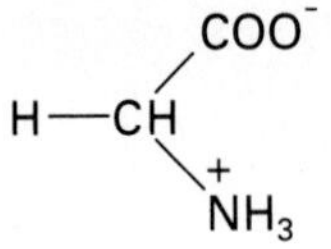 $H-CH$, COO^-, $\overset{+}{N}H_3$	Aliphatic
Alanine	Ala	A	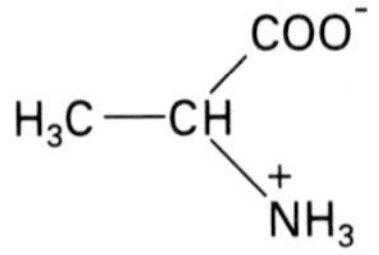 H_3C-CH, COO^-, $\overset{+}{N}H_3$	Aliphatic
Valine	Val	V	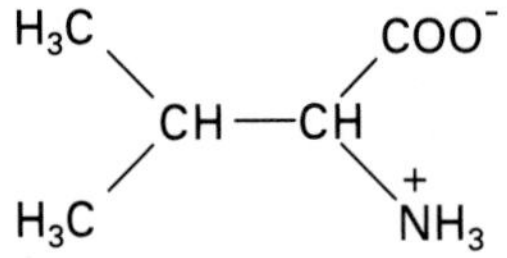 H_3C, H_3C, $CH-CH$, COO^-, $\overset{+}{N}H_3$	Aliphatic
Leucine	Leu	L	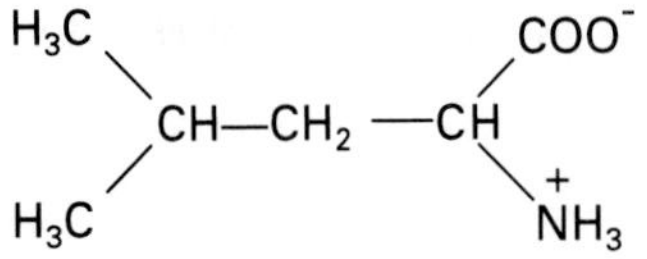 H_3C, H_3C, $CH-CH_2-CH$, COO^-, $\overset{+}{N}H_3$	Aliphatic
Isoleucine	Ile	I	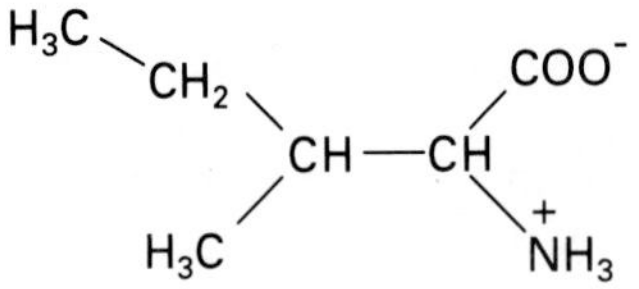 H_3C, CH_2, H_3C, $CH-CH$, COO^-, $\overset{+}{N}H_3$	Aliphatic
Serine	Ser	S	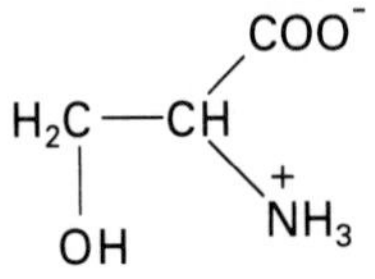 H_2C-CH, OH, COO^-, $\overset{+}{N}H_3$	OH group
Threonine	Thr	T	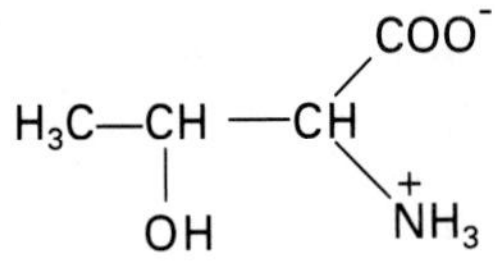 $H_3C-CH-CH$, OH, COO^-, $\overset{+}{N}H_3$	OH group
Tyrosine	Tyr	Y	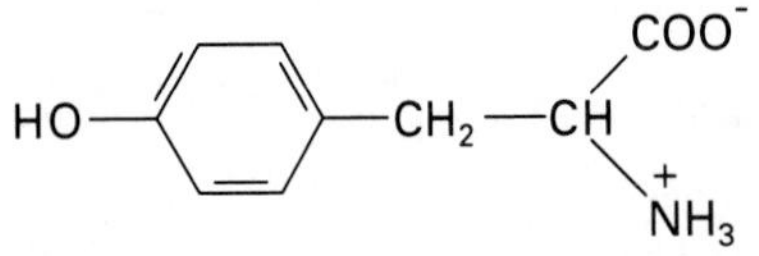 $HO-\langle\rangle-CH_2-CH$, COO^-, $\overset{+}{N}H_3$	OH group and aromatic

Figure 3-1. The twenty encoded amino acids found in proteins.

Name	Abbreviation		Structural Formula	Chemical Nature of Side Chain
	Three-Letter	One-Letter		
Cysteine	Cys	C	H_2C—CH with COO^-, SH, $\overset{+}{N}H_3$	Sulfur
Methionine	Met	M	H_2C—CH_2—CH with COO^-, S—CH_3, $\overset{+}{N}H_3$	Sulfur
Aspartate	Asp	D	^-OOC—CH_2—CH with COO^-, $\overset{+}{N}H_3$	Carboxyl anion
Asparagine	Asn	N	H_2N—$\overset{O}{\overset{\|}{C}}$—$CH_2$—$CH$ with COO^-, $\overset{+}{N}H_3$	Amide group
Glutamate	Glu	E	^-OOC—CH_2—CH_2—CH with COO^-, $\overset{+}{N}H_3$	Carboxyl anion
Glutamine	Gln	Q	H_2N—$\overset{O}{\overset{\|}{C}}$—$CH_2$—$CH_2$—$CH$ with COO^-, $\overset{+}{N}H_3$	Amide group
Arginine	Arg	R	HN—CH_2—CH_2—CH_2—CH with COO^-, $\overset{+}{N}H_3$; $\overset{\|}{C}$—NH_2, $\overset{+}{N}H_2$	Cationic group
Lysine	Lys	K	CH_2—CH_2—CH_2—CH_2—CH with COO^-, $\overset{+}{N}H_3$; $^+NH_3$	Cationic group

Figure 3-1, cont'd. The twenty encoded amino acids found in proteins. *Continued.*

Name	Abbreviation Three-Letter	Abbreviation One-Letter	Structural Formula	Chemical Nature of Side Chain
Histidine	His	H		Cationic group and aromatic
Phenylalanine	Phe	F		Aromatic
Tryptophan	Trp	W		Aromatic
Proline	Pro	P		Imino acid

Figure 3-1, cont'd. The twenty encoded amino acids found in proteins.

+ 2 H. Glutathione is a reducing agent of special importance in erythrocytes (discussed later). Other functions include its use (i) in the liver to conjugate compounds before they are excreted in bile; (ii) in the pancreatic formation of insulin; and (iii) as a constituent of leukotrienes.

Thyrotropin-releasing hormone

Thyrotropin-releasing hormone (TRH) is another tripeptide. Because tripeptides are so small, they, and their biological activities, have long remained undetected. TRH originates in the hypothalamus and is then transported to the pituitary, where it stimulates the release of TSH (thyroid-stimulating hormone), which, in turn, activates the thyroid gland to elaborate thyroxine. TRH was the first releasing hormone to be identified, purified, and synthesized. Other releasing, or regulating, hormones (RH) of the hypothalamus include adrenocorticotropic hormone-RH, growth hormone-RH, gonadotropin-RH, and prolactin-RH.

Endorphins

Endorphins are polypeptides (17-31 amino acids long) with strong analgesic potencies (18-30 times more powerful than morphine). They bind to opiate receptors in the brain, and are involved in endogenous control of pain perception.

Hormones

Many hormones are peptides; for example, antidiuretic hormone and oxytocin are nonapeptides synthesized in the hypothalmus and stored in the posterior pituitary, with quite homologous structures and therefore partially overlapping functions (Figure 3-3).

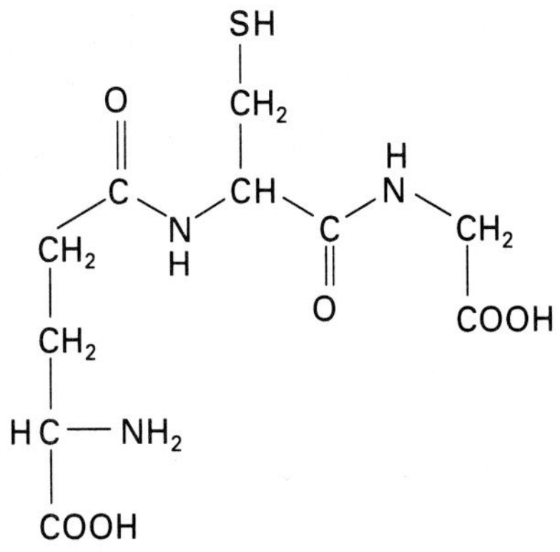

γ-Glutamyl-cysteinyl-glycine (GSH)

$$GSH + GSH \rightleftharpoons GSSG + 2H$$

Figure 3-2. Glutathione.

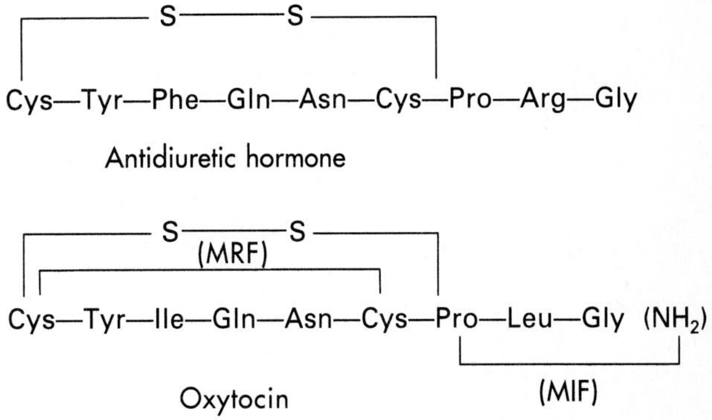

Figure 3-3. Homologous structures of antidiuretic hormone and oxytocin. The ring structure of oxytocin may be the source of melanocyte releasing factor (MRF), and the tripeptide side chain the source of melanocyte inhibiting factor (MIF).

Structure of proteins

Proteins are large macromolecular complexes with molecular weights ranging from 10 to 1,000 kilodaltons (kDa). Molecular weights can be determined by various methods, including: (i) ultracentrifugation (sedimentation rate); (ii) electrophoresis (charge/mass ratio); and (iii) molecular sieving through gel or filter pores that exclude proteins larger than the pore size. Usually some proteins of known molecular weights are included in an assay to serve as standards.

All proteins contain one or more polypeptide chains and practically all contain one or more of the following: carbohydrates, lipids, nucleic acids, heme, and minerals. Though chemically a distinction can be made between the protein moiety and the adsorbed ligands, physiologically that distinction does not make sense, since only the protein-ligand combination has a defined function.

Primary structure

The peptide chain of amino acids is genetically coded and then modified posttranslationally (discussed later). The primary structure is the only thing that is genetically coded. All other structural elements follow the laws of chemistry and physics: the "system" will find the lowest free energy state under a given set of environmental conditions (pH, redox potential, temperature, and ionic strength and composition), and that state of maximal stability is reflected in the stable, characteristic, three-dimensional shape (structure) of the protein molecule.

Secondary structure

Peptide chains exist as coiled helices, as sheets of antiparallel-oriented chains, or in random coil configurations. Formation of those structures establishes a large number of hydrogen bonds between different amino acids (Figure 3-4) that lower the free energy of the system and thus stabilize it.

Tertiary structure

The secondary structures are folded and intertwined (Figure 3-5). Disulfide bonds between cysteine residues, located on either the same or different peptide chains, are chief tertiary structure determinants. The sensitivity of disulfide bond formation to oxidation and reduction requires homeostatic control of the body's redox potential (discussed later).

Ionogenic bonding shapes peptide chains by bringing opposite charges together. This makes the stability of proteins dependent on the homeostatic control of pH, ionic strength, and ion composition in their environment.

Hydrophobic interactions between nonpolar amino acid residues in a protein (cf., oil droplets) contribute to stabilizing the tertiary protein structure. Aggregation of nonpolar amino acid residues forms oily pockets that allow interaction of the protein with lipids (see Figure 3-5).

Quaternary structure

Many proteins possess no more than a tertiary structure; they are monomers. Arranging monomeric subunits (in some cases more than 10 of them) in a

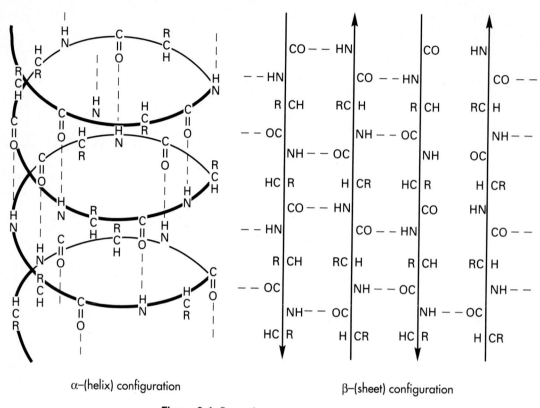

α–(helix) configuration   β–(sheet) configuration

Figure 3-4. Secondary structure of proteins.

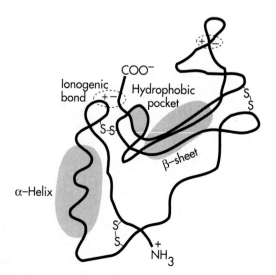

Figure 3-5. Tertiary structure of a protein. A single (hypothetical) peptide chain is diagrammed as a line connecting the α-carbons of amino acids from the amino ($-NH_3^+$) to the carboxy ($-COO^-$) terminal. A region of α-helix and one of pleated sheet are shaded; the rest of the chain is a random coil. The chain is cross-linked by disulfide bridges between cysteine residues at the indicated positions; also ionogenic bonding and hydrophobic interactions contribute to the tertiary structure.

quaternary structure produces the final, functional shape of polymeric proteins (e.g., many enzymes, hemoglobin, ferritin). Often, monomers of different kinds are combined.

In summary, a protein's structure may look capricious at first glance, but, in fact, it is totally fixed and characteristic under given environmental conditions.

Relation between structure and function of proteins

A listing of protein functions includes the following items, most of which will be discussed later.

- Enzymes (all enzymes are proteins).
- Receptors in membranes.
- Certain hormones and most cellular receptors that recognize hormones are proteins or (poly)peptides.
- Proteinaceous factors control transcription and translation processes by which the genetic code is expressed.
- Structural elements in the body (collagen, cytoskeleton)
- Lubricants (mucus)
- Transport of ligands in blood, in cells, and across cell membranes
- Immune defense system
- Blood-clotting factors
- Fluid retention

In first instance, these functions rely on a perfect protein structure that requires a functional gene and fidelity in the transcription and translation of the genetic message. Lacking those prerequisites leads to an altered primary structure of the protein, which may or may not be accompanied by a loss of function (discussed later). In addition to genetics, environmental factors may profoundly affect the functioning of a protein.

Denaturation of proteins

A protein may lose its biological activity as a result of structural reformation induced by changing the environment. The protein finds temporarily (reversible, when the environment returns to its original state) or permanently (irreversible) a different structure of lowest free energy in response to the altered environment.

Nature guards against involuntary changes in protein structure by the homeostatic control of the body's internal environment (pH, redox potential, temperature, ionic strength, and ion composition). In some instances, where it is nature's intent to denature a protein, the environment is accommodated to do so; for example, digestion in the stomach or in lysosomes.

For experimental purposes of separating protein mixtures, or isolating and characterizing proteins, it is often advantageous to use a method of controlled denaturation. Such methods include boiling, salting, dehydration, H-bond disruption by urea, acidification, and isoelectric precipitation.

Reversible changes in protein structure caused by ligand binding

Many protein functions relate to transport: the protein binds small molecules (ligands) at one site in the body where certain environmental conditions prevail. The protein-ligand complex then assumes its characteristic (lowest free energy) structure, and in that shape it transports the ligand to its destination. At the site of destination, different environmental conditions may prevail; hence, the protein may assume a different tertiary structure, which then frees the ligand for delivery. Protein-ligand binding helps regulate the physiologic effects of an active compound, since in its unbound form, it can enter cells because of its smaller size. Catabolism of unbound ligand allows an equilibrium shift toward dissociation of additional ligand at the site of its metabolic use.

The following are examples of reversible ligand binding:

- Hormone transport by serum proteins
- Oxygen transport by hemoglobin
- Lipid transport by lipoproteins
- Bilirubin transport by serum albumin
- Substrate binding to enzymes

PROTEIN BIOSYNTHESIS: GENETIC CONTROL

This section starts with a review of how genetic information contained in nuclear DNA is copied and transferred to future generations of cells. Following this is a look at a given cell that must obey the genetic masterplan contained in its DNA. Genes must first be transcribed in the form of RNA before their message can be imparted upon protein biosynthesis. The initial RNA transcript of a gene contains noncoding sequences that are "edited out" in the nucleus, giving rise to different species of RNA (e.g., ribosomal-, transfer- and messenger-RNA) each fulfilling a well-defined function in protein synthesis. Messenger RNA is exported into the cytoplasm where it is translated on ribosomes into a protein. That protein can then be altered posttranslationally to suit the needs of the cell or be exported from the cell. Despite refined control over the maintenance of pristine DNA, the fidelity of gene transcription and translation, and the quantity and quality of protein synthesis, errors do occur that introduce mutations. A detailed picture of molecular genetics is emerging, thus allowing the scientific community to development means (antibiotics, chemotherapy) by which to cripple unwanted growth and to recognize and rectify faulty genetic traits.

To avoid getting lost in the molecular details of this fascinating topic, the text will adhere to its objectives (ability to read professional literature and apply that to related fields) and focus especially on the following:
- Genetic control of cell structure and metabolic functioning
- Mutations: inborn diseases and gene modifying influences
- Genetic engineering (recombinant DNA, reverse transcriptase)
- Antibiotics acting by interference with protein biosynthesis

In what follows, many of the items listed should be familiar from previous training. If needed, the use of a textbook is recommended to review certain topics. The following abbreviations will be used for the bases that make up the structures of nucleic acids: A = adenine; G = guanine; C = cytosine; T = thymine; and U = uracil.

DNA and transfer of genetic information
Functions of DNA

There are two main functions of DNA:
- It is replicated so genes are inherited by offspring.
- It serves as a blueprint for the synthesis of various classes of RNA and proteins.

Structure of DNA

The DNA helix consists of two strands, oriented in an antiparallel way and held together by H-bonding between the complementary base pairs A—T and C—G (Figure 3-6). The backbone of each strand consists of a sugar-phosphate chain in which deoxyribose units are linked in their 3′ and 5′ positions by phosphate diaster bonds; hence, a DNA strand has a 3′ and a 5′ terminal.

Occurrence of DNA

Eukaryotic cells (found in all animals and plants) have a membrane-bounded nucleus in which DNA, associated with about an equal weight of proteins in a chromatin structure, is contained in multiple chromosomes. Prokaryotic cells (e.g., bacteria), in contrast, contain only one chromosome that is not well demarcated in the cytoplasm. In eukaryotic cells, all genetic information is carried by DNA, predominantly in the nucleus, but some in mitochondria.

The number of chromosomes varies with animal species. The human genome consists of 6.4×10^9 base pairs of DNA contained in 23 pairs of homologous chromosomes during the stable gap-1 phase of the cell cycle (Figure 3-7). Having pairs of chromosomes, each one derived from one parent, is termed diploidy. As the stretched-out length of all DNA in a chromosome is approximately 47 mm, the length of DNA must be compressed about 8000-fold to fit inside the chromosome. This "packing" is initially accomplished by the DNA wrapping itself around clusters of histone molecules, thus forming nucleosomes. Histones are positively charged proteins due to their high contents of lysine and arginine; histones and nonhistone proteins associated with DNA have regulatory control over DNA activity. Nucleosomes arrange themselves in coiled strings and those strings then wind around themselves, forming supercoils. In DNA replication, rapid uncoiling of DNA must occur.

Nuclear DNA is a heterogenous mixture, most of which does not code for a protein molecule. About 70% consists of unique sequences (few copies or only one per genome), which include the ones that encode the major cell proteins; these coding sequences (exons) are interspersed with intervening sequences (introns) that are copied but then "edited out" of the final transcript (per below). The unique sequences are separated by various kinds of highly (millions per genome) and moderately (hundreds per genome) repetitive sequences of 2-300 base pairs in length that are not transcribed. Moderately repetitive (over 100 copies per genome) are the DNA sequences that code for transfer RNA and ribosomal RNA species, and for histones; those repetitions are sequential so that, for example, all histones are transcribed in tandem.

Mitochondrial DNA is a double-stranded, circular molecule of about 15,000 base pairs that codes for several mitochondrial proteins. The mitochondrial genetic code contains four codon assignments for amino acids and chain termination signals that differ from those in the nucleus of animal and plant cells. Proteins encoded in mitochondrial DNA are synthesized on ribosomes inside mitochondria. Over 90% of

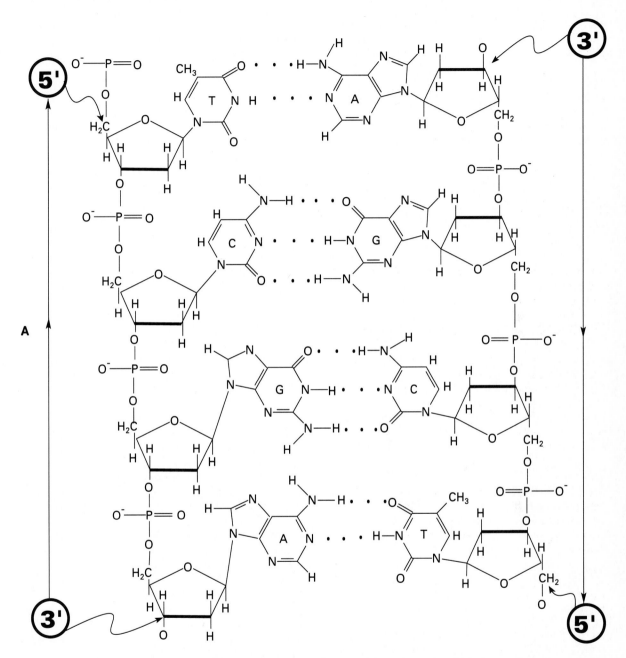

Figure 3-6. Structure of DNA. **A,** Two antiparellel strands are shown in which the continuous chains of deoxyribose-phosphate are linked via hydrogen bonds between the base pairs A-T and C-G.

Continued.

B

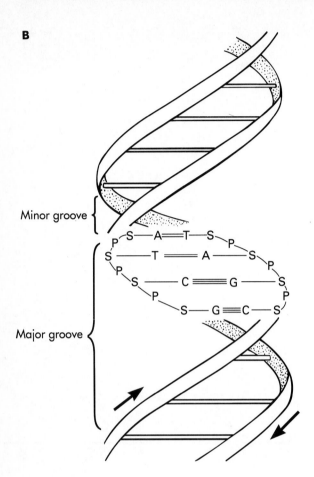

Figure 3-6, cont'd. B, Diagram of a portion of a DNA double helix in which the sugar- *(S)* phosphate *(P)* chains are shaded.

Figure 3-7. Cell cycle. In the life cycle of a cell four phases are discernible: gap-1 *(G₁)*, a phase of reproductive inactivity when diploid chromosomes are present; synthetic (S) phase in which DNA replicates; gap-2 *(G₂)* when cells contain twice the amount of DNA as during G_1 because each chromosome has split into two identical sister chromatids; and mitosis (M) in which the two daughter cells part.

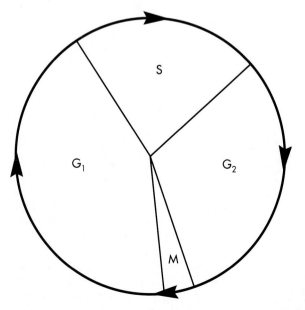

mitochondrial proteins, however, are encoded in the nucleus and imported from the cytoplasm.

Synthesis of nuclear DNA

During the synthetic phase of the cell cycle, DNA is replicated in a semiconservative manner. Each of the two strands serves as a template for replication via base pairing; hence, a daughter DNA molecule consists of one parental and one new strand (Figure 3-8).

In eukaryotic cells, four different species of DNA polymerase have been identified, one of which is for mitochondrial DNA synthesis and one for DNA repair. DNA polymerase α functions in the replication of nuclear DNA. DNA replication by DNA polymerase α proceeds only in the 5' to 3' direction; thus, one strand is oriented such that on one primer a long daughter sequence, termed the leading strand, is replicated continuously. In the complementary strand of parental DNA, replication seems to go in the opposite (3' to 5') direction. This feat is accomplished by 5' to 3' replication of small (100-200 nucleotides) sequences for each, which require short (4-10 bases long) primer sequences of RNA synthesized by a special RNA polymerase, or primase, enzyme (Figure 3-9). An RNA primer is attached by base pairing to a parent DNA and then DNA polymerase adds a daughter-chain fragment of DNA to the primer. These DNA fragments are about 100-200 base pairs long and are called Okazaki pieces, after their discoverer. The RNA primer sequence is then enzymically degraded and replaced by DNA bases, after which adjacent DNA fragments are joined to the lagging strand of daughter DNA by DNA ligase.

During DNA synthesis, newly replicated DNA is constantly subjected to "proofreading," "editing," and replacement of incorrect bases by special enzymes that work in tandem with DNA polymerases.

Before replication can begin, the supercoiled structure of DNA must first be unwound. A DNA helicase enzyme uncoils DNA and pries the chains apart at the site of a replication fork, while a special protein binds to the single strands of unwound DNA to prevent their reannealing. This gives rise to replication bubbles during DNA synthesis. Ahead of a replication fork, DNA gyrase removes twists that the unwinding process had introduced.

Uncoiling of DNA, synthesis of histones, formation of nucleosomes, and recoiling of new DNA must keep pace with replication, and, therefore, slow the process down. Two factors in particular help to speed

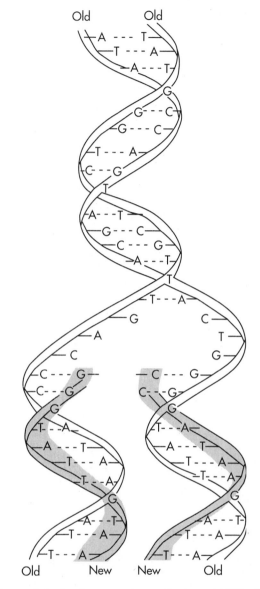

Figure 3-8. Semiconservative replication of DNA. *Redrawn with permission from Watson JD: Molecular biology of the gene, ed 4, p. 283, Menlo Park, CA, 1987, Benjamin/Cummings.*

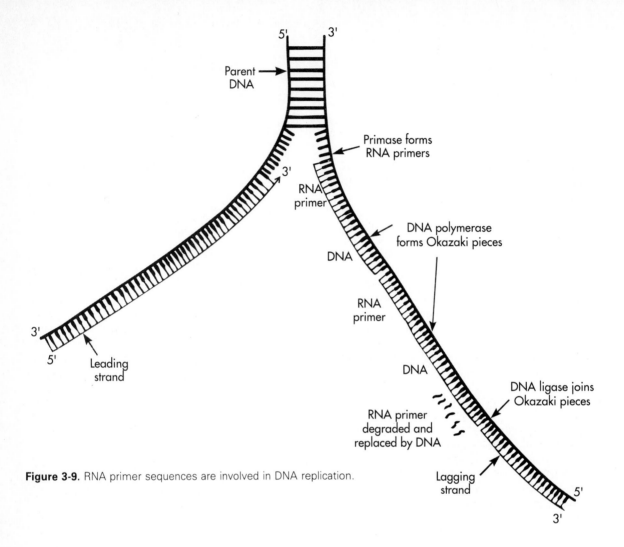

Figure 3-9. RNA primer sequences are involved in DNA replication.

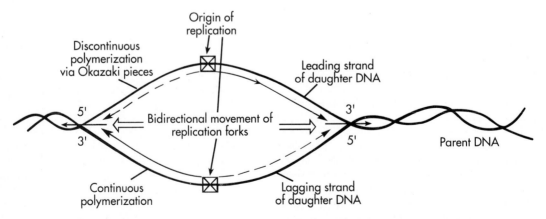

Figure 3-10. Bidirectional movement of replication forks on DNA. In a replication bubble, continuous polymerization of leading strand and discontinuous formation of lagging strand of daughter DNA occurs.

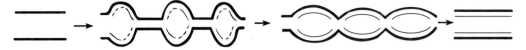

Figure 3-11. Multiple replication origins on a chromosome.

up DNA synthesis: (1) replication forks move bidirectionally from each origin (Figure 3-10); and (2) multiple origins of replication are present on each chromosome so that DNA replication starts at multiple sites simultaneously (Figure 3-11).

Transcription of DNA: RNA synthesis and processing

DNA is not directly involved in protein synthesis; rather, the genetic message is transcribed and edited in the nucleus and then conveyed by RNA to the cytoplasm, where the message is translated into the primary structure of proteins at the site of ribosomes. Several RNA species are involved in protein synthesis: messenger RNA (mRNA) carries the genetic message to ribosomes, where ribosomal RNA (rRNA) is involved in assembling the polypeptide chain by bringing mRNA in contact with transfer RNA (tRNA) molecules that carry encoded amino acids.

Some major features are common to all RNA structures. Ribose, not deoxyribose, is the sugar moiety. In RNA, the base thymine (T) does not occur; uracil (U) is found instead; hence, tritium-labeled T is used in research as a specific marker for DNA, and U is used for RNA. RNA occurs as a single strand, albeit pairing of complementary base sequences may bring distant segments of that strand in apposition, thus, creating loops.

Mechanism of RNA synthesis by DNA transcription

While in DNA synthesis both strands are replicated, in RNA synthesis, only one of the two DNA strands serves as the template (or coding strand) for transcription of a given gene, while for that gene, the other strand (antitemplate or noncoding strand) is not transcribed; for a different gene, the roles of the DNA strands may be reversed.

The different RNA species are all transcribed from DNA genes, for which purpose there are three classes of DNA-dependent RNA polymerase, and are indicated by Roman numerals. RNA pol I transcribes rRNA in the nucleolus region; in the nucleoplasm, RNA pol II transcribes mRNA and RNA pol III transcribes tRNA.

The process of transcription (Figure 3-12) starts at a promoter site; that is, a short string of bases within which a characteristic sequence that starts with T,A,T,A (the **TATA box**) is found. With the aid of one of its protein subunits, sigma factor, a polymerase is linked to the TATA box. Each class of RNA polymerase recognizes a specific type of promoter. The polymerase pries the two DNA strands apart and at the initiation site, a few bases downstream from the promoter site, it begins transcribing RNA from a template DNA chain in 3′ to 5′ direction by the rules of base pairing, whereby the RNA transcript is formed in antiparallel fashion from 5′ to 3′; the sigma factor dissociates. The process of RNA chain elongation continues until a termination signal on the DNA chain is encountered and recognized (probably with the help of a termination factor such as rho factor, as in prokaryotes), whereupon DNA, rho factor, and the primary RNA transcript disengage.

Allosteric sequences on DNA are found where environmental or chemical factors may either stimulate or inhibit transcription. Depending on their effect, these sequences are called **enhancers** or **silencers.** Those sites may be thousands of bases removed from the promoter site in either the upstream or downstream direction and may be oriented in either the 5′ to 3′ or 3′ to 5′ direction; however, they must be located on the same chromosome (which is taken as evidence that their effect is not chemically mediated).

Other influences on transcription are exemplified by thyroid or steroid hormones. Specific receptors in the cytoplasm of a cell bind those hormones and consequently change the tertiary structure of the protein receptor. Those receptor-hormone complexes then enter the nucleus, where they are recognized by a specific receptor-recognition site on DNA, a hormone responsive element (HRE), a few hundred bases proximal from where the transcription of steroid-responsive genes starts. An HRE in a gene may either stimulate or inhibit transcription. Stimulation of the gene for a rate-controlling enzyme in gluconeogenesis (phosphoenolpyruvate carboxykinase [PEPCK]) by glucocorticoids is a good example, as attachment of

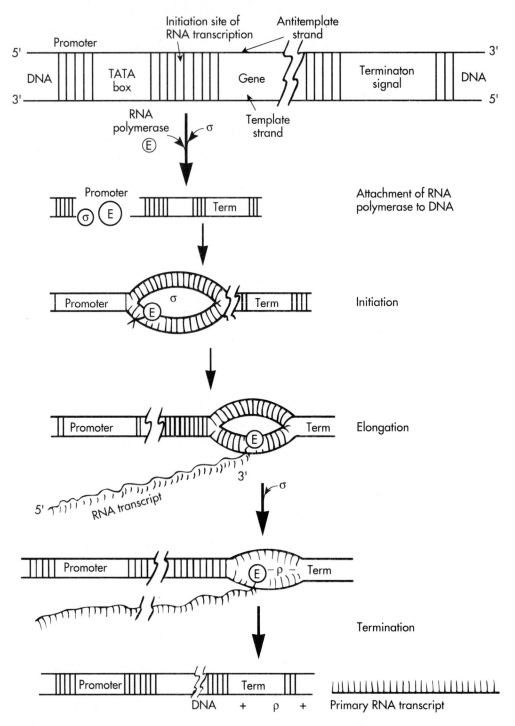

Figure 3-12. Synthesis of a primary RNA transcript from DNA. The various phases of transcription are indicated. Involvement of ρ factor in the termination phase in eukaryotes is speculative.

the glucocorticoid-receptor complex to its receptor-recognition site on the DNA converts the HRE into an active enhancer element. The gene for PEPCK holds, in addition, a 15-base sequence that responds to insulin by inhibiting PEPCK transcription; the insulin effect overrides that of glucocorticoids.

RNA processing

Different RNA species (mRNA, tRNA, rRNA) are involved in protein synthesis; all are transcribed from nuclear DNA. The primary transcript of DNA is hnRNA, heterogeneous nuclear RNA. In most cases, this transcript has to be processed to produce RNA molecules that can function in protein synthesis. Processing takes place in the nucleus. Some seg-

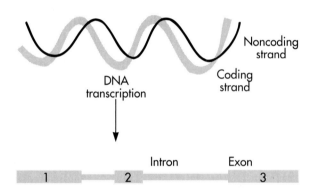

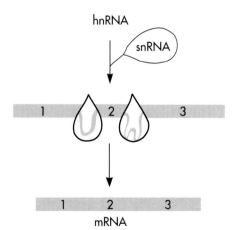

Figure 3-13. Posttranscriptional processing of RNA. Introns are excised from the primary heterogeneous nuclear RNA transcript *(hnRNA)* with the help of enzymic activity associated with small nuclear RNA (snurps), which also joins the exons.

ments of RNA may have to be trimmed at the ends by exonuclease enzymes; some bases may have to be added or chemically altered (e.g., methylated). Heterogeneous nuclear RNA contains coding sequences, or **exons,** which may be separated by large stretches of **introns.** The latter are excised and then the exons are joined (Figure 3-13). This splicing of hnRNA is performed by small nuclear RNA (snRNA, alias "snurps") that has enzyme activities even though it is devoid of protein. Snurps, being both genetically and enzymically active, are considered by some to be potential primordial molecules, though this topic is controversial.

Different RNA species

Messenger RNA (mRNA) carries the genetic message for protein synthesis in the form of codons to be translated in the cytoplasm. Eukaryotic mRNA is **monocistronic,** that is, it codes for a single polypeptide chain. After processing its primary transcript, mRNA leaves the nucleus with its 5′ head marked by a unique base, methylguanidine, together with methylated ribose, that serves as a recognizable cap (Figure 3-14). In addition, mRNA often has a 3′ polyadenylate tail of variable length. These alterations on both ends may lend stability to the RNA molecule by increasing its resistance to mRNA-ase. The cap may further be involved in the attachment of mRNA to the small 40 S (Svedberg units) ribosomal subunit during translation of mRNA into proteins.

Ribosomal RNA (rRNA) is involved in ribosomal functioning during the translation of mRNA into proteins. There exist four different types of rRNA, three of which are in the larger (60 S) ribosomal subunit and one in the smaller (40 S) subunit. There are over 100 rRNA genes in a genome. The genes associated with nucleoli produce a transcript of three of the rRNA types in tandem; that transcript is cleaved and then further trimmed into three unequal, functional rRNA molecules. The fourth rRNA type is produced in the nucleoplasm.

Transfer RNA (tRNA) is an adaptor molecule. When on a ribosome the genetic message encoded in triplets of bases (codons, discussed in the section on genetic code) on mRNA is translated into a peptide chain; the peptide chain itself does not come in contact with mRNA. Rather, tRNA contains two specific binding sites to fulfill its adaptor role. On one site it binds a specific amino acid that it transports to a ribosome, and on a distant second site on the molecule, tRNA contains a triplet of bases (anticodon)

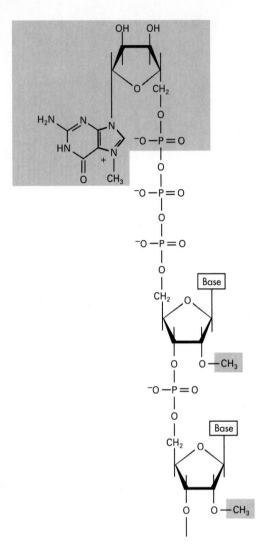

Figure 3-14. The 5' cap of eukaryotic mRNA.

size (75-85 nucleotides in length), but not in their L shaped tertiary structure (Figure 3-15, A) obtained by bringing the two side-arms in close apposition.

Though tRNA is single stranded, its secondary structure has a characteristic cloverleaf shape (Figure 3-15, B) featuring three loops and an extra arm that result from internal base pairing. The ACC terminal of its acceptor arm is where the particular amino acid attaches, and the anticodon loop contains the unique base triplet that binds the tRNA–amino-acid complex to the mRNA's specific codon. The other loops involved in the temporary attachment of tRNA to the ribosome and in the loading of the amino acid onto tRNA are named after the occurrence of unusual bases within them: the D loop after dihydrouridine, and the T-Psi-C loop after ribothymidine and pseudouridine. Several other unusual bases occur in tRNA, resulting from the posttranscriptional processing of bases. The extra arm is variable in length in different tRNA species.

Transcription of tRNA yields a long percursor RNA chain that often contains several different tRNA molecules transcribed in tandem. The precursor chain is **processed** whereby different tRNA molecules are separated, trimmed by exonucleases, and often rid of an intron by snurps. Then the ACC terminal is added and some of the bases are modified before the functional tRNA molecule is obtained. As tRNA is not stable in eukaryotes, constant production is required for which the genome contains hundreds of repetitive sequences.

Translation of messenger RNA; genetic code; protein synthesis

Having reviewed various classes of RNA, the text will now introduce some of the major features of ribosome structure and the genetic code before putting it all together functionally in the process of protein synthesis. Finally, the method by which posttranslational processing adapts a protein to its function and allows it to reach its destination will be examined.

Structure of ribosomes

The genetic message encoded on mRNA is read by amino acid–carrying tRNA and translated into a peptide chain on the **ribosome,** an agglomerate of different rRNA and protein species. As ribosomes are quite stable in the cytoplasm, they can perform many translations. Ribosomes occur in cytoplasm either in a free form for the synthesis of proteins of local importance, or attached to rough ER to produce proteins

that is complementary to the codon on mRNA to which it binds by base pairing; this triplet specifies the next amino acid to be incorporated onto the growing peptide chain elsewhere on the ribosome. With its anticodon still connected to the codon on mRNA, tRNA then adds that amino acid to the peptide chain before leaving the ribosome for another round of duty. Each cell contains over 30 different tRNA species, each one carrying a unique combination of anticodon and amino-acid specificity. These tRNA species differ in their primary structure (i.e., base sequence) and

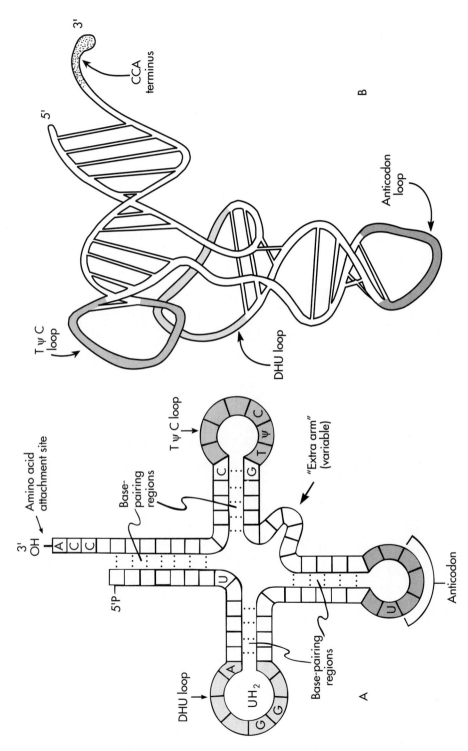

Figure 3-15. Structure of a tRNA. **A,** Common features of the secondary structures of different species of tRNA. **B,** Tertiary structure of yeast phenylalanin tRNA, after a drawing by Dr. Sung-Hou Kim. In **A** and **B,** corresponding loops have been similarly shaded. *Modified and reproduced, with permission, from Stryler L: Biochemistry, ed 2, pp 647-648, New York, 1981, Freeman & Co.*

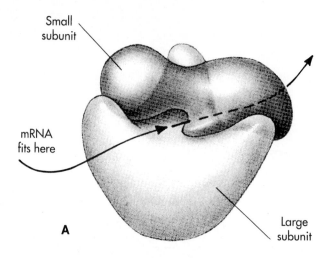

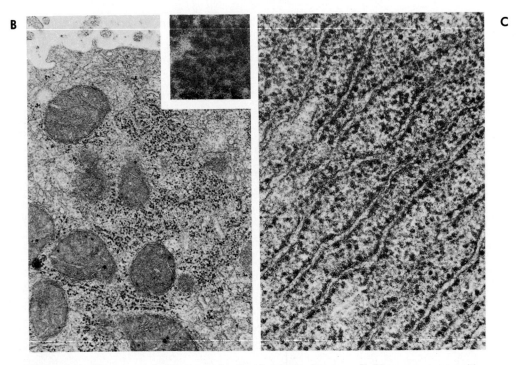

Figure 3-16. Ribosomes. **A,** The two subunits of a single ribosome. **B,** Ribosomes occur either in the free form (panel **B,** with enlarged inset) or attached to the endoplasmic reticulum (panel C). Electron photomicrographs of a rat hepatocyte. **A** *Reproduced with permission from Martini F: Fundamentals of Anatomy and Physiology, p 56, Englewood Cliffs, NJ, 1989, Prentice-Hall.* **B** *Courtesy Dr. Rick A. Rogers, Harvard School of Public Health.*

for export or for cell organelles. Polyribosomes or polysomes are strings of individual ribosomes attached to one mRNA molecule, producing multiple protein copies by the translation of a single mRNA message (Figure 3-16). Eukaryotic ribosomes have a sedimentation coefficient of 80 S and a molecular weight of about 4,200 kDa. They consist of a small (40 S) and a large (60 S) subunit. The subunits exist as separate entities, but they unite after protein synthesis has been initiated on the small subunit. Mitochondria synthesize a small fraction (less than 10%) of their proteins on ribosomes that resemble the smaller (70 S) prokaryotic ribosomes.

Ribosomes contain about 60% of their weight in the form of four different rRNA species; the rest of their weight consists of a mixture of around 85 different ribosomal proteins. All of these constituents are synthesized in coordinated fashion; for example, three of the rRNA species are transcribed as one sequence and then split up. Though the functions of all constituents are not known, it is certain that they provide the ribosome with (i) binding sites for mRNA; (ii) the complex of tRNA with its amino acid; (iii) GTP; (iv) the special factors involved in the translation process; and (v) attachment to membranes of the endoplasmic reticulum.

Genetic code

Only four different bases are found in DNA and, thus, only four complementary bases have been transcribed into mRNA. These nucleotides on mRNA are grouped in three-base code words (triplets) called codons. As there are 4^3 ($=64$) possible permutations and combinations in picking groups of three bases out of a pool of four different ones, the genetic code consists of 64 codons (Table 3-1). Three codons (termed **nonsense codons** as they do not encode an amino acid) are used in the cell as termination signals for the translation of a peptide chain. As there are no anticodons for these termination codons, their message is read by proteinaceous termination factors that release the peptide from the mRNA. That leaves 61 codons for 20 amino acids, meaning that more than 1 codon can specify the same amino acid: the code is said to be **degenerate**. It is important to note the following: several bases code for the same amino acid (degeneracy), but a given codon only codes for one amino acid; the code is not ambiguous. The codon AUG is part of an initiation signal on mRNA, but the same codon defines an internal methionine residue in the peptide chain. There is no punctuation

Table 3-1   The genetic code

First base (5′ end)	Second base				Third base (3′ end)
	U	C	A	G	
U	Phe	Ser	Tyr	Cys	U
	Phe	Ser	Tyr	Cys	C
	Leu	Ser	Stop	Stop	A
	Leu	Ser	Stop	Trp	G
C	Leu	Pro	His	Arg	U
	Leu	Pro	His	Arg	C
	Leu	Pro	Gln	Arg	A
	Leu	Pro	Gln	Arg	G
A	Ile	Thr	Asn	Ser	U
	Ile	Thr	Asn	Ser	C
	Ile	Thr	Lys	Arg	A
	Met	Thr	Lys	Arg	G
G	Val	Ala	Asp	Gly	U
	Val	Ala	Asp	Gly	C
	Val	Ala	Glu	Gly	A
	Val	Ala	Glu	Gly	G

Individual bases of a triplet codon are presented 5′ to 3′ with first base left, second base at the top, and third base on the right; for example, UGG is the codon for tryptophan only and AGU represents serine. Three codons, labeled Stop, dictate termination of the peptide chain. AUG is part of the chain-initiation signal but otherwise codes for methionine wherever it occurs in the peptide chain.

in the genetic code: the message on mRNA is read as an uninterrupted string of successive codons from chain-initiating to chain-terminating codon. With the exception of four different codon assignments in mitochondria, the genetic code is universal in all forms of life.

In the recognition of a codon by an anticodon, tRNA orients itself towards mRNA in a manner so that the three bases of the anticodon run antiparallel to the base triplet of the codon. The first two bases of the codon and the last two bases of the anticodon combine by the rigid base-pairing rules; however, the matching of the third codon base with the first anticodon base allows flexibility or **wobble**. A consequence of wobble is that a tRNA molecule can pair its anticodon with more than one codon on mRNA, provided those codons only differ in their third-base positions. In the encoding of several amino acids, the third base of the codon is immaterial (Table 3-1) due to degeneracy of the genetic code. Therefore, wobble never introduces ambiguity, as it only occurs in cases in which the third base in the codon is inconsequential. Wobble diminishes the number of tRNA species needed to match all codons; hence, fewer than 61 different tRNA species exist.

The translation process

A key consideration in the entire process of transferring genetic information from DNA in the nucleus (or mitochondrion) to the synthesis of a protein on a ribosome in the cytoplasm (or mitochondrion) is fidelity, for the consequences of low fidelity can lead to lethal or crippling mutations or to the production of nonfunctional or harmful proteins. Already this text has considered the rigid rules whereby DNA is replicated and the various species of RNA are transcribed, proofread, corrected, and edited in the nucleus, and has reviewed the criteria for matching codons on mRNA with anticodons on an amino acid–tRNA complex at the site of a ribosome.

What follows is a review of the translation process with the linking of an amino acid to its specific tRNA. Amino acids are first activated by ATP and then bound to tRNA in a two-step reaction catalyzed by an aminoacyl-tRNA synthetase that is unique for a given amino acid. That enzyme has a very responsible function: an error such as joining an amino acid with the wrong tRNA (one that carries an incorrect anticodon for that particular amino acid) would lead to translation of an amino acid that the codon on mRNA had not intended to be there. The synthetase enzyme, therefore, also proofreads its work and, when found in error, hydrolyzes the amino acid–tRNA complex before it enters into the translation process. Thus a specific enzyme and a specific tRNA are involved for each individual amino acid, and those specificities add to measures that safeguard the fidelity of translation.

Translation of the genetic message transcribed on mRNA takes place in the cytoplasm (or in mitochondria). It progresses in the 5′ to 3′ direction of mRNA through steps that are characterized by **initiation, elongation,** and **termination** of a peptide chain. Each of these steps involves specific factors whose activities are absolutely crucial for translation. Absence or chemical alteration of just one of the multitude of factors stops protein synthesis.

- Initiation is directed by initiation factors as described herein. An mRNA attaches with its cap to the smaller ribosomal subunit; it contains an initiation signal sequence with an AUG coding for methionine. As the message on mRNA may code for additional methionine residues, there are two different tRNA molecules that recognize AUG: an initiator tRNA and a tRNA for internal AUG codons. A complex consisting of methionine and its initiator tRNA links its anticodon to the chain-initiating AUG codon on the mRNA. The larger ribosomal subunit now joins, thus completing the initiation phase having an intact ribosome connected to an mRNA (Figure 3-17). The first (chain-initiating) codon on mRNA is occupied by the methionine-tRNA complex, and one of the arms of the cloverleaf structure of the tRNA is simultaneously attached to the peptidyl-tRNA binding site (P site) on the ribosome. The P site is where, during later phases of translation, the growing peptide chain is attached via the tRNA belonging to the most-recently coded amino acid. Adjacent to the P site is the A site, where the next codon is signaling for the next aminoacyl-tRNA complex.

- Elongation requires elongation factors as are described herein. A complex of an amino acid with its tRNA binds to the signaling codon at the A site (Figure 3-18). Next, the growing peptide chain detaches from its tRNA on the P site and is linked by peptidyl transferase to the just-arrived amino acid positioned with its tRNA at the A site, while the previous tRNA vacates the P site. The newly elongated peptidyl-tRNA complex is translocated to the vacated P site, leaving the next codon on the reopened A site ready for a new round of elongation as the ribosome rolls along the mRNA.

- Termination occurs when a chain-terminating codon appears on the A site (Figure 3-19). As there is no tRNA with an anticodon complementary to a chain-terminating codon, cooperation of a releasing factor and peptidyl transferase dissociates the finished peptide chain and the last tRNA from the mRNA; the two ribosomal subunits separate.

The polarity of protein synthesis is such that the first amino acid translated (methionine) is the amino terminal of the peptide chain, and the last amino acid translated before the chain is released constitutes the carboxyl terminal. Energy for the various reactions involved in translation is provided by GTP. Translation proceeds amazingly fast: on 1 ribosome, some 100 codons are translated per minute, that is, a peptide of about 10 kDa.

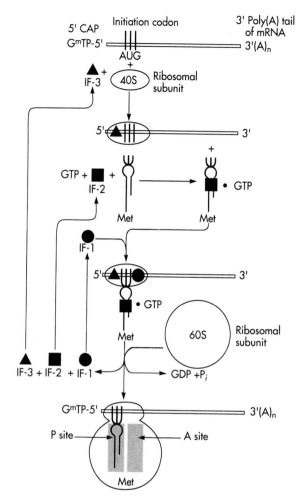

Figure 3-17. The initiation step of protein synthesis. The mRNA template is shown as a bar with a 5' cap and poly(A) tail. Three initiation factors *(IF)* participate, together with GTP, the ribosomal subunits, and the complex of methionine to initiator tRNA (hairpinlike structure). The P site and the A site represent the peptidyl-tRNA and aminoacyl-tRNA binding sites of the ribosome, respectively. *Reproduced, with permission, from Murray RK, et al: Harper's bio-chemistry, ed 21, p 421, Norwalk, CN, 1988, Appleton & Lange.*

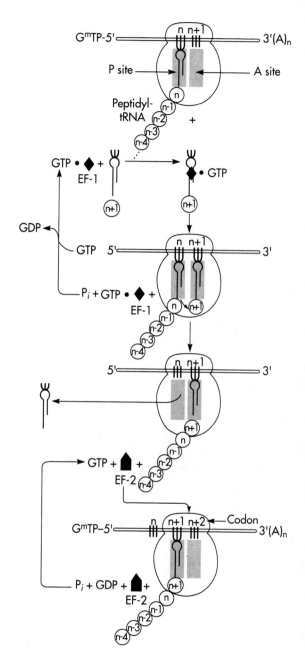

Figure 3-18. The elongation step of protein synthesis. Two elongation factors *(EF)* participate. The small circles labeled n − 1, n, n + 1, etc., represent amino acid residues of the newly formed protein molecule. *Reproduced with permission from Murray RK, et al: Harper's bio-chemistry, ed 21, p 423, Norwalk, CN, 1988, Appleton & Lange.*

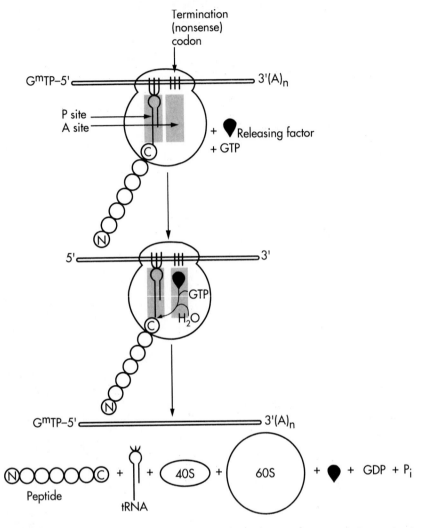

Figure 3-19. The termination step of protein synthesis. *N* and *C* represent the amino- and carboxy-terminal amino acids of the peptide chain, respectively. *Reproduced with permission from Murray RK, et al: Harper's bio-chemistry, ed 21, p 424, Norwalk, CN, 1988, Appleton & Lange.*

Posttranslational processing

The attachment of several ribosomes to an mRNA (polyribosome or polysome) allows multiple translations of the same message. Ribosomes belonging to a polysome continue to move along the message until the mRNA is enzymically degraded (Figure 3-20).

Proteins synthesized on ribosomes in the cytoplasm of the cell can function within the cell. For the production of other intracellular proteins and export proteins, ribosomes, after linking to mRNA and assembling their subunits, attach themselves to membranes of the endoplasmic reticulum (ER) of the cell, forming rough ER. The initial chain that is translated constitutes a leader sequence or signal peptide, a string of 20 apolar amino acids that allows the growing peptide chain to traverse the hydrophobic (lipid) interior of the ER membrane (Figure 3-21). In the ER, signal peptidase clips off the leader sequence, while the translation process continues to extrude more of the growing peptide into the lumen of the ER.

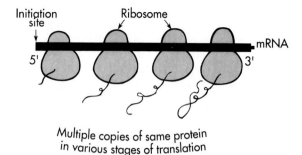

Figure 3-20. Polysomal mRNA translation.

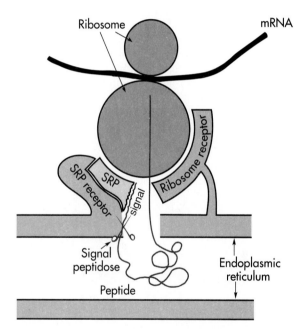

Figure 3-21. A signal sequence aids a newly translated peptide chain to penetrate into the endoplasmic reticulum. A signal recognition particle *(SRP)* is bound tightly to the ribosome by a newly translated signal sequence of some 20 amino acids, and elongation is halted temporarily. The ribosome-SRP complex then binds to a SRP receptor (alias docking protein) located on the ER, whereupon SRP dissociates from the ribosome. Elongation now resumes, the signal sequence penetrates the ER membrane and is clipped off by signal peptidase, while the remainder of the protein is gaining access to the ER. Additional ribosome receptors on ER may be involved.

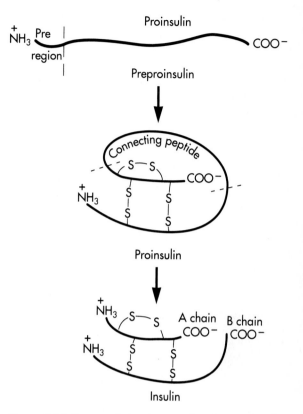

Figure 3-22. Posttranslational processing of preproinsulin. The pre region (signal sequence) and, later on, the connecting peptide chain are removed.

Posttranslational processing of the newly synthesized protein continues in the ER lumen, where glycosidic chains may be attached to the protein. In the Golgi apparatus, more changes in the glycosidic chains of glycoproteins are made; for example, lipid complexes may be added (lipoproteins), more amino acids may be cleaved off, and special groups may be added to target the proteins to their final destination.

Posttranslational alterations include hydroxylations of lysine and proline in some proteins, methylation of histidine in muscle proteins, conversion of zymogens (proenzymes) into active enzymes (e.g., pepsinogen to pepsin), and oxidation of certain amino acids (e.g., in procollagen to allow cross-linking of peptide chains for increased strength in collagen). Posttranslational processing will be exemplified with insulin and collagen because of the unique importance of these compounds.

Structure of insulin. Insulin is produced in β cells of the pancreatic islets of Langerhans (Figure 3-22). The original transcript codes for preproinsulin; upon lation, the "pre" sequence (signal) is clipped off, leaving one chain of 94 amino acids (proinsulin) that is coiled by the formation of three disulfide bridges between distantly located cysteine residues. Depending on conditions prompting pancreatic response, a portion of the proinsulin is converted to insulin by editing out a 33–amino-acid connecting peptide from the middle of the molecule, leaving a 21–amino-acid segment (A-chain) and a 30–amino-acid segment (B-chain) connected only by disulfide bridges.

Structure of collagen. Collagen constitutes over one third of all animal protein. Its strong, ropelike fibers are the structural elements of the organic matrices of bones, cartilage, tendons, skin, heart valves, placenta, and uteri. Collagen also occurs as sheets, for example, in the skin and basement membranes of epithelial and endothelial cells (blood vessels, glomeruli). Collagen strands are dispersed in interstitial spaces. Collagens of bones and tendons regularly undergo remodeling by lysosomal collagenase degradation and resynthesis in connective tissue cells in response to strenuous physical activity, such as athletic training, to better meet the stresses placed upon them.

The basic building block of collagen is a peptide (α chain) that originates as preprocollagen, which is extensively modified posttranslationally. During entry into the endoplasmic reticulum, the leader sequence is clipped off, whereupon hydroxylations of prolyl and lysyl residues occur, as well as glycosylations, disulfide bond formations, and finally the intertwining of three α chains into a strand of procollagen, which is exported by way of the Golgi apparatus. Outside of the fibroblast, aminopeptidase and carboxypeptidase remove nonhelical portions, leaving tropocollagen (Figure 3-23). Fibrils of tropocollagen undergo oxidation of hydroxylysyl residues to aldehydes, which then cross-link with amino groups of lysyl residues; in this way bridges are formed within tropocollagen fibrils and also between fibrils so that fibrils band together to form a sturdy collagen fiber.

Seven genetically different α chains are contained within five types of collagen present in various tissues. Though tissue distribution and physical appearance (fibrils, sheets) varies, the following common denominators in the amino acid constitution of collagen exist.

- Every third amino acid in an α chain of the helical portion of collagen is glycine; hence, glycine can be growth-limiting in young animals.

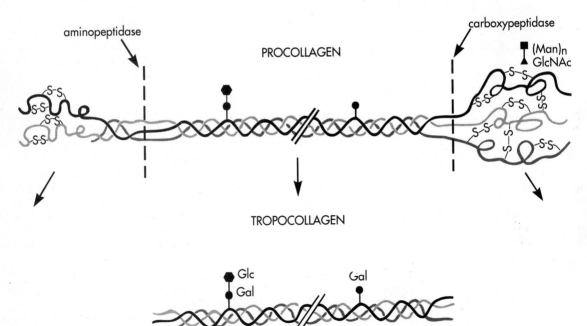

Figure 3-23. Posttranslational processing of collagen. Procollagen, consisting of a helical aggregate of three α chains, is converted to tropocollagen. *Man,* Mannose; *Gal,* galactose; *Glc,* glucose; *GlcNAc,* N-acetylglucosamine.

The small molecular size of glycine makes the tight coiling of α chains possible.

- Several essential amino acids are either present in low concentrations or absent (tryptophan), making collagen a low-quality protein in terms of its nutritional value.
- About 25% of the amino acids contained in collagen are proline or hydroxyproline. The hydroxylation reaction of proline requires ascorbic acid, which derives its name from the fact that diets deficient in it lead to *scorbutus* (scurvy), a lethal condition in which formation of functional collagen is defective. This condition once decimated the ranks of the merchant and military marine, which led to inclusion of citrus fruits in the seafarers' ration.

Different kinds of heritable defects in collagen structure have been reported in mankind, dogs, cats, sheep, and cattle. Some genetic mutations give rise to abnormal α chains, while other genetic disorders stem from the absence of the necessary posttranslational enzyme activities; both lead to nonfunctional collagen and death. Nutritional deficiencies may also cause collagen disorders; not only a lack of vitamin C, but also defective copper metabolism (reported in pigs). Copper is required in oxidase activities such as cytochrome oxidase and the oxidase involved in the oxidation of hydroxylysyl residues, needed for collagen cross-linking. Collagen disorders are characterized by abnormal bone formation (*osteogenesis imperfecta*), slow wound healing, and a hyperextensible, fragile skin that tears (*dermatosparaxis*), causing bleeding and infections.

Control of protein synthesis

Research on bacteria has laid the foundation, and continues to be of paramount importance, to the understanding of what controls protein biosynthesis. It also has coined much of the jargon in the field of physiological chemistry, since the mechanisms of protein synthesis in prokaryotes and eukaryotes are quite similar.

When *E. coli* is cultured in a medium that contains both glucose and lactose as nutrients, it first depletes the glucose supply; then the growth rate of the bacteria is interrupted while lactose transporting and metabolizing enzymes are synthesized; growth continues, fueled by lactose. The molecular basis for this control over protein synthesis centers around the lac operon, a stretch of DNA with these functional subdivisions:

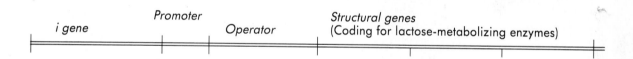

The promoter is the site where DNA-dependent RNA polymerase attaches; this is the enzyme that transcribes the structural genes of three enzymes required for lactose metabolism. During glucose feeding, the operator site is occupied by a repressor substance that is encoded in the i gene and constitutively manufactured; occupation of the operator site represses transcription. Lactose frees the operator site of the repressor substance, so that the RNA polymerase is allowed to transcribe the structural genes. With lactose serving as an inducer, the gene has been derepressed.

In eukaryotes, matters are complicated by (i) the presence of a nucleus with nuclear membranes separating transcription from translation, (ii) introns that have to be excised from hnRNA transcripts, and (iii) a huge genome compared to that of prokaryotes. Control of protein biosynthesis in animals is, therefore, much more intricate than that in bacteria, and, thus, is less well understood. Though it is fair to say that gene expression in eukaryotes is primarily controlled by the amount of mRNA made available for translation, at every step of the way control mechanisms are working, from nucleus to cytoplasm, from the processes of DNA replication, chemical modification, repositioning in chromosomes, and activation by inducer substances through transcriptional RNA synthesis, posttranscriptional processing, degradation, and translation into protein. This train of events is followed in reviewing the control of eukaryotic protein synthesis.

Large portions of DNA are never transcribed, and some segments of DNA are constitutively (i.e., continuously) transcribed; between these extremes lie the genes whose transcription is controlled according to need.

Repression of operators may account for cell differentiation; starting with the identical genome in each cell, different genes are repressed in the various cells. Derepression then leads to dedifferentiation of cells; for example, the manifestation of glucose-6-phosphate dehydrogenase (oxidative pentose shunt) activity in dystrophic, but not in normal muscle cells. Derepression can be brought about by metabolic inducers, such as when a given enzyme is needed, or in pathological cases when uncontrolled transcription may occur, for example, activation of an oncogene by a carcinogen, leading to cancer.

A major influence on the time, locus, and rate of transcription is exerted by chemical changes in chromatin, resulting from reversible (on/off) methylations, acetylations, and phosphorylations of histones and nonhistone proteins that affect the activity of the DNA with which those proteins are associated.

Another major chemical effect on chromatin structure, inhibiting DNA transcription, results from the methylation of deoxycytidine residues in DNA. Mammalian DNA contains an average of about 4% of its cytosine base in the methylated form (5-methylcytosine), but that methylated cytosine is unevenly distributed. Genes that are highly methylated are not transcribed in many cases; for example, (i) only the unmethylated ribosomal genes are expressed in mouse liver; (ii) of the two X chromosomes in the somatic cells of women, only one is transcriptionally active; the inactive X chromosome is the more highly methylated, and experimental demethylation leads to its increased expression.

Thus far, transcriptional control by covalent chemical changes in either the protein or DNA moiety of chromatin has been considered. In many genes, allosteric sequences on DNA exist where signaling by environmental or chemical factors may dramatically affect transcriptional activity. These enhancer elements (stimulatory) or silencer elements (inhibitory) may be thousands of bases removed from the promotor site in either the upstream or downstream direction, and may be oriented in either the 5' to 3' or reverse direction; however, they must be located on the same chromosome to affect initiation of transcription at the promoter (which is taken as evidence that their effect is not chemically mediated). Activation of an enhancer element stimulates not only the gene to which it belongs, but also various promoters in remote genes on the same chromosome.

Another signaling interaction with nucleoproteins, previously mentioned, relates to the mode of action of steroid hormones, such as cortisol (glucose metabolism), estradiol, progesterone, testosterone (sex hormones), aldosterone (mineral balance), and the hormone derived from vitamin D, 1,25-dihydroxycholecalciferol (calcium and phosphate balance). These hormones, like thyroid hormones, enter the cell and combine with a receptor in the cytoplasm, causing a change in the tertiary configuration of that receptor. The steroid-receptor complex travels into the nucleus where it associates with a receptor on chromatin, which in turn affects a hormone responsive element (HRE) on DNA, located a few hundred bases proximal from where transcription of steroid-responsive genes starts. An HRE in a gene may either stimulate or inhibit transcription. As previously discussed, stimulation of the gene for a rate-controlling enzyme in gluconeogenesis (phosphoenolpyruvate carboxykinase; PEPCK) by glucocorticoids is a good example, as attachment of the glucocorticoid-receptor complex to its receptor recognition site on DNA converts the HRE into an active enhancer element. The gene for PEPCK holds, in addition, a 15-base sequence that responds to insulin by inhibiting PEPCK transcription; the insulin effect overrides that of glucocorticoids.

An effective adaptation to an increased demand for a gene product is to physically make more genes for that product available. There are two manners in which cells do just that. One is by repetitive DNA sequences: for example, there are hundreds of copies of rRNA and tRNA genes in the genome of animal cells, and that same repetitive genome is inherited from generation to generation. The other manner in which cells can produce an increased number of copies of a specific gene is by amplification of one preexisting gene. This adaptation occurs within one generation. Gene amplification during DNA synthesis is the result of repeated initiations of the replication of a given gene (Figure 3-24). The many copies of one amplified gene then provide multiple sites for transcription of that gene's product, which is temporarily in high demand in the cell. The classic example is amplification of the chorion gene-coding for eggshell protein during oogenesis in the fruit fly. Another example is the 200-fold amplification of the gene for dihydrofolate reductase in response to administering an inhibitor of that enzyme (methotrexate, an anticancer drug).

Another form of physical control over DNA transcription is relocation of genes. In germ cell lines, the genes that encode antibody proteins are divided into segments that are widely separated in the ge-

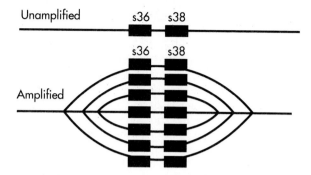

Figure 3-24. Gene amplification of chorion protein genes s36 and s38 produces compounded replication bubbles. *Reproduced with permission from Chrisholm R: Gene amplification during development, Trends Biochem Sci, 7:161-162, 1982.*

nome, and are inactive. During the development of an antibody-producing cell, the separate pieces of the antibody genes are relocated near each other, so that they can be transcribed as a single mRNA precursor under one promoter.

Gene relocation control should not be confused with control by gene rearrangement, which is a post-transcriptional mechanism. Gene rearrangement is possible by combining exons in different sequential orders after introns have been excised from the primary transcript. This allows an immense variety of final transcripts from a limited amount of DNA. An enlightening example is provided by the low-density lipoprotein (LDL) receptor, which is a glycoprotein located on the plasma membranes of cells. In its mature form (after a signal sequence of 21 amino acids has been clipped off) the receptor consists of 839 amino acids. With 3 bases per codon, only some 2500 bases would have to be in the message; yet, the original gene in DNA is more than 45,000 bases long. It contains 18 exons, of which 13 encode protein sequences that are homologous to sequences in other proteins with totally unrelated functions (epidermal growth factor, blood clotting factors, and an immuno-complement factor). Thus, the LDL receptor is a mosaic protein in which exons shared with different proteins have been rearranged.

Other forms of posttranscriptional control of protein synthesis center around RNA. The stability of mRNA in the cytoplasm, meaning its resistance to enzymic degradation, may be related to its 5' cap or 3' poly(A) tail. As there are more mRNA primary transcripts in the nucleus than there are mRNA molecules in the cytoplasm, there must exist in the nu-

cleus a mechanism for differential processing of mRNA, determining which mRNA will be translated and which one degraded.

At the level of translation, many questions still need to be answered; for example, What are the relative priorities and differences in rates with which various incoming mRNA messages are translated in the cytoplasm? An initiation factor of translation (eIF-2) exists in an inactive (phosphorylated) and active (dephosphorylated) form that are interconvertible and, thus, must be controlled. Elongation factor eEF-2 is inactivated by association with ADP-ribose (from NAD) under the influence of diphtheria exotoxin.

Damage and repair of DNA; mutations

Some of the many safeguards that guarantee the fidelity of replication of the DNA structure and transmittal of its genetic information have been reviewed. Such fidelity is needed to preserve both the identity of a species and the well-being of an individual, as mistakes will cause changes in the genome (i.e., mutations). The consequences of mutations may well go unnoticed; or else, they may be beneficial to the species (evolution), or deleterious to it. The following passages describe the molecular basis underlying mutations, identify some of the factors and conditions that can cause mutations by damaging DNA structure, and, finally, examine the unceasing DNA repair efforts with which nature protects DNA integrity.

Mutations

Mistakes are common in DNA replication and the further processing of genetic information; also the composition of DNA is under constant attack by chemical and environmental factors. Fortunately, proofreading mechanisms are always active, detecting practically all errors in base composition, and an active DNA repair system makes amends. The astonishing efficiency of these systems that protect the body's genome is attested by the fact that in a single cell generation, on average approximately one mutation occurs per billion base pairs of DNA. Low as that rate may be, eventually lasting changes in the genome do occur. In mature cells, this may cause ineffective control over cell functioning and lack of adaptation to a changing environment. For instance, instead of functional enzyme proteins, altered, worthless proteins may be synthesized. Those changes become all the more probable with increasing length of time; hence, herein lies a mechanism that contributes to the aging of cells. Alternatively, mutations may help a cell or species to adapt to a permanently changed environment and, thus, be a basis for evolution.

In most cases, errors in structure or copying of DNA go unnoticed, since the vast majority of cells continues to function normally and to fulfill the needs of the organism. But in areas of rapid cell growth, where stem cells or blast cells are damaged (e.g., by radiation or drugs), the effects are more easily discernible: loss of hair, loss of intestinal mucosal cells (malabsorption, bleeding, diarrhea), or shortage of formed elements in blood (low red and white cell counts). There are two instances of particular concern: (i) oncogenes may become activated so that cells are produced with uncontrolled growth (cancer); and (ii) the genome of germ cells may be altered, threatening the survival of the offspring or else giving rise to damaging mutations.

A mutation is defined as a change in the nucleotide sequence of either a gene or a transcript. Changing a single base on mRNA will give rise to an altered codon (Figure 3-25). If the third base of the codon is changed, chances are that the amino acid normally encoded will still be translated because of degeneracy of the genetic code; this is known as a **silent mutation.** Changes in first or second nucleotide are more deleterious (missense mutations), since they cause substitution of an anomalous amino acid in the primary transcript. In that case, (i) either there is no detectable effect, for example, when the normal amino acid was still encoded, or when a functionally similar amino acid is substituted, such as Glu for Asp or Leu for Val; or (ii) there is a detectable effect. A detect-

able effect may be partially acceptable (decreased functionality of the protein) or unacceptable (loss of functionality). Examples of all of these mutations have been characterized in the hemoglobins.

It is an extreme case of unacceptability when a mutation generates an untimely chain-terminating codon. Other extremely damaging mutations come about by either the insertion of an extra base or the deletion of a single base. Reading through the encoded genetic message, every codon up to the frame shift will be normal and give rise to a normal sequence of amino acids; but distally from the frame shift every codon will have been altered, so that different amino acids and different chain termination will result (see Figure 3-25).

The above may be compared with an English message written in a string of three-letter words:

... **XXX XXX NOW THE DOG RAN FOR THE FOX CUT XXX** ...

Normally, translation starts with the initiating word (NOW) and terminates on CUT. Deletion of the N of RAN would translate into nonsense:

... **XXX XXX NOW THE DOG RAF ORT HEF OXC UTX XX** ...

The phrase is left with nonexisting words and no sentence termination due to the frame shift mutation. A three-letter deletion (or insertion) would have been tolerable; for example, when one, or both, of the THEs had been cut (or inserted at their proper places); but if DOG had been cut, the message would also have lost its meaning.

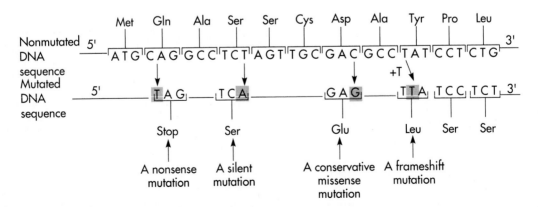

Figure 3-25. Molecular basis of mutations. *Reproduced with permission from Colby DS: Biochemistry: a synopsis, p 194, Los Altos, CA, 1985, Lange Medical Publications.*

Causes of DNA damage; mutagens

In addition to errors made in DNA synthesis, there is a great variety of environmental, physical, and chemical factors that threaten the integrity of the DNA structure. Damaged DNA is usually easily detected by the proofreading mechanisms and then either repaired, that is, replaced by native DNA, or else retained, in which case there is permanent mutation if not cell death. In some cases, DNA structures are modified intentionally; for example, to introduce a lethal mutation in a microorganism by the action of certain antibiotics; or to study molecular genetics experimentally, using mutagens to introduce base changes in DNA. The types and extents of structural damage inflicted upon DNA vary a great deal, as the following abbreviated summary illustrates.

Heat energy suffices to dupurinate DNA by dissociation of the adenine and guanine bases from their deoxyribose at a daily rate in the thousands per cell; it also deaminates the cytosine and adenine bases. Deamination of cytosine yields uracil (a foreign base in DNA) that upon replication, pairs with adenine, thus causing a mutation if the defect is not excised promptly. Alkylation of bases, occurring due to toxic substances such as mustards, is also effected experimentally with the aid of alkylating agents (e.g., ethylmethane sulfonate). These are powerful mutagens, some of which link two bases in either the same strand or between the two strands, while others cause predictable changes in base pairings. Many other chemical mutagens cause changes in base pairings; for example, (i) nitrous acid, oxidatively removing —NH₂ and substituting —OH groups on C, A, or G; and (ii) hydroxylamine, modifying C so it will only pair with A. Experimentally, the DNA structure can be altered and frame-shift mutations introduced by insertion or deletion of nucleotides, or by agents (e.g., acridines) that possess flat molecular structures, which they can intercalate between the complementary bases of a DNA chain. Much-used to introduce mutations in DNA, especially for the purpose of producing antibiotics, are base analogs, look-alikes of real bases that are incorporated into DNA and then pair with predictable, incorrect bases.

In addition to these chemical mutagens, there are physical influences from the environment that can damage DNA. Ionizing radiation may cause chain breaks. Dimerization of two adjacent thymine or cytosine bases may occur under the influence of ultraviolet light (Figure 3-26). These dimers may be excised or they may be cleaved and restored to the monomers under the influence of visible light by a photoreactivating enzyme.

DNA repair

Excision-repair of most of the aforementioned mutations in one strand of DNA is a two-step process. First the defect is recognized by proofreading and marked as aberrant DNA; and then the defect is ex-

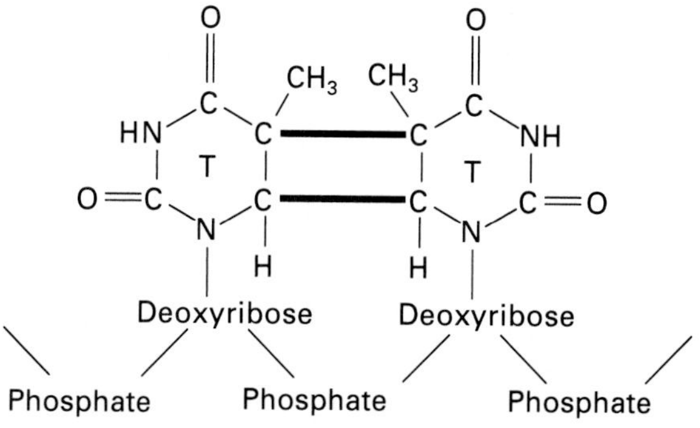

Figure 3-26. Thymine-thymine dimer on DNA.

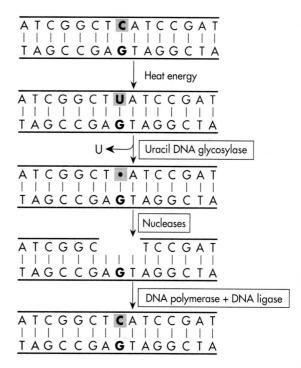

Figure 3-27. Excision-repair of mutated DNA. *Courtesy Dr. B. Alberts. From Murray RK et al: Harper's biochemistry, ed 21, Norwalk CT, 1988, Appleton & Lange.*

cised and replaced by native DNA via the rules of base pairing with the complementary copy on the undamaged strand. Figure 3-27 diagrams excision-repair of a U base formed by deamination of the native C base. The aberrant base U is detected and excised by a specific glycosylase; then, endonuclease activity cuts out additional bases on either side of the now-open site; DNA polymerase pairs the proper bases with the intact complementary strand, and finally DNA ligase reseals the sugar-phosphate "backbone" of the DNA strand.

Antibiotics

A clinically useful (nontoxic) antibiotic is one that cripples multiplication of microorganisms without interfering with the mammalian host cells. For survival, any cell depends on DNA replication and protein synthesis. These are multifactorial processes that can be interfered with at the level of DNA synthesis, and mRNA transcription and translation. Even though great similarities exist between protein-synthesizing processes of prokaryotes and eukaryotes, there are some differences (e.g., different composition and size of ribosomes) on which nature and the pharmaceutical industry capitalize to manufacture prokaryote-specific antibiotics.

The DNA structure can be modified by administering base analogs that are incorporated into DNA and lead to either nonfunctional DNA or incorrect base pairings, resulting in lethal mutations. Examples are (i) 5-fluorouracil or 5-bromouracil, which are mistaken for cytosine and, thus, pair with guanine (Figure 3-28); (ii) thiobases in which amino groups have been replaced by —SH groups; and (iii) azapurines in which a carbon is replaced by a nitrogen, such as azaguanine.

Similar forgery tactics are used to modify RNA

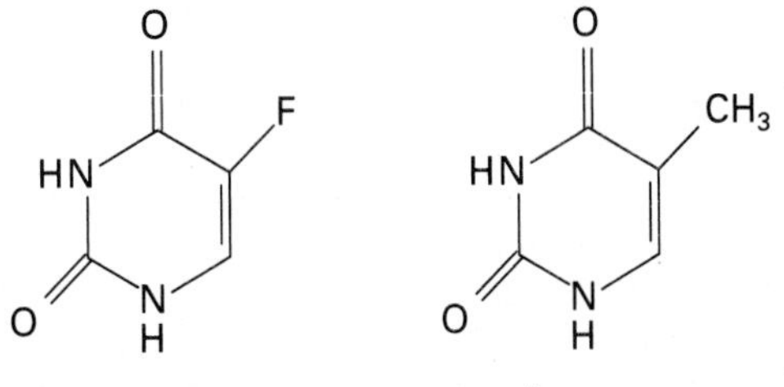

molecules; for example, the ribose moiety of nucleosides can be replaced by arabinose, another pentose, or by a thioribose. A classic example of base fakery is the use of puromycin, resembling the amino end of the tyrosine-tRNA complex (Figure 3-29). Puromycin binds to a ribosome at the A site so that the entry of aminoacyl-tRNA complexes is barred and the incomplete peptide with puromycin at its C terminal leaves the ribosome. Puromycin inhibits protein synthesis in both prokaryotes and eukaryotes.

Antibiotics that inhibit transcription in prokaryotes include rifampicin, which inhibits the movement of RNA polymerase along the template strand of DNA, and rifamycin, which blocks the advent of the first RNA base at the initiation site of transcription.

Antibiotics that inhibit translation center their activities around ribosomes. Mitochondria contain 70 S ribosomes similar to those of bacteria but different from the 80 S ribosomes of eukaryote cytoplasm. A number of antibiotics, such as chloramphenicol, erythromycin, and tetracycline, inhibit 70 S but not 80 S ribosomes and, thus, are safe for mammalian hosts. In contrast, cycloheximide only works in eukaryotic cells, which makes it a good research tool, but of no clinical value. Puromycin and sparsomycin are examples of antibiotics that cripple protein synthesis in both eukaryotes and prokaryotes. The modes of action of these antibiotics on the translation process of protein synthesis range from inhibiting the initiation phase to interfering with elongation, by inhibiting the binding of aminoacyl-tRNA complexes to ribosomes and inactivating enzymes and factors involved in shuttling the peptide chain between the A and P sites on the larger ribosomal subunit.

Several bacterial and plant toxins are antibiotics in that they cripple protein synthesis, often by chemically rendering one of the translation factors ineffective. An example is diphtheria toxin, which inactivates elongation factor-2 in mammalian cells.

While on the topic of antibiotics, it would be shortsighted to restrict the discussion to only genetics and protein synthesis. Other antibiotic strategies, which shall be returned to in later chapters, aim at crippling energy metabolism (oxidative phosphorylation) or depriving the microorganism of a vital vitamin by administering a look-alike compound that takes the vitamin's position in a metabolic process, but does not function as a vitamin. For example, sulfanilamide "falsely imitates" dihydrofolic acid, an essential B-vitamin for many microbial cells and also for animals. Sulfanilamide was used before the advent

Figure 3-28. 5-Fluorouracil, a xenobiotic DNA base analog of thymine.

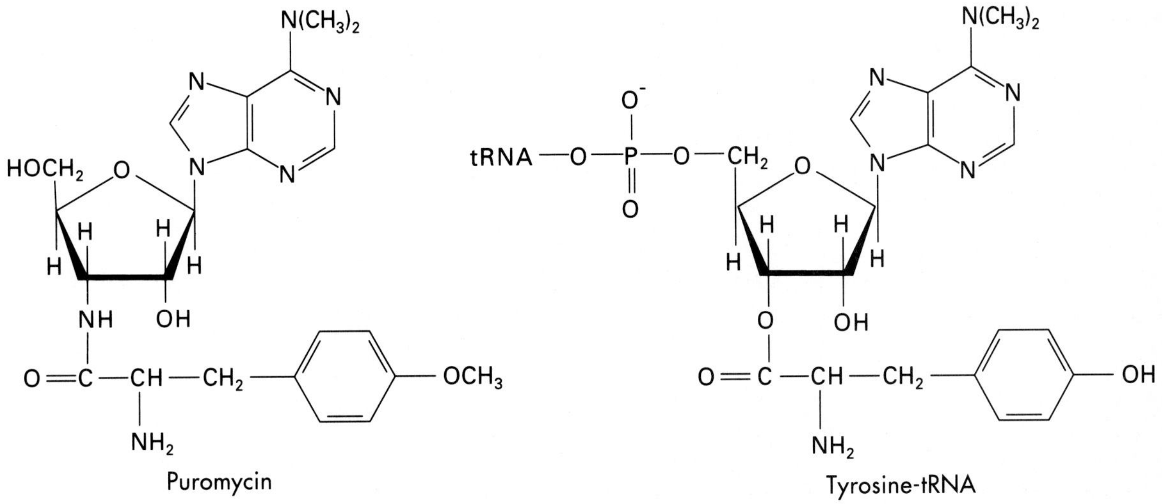

Figure 3-29. Puromycin resembles the 3' end of tyrosine-tRNA complex.

of penicillin, and is still prescribed in cases of hypersensitivity toward penicillin. (Penicillin acts by crippling the synthesis of cell wall mucopolysaccharides.) Another false imitator of dihydrofolic acid, methotrexate, is used in medicine as an anticancer agent; understandably, it is very toxic.

Interferons are a class of glycoproteins elaborated by leukocytes and fibroblasts in response to viral infection. The minute amounts of interferon elaborated render the body resistant to simultaneous infections by different viruses. This antiviral state of cells derives from inhibition of viral multiplication. Interferons also inhibit cell growth; this is why they are being pursued as anticancer agents. Interferons act by inhibiting protein synthesis at mRNA translation in two different ways: (i) by activating mRNA-ase activity; and (ii) by phosphorylating, and thereby inactivating, initiation factor-2.

Genetic engineering

This section illustrates some medically relevant applications in the area of molecular genetics.

The process of transcription, as discussed above, involves a DNA-dependent RNA polymerase enzyme that transcribes DNA into a complementary RNA copy. In certain viruses, the retroviruses (e.g., acquired immunodeficiency syndrome, feline infectious peritonitis, and feline leukemia virus), a reverse transcriptase (RNA-dependent DNA polymerase) reverses transcription; That is to say, using RNA as a template, this enzyme produces a single complementary DNA strand (cDNA). For reproduction of the virus, the cDNA strand is first paired, and then double-stranded DNA, carrying the viral code, is incorporated into the host cell's genome, forcing the host cell to manufacture more viral RNA. Certain retroviruses (RNA tumor viruses) are used in genetic engineering when one wants to produce substantial amounts of a precious protein, or the gene or the mRNA of that protein. First the amino acid sequence of the protein is determined; then an mRNA coding for that amino acid sequence is synthesized (or the naturally occurring mRNA of the protein is isolated and purified). With reverse transcriptase, the complementary gene to that mRNA is made, incorporated in the genome of the host cell, and reproduced.

Recombinant DNA technology (Figure 3-30) is used to make bacteria synthesize bulk amounts of rare proteins or genes and mRNA coding for those proteins. **Plasmids,** found in bacteria, are circular double-stranded DNA molecules that replicate autonomously. A **restriction endonuclease** is an enzyme that splits a DNA chain at a specific sequence of bases (e.g., between G and A of the sequence GAATTC). Large numbers of these enzymes, each one specific for a given base sequence, have been isolated from bacteria and are commercially available. Now, if a plasmid is opened by this restriction endonuclease, the "outer" circular strand of the plasmid DNA will leave the sequence TTAA exposed, which is complementary to the "inner" circle's exposed AATT. The two ends are like two pieces of velcro and are called **sticky**

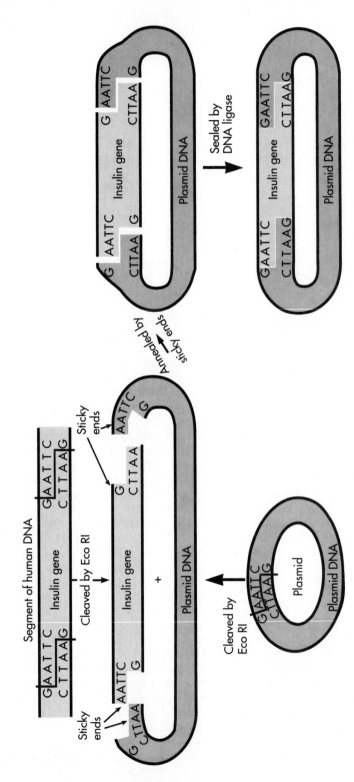

Figure 3-30. Recombinant DNA formation. Using a restriction endonuclease (Eco RI) to open up a bacterial plasmid DNA ring, and then using the same enzyme to excise a segment of human DNA that contains the insulin gene, matching sets of sticky ends are generated that allow annealing and sealing of the plasmid with the human-DNA insert. The chimeric DNA thus produced is inserted back into bacteria, where it will reproduce. The cloned human-DNA sequence can then be excised by using the same endonuclease as before.

ends. When the same restriction endonuclease is used to excise a segment of an animal's genome, which contains a useful gene (e.g., the gene coding for insulin), that gene will have the identical sticky ends as the open plasmid. The insulin gene, therefore, may seal the plasmid by including itself, thereby enlarging the circle of plasmid DNA. The hybrid plasmid is inserted back into the bacteria, where it will be reproduced continuously. Expressed in the jargon of the field: recombinant DNA, consisting of a **donor** gene (insulin) and a **vector** (plasmid DNA), is introduced into a host cell where it allows **cloning** of the donor gene. With the aid of the same restriction endonuclease, the segment of donor DNA with the insulin gene, produced by the bacteria, can be cleanly excised and then harvested. Also, one can have the bacteria translate the genetic message into insulin production.

Similar recombinant DNA methodology is used to induce bacteria to produce bulk quantities of antisense mRNA. Antisense mRNA, the product of transcribing the noncoding DNA strand for that mRNA, is complementary to sense mRNA with which it can combine (by base pairing) to form an mRNA complex that cannot be translated into a protein. By using antisense mRNA, therefore, one can suppress the synthesis of undesirable proteins in a cell. This approach, still in its infancy, promises to be of future use to fight viral diseases; meanwhile, it serves to probe the functions of individual genes and to create controlled mutations for the study of genetic diseases.

The following application of the knowledge of genetic control enters into the area of ethics. Metallothionein is an intracellular protein that binds and transports bivalent cations, such as zinc, copper, or cadmium. Transcription of the gene for that protein is inducible by demand for its function, that is, by administering these metal ions. This induction works at the level of the metallothionein promoter region. In an experiment, splicing this region out of the DNA, then linking it to the structural genes of growth hormone, and injecting this DNA hybrid into a fertilized mouse ovum (which was then placed in the uterus of a surrogate mother to develop) yielded a mouse that responded to supplementation of zinc or cadmium in its drinking water by increased transcription of its growth hormone gene. Thus a mouse became double the size of its litter mates that either had not been genetically treated or, when treated, did not receive the metal ions. Similarly, treating fertilized mouse eggs with chimeric DNA that contained the metallothionein promoter region linked to the struc-

tural genes of the LDL receptor produced mice that could clear their bloodstream of intravenously injected low-density lipoprotein 8 to 10 times more rapidly than could normal mice. It is necessary to realize that these examples of genetic engineering produced animals with an altered genome (transgenic animals) that became a new inborn trait in this species. This demonstrates the awesome potential scientists now possess to permanently alter nature's creation!

STUDY QUESTIONS

1. Which of the following hormones are small peptides (as opposed to proteins or hormones not containing amino acid): (A) Glucagon; (B) ADH; (C) Corticosteroids; (D) Thyroxine; (E) TRH?

2. *a.* List a peptide connecting the signaling of a hypothalamic nervous receptor with the release of a pituitary hormone.
   b. List the hormone and gland that intermediate between hypothalamic TRH and thyroid gland hormone releases.

3. Name a group of peptides that acts as analgesics.

4. For what determinant of protein structure is it necessary that the redox potential be homeostatically controlled?

5. *a.* Exemplify posttranslational processing of proteins; and
   b. List the subcellular organelle where the final product is targeted toward its ultimate destination.

6. Give the technical term and function of the amino acid sequence removed from preproinsulin in the formation of proinsulin.

7. Where in the cell is posttranslational glycosylation of (glyco)proteins started and where is it completed?

8. *a.* All proteins are synthesized on rough ER. (True/False)
   b. Mitochondria contain ribosomes such that they can synthesize their own proteins. (True/False)

9. List the pyrimidine base that is part of DNA's composition, but is absent from RNA.

10. Given the composition of the helical backbone of DNA, and the peculiar amino acid composition of histones, list a force that binds DNA to histones.

11. *a.* List the technical term for the copying of RNA from DNA.
    b. In what manner does the "cap" on mRNA aid in the initiation phase of translation?

12. Name the compound that carries anticodons.

13. Explain the term "wobble" used to indicate that several codons may exist for one amino acid.

14. Are all of the following needed for translation: 40 s ribosomal subunit, GTP, and elongation factor-2?

15. How is the message "end of peptide chain" conveyed to the protein-synthesizing machinery?

16. Name the segments of hnRNA that must be excised so a functional mRNA is formed.

17. As the first codon to be translated on a ribosome calls for methionine, why don't all of the body proteins' primary structures start with methionine?

18. *a.* List the function of snRNA (snurps) in the nucleus.
    b. What is unique about snurps?

19. A given mRNA sequence can only be translated once. (True/False)

20. If an agent inhibited mRNA-ase activity, would that agent be: (A) a potential carcinogen; or (B) a possible anticancer drug?

21. *a.* List the DNA locus where attachment of DNA-dependent RNA polymerase regulates transcription of structural genes.
    b. List the DNA locus stimulated by glucocorticoid hormones, so that a promoter on the same DNA strand becomes activated and appropriate enzyme codes on DNA are transcribed.

22. List the technical term for activation of the genome of liver cells to produce gluconeogenic key enzymes in response to hypoglycemia.

23. *a.* List the connection between interferon phosphorylating initiation factor-2 and the fact that interferon is a promising anticancer agent.
    b. List the mode of antibiotic action of valinomycin and gramicidin.
    c. By what mechanism does puromycin function?
    d. Certain bacterial (diphtheria) and plant (ricin) toxins cripple protein synthesis by what mode of action?

24. *a.* In the recombinant-DNA technique (e.g., for insulin production), what risk is associated with the fact that a restriction endonuclease always excises more DNA than just the segment that codes for insulin?
    b. Why must the identical restriction endonuclease be used to clip the insulin gene from donor DNA and to splice that gene onto bacterial plasmids?

25. What may happen when the promoter sequence of metallothionein linked to the structural gene of triglyceride lipase (the enzyme that breaks down our fat stores) is inserted into the embryonal genome of a mouse, and then, later in its life, Zn^{++} ions are added to the animal's drinking water?

26. *a.* What is the function of reverse transcriptase in retroviral diseases such as acquired immunodeficiency syndrome?
    b. How can that enzyme be utilized to produce sizeable amounts of mRNA coding for a precious protein?

27. Explain why a mutation in DNA does not alter the primary protein structure in some cases.

28. *a.* List the purpose of ongoing DNA synthesis outside the S-phase of a cell cycle.
    b. Why is DNA damage caused by radiation often irreparable, in contrast to depurination damage?

29. Explain how a seemingly infinite variety of antibody proteins can derive from a finite genome.

30. If it is true that the disease scrapie in sheep is transmitted by an agent (prions) that contains no nucleic acids but consists solely of proteins, then suggest a plausible way in which that agent might multiply in the host cell.

31. *a.* List the molecular genetic term (derived from the operon concept) denoting that a cell does not express a portion of its genetic blueprint (cell differentiation).
    b. List an example.

32. What is an oncogene?

4 Enzymes

NEED FOR ENZYMES

Chemists make use of the following conditions to stimulate chemical reactions: high concentrations of reactants; extremes of pH, temperature, and pressure; anhydrous media; and agitation. But in the body, mild conditions prevail: aqueous medium; temperature at 37° C; pH 7.4; and low concentrations of reactants. Hence, the body employs enzymes instead of chemists.

Enzymes speed up reactions (catalysis), boost efficiency of reactions, give direction to reactions, and allow rate control over reactions. However, enzymes are not miracle workers: they can only catalyze reactions that go downhill, energetically speaking. Any seemingly uphill process is driven by a downhill one that takes place simultaneously, as illustrated in the following equation:

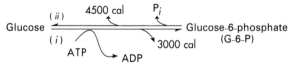

Step 1 is catalyzed by glucokinase or by hexokinase; step 2 by glucose 6-phosphatase, (G-6-P-ase).

An energy profile (Figure 4-1) shows that 4500 cal (of ATP's 7500) are used to boost the free-energy level of glucose to that of G-6-P, while the remaining 3000 cal are irretrievably lost as heat. The reaction is therefore irreversible.

When both glucokinase and G-6-P-ase are active at the same time, a futile cycle is established in which the G-6-P formed is immediately hydrolyzed again, and heat is produced from the disposal of energy contained in ATP. In warm-blooded animals, such futile cycles do indeed exist (in fact, four different cycles

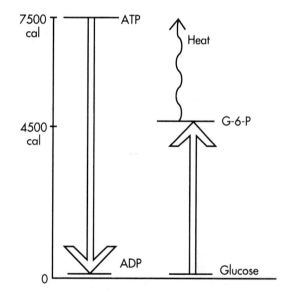

Figure 4-1. Energy profile of the glucokinase reaction in hepatocytes.

will be discussed later). But there is always a net direction of these reactions. For instance, conditions stimulating glucokinase (such as high levels of glucose and insulin occurring after a meal) inhibit G-6-P-ase, and vice versa.

Nature of Enzymes
Definitions

An enzyme is a catalyst, speeding up reactions that are energetically feasible. An enzyme may consist of an apoenzyme (protein) plus a coenzyme that renders the complex enzymically active. Examples of coenzymes include B vitamins (discussed below).

Physiology deals with enzyme activities rather than with purified enzyme molecules. Different kinds of enzyme protein molecules that exhibit similar activity are called **isoenzymes** or **isozymes.** Glucokinase and hexokinase are isozymes when glucose is used as substrate. Of clinical significance are the five isozymes of lactate dehydrogenase (LDH), all of which catalyze the following reversible reaction:

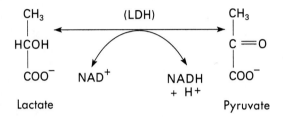

In the clinical laboratory, these five isozymes are readily separated by electrophoresis, with each organ or tissue containing it having a characteristic proportion of isozyme. High concentrations of LDH are found in liver, cardiac and skeletal muscle, erythrocytes, gut, and renal cortices. Although assay of total serum LDH activity is by no means tissue specific, appearance of specific LDH is frequently diagnositic for liver or heart damage (Figure 4-2).

Common names for enzyme activities usually have "-ase" attached as a suffix to either the name of the substrate or the kind of enzymic activity: for instance, G-6-P-ase; phospholipase; pyruvate dehydrogenase; and cholesterol esterase.

An active site (isosteric site) and allosteric sites may be located on an enzyme protein molecule. An isosteric site is where a substrate fits and a reaction is catalyzed. Isosteric sites may be permanent (as in constitutive enzyme activities), or they may be induced by need for an enzyme activity (adaptive enzyme activity). Factors that may induce enzyme activity include substrates and second messengers of the neuroendocrine system. Allosteric sites on enzyme proteins are loci where compounds may attach to control isosteric activity by causing changes in the tertiary structure of the enzyme molecule. Activation or inhibition of enzyme activities can be allosterically enacted. As illustrated, attaching a compound to an allosteric site may modify the structure of the isosteric site and inhibit the enzyme activity (Figure 4-3).

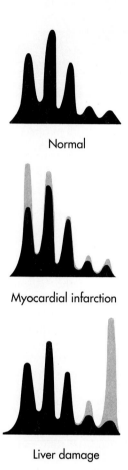

Figure 4-2. Normal and pathologic pattern of lactate dehydrogenase isozymes in human serum.

Chemical nature of enzyme reactions

A large variety of reactions are catalyzed by enzymes (e.g., hydrolysis, group transfers, oxidation-reduction reactions, and phosphorylations).

Substrate specificity ranges from very strict to relaxed. Example of absolute specificity: only L-amino acids and D-sugars are metabolized. Example of more relaxed specificity: group specificity occurs in the intestinal aminopeptidase and carboxypeptidase activities that attack dietary peptides from the amino and carboxy terminals, respectively, biting off one amino acid at a time until the entire peptide is broken down.

Coenzyme specificity also ranges from very strict to relaxed. For example, glucokinase requires ATP, Mg^{++}, and K^+; substituting other high-energy compounds or minerals causes loss of enzyme activity.

ADAPTIVE MODIFICATIONS OF ENZYME ACTIVITY

GENETIC CONTROL

New enzyme synthesized
Activation and inhibition of enzyme synthesis
Molecular diseases

PHYSIOLOGIC CONTROL

1. Competitive inhibition; pharmaceutical
2. Noncompetitive inhibition
   Allosteric effects (negative feedback loops;
       parasites; colostrum)
   Isosteric effects
3. Activation
   Allosteric effects (induction; feed forward)
   Cooperativity
   Pharmaceutical
4. Proenzyme activation; positive feedback
5. Covalent enzyme modification (protein kinases
   and protein phosphatases)
6. Controlling reactant availability
   Cell compartments; shuttles
   Macromolecular complexes of enzyme pathways
   Protein binding of reactants
   Transport of reactants to enzyme site
7. Organismic neuroendocrine control

Control of enzyme concentration

Genetic induction mechanisms regulate cellular metabolism through enzyme synthesis. Genetic induction may take the form of a temporary and reversible induction of enzyme synthesis, or a more permanent and nearly irreversible differentiation of cells.

Differentiation of cells occurs in spite of the fact that all cells have the same genetic blueprint. This feature reflects repression of different portions of the genome in various cells. Cells in culture may dedifferentiate because of induction of certain enzyme activities.

Induction of enzyme synthesis at the time when that enzyme's function is needed may lead to a 2- to 1000-fold increase in enzyme concentration. The following are examples of inducible enzymes:

- Glucokinase in the liver responds to dietary glucose; as the microbial flora in the rumen digests nearly all glucose, the ruminant's liver does not need, and hence practically lacks, glucokinase activity;

- Arginase (see above);
- Sucrase in the gut is induced by long-term sucrose feeding; lactase, on the other hand, is only mildly induced by long-term milk ingestion;
- Penicillinase in bacteria is inducible, which causes drug resistance to long-term penicillin treatment.

Enzymes whose activities in cells are independent of induction are called constitutive enzymes (e.g., hexokinase); they are of lesser importance in the control of metabolism.

It is important to distinguish induction of enzyme synthesis (genetic) from induction of enzyme activity (physiologic).

Molecular diseases

Molecular diseases (inborn errors of metabolism) are transmissible defects resulting from genetic mutations leading to nonfunctional (enzyme) proteins. The following are examples.

- **Phenylketonuria (PKU).** The enzyme that converts phenylalanin to tyrosine is lacking; excess phenylalanine is then converted to phenylpyruvate, phenylacetate, and phenyllactate, which affect brain development in infants.
- **Galactosemia.** Lack of an enzyme needed to metabolize galactose causes the sugar to accumulate; in the eye, it may be reduced to galactitol causing cataracts.
- **Glycogen storage disease.** Lack of one of the enzymes that catabolizes glycogen into free glucose (e.g., glucose 6-phosphatase) leads to glycogen accumulation when blood sugar levels are critically low.
- **Sickle cell anemia.** A substitution mutation of one amino acid in hemoglobin diminishes oxygen carrying capacity.

When a molecular disease is present, genetic control over enzyme activity is slow: several hours must be allowed for synthesis of new protein molecules. It is especially important, therefore, that adaptations be made to chronic changes in conditions such as diet, climate, growth, or pregnancy. For adaptations to acute changes, however, the physiologic mechanisms used to modify the activities of already existing enzyme molecules are needed.

Physiological modifications of enzyme activity

Competitive inhibition of enzyme activity

A look-alike (fake) of either the substrate or a cofactor (vitamin, mineral, high-energy compound) competes with the real substrate or cofactor at the isosteric site of the enzyme. Characteristic of this fast-acting control is that K_m is increased by the presence of the fake, but V_m is unaffected, as the fake may be drowned out by higher concentrations of the real substrate (Figure 4-9).

Examples of competitive inhibition follow:

- Malonate fakes succinate in the succinic dehydrogenase reaction. The fake binds with its two carboxyl groups to the enzyme, but no reaction can occur with it (Figure 4-10).
- Antibiotics, e.g., puromycin (see above).
- Growth requires DNA synthesis, which entails methylation and reduction of uracil to thymine. This U to T conversion involves a methylated derivative of the cofactor tetrahydrofolate and produces dihydrofolate. The enzyme that converts dihydrofolate back to tetrahydrofolate can be inhibited by fakes of dihydrofolate (Figure 4-11), which are therefore used as drugs to suppress unwanted growth; for example, aminopterin and methotrexate to combat cancer, and sulfanilamide, a look-alike of the central portion of the dihydrofolate structure, as an antibacterial drug.

Chemical engineering of new pharmaceutically active fakes is one of the mainstays of the drug industry, as all kinds of bacteria and insects develop drug-resistant mutations after the same drug has been administered for an extended period of time.

Competitive inhibition is a reversible control over enzyme activity, since it is usually possible to crowd the fake out with real substrate or cofactor.

Noncompetitive inhibition

A competitor substance binds allosterically or isosterically to an enzyme molecule and thereby changes the enzyme's tertiary structure, so that the isosteric site for attachment of the substrate is lost. This form of inhibition can be irreversible (e.g., lead poisoning).

By losing active enzyme molecules, V_m decreases, while K_m remains unchanged (Figure 4-12). This, too, is a fast-acting control over enzyme activity.

Negative feedback is a reversible form of noncompetitive allosteric control in which a distant end product of a biosynthetic pathway inhibits the activity of a rate-controlling ("key") enzyme at an early step in the pathway (Figure 4-13). The step under negative feedback control (B→C) is usually irreversible, and one that commits its product (C) to the remainder of the pathway. When the step from B to C is al-

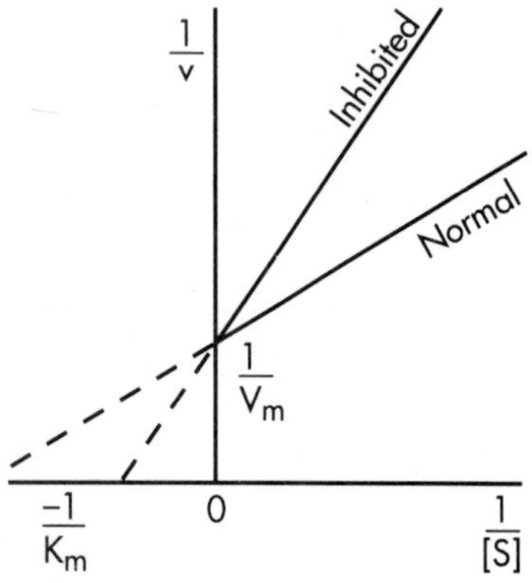

Figure 4-9. Competitive inhibition of enzyme activity. The inhibition increases K_m but does not affect V_m.

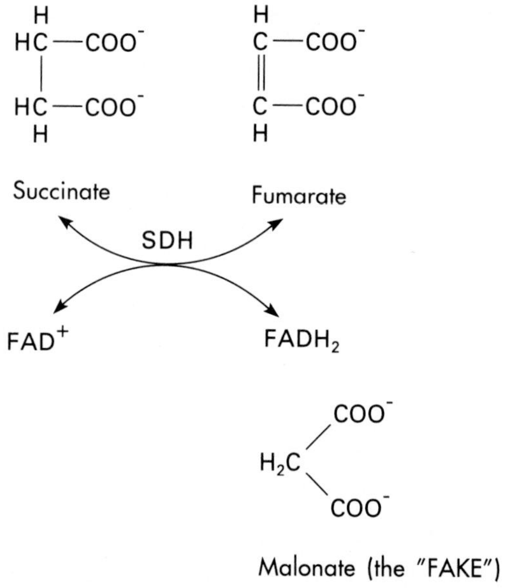

Malonate (the "FAKE")

Figure 4-10. Competitive inhibition of succinate dehydrogenase (SDH) by malonate. Note intermediation by the B vitamin flavin as flavin-adenine dinucleotide (FAD).

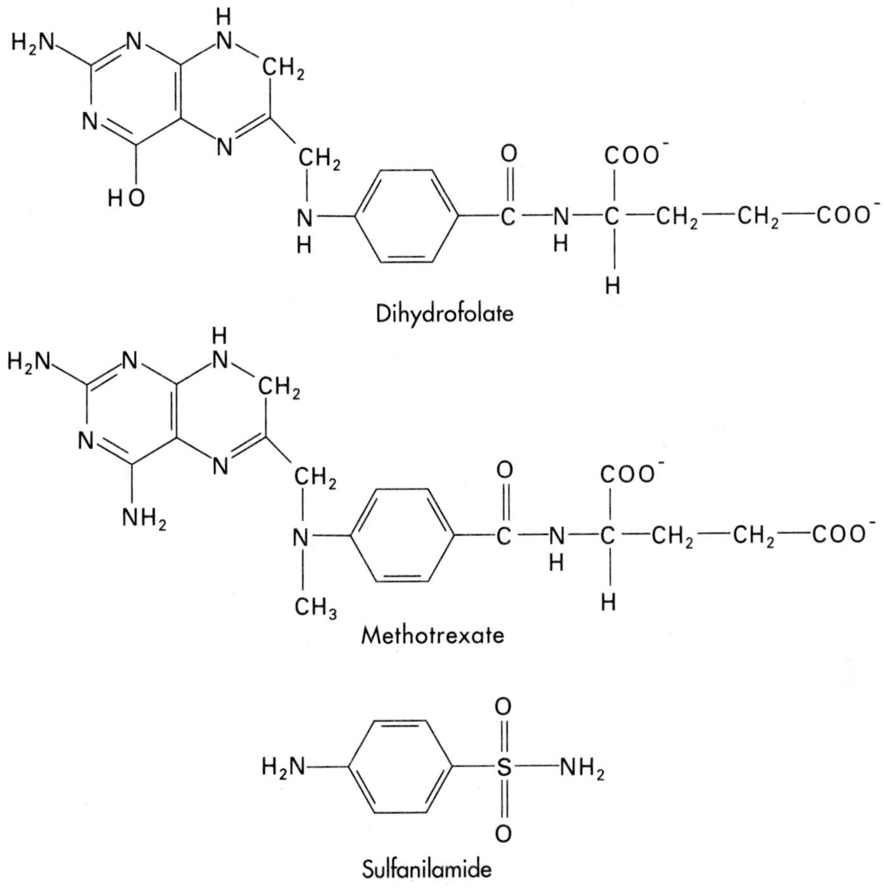

Dihydrofolate

Methotrexate

Sulfanilamide

Figure 4-11. Drugs that suppress growth by competitive enzyme inhibition. Replacing in methotrexate the *N*-bound methyl group by H yields the structure of aminopterin.

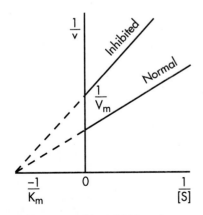

Figure 4-12. Noncompetitive inhibition of enzyme activity. The inhibition decreases V_m without affecting K_m.

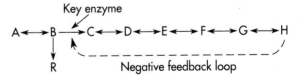

Figure 4-13. Allosteric control of a metabolic pathway (from A to H) via negative feedback of a distant product (H) on an early key enzyme.

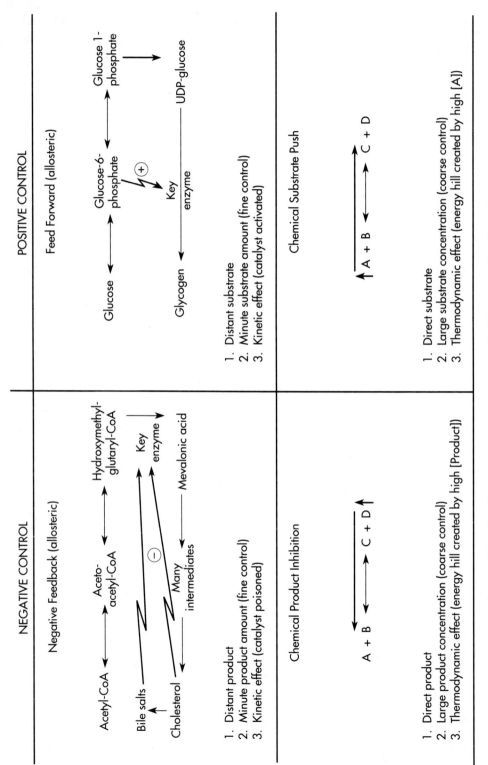

Figure 4-14. Control of reactions by allosteric effects on key enzymes compared with mass-action effects by reactants.

losterically inhibited, intermediate B can go back to A or proceed to R.

It is important to understand that allosteric inhibition is **not** the same thing as product inhibition. The latter requires a high concentration of product and then inhibits the immediate reaction that formed it; in Figure 4-13, if high D would inhibit the conversion of C to D, then that would be product inhibition. In contrast, negative feedback control only requires very minute amounts of an inhibitor, since the enzyme (which is also present in minute amounts) is inactivated by attaching one inhibitor molecule per enzyme molecule. Therefore, since the end product is not immediately removed by metabolism, it can allosterically attach to the rate-limiting enzyme and, thus, block continuation of its own biosynthesis. To understand the sensitive control over key enzyme activities in metabolism, allosteric effects on enzyme kinetics must be clearly distinguished from thermodynamic mass-action effects of reactants in inhibition and stimulation of a reaction (Figure 4-14).

Not only is negative feedback control extremely sensitive, it is also rapid, compared to the slow genetic repression by product. Negative feedback is one of the most important factors in establishing homeostatic control over the concentration of various compounds in tissues and the bloodstream. Examples of negative feedback control are the rates of biosynthesis of fatty acids, cholesterol, and the bases of nucleic acids.

Lack of negative feedback control over the purine bases (adenine and guanine) causes gout. Oxidation of these bases leads to overproduction of uric acid, manifesting itself in the form of arthritic swellings of joints and of kidney stones. The uric–acid-forming enzyme can be competitively inhibited with the drug allopurinol, which fakes out the natural substrate hypoxanthine (Figure 4-15).

Another example of noncompetitive inhibition is the trypsin inhibitor of colostrum that allows a suck-ling to obtain intact proteins (immune factors) from its mother's milk. Intestinal parasites may also be equipped with inhibitors to intestinal enzymes that could otherwise digest them, in addition to often having indigestible outer constituents.

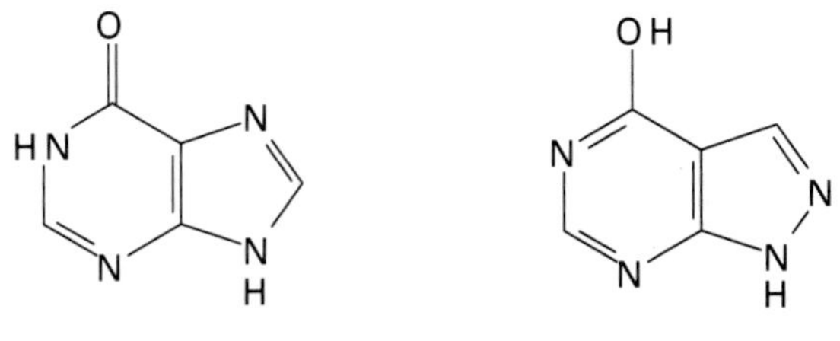

Activation of enzyme activity

Cooperativity (either inhibitory or stimulatory) occurs when allosteric or isosteric attachment of substrate or product to an enzyme protein causes a tertiary structural change in that protein, so that the K_m of the reaction is affected. The result is a sigmoid curve for velocity versus substrate concentration, as is illustrated for oxygen binding to, or unloading from, hemoglobin (Figure 4-16). It is important to realize the physiologic significance of the sigmoid curve: easy unloading of oxygen is possible at sites where the oxygen tension is low, as in body tissues.

Allosteric activation is equally important as is allosteric inhibition. It is fast, compared to slow genetic induction of enzyme activity, and reversible.

A key enzyme may be present in dormant form; it is then quickly activated by either the direct substrate or an indirect (distant) substrate. The following are examples:

- Glucokinase is activated by glucose, its direct substrate.
- Glucose 6-phosphate activates glycogen synthase, though it is not the direct substrate for it; this activation, called feed forward, directs the distant substrate glucose into the pathway of glycogenesis (see Figure 4-14).

To summarize, a comparison should be made between the following: (i) negative feedback (minute

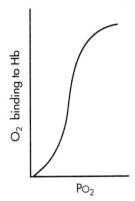

Figure 4-16. Cooperativity. Binding of oxygen to hemoglobin *(Hb)* in relation to oxygen tension *(PO₂)*.

Hypoxanthine

Allopurinol

Figure 4-15. Allopurinol resembles hypoxanthine.

amounts of distant product inhibit the key enzyme located early in the pathway, so that no more product is formed); (ii) feed forward (minute amounts of distant substrate activate the key enzyme, thereby sustaining the formation of ultimate product); (iii) product inhibition (large amounts of the direct product of a reaction drive the reaction backwards); and (iv) pushing a reaction forward with large amounts of the direct substrate.

Experimentally, one can distinguish between genetic and allosteric activations by adding a protein-synthesis inhibitor (e.g., puromycin or actinomycin D) concurrently with the activator substance. Then, any activation observed is not genetic.

Proenzymes (zymogens)

Proenzymes are the direct product of translation after a leader sequence has been clipped off. They are inactive forms of enzyme proteins. Storing zymogens protects tissues from self-destruction. When the enzyme activity is needed, zymogens are rapidly, and irreversibly, activated by proteolytic cleavage. For instance, if pancreatic cells were to store trypsin, chymotrypsin, and carboxypeptidase, the cells would digest themselves. The activation of pancreatic digestive enzymes, and of gastric pepsinogen, is an autocatalytic process, brought about by positive feedback (which is rare in nature); for instance, a small amount of stomach acid (HCl) converts some pepsinogen to pepsin, and pepsin, in turn, converts more of the zymogen by proteolytic removal of a peptide segment.

In parallel fashion to storing zymogens, blood-clotting factors are stored as inactive precursors; thus, when the need for hemostasis arises, prothrombin is rapidly converted to active thrombin which, in turn, activates conversion of fibrinogen into fibrin. Also, hormones are, in some cases, stored as inactive prohormones (e.g., preproinsulin and proinsulin). However, proinsulin does possess some insulin-like activity.

Enzyme activation by changing quaternary structure

Quaternary compilation of from two to more than ten monomeric subunits is an activation mechanism of many enzymes whose activities adapt to need by rapid (and reversible) association/dissociation equilibria of prefabricated subunits (e.g., muscle phosphorylase; hepatic pyruvate dehydrogenase complex).

Covalent modification of enzyme protein

In many cases, an enzyme protein has to be phosphorylated or dephosphorylated to become enzymat-

ically active. This is a very rapid and reversible modification of enzymic activity. Many key enzymes are controlled in this way, such as (i) phosphorylase, key bearer to the body's glycogen store; and (ii) adipolytic triglyceride lipase, key bearer to the fat stores.

These pivotal phosphorylations and dephosphorylations of key enzymes are directed by a cascade of interlocking controls, involving enzymes (protein kinases and phosphatases) whose activities are regulated by hormones (via their second messengers) that in turn respond to signals from the nervous sytem.

Controlling availability of reactants

Structural and organismic features of cells may control accessibility of enzymes to substrates and cofactors.

- Compartmentalization of enzymes in subcellular particles may limit enzyme activities, since substrates and cofactors must be shuttled across membranes toward those subcellular sites; for example: shuttling fatty acids from cytoplasm, where they are stored, into mitochondria, where they are combusted.

- A macromolecular complex, containing all the enzymes of a given pathway in one unit, forms a bucket brigade. The substrate enters and is held until it is released by the last enzyme of the pathway as the finished product. This is the advantage: though macroscopically the substrate concentration may be extremely low, it remains high at the site of the enzyme throughout the entire pathway, and, thus, the reaction velocity remains high (examples: cytoplasmic fatty acid synthesis; mitochondrial oxidative phosphorylation).

- Protein binding of reactants may leave only a small amount of unbound reactant available for the enzyme reaction. The larger, protein-bound reservoir of reactant serves as a buffer: it delivers free reactant as soon as the reaction demands more substrate. For example, various hormones are carried protein-bound in the bloodstream (e.g., thyroxine); so are free fatty acids, vitamin B_{12}, calcium, and iron. An added advantage of protein binding is that small hydrophobic molecules escape loss from the body by glomerular filtration in the kidneys.

- Transport across cell membranes is required for entry of compounds from the interstitial fluid into cells.

Organismic control

The following is a brief review of how the adaptive rate modifications of enzymes are integrated in the body.

Homeostasis does not mean that the level of a substance in the blood or cells remains absolutely constant at all times. On the contrary, variations are the order of the day. But a decrease in the level of a substance causes an increase in the activity of the key enzyme responsible for the production of that substance; just as an increased level of that substance causes allosteric inhibition of that key enzyme. These corrective adaptations of the activities of key enzymes direct pathways of metabolism toward maintaining the status quo in the body.

One might ask, why all the emphasis on key enzymes? It is because a distinction must be made between constitutive and adaptable enzyme activities. Most enzyme activities in the body are plentifully available at all times (i.e., constitutive). Constitutive enzyme activities are dictated by the amounts of metabolic intermediates "shoved" on their way by the finely controlled activities of adaptable (key) enzymes. This system may be likened to house plumbing, where water flow through the pipes (which are constitutive) is dictated by the opening and closing of adaptable faucets (Figure 4-17).

No matter how ample the capacity of the constitutive portion of the enzyme pathway, the flow of metabolic intermediates is controlled by the extent to which the key enzyme activity is activated. In the sketch (see Figure 4-17), two "faucets" are almost closed (enzymes 6 and 11) so that the rates of formation of potential products A and C are down to a trickle; but faucet enzyme-2 is wide-open at the moment, allowing a stream of metabolic intermediates to go all the way through enzyme-5; then, with key enzyme-6 closed but key enzyme-9 open, metabolism

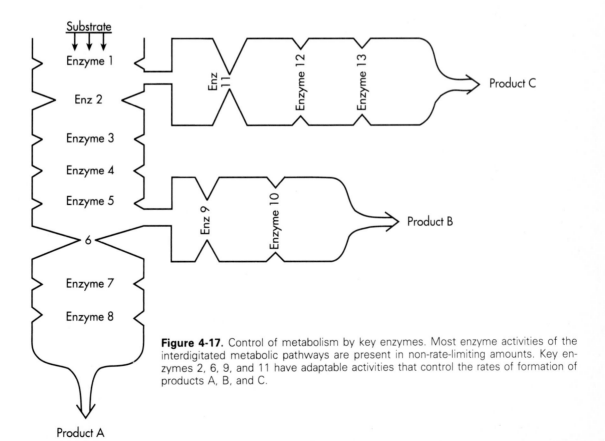

Figure 4-17. Control of metabolism by key enzymes. Most enzyme activities of the interdigitated metabolic pathways are present in non-rate-limiting amounts. Key enzymes 2, 6, 9, and 11 have adaptable activities that control the rates of formation of products A, B, and C.

is directed toward formation of product B. This example shows how adaptive modifications of just a few key enzymes does two things at once: (i) it directs metabolism, so that one product gets formed while other products are not formed at a given time; and (ii) it determines the rate of formation of that product by activating only the desired quantity of key enzyme (enzyme-9 in the sketch). Probably product A feeds back on the activity of enzyme-6, and the presence of a high enough level of product C allosterically inhibits the activity of key enzyme-11. To exemplify the need to control rate and direction of metabolism, a scheme is presented that depicts alternative metabolic routes for dietary glucose entering the liver (Figure 4-18).

The discussion on metabolism spends little time with the nonadaptable enzymes; animals must be assumed to possess all those enzymes, or else they would not be alive. For medical physiology it is only important to diagnose that something is wrong with the direction of a pathway or the extent to which it goes, and then institute treatment geared to adjust the activity of the key enzyme involved to the proper level. Focus shall, therefore, be on key enzymes.

In general, only key enzymes are allowed to exist in one form of dormancy or another. That makes sense, for, with the time-consuming protein synthesis already completed, activation of a dormant enzyme is extremely rapid, so that there can be a quick adaptive response to an established need for that key enzyme's activity. Dormant enzyme activities can be awakened by neuroendocrine signals, allosteric activation under the influence of substrate, proteolytic activation of zymogens, polymerization of inactive monomers, or the addition or removal of a phosphate group.

If key enzymes, such as phosphorylase (controlling glycogen stores) and adiopolytic triglyceride lipase (controlling fat stores) would not occur in dormant forms, but, instead, be continually active, how then would it ever be possible to build up glycogen and fat stores after a meal? Obviously, these key enzymes that literally hold the keys to our energy stores must be kept dormant through the time (after a meal) of glycogen and fat deposition, and they must be activated reversibly when the need for the stores' contents arises.

Physiologic control over metabolism, thus, is achieved by regulating the activities of key enzymes and inducing or repressing the synthesis of enzymes. Certain dietary ingredients may modify key enzyme activities either by allosteric effects or via hormonal responses to their presence. Hormones affect metab-

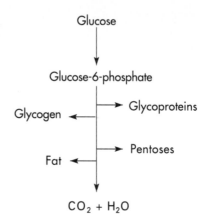

Figure 4-18. Alternative pathways for glucose metabolism in the liver.

olism not only be modifying activity and synthesis of key enzymes, but also by controlling transport of substrate molecules across cell membranes to enzyme sites. Secretion of hormones, in turn, is partially under the control of the nervous system, as is the direct activation of certain key enzymes. Nervous controls are very sensitive to minute changes in the body's equilibria, and their adaptive responses to those changes are extremely rapid and reversible.

CLINICAL USE OF ENZYMES

Clinical laboratory analysis of tissues and body fluids has given physiologists a fair idea of which constituents should be present in various tissues and body fluids (e.g., plasma), and how much of each of those constituents should normally be there. Many enzymes are contained in tissue cells and should not be found in plasma at all, unless the tissue is damaged, cells are destroyed, and the enzymes are released into the plasma. Clinical analysis for the presence and concentration of these tissue enzymes in plasma has become a common diagnostic tool. Examples follow:

- Lactate dehydrogenase (LDH) isozymes in plasma may be diagnostic for heart or liver damage (see Figure 4-2).
- Arginase, a key enzyme in urea production: since urea formation is rather specific for liver cells, arginase activity in blood is diagnostic for liver damage.
- Creatine phosphokinase (CPK): muscle has a unique energy store in the form of phosphocreatine; its high-energy phosphate is transferred by CPK to ADP, forming ATP needed for muscle contraction. Normally, only a little CPK is pres-

ent in the blood; a significant increase in CPK, then, can confirm a diagnosis of disorders affecting skeletal or heart muscles.

Determing levels of various organic compounds in body fluids is another clinical use of enzymes. For example:

- Glucose oxidase is specific for oxidizing glucose: the electrons taken from glucose are absorbed by a reduction-oxidation indicator which, when reduced, turns blue. One can test for the presence of glucose in urine (glucosuria) with a commercially available dip stick that is impregnated with glucose oxidase and redox indicator. Some commercial dip strips also indicate ketone bodies and protein in urine.
- Lactic acid can be assayed with LDH.
- Urea in the urine or blood can be assayed with urease.

Enzyme therapy is also an area of current interest. A problem associated with intravenously injecting enzymes is that the recipient makes antibodies against them. Methods to obviate this problem include: (i) injecting the enzyme encased inside a liposome (to combat lipidoses caused by deficiencies of lysosomal enzymes); and (ii) by means of an indwelling cannula, releasing the enzyme at the site where its activity is needed (e.g., streptokinase to dissolve blood clots in coronary arteries).

For clinical, research, and industrial purposes, enzymes are being used to synthesize compounds which, by classical means of organic chemistry, are hard to obtain. Expecially promising is the manufacturing of compounds with biocatalytic properties made to order.

In summary, enzymes can speed things up, but they are not miracle workers. Reactions must obey the laws of energy economy. Having considered how reactions are executed when feasible, the text will now explore why things move in given directions, bringing up the topics of bioenergetics and receptors.

STUDY QUESTIONS

1. Name the compound that makes the uphill process of glucosephosphate formation energetically feasible.

2. What would the net result be of a futile cycle consisting of the reactions when glucokinase is added to glucose 6-phosphatase?

3. *a.* List by name (not abbreviation) a B vitamin involved in an enzyme reaction.
   b. List two B vitamins involved in shuttling electrons.

4. Due to narrow enzyme specificities, the body can only metabolize the D / L (choose one) form of sugars and the D / L (choose one) form of amino acids.

5. Other than essential amino acids (that are needed for enzyme protein synthesis), list an organic and an inorganic class of nutritional ingredients that must be present in the diet for proper enzyme functioning.

6. *a.* Does genetically inducing an enzyme's synthesis increase V_m, K_m, both, or neither?
   b. The K_m expresses the maximum velocity of an enzyme reaction with a given substrate. (True/False)
   c. At a branching point in a metabolic pathway, substrate present at a low concentration engages in the reaction that has: high K_m; low K_m; high V_m; low V_m. (Choose one.)

7. The body's enzymes, in general, have their maximal activity at physiologic pH. (True/False)

8. Exemplify a pharmacologic use of competitive enzyme inhibition.

9. *a.* What structure-determining element of an enzyme protein is lost by lead poisoning?
   b. Exemplify an enzyme activity regulated by changing quaternary structure.

10. *a.* What is the general mode of action of drugs such as methotrexate and sulfanilamide?
    b. What mode of enzyme activation is indicated when the activation is abolished in the presence of puromycin?

11. The action of steroid hormones regulating certain key enzyme activities, is by (choose A or B): (A) increasing enzyme synthesis in cells; or (B) allosterically activating existing enzyme.

12. *a.* Why is negative feedback control infinitely more sensitive than chemical product control?
    b. List an example of this kind of control.
    c. Name a disorder caused by a lack of this kind of control.

13. Enzymically, explain the cause and development of glycogen storage disease.

14. Exemplify a pancreatic and a gastric zymogen whose activations are under positive feedback control.

15. *a.* List an enzyme whose presence in the bloodstream is indicative of liver damage.
    b. List an enzyme whose isozyme typing in serum can be diagnostic for a heart infarct.

16. List a practical diagnostic use of enzymes in detecting glucosuria.

17. What is the practical consequence of the fact that penicillinase in bacteria is inducible?

18. Give an advantage of having an entire metabolic pathway contained in one macromolecular enzyme complex (e.g., fatty acid synthesis).

19. List a putative enzyme-related function of microtrabecular network in cytoplasm.

20. For what purpose is arginase induced by glucocorticoids?

21. List a process by which certain key enzymes are quickly activated from their dormant state when their activities are needed.

22. List the protein that combines with calcium intracellularly and then functions to activate key enzymes.

23. *a.* What does a protein kinase do to affect enzyme activity?
b. What, in turn, regulates protein kinase activity?
c. List a key enzyme under protein kinase/phosphatase control.

24. How do proteins in colostrum escape trypsin digestion in the gut of newborns?

25. List a possible reason for the use of liposomes as a means of intravenously injecting an enzyme into an animal with a molecular disease.

26. Definitions and terminology:
a. Give the technical term denoting different enzymes that are capable of catalyzing the same chemical reaction, and name a clinical method used to separate such enzymes.
b. Any part of an enzyme's protein structure that is not the active site is denoted technically by which term?
c. List the technical term denoting that an enzyme's activity can be rapidly increased to meet a sudden demand for it.
d. List the technical term denoting that an enzyme's activity is present in non–rate-limiting amounts at all times.
e. Define and exemplify a molecular disease.
f. Give the technical term for the fact that the distant substrate glucose 6-phosphate activates the key enzymes of glycogenesis.
g. List the technical term denoting that a distant end product regulates the rate of its biosynthesis by controlling an early key enzyme in the pathway.

Physical-chemical features of biological transport

ENERGY
Different forms of energy
Energy and entropy

Energy may be defined as the capacity to do work or serve as a source of heat. Energy takes on different forms, such as electrical energy, chemical energy, and heat. In general, different forms of energy are interchangeable; the chemical energy contained in food can be commuted into work or heat. However, every energy transaction is accompanied by an irretrievable loss of some of the available energy. This loss, due to a change in entropy of the system, may be caused by friction or by an increase in randomness. One may popularize the entropic energy loss by calling it the house percentage; the price of doing business; or the taxes deducted from gross income before arriving at spendable, net income. In keeping with the latter analogy, free energy, G (i.e., spendable energy), is defined as the difference between total available energy, H, minus loss of energy caused by increased entropy ($T \cdot \Delta S$; in which T stands for absolute temperature and S for entropy). So, when a system changes (e.g., glucose is metabolized to lactate), the amount of free energy available to do work (ΔG) equals the total energy change (ΔH), minus the entropy gain (ΔS), multiplied by body temperature (T).

$$\Delta G = \Delta H - T \cdot \Delta S$$

The following comments may be attached to that formula:

- The inescapable, and irretrievable, entropic energy loss that is associated with any energy transaction, makes all processes irreversible in principle. For instance, the pendulum on a grandfather clock converts kinetic energy into potential energy as it swings upward, and potential energy back into kinetic energy as it swings downward; all the while, though, it is losing a bit of total energy in the form of entropic heat loss caused by friction at the fulcrum. There is no such thing as mobile perpetuum. Eventually all available energy on this earth will have been spent on entropy changes; everything will then be randomized; so there will no longer be differences in height (e.g., mountains), atmospheric pressure, electrical voltage, temperature, etc. This far-distant scenario is referred to as entropic death of the universe.
- Spontaneous (passive) processes go downhill, that is, they are characterized by a negative value for ΔG. According to the formula, a negative ΔG may result from a negative ΔH (energy-driven processes), or from a positive ΔS at constant body temperature (entropy-driven processes). An example of an energy-driven process is an avalanche of snow coming down a moun-

79

tain or the formation of water from hydrogen and oxygen gases. One entropy-driven process is solubilization of a salt crystal in water (increased randomness). Spontaneous processes proceed downhill along a gradient. A gradient is a force, such as an electrical gradient directing ions or electrons, or a chemical gradient moving compounds in the direction of the lower concentration. A passive process continues as long as the gradient exists; ultimately the process will wipe out its gradient (e.g., air flow from a punctured tire). At that instance, the tendency (force) driving a compound in one direction is offset by an equal force driving the compound in the opposite direction; equilibrium has been reached; ΔG now equals zero; the reaction stops.

- Processes that require input of energy are called uphill or active processes. Though one can isolate an active process philosophically (e.g., fatty acid synthesis from acetyl-CoA), an active process only occurs in nature if it is coupled with a passive process that provides enough energy for uphill movement; for instance, the uphill fatty acid synthesis after dinner is possible because of a larger downhill energy release from the breakdown of glucose. This metabolic example compares with the situation where a child comes rolling down a steep hill on a bicycle, thus generating enough energy to climb a lesser hill without pushing the pedals. Also, in a siphon, water may move uphill in one compartment because there is a larger downhill drop in a subsequent compartment.

In sum, energy and entropy changes must be considered to determine whether a reaction is energetically feasible; that is to say, active or passive. As the entire flow of nature is downhill, for each isolated active process there is a downhill process that "pays the energy bill."

Energy input; activation energy

In light of the discussion about spontaneous processes, How can nature allow unstable states (nonequilibrium) to continue? Why, for example, are gradients allowed to exist? Why does a glucose molecule exist (instead of its breakdown products)?

There are two answers to these questions:

- Constant input of energy maintains the unstable situation of life (nonequilibrium) (e.g., food intake; Na^+/K^+ pump in cells).

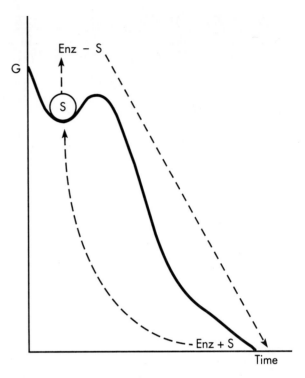

Figure 5-1. Activation energy. An enzyme *(Enz)* lifting a substrate *(S)* over the activation energy hump releases free energy *(G)*.

- Activation energy barriers must be overcome. For example, when a stone clings to a hillside, kept in that unstable situation by a little ridge of dirt preventing it from sliding down, either the dirt must be removed or the stone lifted above the ridge, so that the stone can roll downhill. The same is true for life processes; molecules may be barred from going downhill by an activation energy barrier; the combination of substrate with an enzyme lifts the substrate above the activation energy barrier, so the reaction becomes possible (Figure 5-1).

Commuting one form of energy into another

One form of energy can be converted into another; for instance, chemical energy (food, ATP) can be commuted into muscle contraction or a Na^+/K^+ pump. Each conversion, though, demands its entropy price, usually in the form of heat loss. The more useful energy (work, ATP) one harvests from a given energy transaction, the smaller the heat loss. In a warm-blooded animal, the sum of metabolic heat losses contributes to the maintenance of body temperature.

Kinetic considerations; transport
Energetics and kinetics

Energy considerations do show the extent and direction of processes, and whether energy is released or required. However, energy considerations do not show how fast a process will go and which route it will take. To learn about the velocity and pathways of processes, transport kinetics must be taken into account.

Different forms of transport

Different needs for transport create different forms of transport processes; for example:

- Shuttling of fatty acids, pyruvate, amino acids, and ketone bodies between cytoplasm and mitochondria is one of the factors that regulate oxidative metabolism.
- Other intracellular shuttles involve getting substrates to enzymes, or hormones into the nucleus.
- Cellular uptake of nutrients from the circulation (e.g., transport across the blood-brain barrier; glucose entry into fat cells aided by insulin).
- Targeting certain compounds (hormones, drugs) to specific cells.
- Different transport mechanisms for lipids and water-soluble substances from the intestine.
- Protein carriers exist with varying specificities for transport of different compounds in the bloodstream.
- Specific mineral pumps exchange Na^+, K^+, Ca^{++}, Mg^{++}, and H^+ cations and various anions across the plasma membrane, and intracellularly to and from subcellular organelles.
- Various transport systems exist for excretion of compounds into bile and urine.

Presently, transport, an item of general physiologic importance, shall be examined. This chapter deals with the physical-chemical characteristics and biological applications of diffusion, osmosis, and Donnan equilibria. In the next chapter, some uniquely biological transport phenomena (modes of passive, active, and carrier-mediated transport across cell membranes; receptors; hormone action; conveying environmental messages to cell interiors) are highlighted in the context of cell surface phenomena.

DIFFUSION
Definition

Diffusion is the spontaneous movement of particles (ions, molecules, aggregates) along a concentration gradient. The driving force is randomization of particle concentrations, or entropy gain.

Rate of diffusion

Three factors determine the rate of diffusion at any given temperature: (i) the concentration gradient: the steeper the gradient, the faster the movement; (ii) the surface area across which diffusion is taking place: the larger the surface, the more substance moves across it per given amount of time; and (iii) the diffusion constant (F) of a compound: small, streamlined particles diffuse faster than large, odd-shaped ones; their diffusion constant is high. Combining these three factors:

Diffusion Rate =
F × Surface Area × Concentration Gradient

This formula should be written as a differential equation, since the concentration gradient steadily diminishes because of diffusion. Only at the expense of energy input can a concentration gradient be maintained.

Physiological considerations

Stirring expedites diffusion (e.g., peristalsis in the intestine). To increase diffusion effectiveness, surface areas of cells are enlarged microanatomically in the form of microvilli (e.g., gut mucosa; parenchymal liver cells; renal tubular cells). To aid diffusion, where needed, concentration gradients are maintained at the expense of energy input; for example, NaCl and urea gradients in the kidneys help regulate water conservation.

OSMOSIS
Definition; semipermeable membranes

For the movement of water to occur in body fluids, there must exist a gradient for its movement. Thus, water will diffuse from an area of higher water concentration (i.e., water containing less solute), to an area of lower water concentration (i.e., water containing more solute). This process of water movement, referred to as osmosis, occurs across membranes permeable to water but not to particular solutes (e.g., proteins). Therefore, for osmosis to occur, two different concentrations of a substance dissolved in water must be separated by a semipermeable membrane. In physiology, this is generally called osmotic water movement across capillary membranes and cell membranes, both being relatively impermeable to proteins.

Osmotic pressure; osmolarity

The three factors dictating the diffusion rate of solutes also apply to osmotic water movement (diffusion constant; surface area; and concentration gradient). However, because of the semipermeable membrane, a distinction must be made between movements of solute and water molecules. Therefore, consider the following example:

A Thistle tube (an upside-down funnel) is closed off by a semipermeable membrane (Figure 5-2). Small salt ions are free to move in and out, but adding to the funnel compartment a protein, too large to cross the membrane, sets up a water gradient directed toward the inside of the tube: Water moves in (osmosis). This pushes the meniscus up against gravity: the protein gradient inside the tube is using water to do work.

The force that allowed the water to do this work is called the **osmotic pressure** of the solution. The osmotic pressure, at a given temperature, is determined by the concentration of particles. The nature of the semipermeable membrane does not matter; in fact, no membrane needs to be present; one speaks of the osmotic pressure of a solution regardless of the presence of or lack of a membrane. Also, the nature of the particles does not matter; only the number of particles in solution counts. Therefore, a Na^+ (atomic weight 23) exerts the same osmotic pressure as a protein molecule of molecular weight 200,000.

The following are two ways of expressing the concentration of particles in solution: (i) osmolarity: the number of osmoles per liter of solution; and (ii) osmolality: the number of osmoles per kilogram of water. In analogy with the pressure-volume relationship of ideal gases [$P \cdot V = R \cdot T$], the osmotic pressure of a solution equals $R \cdot T \cdot C$, in which C is the concentration of solute expressed in osmoles per liter. Thus, the osmotic pressure of one osmole in a liter, at zero centigrade, equals 22.4 atmospheres ($= 22.4 \cdot 76$ cm Hg $= 22.4 \cdot 76 \cdot 13.6$ cm H_2O); that is, a water column of 770 feet exerts the equivalent pressure of a 1 osm solution.

In a body tissue, fluid compartments (e.g., intracellular and extracellular fluids) are separated by semi-

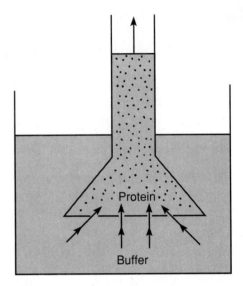

Figure 5-2. Thistle tube containing a protein solution separated from surrounding buffer by a semipermeable membrane demonstrates osmotic work.

permeable membranes. These membranes are selectively permeable to small solutes (e.g., Na^+ and Cl^- ions) but not to proteins. Hence, proteins are quite unevenly distributed (being concentrated in cells), whereas the small salt ions tend to distribute more evenly except for Donnan equilibrium effects (discussed later in chapter) and for the intervention by active processes, such as the Na^+/K^+ pump. When considering total osmotic pressure, the small salt ions are by far the chief determinants. But when considering osmotic pressure differences between compartments, the permeable salt ions do not contribute much; these differences are determined by the proteins' uneven distribution. The osmotic pressure attributable to macromolecules (proteins) is called **oncotic pressure,** or **colloid osmotic pressure.**

Quantitative

Representing plasma as a 0.9% NaCl solution with 6% protein (with mean molecular weight = 120,000), 1 l of plasma contains 9 g of NaCl (i.e., 150 mmoles, equal to 300 mosmoles); and 60 g of protein (i.e., 0.5 mmole, or 0.5 mosmole). The oncotic pressure, thus, is less than 0.2% of the total osmotic pressure of plasma, yet is of vital importance for the distribution of body fluids.

Relation of oncotic pressure to distribution of body fluids

One of the vital functions of plasma proteins is to maintain osmotic gradients between the bloodstream and interstitial fluid. Those gradients establish fluid movements that are essential in the exchange processes of nutrients from the blood to the tissues and waste products from the tissues back to the blood. Once more, it is essential to realize that from the total osmotic pressure of plasma (about 5000 mm Hg), the oncotic pressure accounts for only about 0.2% (about 25 mm Hg). In living systems, this oncotic component consists almost entirely of proteins. Because of the semipermeability of biological membranes, the electrolyte concentration in interstitial fluid is about equal to that in plasma, but the protein concentration is much lower; the oncotic pressure of interstitial fluid is about 10 mm Hg. Therefore, there exists a net osmotic gradient between plasma and interstitial fluid of 15 mm Hg, which can be attributed to a difference in protein concentrations in the two fluid compartments. This oncotic gradient pulls fluid into the bloodstream. On the arterial side of the blood circulation, the blood pressure more than offsets the oncotic pull, so that there is a net filtration pressure that drives fluid out of arterial blood (Figure 5-3). On the venous side, however, the blood pressure is low, so that the oncotic pressure wins out, and there is a net absorption pressure that pulls fluid into venous blood. The outcome of it all is that tissue cells, bathing in interstitial fluid, are supplied with nutrients that filter in with the fluids from the arterial side, and that wastes from those cells are carried away and absorbed with the fluid drain on the venous side. The liver and kidneys, then, remove wastes from blood, decide whether or not some of those waste products can be recycled into usable compounds, and, if not, eliminate them into bile or urine.

Following are notes to the above process:
- The four forces that determine net fluid movement in or out of a blood vessel (see Figure 5-3) are referred to as **Starling's forces** (named for the physiologist who first detailed their functions).
- Together, hydrostatic and oncotic pressures maintain a constant distribution of fluid in plasma and interstitial spaces. On the other hand, the total amount of body water is determined by the total osmotic pressure, and thus, by the electrolytes present in body fluids. Regulation of the body's electrolyte content and composition, therefore, exerts control over total water balance in the body; this is one of the important functions of the kidneys.
- Edema is fluid accumulation in interstitial fluid spaces, caused by any one of the following:
  - Enhanced venous pressure (right-sided heart failure, venous obstruction).
  - Decreased plasma oncotic pressure (liver disease, hemorrhage, nephrosis, starvation, and the like).
  - Increased interstitial fluid oncotic pressure (tissue damage).
  - Increased capillary permeability (histamines, kinins, and the like).
  - Lymphatic obstruction.
- Protein reservoirs in tissues can be broken down and serve for the hepatic production of glucose and plasma proteins; or the tissues can deposit excess proteins. Thus, tissues serve as a buffer to guard against fluctuations in plasma protein; that is, they buffer the plasma oncotic pressure.
- Calamities may arise that overburden the tissues' protein buffering capacity; for example, (i) acute, large loss of albumin caused by nephrosis or burns; or (ii) starvation or chronic malnutrition, in which case a lack of essential amino acids finally leads to lowered plasma protein levels and, in turn, to fasting edema. Feeding infants grain starches exclusively produces lysine and methionine deficiencies and thereby the protein-deficiency syndrome of kwashiorkor, characterized by edema and fatty liver.
- Fluid therapy: 1 g of albumin holds about 18 ml of fluid in the bloodstream. Infusion of concentrated albumin (25 g per 100 ml) is equivalent in oncotic effect (i.e., fluid retention) to about 500 ml of plasma. This effect is beneficial when restoration of a critically low plasma volume is needed; for instance, to prevent or treat hypovolemic shock.

Tonicity
Physiological buffers

The term **isotonic** (and by contrast hypotonic and hypertonic) is used in physiology to denote that a solution has not only quantitatively the proper osmolarity, but also qualitatively contains the proper life-supporting ingredients. Tonicity thus describes the effective osmotic pressure of a solution relative to plasma. A typical isotonic buffer contains the right

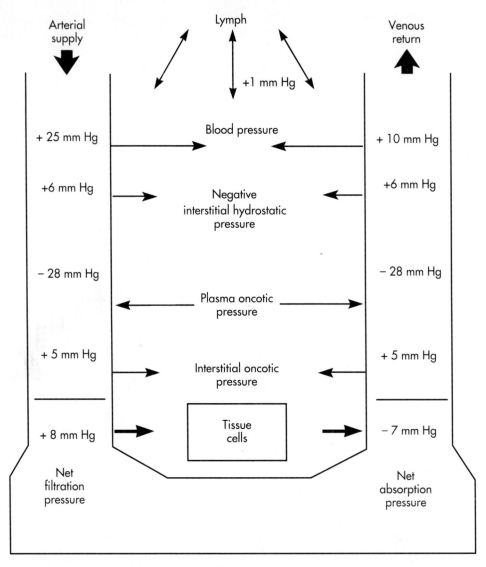

Figure 5-3. Role of oncotic pressure in body fluid distribution. Starling forces control fluid movement in an arterial-venous loop. Interstitial fluid hydrostatic pressure tends to move fluid outward through the capillary membrane into the interstitium when it is negative, and inward toward the capillary bed when it is positive. Interstitial hydrostatic pressure apparently varies from one organ to another; and although there is some controversy, it is thought to be subatmospheric (i.e., a semivacuum or suction pressure) in subcutaneous tissue (as shown here), yet positive in the liver, kidney, and brain. The subatmospheric nature of the interstitial fluid pressure could be thought of as drawing fluid out of the blood on the arterial side (shown here as a +8 mmHg), and also (in some places) serving as a means of holding tissues together. The lymphatic pump would help to establish and maintain a negative interstitial fluid pressure. The absolute difference between the net filtration pressure and the net absorption pressure (i.e., +1 mmHg) is additional pressure used to drive lymph flow, which accounts for about 10% of the fluid filtered on the arterial end of the capillary.

total osmolarity, pH, Na^+, K^+, Mg^+, Ca^{++}, HCO_3^-, Cl^-, $H_2PO_4^-$, and nutrients (such as glucose, vitamins, amino acids), and may be oxygenated. Optimal solutions for incubating certain tissues in vitro for cell culture, or for life-supporting infusions, are named after their originators: for example, Krebs-Ringer, Krebs-Henseleit, and Tyrode's buffers.

When only osmolarity is considered, without paying attention to the ionic species that make up a solution, the terms iso-osmolar, hypo-osmolar, and hyperosmolar are used. The calculated osmotic concentration of a solution will not, however, predict its effects on the movement of water across cell membranes. This is determined by the type of solute, and the permeability of the membrane to that solute. The following examples will illustrate this concept:

- A 300 mOsm solution of NaCl is iso-osmotic to body fluids. When a cell is placed in this solution, it does not change size. Therefore, this solution is isotonic, with the cell membrane being effectively impermeable to NaCl.
- A 300 mOsm solution of urea is also iso-osmotic to body fluids. However, when a cell is placed in this solution, it swells and bursts. Therefore,

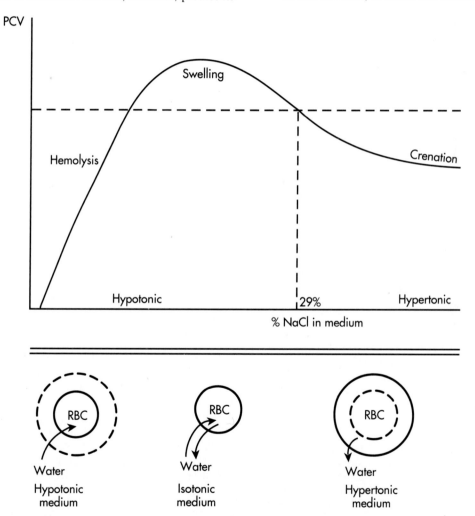

Figure 5-4. Effect of environmental tonicity on erythrocytes. The packed cell volume *(PCV)* of red blood cells *(RBC)* responds to the salt concentration in the medium.

this solution is hypotonic. The cell membrane is permeable to urea, therefore urea exerts no "effective" osmotic pressure, and water moves down its concentration gradient into the cell.

These are the differences between osmolarity and tonicity, and also the realities of water movement in physiological systems.

Hemolysis and crenation of erythrocytes

Erythrocytes, suspended in a hypotonic medium, take in water, swell, and may burst (hemolysis). In a hypertonic medium, they lose water and shrink (crenation).

These effects are followed in microhematocrit tubes in which a volume of blood is centrifuged and the hematocrit, also termed **packed cell volume (PCV),** is measured as a fraction of the total volume. In most domestic animal species a PCV of 23 to 47% is normally observed; hypotonic swelling increases this value, and either hemolysis or crenation decreases it (Figure 5-4).

Physiologic control of tonicity; outline

Osmotic pressure, being such a large force, must be narrowly controlled to ensure proper body functioning. The nervous system provides osmoreceptors that face the bloodstream and respond to osmolarity changes within a range of 2% around the norm. Endocrine responses (aldosterone, antidiuretic hormone, atrial natriuretic factor, renin-angiotensin) then instruct the kidneys to conserve water, Na^+, etc., or to let those pass into the urine. These topics will be detailed later.

Dialysis

The principle behind dialysis is that by enclosing a protein solution in semipermeable tubing bathed in a medium, one can exchange small ions, while retaining the protein. The kidney functions by dialysis: large protein molecules cannot dialyze through the semipermeable (glomerular) blood vessel, but small ions and wastes can.

The artificial kidney apparatus consists of a long stretch of semipermeable tubing suspended in a temperature-controlled physiological buffer bath; this substitutes for a defective kidney. The patient's blood passes through the tubing, and small metabolic wastes (e.g., urea) are dialyzed out, while the blood is equilibrated with the proper pH, nutrients, and minerals contained in the bathing fluid.

DONNAN MEMBRANE EQUILIBRIA
Equation showing equivalence of electrical and chemical energy
Definitions

In view of the semipermeability of the blood capillaries, it could be expected that the qualitative and quantitative electrolyte composition (the so-called electrolyte framework) of interstitial fluid is the same as that of plasma. However, it must be remembered that (i) most protein molecules cannot traverse the capillaries, and (ii) those proteins, at pH 7.4, carry a net, negative charge. Electroneutrality of plasma is maintained by the presence of satellite cations. Hence, because of the presence of a semipermeable membrane between two fluid compartments, of which one contains more anionic protein than the other, the distribution of cations over the two compartments is uneven. This is one feature of Donnan equilibrium. The other feature is that an electrical potential difference is established between the two compartments.

Deriving the equation

There is equilibrium in situation A (Figure 5-5). Adding a negatively charged protein accompanied by satellite cations (for electroneutrality) produces situation B, in which Na^+ wants to travel along its concentration gradient (i.e., from compartment 2 to 1) but Cl^-, which has to accompany the Na^+ for electroneutrality, does not want to go, since it is already evenly distributed. The large Na^+ gradient prevails, though, so that one Na^+ ion (accompanied by one Cl^- ion) moves from compartment 2 to 1. This sets up situation C in which there is equilibrium. One way to ascertain whether or not equilibrium indeed exists is to realize that the tendency for Na^+ to continue traveling along its gradient [free energy loss $= RT \cdot \log([Na_2^+]/[Na_1^+])$] is exactly offset by the tendency of Cl^- wanting to travel the other way [free energy loss $= RT \cdot \log([Cl_1^-]/[Cl_2^-])$]. This is so because the ratio of Na^+ concentrations ($9:6 = 1.5$) equals the ratio of Cl^- levels ($6:4 = 1.5$). Thus, the total free-energy change of those ion movements would be zero; that is, equilibrium.

Another way to look at the Donnan equilibrium is from the viewpoint of only the Na^+ ion or the Cl ion (Figure 5-6). At equilibrium, the energy obtained by moving Na^+ from compartment 2 to 1 along its chemical gradient is exactly offset by the energy obtained from moving Na^+ in the opposite direction along the electrical gradient (ΔE). As a result, the

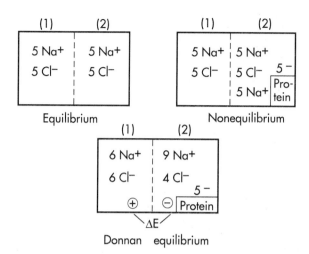

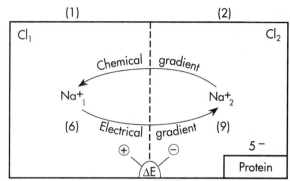

Figure 5-6. Electrochemical gradient.

Figure 5-5. Donnan equilibrium between two compartments is characterized by an uneven mineral distribution balanced by an electrical voltage gradient (ΔE).

net electrochemical gradient is zero, and there is no net Na^+ movement in either direction. Mathematically, that Na^+ equilibrium can be formulated:

$$\text{Electrical energy} = \text{Chemical energy}$$
$$n \cdot e^- \cdot \Delta E = RT \cdot \ln ([Na_2^+]/[Na_1^+])$$
$$\Delta E = \frac{RT}{n \cdot e} \ln ([Na_2^+]/[Na_1^+])$$

For Na^+, at 30° C: $\Delta E = 0.06 \log ([Na_2^+]/[Na_1^+])$

For Cl^-, $\Delta E = 0.06 \log ([Cl_1^-]/[Cl_2^-])$, yielding, of course, the same ΔE as for Na^+. With $\Delta G_{Na} = \Delta G_{Cl}$, the sum $\Delta G_{(Na+Cl)}$ equals zero, which means equilibrium: so there is no more net movement of Na^+ and Cl^- ions.

In summation, the equation for the Donnan potential relates the uneven distribution of ions to the occurrence of a transmembrane potential difference and expresses the equivalence of chemical and electrical energy.

Physical considerations

It is not difficult to translate the above theoretical model into physiological reality where there is a plethora of different fluid compartments separated from one another by semipermeable membranes. These fluid compartments in the body (or within subcellular structures) have grossly different protein concentrations. Hence, there are Donnan equilibria everywhere. Let us briefly pause at some of the important

consequences of Donnan equilibria on physiological systems.

Oncotic pressure is accentuated

Due to the uneven distribution of proteins among neighboring fluid compartments, satellite ions (though diffusible through the semipermeable membrane) are also unevenly distributed. The satellite cations are held in the protein-rich compartment for the purpose of electroneutrality, and the osmotic contribution of these ions adds to the oncotic pressure of the protein. (See Figure 5-5 of Donnan equilibrium: there are 14 particles in compartment 2, compared to only 12 in compartment 1.) The plasma oncotic pressure is approximately 25 mmHg, with 18 mmHg of this caused by dissolved protein and 7 mmHg by cations held in plasma by the negatively charged protein molecules.

Electrical potential difference

Inside the cell, a negative potential exists relative to the outside, which is caused by a higher intracellular concentration of anionic protein. This potential difference is measured by impaling the cell with a microelectrode and reading its potential, relative to the extracellular reference electrode, with a voltmeter. Typical values for ΔE in muscle cells are in the 70 to 90 mV range.

The electrical potential difference is also measured indirectly, by substituting measured values of intracellular and extracellular K^+ and Cl^- in the Donnan equation for ΔE.

Here are examples: With intracellular $[K^+] = 140$ milliequivalents/L and extracellular $[K^+] = 5$ meq/L, we derive the following:

$$\Delta E = 0.06 \log(140/5) = 0.087V \ (= 87 \ mV).$$

Similarly, $[Cl^-]_{out}/[Cl^-]_{in} = 125/9$ which yields this equation:

$$\Delta E = 68 \ mV.$$

Obviously, there exists only one value for ΔE. Therefore, the measured values of K^+ and Cl^- ion distributions indicate that both of those ions are close to Donnan equilibrium, but neither is exactly in equilibrium. In fact, no ion is exactly in equilibrium in living systems, but when the combined distributions of all ions (except Na^+) is considered, their sum is in close accord with the observed ΔE. As discussed below, the Na^+ ion distribution is maintained in a state of nonequilibrium by energy-requiring means.

Importance of K+ homeostasis

Nerve and muscle membrane resting potentials are mainly due to the diffusion of K^+ from a solution of higher K^+ concentration (the cytoplasm), to one of lower concentration (extracellular fluid). Since K^+ is the major permeant cation in the resting state, electrical work is approximately equal in magnitude and opposite in sign to the concentrative work for K^+, and there is only one unknown quantity in the equation, namely ΔE (electrical, or equilibrium potential). Thus ΔE can be approximated from measured intracellular and extracellular concentrations of K^+. Physiologically, this is of enormous importance. Considering that the processes of muscle contraction and conductance of nerve impulses depend on the value of ΔE, these vital processes depend on homeostatic maintenance (buffering) of the ratio $[K^+]_{in}/[K^+]_{out}$. This point is best illustrated by the following examples.

In a muscle cell with a normal resting potential (ΔE) of 80 mV relative to the extracellular fluid, an incoming nerve impulse, signaling the muscle to contract, changes the relative conductance of Na^+ and K^+ in the muscle cell membrane and thereby drops the ΔE below 60 mV, a threshold value at which a positive feedback cascade occurs that leads to contraction. Now the vital role of K^+ in this process can be ascertained by considering the following three cases (Figure 5-7):

- Normal: $[K^+]_{in}/[K^+]_{out} = 140:5$ and thus, according to its Donnan equilibrium, K^+ contributes 87 mV to the overall resting membrane potential. Nerve signals cause ΔE to drop under 60 mV, so contraction occurs: muscular activity is under nervous control.
- Hypokalemia: For instance, $[K^+]_{in}/[K^+]_{out} = 150:3$, K^+ contributes 102 mV to the overall membrane potential. This contribution raises the resting membrane potential to such an extent that even a large nerve impulse cannot drop it below threshold. The muscle is now refractory (insensitive) to nerve signals. Muscle paralysis or at least severe muscle weakness is observed. Respiration may stop due to muscle paralysis. Also, when K^+-wasting diuretics are administered, muscle weakness may be observed unless K^+ is supplied.
- Hyperkalemia: For instance, $[K^+]_{in}/[K^+]_{out} = 90:9$ to which belongs a Donnan potential of 60 mV. This fact alone, without nervous input, causes the resting membrane potential to move toward the threshold value. This results in hyperexcitability and uncontrolled muscular contractions. Applied to the heart muscle, one observes arrhythmia followed by cardiac arrest. Rapid K^+ injection quickly kills an animal.

K^+ homeostasis. The above examples bring out the vital need for homeostatic control of the $[K^+]_{in}/[K^+]_{out}$ ratio. The $[K^+]_{out}$ is especially crucial: its value is so small (about 4 meq/L) that a tiny variation in it (e.g., 1 meq/L) immediately changes the ratio tremendously (by 25%). Conversely, a 1 meq/L rise in the $[Na^+]_{out}$ (about 140 meq/L) changes the $[Na^+]_{in}/[Na^+]_{out}$ ratio nominally. Thus, it is no wonder that much of the physiological control machinery is made to bear upon the plasma K^+ level. Nervous sensors (receptors) activate several endocrine systems in brain, adrenals, and kidneys, and under those influences, kidney function is directed toward either conserving or voiding K^+ ions.

Importance of H+ homeostasis

The text has already examined the need for pH homeostasis with respect to the regulation of enzyme activities in the body. It will now cover the effect of pH on Donnan equilibria and the physiological consequences thereof.

During acidosis, cells take up hydrogen ions; these ions combine with dissociated carboxyl groups on proteins, and thus, intracellular proteins lose some of their negative charge. As these proteins get closer to their isoelectric pH, intracellular cations are no longer needed for electroneutrality and, therefore, leave

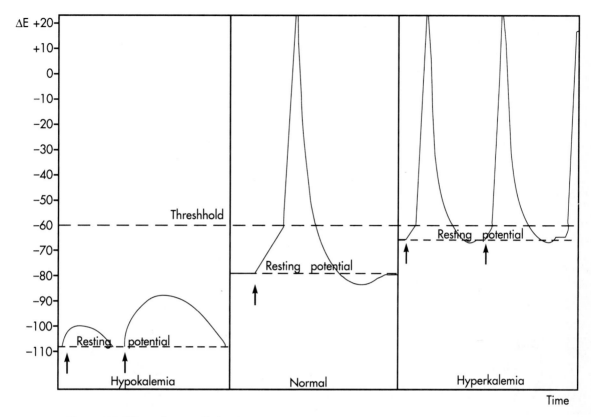

Figure 5-7. Effect of serum K^+ levels on muscle contraction. In the case of hyperkalemia, graded responses to nerve impulses are observed, but the muscle remains unexcitable. During hypokalemia, most nerve impulses give rise to action potentials so that hyperexcitability ensues. Arrows indicate time of nerve impulse.

cells. The result may be hyperkalemia with its associated dangers.

With lowered pH comes decreased charge on proteins and, thus, diminished Donnan effects. The distribution of mineral ions between the interior and exterior of the cell is altered. Oncotic pressures are affected because of lower satellite cation concentrations. Electrical potential differences over cell membranes are diminished, and this, in turn, affects transport processes, muscular contraction, and excitability by nervous stimulation.

ACTIVE TRANSPORT
Definition

Active transport is transport against an electrochemical gradient. Energy for active transport comes from the hydrolysis of ATP by ATP-ases. Most membranes are rich in ATP-ase activities. It is important to note

the following: to determine whether a transport process is active or passive, the chemical (concentration) gradient must be considered, as must the electrical gradient for charged compounds.

The Donnan equation is used to gauge whether a transport process is active or not. For instance: for the K^+ distribution, a ratio of 140:5 was found, from which a ΔE value of 87 mV was derived. If a ΔE of 70 mV were now measured, then it could be concluded that lowering the calculated ΔE should be a spontaneous (passive) process; such a lowering would occur if K^+ left the cell, and thus, movement of K^+ out of the cell would, in this case, be passive; hence, cellular K^+ uptake is active.

The Na^+ ion

The Na^+ concentration is high in plasma (ca. 140 meq/L) and low in cells (ca. 10 meq/L). This is a nonequilibrium situation; both chemical and electrical gradients are pointing toward the cell interior. Hence, cells are constantly being assaulted by Na^+ ions from outside; and cells have to bail out that Na^+ non-stop. The bailing out is an active process, requiring a great deal of energy (ca. 25% of the human body's caloric requirement at rest is spent on the Na^+ pump). The hardware of the sodium pump is a Mg^{++}-activated ATP-ase enzyme, located in the plasma membrane of nearly all cells, which releases Na^+ to the outside and brings K^+ inside the cell.

Active transport of organic compounds

If the body were to rely on passive transport to absorb glucose from the gut, it would lose a large amount of it because of incomplete absorption against a glucose gradient of 100 mg/dl in the bloodstream. Fortunately, in most animal species, intestinal glucose absorption is an active process, and thus, is independent of glucose levels in the gut and blood.

The large Na^+ gradient, directed toward the cell interior, functions as the driving force behind active transport of glucose across the cell membrane of gut mucosa and for amino acid transport in the gut, liver, kidney, and other tissue cells.

A model for active glucose absorption from the gut (Figure 5-8) shows symport (or coupled transport) of

glucose and Na^+ into the mucosa followed by antiport exchange of Na^+ for K^+. Crippling ATP production in mucosal cells, for instance, by blocking oxidative phosphorylation, abolishes Na^+-coupled active absorption of glucose.

Facilitated transport

Thus far, active transport (energy-requiring) and passive transport (diffusion downhill along an electrochemical gradient) have been considered. A third form of transport must be distinguished; namely, facilitated transport. In this case, a compound travels downhill along its electrochemical gradient, but in doing so, it is assisted by a carrier that shuttles the compound across a membrane. For instance: the transport of glucose across plasma membranes of adipose and muscle cells is facilitated by a specific glucose transporter. The major feature that distinguishes active transport and facilitated diffusion from simple diffusion is that both active transport and facilitated diffusion are saturable processes (since they are carrier mediated).

STUDY QUESTIONS

1. How are activation-energy barriers overcome in a cell?

2. The reason why our glycogen stores can exist has to do with:
   a. Need for activation energy.
   b. Dormancy of key enzyme.
   c. Constant investment of energy ("pushing").
   d. All of the above.

3. Exemplify an entropy-driven process.

4. a. Name a microanatomical feature of parenchymal liver cells that aids in diffusional uptake of metabolites from the blood-stream.
   b. List two adaptations whereby the gut mucosa increases diffusion of nutrients.

5. What is the effect of a mild hypotonicity of plasma on the hematocrit?

6. a. What is the concentration of "physiologic" saline?
   b. Roughly, what is the PCV in dogs?
   c. When oxalate-treated blood is centrifuged and the clear supernatant is collected, is the biproduct serum or plasma?

7. a. List the term for osmotic pressure caused by proteins.
   b. About what percentage of total osmotic pressure is due to proteins?

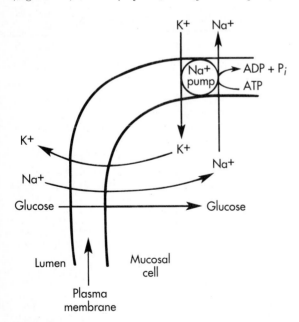

Figure 5-8. Role of the Na^+ pump in glucose uptake by the intestinal mucosa.

8. *a.* List the main determinant (component) of net-filtration pressure that moves fluid out of arteries.

   b. List the main determinant (component) of net-absorption pressure that moves fluid back into the veins.

9. Name the system that can drain proteins from the interstitial spaces between cells.

10. *a.* Which of the following is most important in establishing the total volume of body water: (A) Net filtration pressure; (B) Net absorption pressure; (C) Plasma + tissue minerals; (D) Plasma + tissue proteins?

   b. Though the above considerations determine the total volume of body fluid, what specifically determines the distribution of fluid between different compartments?

11. *a.* List, by its proper medical term, the pathologic effect of lowered oncotic pressure upon body fluid distribution.

   b. List a cause of lowered oncotic pressure.

   c. Why would a diet deficient in lysine cause this condition?

12. The osmoreceptor/ADH system controls: (A) total osmotic pressure; or (B) oncotic pressure.

13. In response to dehydration.

   a. What does ADH instruct the kidneys to do?

   b. What is the whole-body response leading to increased water intake?

   c. What effect has dehydration on the hematocrit?

   d. What effect has dehydration on the oncotic pressure of serum?

14. In fluid therapy of a critically low plasma volume:

   a. Which compound could be infused for vascular fluid retention?

   b. List an ion that should be infused with utmost care to avoid possibly lethal effects.

15. List a waste product that is dialyzed out in an artificial kidney.

16. When an ion is in Donnan equilibrium, its chemical gradient is balanced by its _____ gradient. (Fill in the blank).

17. What causes the transmembrane (Donnan) potential inside the tissue cell to be negative relative to the outside?

18. In a skeletal muscle cell, would the Cl^- level inside the cell have to be higher than, equal to, or lower than the Cl^- level outside the cell (if that ion were in Donnan equilibrium)?

19. *a.* Consider a cell, its predominant cation, and its enviornment, and list the two manifestations of Donnan equilibrium.

   b. Define "active transport" of that cation in relation to those Donnan effects.

20. In a dog, fasting has established a metabolic acidosis because of high levels of ketoacids in the bloodstream. One immediate line of defense against acid-base balance upset is to remove H^+ from the bloodstream in exchange for the chief intracellular cation.

   a. Explain hyperkalemia during acidosis.

   b. List the medical term for the condition when the pH of plasma in a dog is 7.1.

   c. As the body compensates for this condition, these responses are noted: (A) Lungs: _____; (B) Liver: _____; (C) Kidneys: _____; (D) K^+ level in plasma _____. (Complete the responses.)

   d. What effect does this high K^+ level have on the Donnan electrical potential difference between a muscle cell's interior and the surrounding interstitial fluid?

   e. Would this change in Donnan potential bring the muscle closer to or farther away, relative to the point of spontaneous uncontrolled contraction?

   f. Explain cardiac arrest after rapidly injecting a high dose of K^+ intravenously.

21. Why would a drop in pH decrease the oncotic effect of a typical serum protein?

22. A sizeable part of the daily caloric requirement of humans is spent on bailing a certain mineral out of the cells' interiors by a device called what?

23. As cyanide inhibits glucose transport into the gut cells, what kind of transport is indicated?

6 Cell-surface phenomena

FUNCTIONS, COMPOSITION, AND TURNOVER OF CELL MEMBRANES

Classifications

Membranes are classified according to location. Plasma membranes envelop cells. Subcellular membranes are found in the endoplasmic reticulum and around lysosomes, peroxisomes, nuclei, mitochondria, etc. Then there are very specialized membranes, for instance those that form the myelin sheath around nerve axons, and those surrounding milk fat droplets.

Functions of membranes in general

- Structural functions include compartmentalization on a macro- and micro-scale within the body, and protection and shaping of the enclosed entities.
- Signaling to and from environments via receptors on plasma membranes that face the outside of the cell, and the cytoskeleton attached to the cytoplasmic membrane face.
- Aggregation of cells via cell adhesion molecules that face the outsides of plasma membranes.
- Metabolic functions of membranes include (i) guarding import of nutrients and export of wastes, and (ii) enzyme functions; for example, glycosyl transferases, which allow the Golgi apparatus to complete the glycoside chains of glycoproteins, and adenylate cyclase and phospholipases, by which plasma membranes generate second messengers in response to hormone attachment to receptors on the membrane.

- Surface enlargement of cells by microvilli that protrude outward from the plasma membrane and facilitate entry of compounds into a cell.
- Locomotion of isolated cells via cilia and flagellae attached to the plasma membrane, or by chemotaxis, when a cell moves toward a high concentration of a compound to which a plasma membrane receptor of that cell is attracted.

Composition of membranes
Lipids in membranes

In first approximation, a membrane consists of a lipid bilayer. Mostly amphoteric, these lipids align with their apolar fatty acid tails interacting, forming an oily bilayer in the membrane interior, and their polar heads (anionic phosphate and cationic choline ions) directing outward (Figure 6-1, A). The fluid mosaic model of membranes (Figure 6-1, B) embodies current concepts of membrane structure. Proteins overlay, and intrude into, the lipid bilayer. Some proteins, called integral proteins, span the entire width of the membrane; they are involved in signaling to and from the environment. To signal properly, those proteins must be able to move freely in the plane of the membrane, which requires that the lipid bilayer be fluid (oily).

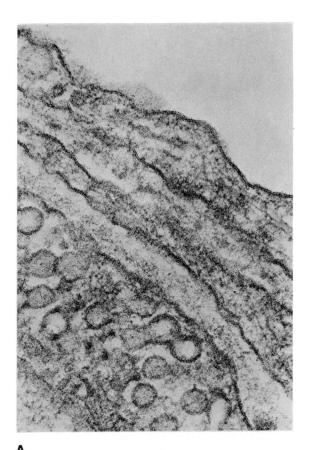

Figure 6-1. A, Sheep type I epithelium. Electron photomicrograph of plasma membrane. Cross section through a membrane appears as a 'railroad track' that sandwiches a more translucent lipid bilayer. **B,** Diagram of the fluid mosaic plasma membrane model shows phospholipid bilayer in which cholesterol and various kinds of protein molecules are embedded. Fluidity of lipid layer is suggested by random configuration of phospholipid tails in interior of membrane; near the polar heads, cholesterol causes rigidity of those tails. Chains of sugars are attached to proteins and lipids facing exterior of cell. *A, Courtesy Dr. Rick A. Rogers, Harvard School of Public Health. B, Reproduced with permission from Bretscher MS: The molecules of the cell membrane, Sci Am 253(4):100-109, 1985.*

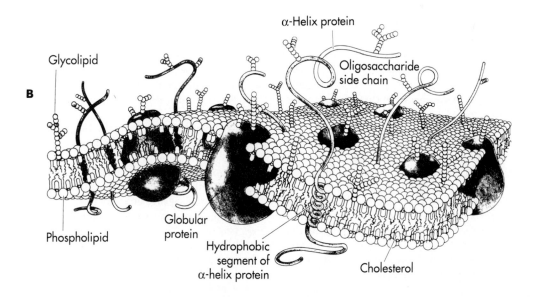

Fluidity of membrane lipids is brought about by the content of polyunsaturated fatty acids (linoleic, linolenic, arachidonic, docosahexaenoic, and eicosapentaenoic acid) in various membrane phospholipids and glycolipids (Figures 6-2 and 6-3). Some polyunsaturated fatty acids are nutritionally essential; that is, their functions are of vital importance, but the body cannot synthesize them, and hence they must be included in the diet. They are easily oxidized and then hardened. Fluidity of the membrane is then lost; the cell can no longer properly respond to its environment and dies. Herein lies one of the causes of cell aging. Vitamins C (water-soluble) and E (lipid-soluble), by being even more readily oxidized, protect polyunsaturated fatty acids. Fluidity is further conserved by constant rejuvenation (turnover) of cell membranes.

Membrane lipids include these classes (see Figure 6-3): phosphatidylcholine, phosphatidylserine, phosphatidylethanolamine, and phosphatidylinositol; cardiolipin (diphosphatidylglycerol); plasmalogens; and glycolipids derived from ceramide, including sphingomyelins, sulfatides, cerebrosides, and gangliosides. Cholesterol occurs in all mammalian membranes in roughly the same concentration as do phospholipids. Cholesterol orients itself with its hydroxyl group in the vicinity of the polar heads of phospholipids; its rigid steroid ring configuration then lends stability and strength to the membrane, while its apolar tail does not interfere with fluidity of the fatty acid tails on phospholipids.

A common denominator in the unending variety of membrane lipids is the fact that their three-dimensional structures are very similar (see Figure 6-3), and thus, in a membrane lipid the polar head is interchangeable with other polar heads; the apolar lipid tails may be interchanged with different apolar moieties. This allows membrane lipids to orient themselves with their apolar moieties in the interior of the membrane and their polar groups directed outwardly.

Proteins in membranes

Proteins overlay and traverse the lipid bilayer. So closely are they interwoven with the lipid matrix that it takes detergents to dissolve membrane proteins. Integral proteins (Figure 6-4) possess characteristic polarity: chains of glycosides are attached to asparagine, threonine, and serine residues located on the part of the protein that sticks out of the cell, and a sequence of some twenty apolar amino acids in the protein's primary structure marks the region where the protein is in contact with the lipid matrix of the membrane. Some proteins have several sequences of apolar amino acids: they traverse the lipid bilayer more than once; twelve times, for example, in the case of the glucose transporter of fat cells. Practically all integral membrane proteins are glycoproteins (Figures 6-4 and 6-5). Their functional components, involved with two-way signaling between cell and environment, include enzymes, receptors, and immunoproteins.

Carbohydrates in membranes

Carbohydrates occur in membranes not only in association with proteins, but also in the form of glycolipids, such as gangliosides (see Figure 6-3). An important function of glycolipids is that they serve as receptors for various hormones. As part of the constant turnover of membranes, glycolipids are broken down in lysosomes. The importance of glycolipids and their lysosomal digestion is seen in brain and other nervous tissues. Myelin, a sheath of isolation material that surrounds nerve axons, is particularly rich in lipids. A large number of lipidoses are known in which inborn lysosomal enzyme deficiencies result in abnormal brain development; Tay-Sachs disease is one such condition (Table 6-1).

Membranes are asymmetric

The sugar chains of glycoproteins and glycolipids face only the outside. Also, the relative concentrations of the different lipid classes in the two membrane faces varies greatly and consistently; no "flip-flop" of these membrane lipids occurs.

Differentiation of membranes, responding to the specific needs of various cells, can take different forms:
- Varying the protein/lipid ratio in membrane composition; most membranes contain about equal amounts of proteins and lipids, but extremes of about 80% lipids (myelin) or about 80% protein (inner membrane of mitochondria) are known;
- Peripheral proteins attached to the membrane; for example, immunoglobulins and cell adhesion molecules;
- Different proteins inserted into the membrane; for example, the electron transfer chain in the mitochondrial inner membrane;
- Large pores in the nuclear envelope to allow passage of macromolecular nucleic acid complexes;
- The many superimposed layers of membrane that form the structure of myelin;
- Membrane protrusions, such as flagellae for cell

Text continued on p. 100.

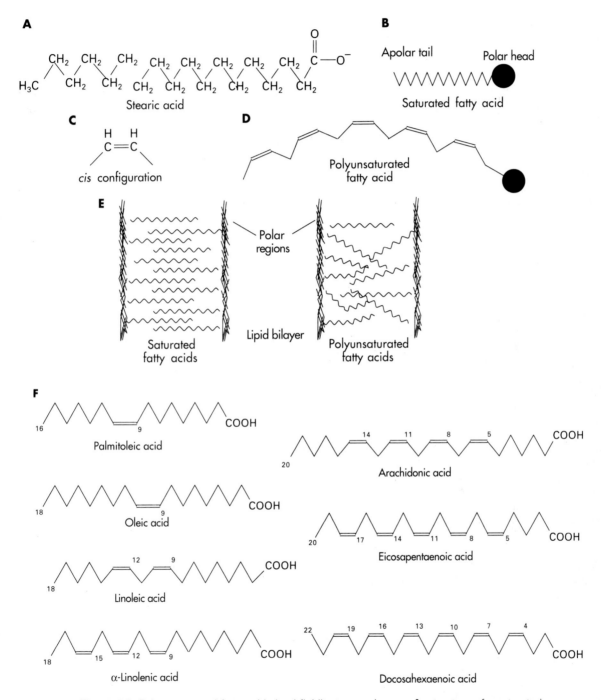

Figure 6-2. Polyunsaturated fatty acids lend fluidity to membranes. **A,** structure of a saturated fatty acid. **B,** Diagram of structure. *Cis*-orientation of carbon chains at a double bond. **C,** brings about a crescent shape of the carbon chains of polyunsaturated fatty acids. **D,** In lipid interior of a membrane, polyunsaturated fatty acids lend fluidity to lipid bilayer as they do not pack as densely as saturated fatty acids. Various saturated **E,** and unsaturated, **F,** fatty acids interchange on membrane lipid molecules.

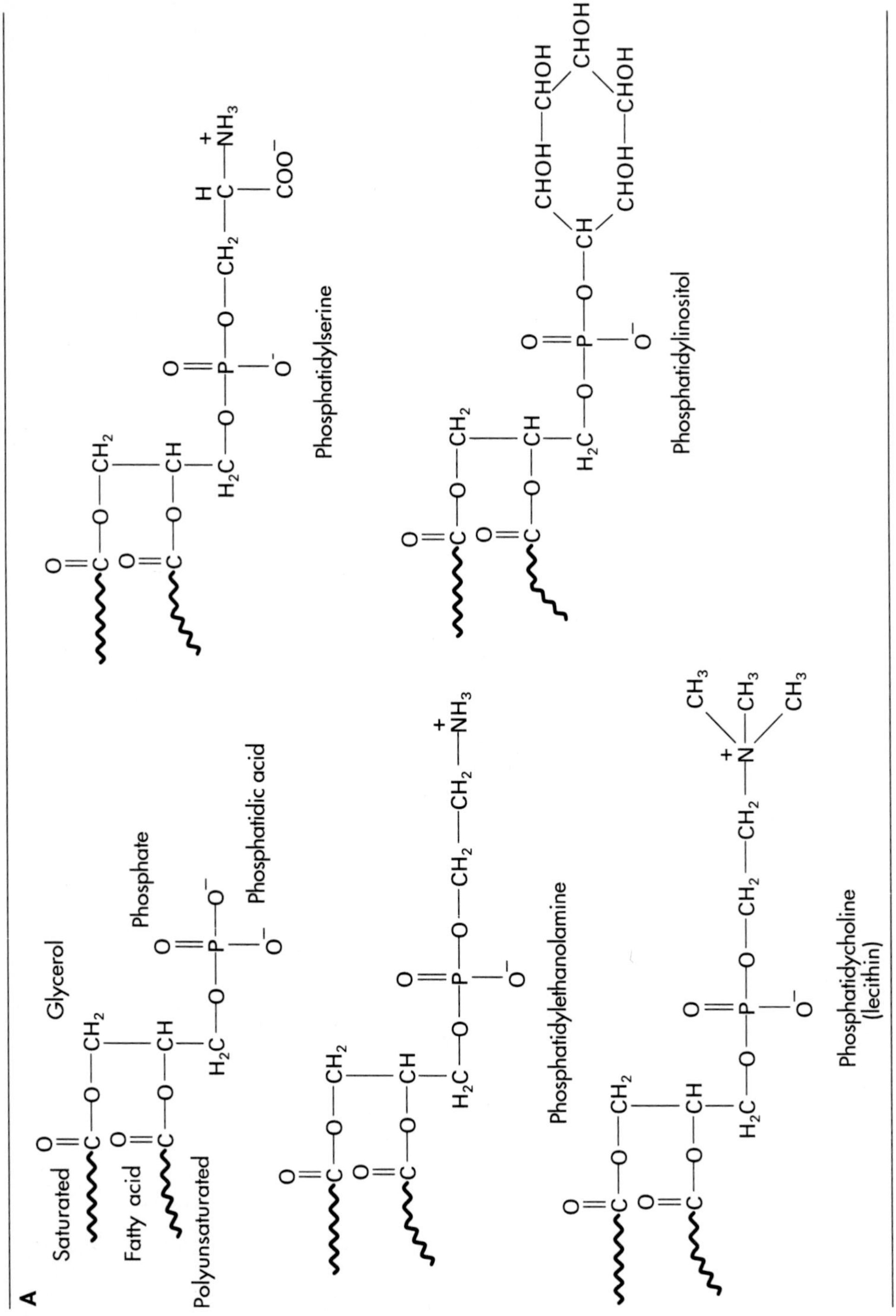
A
Saturated
Fatty acid
Polyunsaturated
Glycerol
Phosphate
Phosphatidic acid
Phosphatidylethanolamine
Phosphatidycholine
(lecithin)
Phosphatidylserine
Phosphatidylinositol

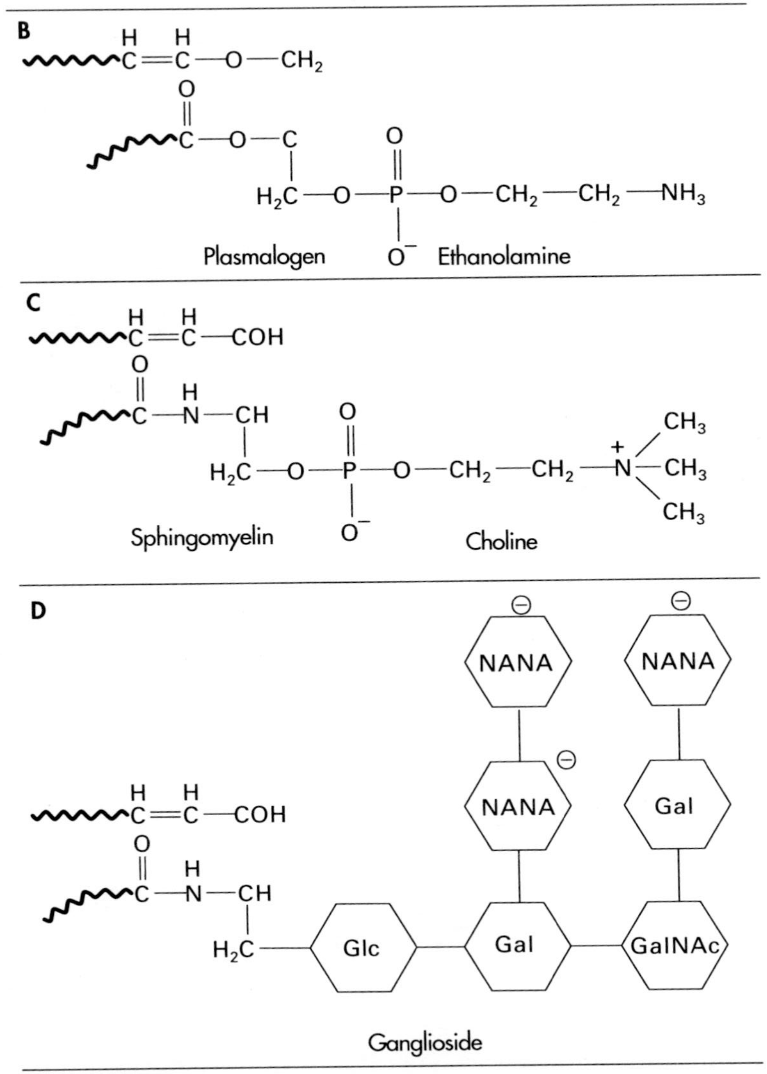

Figure 6-3. Similarity in three-dimensional structure of membrane lipids

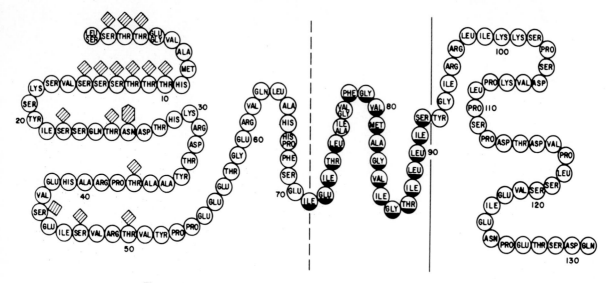

Figure 6-4. Amino acid sequence of an integral membrane protein

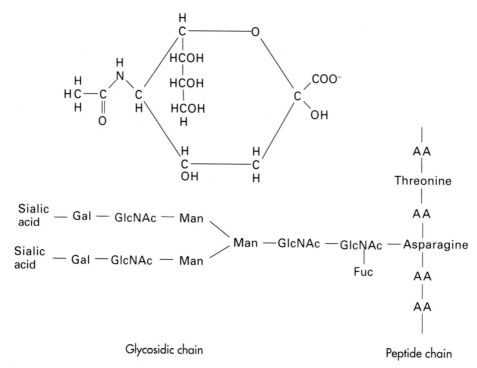

Glycosidic chain

Peptide chain

Figure 6-5. Membrane glycoproteins. A typical sequence of oligosaccharides of an integral membrane protein is shown. Note the chain is attached to the amide group of an asparagine residue provided the asparagine is part of a sequence consisting of asparagine—any amino acid—threonine. Various glycoproteins differ in their proportions of carbohydrates relative to protein, number of antennae on each glycosidic chain, and sugar and aminosugar moieties. In addition, sugars may be attached to the alcohol groups of serine and threonine (Figure 6-4). *AA,* Any amino acid; *Gal,* galactase; *GlcNac, N*-acetylglucosamine; *Man,* mannose; *Fuc,* fucose.

Table 6-1 Sphingolidipidoses in humans

Disease	Enzyme deficiency	Lipid accumulating : Site of deficient enzymatic reaction	Clinical symptoms
Fucosidosis	α-Fucosidase	Cer–Glc–Gal–GalNAc–Gal $\div$ Fuc H-Isoantigen	Cerebral degeneration, muscle spasticity, thick skin.
Generalized gangliosidosis	G_{M1}-β-galactosidase	Cer–Glc–Gal(NeuAc)–GalNAc $\div$ Gal G_{M1} Ganglioside	Mental retardation, liver enlargement, skeletal deformation.
Tay-Sachs disease	Hexosaminidase A	Cer–Glc–Gal(NeuAc) $\div$ GalNAc G_{M2} Ganglioside	Mental retardation, blindness, muscular weakness.
Tay-Sachs variant or Sandhoff's disease	Hexosaminidase A and B	Cer–Glc–Gal–Gal $\div$ GalNAc Globoside plus G_{M2} ganglioside	Same as Tay-Sachs but progressing more rapidly.
Fabry's disease	α-Galactosidase	Cer–Glc–Gal $\div$ Gal Globotriaosylceramide	Skin rash, kidney failure (full symptoms only in males; X-linked recessive).
Ceramide lactoside lipidosis	Ceramide lactosidase (β-galactosidase)	Cer–Glc $\div$ Ceramide lactoside	Progressing brain damage, liver and spleen enlargement.
Metachromatic leukodystrophy	Arylsulfatase A	Cer–Gal $\div$ OSO_3 3-Sulfogalactosylceramide	Mental retardation and psychologic disturbances in adults; demyelination.
Krabbe's disease	β-Galactosidase	Cer $\div$ Gal Galactosylceramide	Mental retardation; myelin almost absent.
Gaucher's disease	β-Glucosidase	Cer $\div$ Glc Glucosylceramide	Enlarged liver and spleen, erosion of long bones, mental retardation in infants.
Niemann-Pick disease	Sphingomyelinase	Cer $\div$ P-choline Sphingomyelin	Enlarged liver and spleen, mental retardation; fatal in early life.
Farber's disease	Ceramidase	Acyl $\div$ Sphingosine Ceramide	Hoarseness, dermatitis, skeletal deformation, mental retardation; fatal in early life.

NeuAc, N-acetylneuraminic acid; Cer, ceramide; Glc, glucose; Gal, galactose; Fuc, fucose.
(From: Brady RO: Sphingolipidoses, Annu Rev Biochem 47:687, 1978)

movement or microvilli, and surface enlargement for better diffusion of compounds into cells.

Cytoskeleton

The cytoplasm between subcellular organelles contains a complex structure (Figure 6-6) consisting of microtubules, intermediate filaments, and microfilaments. This complex, named the **cytoskeleton,** has many important functions, including:

- Allowing the cell interior to respond to outside influences by being attached to the plasma membrane;
- Supporting and shaping the cell interior;
- Attachment of enzyme sequences of metabolic pathways; because of this arrangement, the product of an enzyme reaction is "handed over" to serve as a substrate for the neighboring enzyme; consequently the substrate concentration over the length of the metabolic pathway is high, and the potential rates of enzyme reactions are fast;
- Transport of compounds (e.g., axonal transport in nerve cells) and of cell organelles (mitochondria, lysosomes) along microtubules in both directions causing a constant, stormish commotion throughout the cell interior;
- Directing movement of endocytic vesicles in processes of endocytosis and exocytosis;
- Directing chromosome movement during cell division when microtubules form mitotic spindles;
- Directing not only movements within cells, but also the motility of certain cells themselves (e.g., fibroblasts).

Microfilaments (Figure 6-7, A), about 6 nm in diameter, consist of two intertwined monofilaments of actin, and are mainly involved in cell contractility, often in bundles called **stress fibers.** Microfilaments are often seen forming a mesh underneath the plasma membrane and are connected to integral membrane proteins. Intermediate filaments, 7 to 10 nm in diameter, differ in protein composition and in function; they contribute to cell shaping. Microtubules (Figure 6-7, B), 25 nm in diameter, are a complex of protofilaments each consisting of heterodimers of α-tubulin and β-tubulin; their associated proteins function in intracellular transport and in cell morphology. Microtubules span the distance between perinuclear space and the plasma membrane as a continuous structure. Electron microscopic evidence confirms the existence of a microtrabecular lattice of interconnecting fibers, less than 6 nm in diameter, lending even more structure to the cytoplasm in spaces left by the microtubules and microfilaments.

For the cytoskeleton's function to direct movement, either within cells or of cells themselves, contractile forces are generated by myosin sliding over actin filaments. The protein calmodulin, in the presence of Ca^{++}, holds the sliding filament together, and energy for contraction is derived from ATP under the influence of myosin's ATP-ase activity (cf., muscle contraction; calmodulin is closely related to troponin C in both structure and function).

Several alkaloids impair structural polymerization of tubulin and thus microtubule assembly; e.g., colchicine (used to treat gouty arthritis) and the anticancer agent vinblastine. The polypeptide cytochalasins depolymerize microfilaments. These agents are

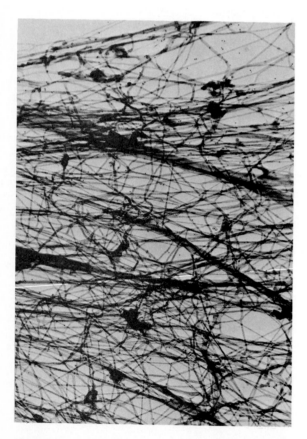

Figure 6-6. Cytoskeleton. Transmission electron photomicrograph of bovine alveolar macrophage cytoskeleton left behind after membranous organelles and the microtrabecular lattice were extracted with a detergent. *Courtesy Dr. Rick A. Rogers, Harvard School of Public Health.*

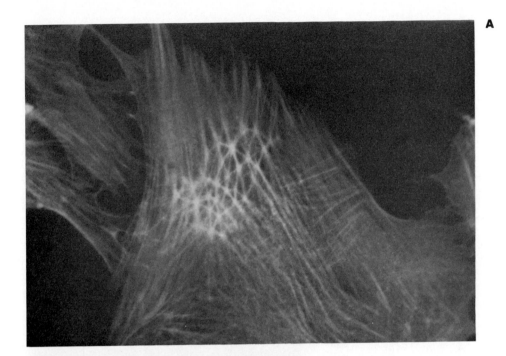

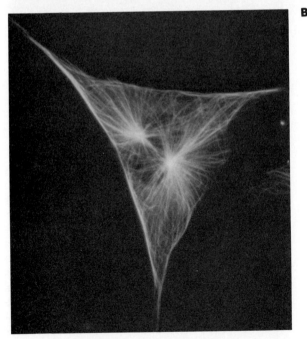

Figure 6-7. Cytoskeleton visualized microscopically after staining with fluorescent monoclonal antibodies against specific proteins. **A,** Microfilaments in a chicken embryo glial cell stained for actin. **B,** Microtubules in a dividing fibroblast from a chicken heart ventricle stained for α-tubulin. *A, Courtesy Dr. Brian S. Spooner, Kansas State University. B, Courtesy Dr. Abigail H. Conrad, Kansas State University.*

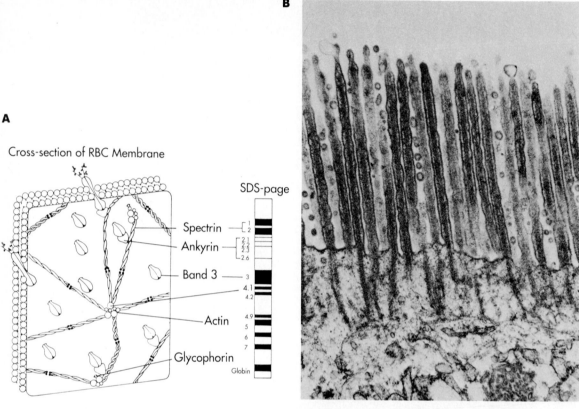

Figure 6-8. Association of cytoskeleton to plasma membrane. **A,** On inner surface of the membrane of a human erythrocyte, a framework of actin and spectrin is associated via ankyrin to integral membrane protein of band III, giving strength and flexibility to the cell. **B,** Microfilaments form scaffolding that stiffens microvilli on surface of sheep intestinal epithelial cell. Cytoskeleton within microvilli is rooted in cytoskeleton of enterocyte. **A,** *Courtesy Dr. Joseph E. Smith, Kansas State University.* **B,** *Courtesy Dr. Rick A. Rogers, Harvard School of Public Health.*

used in research to study involvement of components of the cytoskeleton in various cell functions; for example, cytochalasin cripples endocytosis.

The cytoskeleton is attached to the plasma membrane by specific (and different) proteins in different cells (Figure 6-8). These proteins have been characterized for erythrocytes, intestinal mucosal cells, fibroblasts, and other cells. This attachment is a key link in a two-way communication with the environment.

Biosynthesis and turnover of membranes

Membranes are not synthesized in their mature forms. Rather, the various membrane components are all replaced at their own rates. Thus, membranes rejuvenate, and they do so at an astounding pace; for

instance, some membrane receptor proteins turnover in a matter of minutes.

Constantly, portions of plasma membranes are internalized, digested, and replaced. Phospholipid bilayers are formed on the cytoplasmic surface of the smooth endoplasmic reticulum where they form vesicles that migrate toward the Golgi apparatus. Membrane proteins are synthesized on ribosomes and pushed into the lumen of the rough endoplasmic reticulum, where the leader sequence is clipped and carbohydrate chains are added (Figure 6-9).

A large mannose-rich complex of carbohydrates, bound to the apolar compound dolichol-pyrophosphate, is attached to serine, threonine, or asparagine residues of the protein, the dolichol vehicle comes off, and then the sugar chains are modified by the

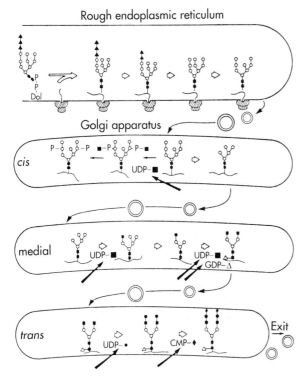

Figure 6-9. Glycosylation of proteins. An oligosaccharide structure, attached to dolichol *(Dol)* is added to newly synthesized protein in the rough endoplasmic reticulum. Subsequent processing in RER and Golgi apparatus is diagrammed. Note the formation of mannose-rich glycoproteins, in addition to the complex ones, in Golgi. ■, *N*-Acetylglucosamine; *O*, mannose; ▲, glucose; △, fucose; ●, galactose; ◆, sialic acid. *Modified and reproduced with permission from Kornfeld R and Kornfeld S: Assembly of asparagine-linked oligosaccharides, Annu Rev Biochem 54:631-664, 1985.*

removal of glucose and mannose and the additions of N-acetyl-glucosamine and N-acetylgalactosamine, galactose, fucose, and sialic acid molecules. Those modifications are started in the endoplasmic reticulum and completed in the Golgi apparatus. The final glycoproteins are mostly characterized by being either rich in branched chains of mannose molecules or by having antennae made up of characteristic sequences of sugars attached to mannose (see Figure 6-4). Sialic acid (also called neuraminic acid), when present, always occupies a terminal position in a sugar chain; it provides anionic charges to the glycoprotein; its significance in glycoprotein turnover is discussed below.

In the distal saccules of the Golgi apparatus, newly formed glycoproteins are sorted, packaged in buds that

are bound by phospholipid bilayers, and modified so as to target them toward their final destination (Figure 6-10). For example, phosphorylation of a glycoprotein's mannose residues targets those enzyme proteins toward lysosomes, since the membrane of prelysosomal organelles contains a receptor (lectin) that is specific for glycoproteins containing mannose 6-phosphate. Other buds emanating from the Golgi apparatus traverse the cell, fuse with the plasma membrane, and then secrete their proteins. For insertion into plasma membranes, the glycoproteins in the Golgi apparatus are embedded in newly synthesized phospholipid bilayer vesicles in such a way that integral proteins, traversing the bilayer, have their sugar chains in the vesicle's interior. Fusion then occurs between lipid bilayers of the vesicle and the membrane, whereby the vesicle opens up (so that the sugar chains of integral proteins face toward the outside of the membrane).

Aside from the constant renewal of membrane lipids by endogenous regeneration, lipid exchange with the environment can modify the lipid composition of membranes (e.g., cholesterol exchange in both directions).

TRANSPORT ACROSS CELL MEMBRANES
Fat-soluble compounds

There is an excellent correlation between the permeability of a compound across biological membranes and that compound's solubility in oil. This stands to reason, since the compound has to traverse the lipid bilayer of the membrane. Lipids and other apolar compounds, and gases such as oxygen, nitrogen, carbon dioxide, and carbon monoxide easily diffuse down their concentration gradients across membranes. Anesthetics often have apolar structures (e.g., halothane, chloroform, ether).

Water-soluble compounds

Because of polar, often ionized, groups that are hydrated, a compound gains water-solubility and loses its ability to permeate biological membranes by simple diffusion. For this reason, drugs that are supposed to work intracellularly have their charged groups shielded; for example, methyl esters are formed from ionizable carboxyl groups. Conversely, the contours of cells in a tissue can be seen under a microscope by perfusing that tissue with a solution of a highly polar, and thus impermeable, fluorescent membrane marker. When a liver cell converts incoming dietary glucose to glucose 6-phosphate, it adds a bulky, polar phos-

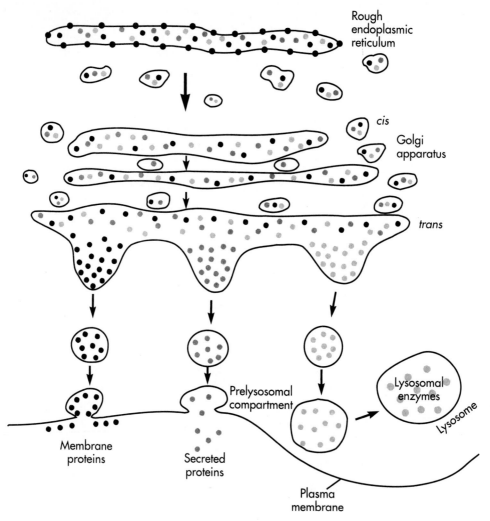

Figure 6-10. Golgi targets proteins to their final destination. Different kinds of glycoproteins are released from the rough endoplasmic reticulum in vesicles that enter the Golgi apparatus, where they are further processed, sorted, and targeted for incorporation into plasma membranes, export in the form of secretory granules, or entry into the prelysosomal compartment.

phate group to the sugar so it can no longer diffuse out of the cell.

Diffusion through ion pores

Plasma membranes contain water-filled channels through which water and hydrated inorganic ions can diffuse. These polar channels across the hydrophobic lipid bilayer are formed by adjacent peptide chains of integral membrane proteins. There are specific channels for Na^+, K^+, Ca^{++}, and Cl^-; the cation pores are lined with negative charges (to repel anions), and the anion channels repel cations by positive charges. Entry of ions through these channels causes transient changes in transmembrane potential. This leads to (i) alternating opening and closing of gates for specific ions, and thus, pulsating ion movements; and (ii) transport of one ion into a cell, affecting the exchange of other ions via their pores; for instance, because of less Na^+ channel blocking, low extracellular calcium levels allow increased Na^+ diffusion into cells, resulting in numbness and cramping in muscles (hypocalcemic tetany).

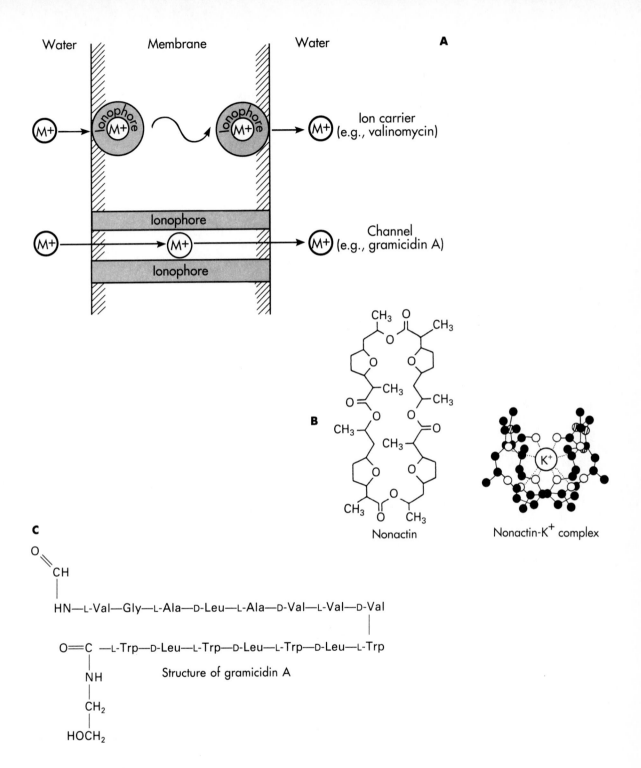

Figure 6-11. A, Action of ionophores. **B,** Ionophore nonactin and its complex with K$^+$. **C,** Gramicidin A. ***A,*** *Reproduced with permission from Ovchinnikov YA: Physico-chemical basis of ion transport through biological membranes: ionophores and ion channels, Eur J Biochem 94:321-336, 1979.* ***B,*** *Reproduced with permission from Finean JB, Coleman R, and Michell RH: Membranes and their cellular functions, 1974, Wiley.*

Because of their small diameter, the polar transmembrane gates only allow passage of inorganic ions and small compounds such as water or urea. However, certain bacterial toxins (e.g., diphtheria) produce large holes in cell membranes, allowing passage of macromolecules.

Ionophores are microbially produced compounds that promote shuttling of ions across cell membranes in one of the following two ways: (i) either they form a basket that envelops the inorganic ion with an inwardly directed polar side and an apolar outer face that allows passage across the membrane's lipid bilayer (e.g., the K^+ ionophores nonactin and valinomycin, and the Ca^{++} ionophore A23187 [Figure 6-11, **A, B**]); or (ii) they form ion channels across the membrane (e.g., gramicidines, a family of decapeptides, and the glycolipid nystatin [Figure 6-11, **C**]). Because of these actions, ionophores are used in medicine as antibiotics and antifungal agents, and in cell research.

The picture of ion transport across cell membranes will be completed later when considering alternative modes of transport. Thusfar, this text has only discussed passive diffusion of ions, for which no energy input is needed; but, in addition, active (energy-requiring) ion exchanges going against electrical and concentration gradients exist (e.g., the Na^+ pump), and so do specific carrier-mediated metal ion transports, such as the routing of dietary iron from the gut via blood to cells, involving special protein carriers and membrane receptors.

Transport of large protein molecules
Endocytosis

There are essentially three forms of endocytosis by which cells internalize large complexes (Figure 6-12).

- Phagocytosis (literally "cell eating"): the plasma membrane extends around and engulfs a foreign body. By this mechanism, particulate matter (e.g., bacteria) is removed from the bloodstream by cells of the reticuloendothelial (mononuclear phagocyte) system.
- Pinocytosis (literally "cell drinking"): the plasma membrane invaginates and then encloses a "gulp" of environmental fluid with all of the compounds that are in it. This occurs in practically all cells.
- Receptor-mediated endocytosis: a compound binds to a specific receptor on the plasma membrane; subsequent enfolding of the membrane brings in the complex of ligand and receptor. This process, in contrast to pinocytosis, allows a cell to discriminate what it ingests. The discussion of endocytosis focuses on the receptor-mediated form.

In the process of receptor-mediated endocytosis, receptors on cell membranes bind to ligands. A ligand (e.g., a hormone or an antibody against a membrane protein) may be multivalent, and thus more than one receptor may move in the plane of the membrane toward the ligand and bind, causing the receptor-ligand complexes to aggregate (Figure 6-13) into patches, which, in turn, are moved toward the tail-

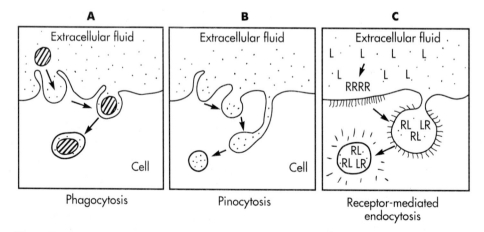

Figure 6-12. Different kinds of endocytosis. **A,** Phagocytosis of a solid particle. **B,** Pinocytosis of extracellular fluid. **C,** Receptor- *(R-)* mediated endocytosis of ligand *(L)* via coated pits. *Modified from Berne RM and Levy MN: Principles of physiology, St. Louis, 1990, Mosby–Year Book Inc.*

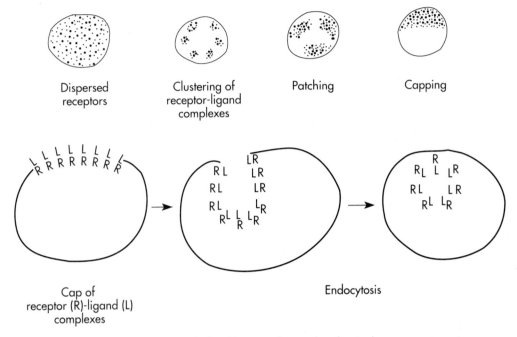

Figure 6-13. Patching, capping, and endocytosis.

end of the cell to form one cap. The cap folds inward, pinches off, and combines with the endosomal compartment of the cell, which is a membrane-bound body of ill-defined shape (discussed below).

Other cell membrane receptors (e.g., low-density lipoprotein receptors and asialoglycoprotein receptors) are clustered in small compartments comprising a total of about 2% of the membrane surface. These compartments are called **coated pits** (Figure 6-14), since they are studded on the cytoplasmic side with an electron-microscopically contrasting layer of a special protein called **clathrin.** Clathrin has a triskelion structure that allows polymerization into a basketlike structure surrounding the coated pit (Figure 6-15). Coated pits are specific for a given receptor and exclude other membrane proteins. The coated pits constantly turn over, regardless of the ligand binding to their receptors (cf., the horses in a carousel that keep on turning irrespective of occupancy). Whether associated with ligand or not, coated pits invaginate, pinch off, and lose their clathrin coat; then several pits combine with an endosome in the peripheral region of the cell (Figure 6-16).

In the endosomal compartment, the pH is lower than in cytoplasm (because of an active H^+ pump in the endosomal membrane), and this causes dissocia-

tion of certain ligand-receptor complexes. Hence, the endosome is synonymously termed **CURL,** an acronym for Compartment of Uncoupling Receptor from Ligand. Receptors of one kind each assemble in curvy outbranches of the endosomal compartment and pinch off allowing the receptors to return to the cell surface for another round of duty. In cases where a receptor-ligand complex does not dissociate, receptors are not returned to the plasma membrane; instead, they are digested with their ligand (see Figure 6-16).

Fusion of endosomal vesicles with primary lysosomes, emanating from the Golgi apparatus, then leads to the formation of secondary lysosomes in which ligand and undissociated receptor-ligand complexes are digested by lysosomal enzymes (see Figure 6-16). Amino acids, monosaccharides, and various lipids (e.g., cholesterol) are released into the cytosol and become available to the cell's metabolism. What remains are residual bodies, the contents of which are exocytosed (literally "vomited" from the cell).

In carrier-mediated transport of ligands, and for some receptors from the cell membrane to lysosomes in the perinuclear regions of the cell, endosomes serve as obligatory intermediates, while the microtubular array of the cytoskeleton directs the traffic. The other endosome function of major physiologic importance

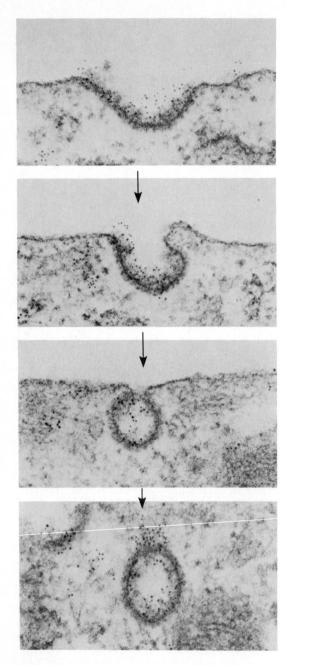

Figure 6-14. Coated pit, involved in process of endocytosis. Note clathrin coat. These electron photomicrographs show the location of low-density lipoprotein receptors on a rat hepatocyte. *Courtesy Dr. Richard G. W. Anderson, University of Texas Sciences Health Center, Dallas.*

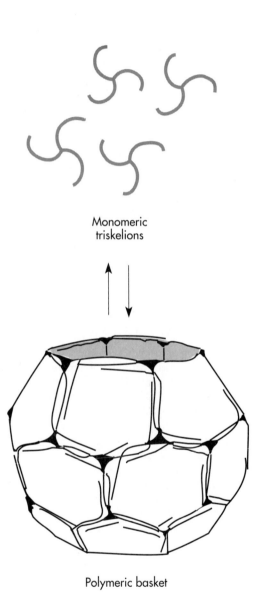

Monomeric triskelions

Polymeric basket

Figure 6-15. Clathrin. The triskelion "basket" structure of clathrin forms coated pits and vesicles.

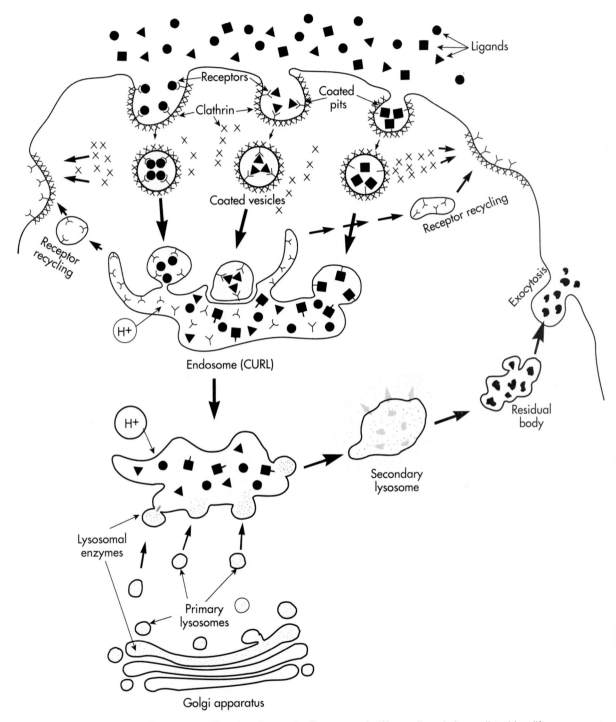

Figure 6-16. Receptor-mediated endocytosis. Transport of different ligands is mediated by different receptors, two of which are shown to form receptor-ligand complexes that dissociate in CURL, while the third one does not dissociate and is digested.

is that the extent of recycling of internalized receptors via CURL to the plasma membrane can be regulated, and, thus, adapted to the need for having that receptor on the cell surface. For instance, a high rate of receptor-mediated endocytosis of low-density lipoproteins (LDL) in hepatocytes makes the continued import of cholesterol undesirable for the cell; the LDL receptors are then tied up in the endosomal compartment, so that recycling of the LDL receptor is inhibited. The receptor is said to be **down-regulated** under these conditions. Many hormone receptors, such as the insulin receptor, are either down-regulated or **up-regulated** by control over endosomal receptor recycling by intracellular products of lysosomal digestion.

Fluidity of membrane lipids is an essential requirement for movement of receptors in the plane of the membrane toward their ligands or coated pits; it is also essential for patching and capping. Lowering environmental temperature, or oxidizing the membrane's polyunsaturated fatty acids, abolishes fluidity of the membrane and, therewith, its responsiveness toward changes in the cell's environment. Also required for the various forms of endocytosis (and for exocytosis) is a functional cytoskeleton to direct intracellular movement of vesicles.

Exocytosis

Movement of large protein compounds out of cells may occur in different forms, depending on the nature and final destination of the compounds. Discussions have already considered certain key functions of the Golgi apparatus in final posttranslational processing of proteins, assembling large molecular complexes, and the targeting of these complexes toward their destination (plasma membranes, lysosomes, export from cells).

Exocytosis is of special importance in the release of endocrine and exocrine substances from glandular cells. In conducting a nerve impulse, exocytosis of neurotransmitter substance from vesicles in a presynaptic neuron into the synaptic cleft propels the impulse toward the postsynaptic membrane of a neighboring neuron.

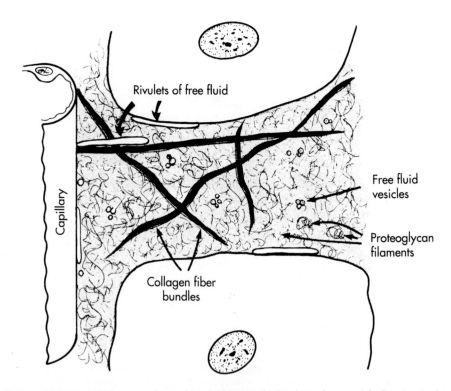

Figure 6-17. Interstitial space. *Reproduced with permission from Guyton AC: Textbook of medical physiology, ed 8, p. 173, Philadelphia, 1991, WB Saunders.*

Special transport systems
Cell-to-cell communication

Individual cells in a tissue are separated by a thin interstitial space filled with a gel matrix consisting of hyaluronic acid and protein in which collagen fibers and some free fluid vesicles are found (Figure 6-17). Though the gel impedes flow of fluid, solutes readily diffuse across it.

Various types of junctions between the plasma membranes of neighboring cells hold cells together within a tissue and allow cell-to-cell communication (Figure 6-18). A desmosome (macula adherens) tightly ties cells together, and a zonula adherens more loosely so; many of these may exist on a single cell membrane. Neighboring cells of epithelial tissues may be connected by a tight junction (zonula occludens) that completely encircles the cells, thereby forming an impenetrable seal barring **paracellular transport,** or passage of compounds from the outside of the tissue to the inside by any route that would bypass the cells. The degree of tightness of tight junctions varies among tissues from the more porous in the gut mucosa to the almost leakproof in liver (forcing **transcellular transport,** which means that compounds must traverse parenchymal liver cells on their way from blood to bile).

To facilitate lateral cell-to-cell communication in a tissue, opposing membranes to the sides of neighboring cells contain areas where many gap junctions are bunched (Figure 6-19, A). A gap junction between two membranes (Figure 6-19, B) consists of a connexon, which is a water pore, bound by a hexagonal array of integral proteins that traverse one membrane and link up exactly with a similar array traversing the neighboring membrane. The continuous, narrow, water pore allows passage of ions and small molecules (sugars, amino acids, nucleotides), but not of proteins or nucleic acids. Connexons open

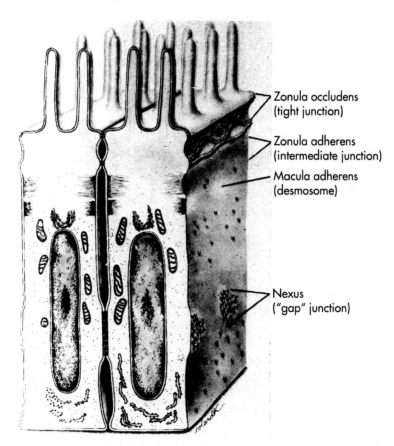

Figure 6-18. Cell junctions. *Reproduced, with permission, from Weinstein RS and McNutt NS: Cell junctions, New Eng J Med 286:521-524, 1972.*

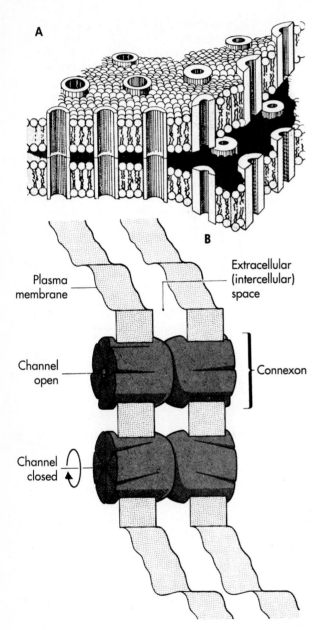

and close gap junctions by sliding their proteins in a manner resembling the diaphragm on a camera lens; the lateral spreading of tissue damage, caused by high Ca^{++} or toxins, for instance, may thus be averted by closing the gap junctions.

Epithelial and endothelial transport

Epithelial cells form a layer that separates internal body compartments or organs from the environment; for example, outer skin; intestinal mucosa lining the lumen of the gut; renal tubular cells; and hepatic parenchymal cells. In their apical region, a barrier consisting of tight junctions separates environmental and internal matter and blocks their exchange via any route other than across the plasma membrane (transcellular), thus, transport by active or diffusional processes can be controlled. In tissues where the junctions are leaky, some water and ions are exchanged via passive paracellular seepage and solvent drag.

Endothelial cells surround blood capillaries and are, in turn, bound by a basement membrane consisting of mucopolysaccharides and collagen fibers (Figure 6-20). These barriers must be overcome by any compound that is taken up by a tissue from the bloodstream. Gases and small apolar compounds can move directly across the capillary membranes. Inter-

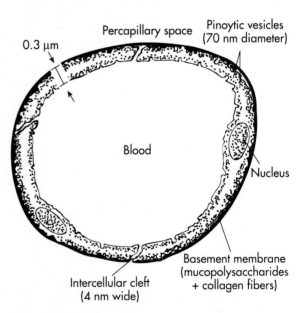

Figure 6-19. A, Cluster of gap junctions. Wide gap junctions between lens cells are formed when narrower hemiconnexons of single membrane bilayers connect. **B,** Gap junctions consist of connexons. **A,** *Reproduced with permission from Brewer GJ: Reconstitution of lens channels between two membranes. In Peracchia C, ed, Biophysics of gap junction channels, Boca Raton, 1991, 314, CRC Press. **B,** Reproduced with permission from Sheeler P and Bianchi DE: Cell and molecular biology, ed 3, 354, New York, 1987, Wiley.*

Figure 6-20. Endothelial wall of a blood capillary in muscle. *Modified and reproduced with permission from Eckert R and Randall B: Animal physiology, mechanisms and adaptations, ed 3, 460, New York, 1988, Freeman.*

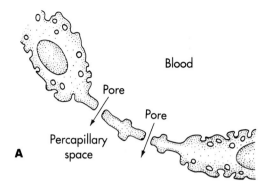

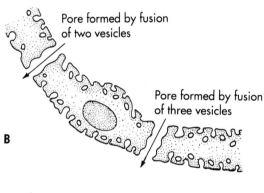

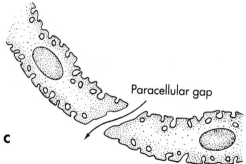

Figure 6-21. Adaptation of endothelial wall to function in various tissues. **A,** Fenestrated endothelium. Note thinning of wall with large pores and a complete basement membrane. These capillaries are found in renal glomerulus and gut. **B,** Pores formed in an endothelium by fusion of a row of vesicles. These pores have been observed in a number of capillary walls, including those of rat diaphragm. **C,** Capillary wall with large paracellular gaps and a broken basement membrane. These capillaries are found in bone and liver and are very permeable. *Reproduced with permission from Eckert R and Randall B: Animal physiology, mechanisms and adaptations, ed 3, 461, New York, 1988, Freeman.*

cellular clefts between endothelial cells allow passage of water and small water-soluble compounds; but larger compounds (proteins) are barred, not only by their size but also by opposing negative charges lining the clefts. Pinocytosis allows transport of larger molecules. Pinocytic vesicles are seen in endothelial cells, and some may unite to form transcellular pores. Large openings across endothelial cells (called windows or fenestrae) are found in renal glomeruli and allow passage of any compound below the size of proteins and particulate constitutents of blood (Figure 6-21). Another adaptation to facilitate transport across the endothelial cell lining of blood capillaries is seen in the liver, where large gaps are found between endothelial cells; also, the basement membrane underneath these gaps is discontinuous.

Blood-brain barrier

The brain is extremely selective in what it takes up from the bloodstream; only those compounds needed for brain metabolism are shuttled across the endothelium. This feature is referred to as the **blood-brain barrier.** Characteristics of the blood-brain barrier are tight junctions found between endothelial cells, an unbroken basement membrane, and specific, carrier-mediated transport systems in brain capillaries for certain compounds, such as glucose, amino acids, choline, adenine, and the excitatory neurotransmitters glutamate and aspartate.

Hepatic transport

To detect and remove circulatory waste materials and excrete them into bile, the liver is equipped with various transport features. Paracellular gaps between capillary endothelial cells and breaks in the basement membrane allow contact of liver parenchymal cells with all soluble components of the blood, including those that are protein-bound. Microvilli stud the blood-facing surface of parenchymal cells and provide an increased surface area for better diffusion (Figure 6-22). In addition, these cells contain receptors for recognition and binding of blood constituents, and carrier-mediated transport systems for passage across the plasma membrane for various compounds (e.g., bile salts, bilirubin, fatty acids, amino acids). Special binding proteins (e.g., ligandin) carry apolar substances across the cells' cytoplasm. Intracellular metabolism (e.g., oxidations, methylations, conjugation with glutathione, amino acids, or glucuronic acid) and packaging (in the Golgi apparatus) into micellar complexes then prepare hepatic products for active excretory transport into bile canaliculi.

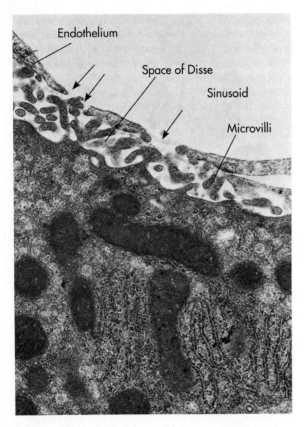

Figure 6-22. Sinusoidal surface of parenchymal rat liver cell. Note small discontinuities in the lining of the sinusoid *(heavy arrows)*. Electron photomicrograph. *Courtesy Dr. Rick A. Rogers, Harvard School of Public Health.*

In addition to the transport systems in parenchymal cells, pinocytic, phagocytic, and receptor-mediated endocytosis of circulatory compounds occurs in the endothelial and reticuloendothelial (Kupffer) cells of the liver.

Transport in blood

Many constituents of plasma are transported in association with proteins. Albumin tightly binds and transports various polar and apolar substances (e.g., nonesterified fatty acids, bilirubin) and delivers these compounds to the liver to be metabolized or excreted into bile. Unbound plasma constituents are filtered in the kidneys' glomeruli and then lost in urine, unless reabsorbed in the renal tubules. Albumin binding also regulates the concentration of unbound, metabolically active calcium ions. Special plasma proteins reg-

ulate transport of iron (transferrin), copper (ceruloplasmin), and vitamin B_{12} (transcobalamine) to their sites of storage or metabolic activity. Hormone binding to proteins in plasma (corticosteroids and progesterone to transcortin, thyroid hormones to thryoglobulin) regulates the concentration of unbound (active) hormones in plasma by a dissociation equilibrium, generates a readily available hormone reservoir, and curtails renal elimination of hormones.

RECEPTORS ON CELL MEMBRANES
General properties and functions

Receptors are a unique class of compounds. They are not enzymes, nor are they hormones. Their function is to recognize and bind a ligand and to direct that ligand to its destination. As with enzymes, the specificity of receptors for ligands varies between groups requiring specific structural configurations.

Chemically, receptors are most often glycoproteins; however, some receptors do not contain proteins; for example, gangliosides (glycolipids) on cell surfaces function as hormone receptors.

Isolation of receptors from cell membranes usually involves dissolving the membrane in a detergent and then selectively binding the receptor on a column that contains an immobilized ligand attached to a neutral support. By this technique (affinity chromatography), all extraneous membrane proteins are washed away, leaving the receptor stuck on the column; finally, the receptor is harvested from the column by elution with a buffer that dissociates the receptor from the ligand, through different pH, a salt concentration, or a higher concentration of competing ligand. This method may be compared with the extraction of a needle from a haystack using a magnet.

Functions of receptors

Receptors on the exterior face of plasma membranes control cell-to-cell interactions (involved in embryogenesis, cell mating, and histocompatibility) and cell-to-ligand interactions (e.g., uptake of nutrients, and cellular responses to nervous and endocrine stimuli). Intracellular receptors are involved with traffic of compounds within cells. All of these receptor functions require an intact cytoskeleton.

Receptors control direction and rate of metabolism in a manner comparable to enzymes. Narrow specificity for the structure of a ligand gives direction to cellular processes; for example, the Golgi produces mannose 6-phosphate containing glycoproteins and targets them to lysosomal receptors. Positive and negative cooperativity help control the rate of ligand binding to receptors. Especially important in rate control over metabolism is the down-regulation of receptors. When a cell is exposed to a high ligand concentration, and it has taken up all the ligand it needs, then many of its receptors are endocytosed; also, their recycling to the cell surface may be inhibited under the influence of intracellular ligand. Thus, the cell surface is denuded of receptors, and the cell is slow to internalize more of the ligand. The cell is then said to be down-regulated. Examples of metabolic control by down-regulation include the following: (i) the number of low-density lipoprotein (LDL) receptors on hepatocytes decreases in response to high LDL levels in plasma, thus preventing them from internalizing more of the LDL's cholesterol than is needed; and (ii) chronic dietary overindulgence, leading to chronic overproduction of insulin, causes the number of insulin receptors on fat cells to decline; cells then become less sensitive to insulin; the levels of metabolites in plasma that stimulate the pancreas to continue its insulin production remain high; the pancreas, thus, may become exhausted (maturity-onset diabetes). In this way, receptors for various hormones (TSH, HCG, LH, ACTH) are down-regulated. Up-regulation increases the number of receptors in response to chronically low levels of their ligands, and, thus, makes the cells more sensitive to those ligands (e.g., prolactin, angiotensin II, LDL).

Lectins

Lectins are a special group of receptors that recognize their ligands only by their carbohydrate moieties. Lectins disregard the remainder of the ligand structure, whether it be a glycoprotein, glycolipid, or cell surface. But, lectins are extremely specific for the exact structure of the carbohydrate chains, and this feature has proven to be most useful. Ligand binding to a lectin on the cell surface leads to mitogenic activity within the cell. For a long time lectins were thought to occur exclusively in plants, from which many lectins were isolated and made commercially available (e.g., wheat germ agglutinin, peanut agglutinin, and concanavalin A). Presently, several lectins have been isolated from the cell surfaces and interiors of mammalian cells.

Examples for the use of lectins:

- Lectins are used for blood typing: Since erythrocytes of a given blood type are characterized by a unique carbohydrate structure on their cell surface, only the lectin that is specific for that structure will bind to those cell surfaces and causes hemagglutination.
- In mammalian physiology, lectins direct whole body and cellular metabolism. Exemplified earlier in the text was a lectin, specific for mannose 6-phosphate, involved in targeting lysosomal enzymes from the Golgi apparatus. Another example derives from the stability of glycoproteins in the bloodstream. Certain glycoproteins possess half-lives of approximately 20 hours; but when sialic acid residues are removed, exposing the penultimate sugar (galactose) of the glycosidic chains, they disappear from plasma with half-lives of less than 2 minutes. The desialylated glycoproteins are endocytosed by liver parenchymal cells, since those cells are the unique location of the lectin that recognizes exposed galactose. Removing this galactose also exposes sugars that are more inward, which are recognized by lectins located on the surface of reticuloendothelial cells (such as Kupffer cells in the liver). Those altered plasma glycoproteins end up in reticuloendothelial cells.
- In affinity chromatography, a lectin can be bound to the stationary phase in the column to retain a specific ligand that can be isolated.
- In medicine, a drug or enzyme can be incorporated in the aqueous core of a liposome; to target that liposome to the intended cell, one might include a glycoprotein that traverses the lipid bilayer of the liposome and is recognized by a lectin on the target cell's surface. Similarly, a liposome that contains an anticancer drug in the aqueous center may be provided with a lectin that is specific for a unique carbohydrate in the glycocalyx of a malignant cell.
- Many of the interactions of cells with other cells or macromolecules are intermediated by lectins.

Cell-to-cell interactions mediated by receptors

- Cell aggregation to form organs occurs in embryogenesis. This can also be shown in vitro in mixed organ cultures of thyroid and heart cells, where cells of the same tissue aggregate. Cell adhesion molecules on different cells either bind directly, or indirectly via a multivalent go-between molecule.
- Platelet aggregation occurs among platelets and with collagen, in hemostasis. Four glycosyl transferases (transferring saccharides between platelets

and collagen, between platelets and glycoproteins, and between platelets) are present in adult platelets. Since the adult platelet no longer manufactures protein, the role of these transferases, found in the plasma membrane, may be adhesion via interactions with lectins.

- Phagocytosis of invading microorganisms by reticuloendothelial cells is preceded by lectin binding.
- Reproduction: the lectin-mediated interaction of sperm with egg cell leads to a change in the plasma membrane of the ovum that prevents multiple fertilizations.
- Bacterial infection: binding of bacteria, via lectins to specific sugars on the surface of host cell is required for colonization and infection of the host. For instance, *E. coli* bacteria have a lectin that recognizes, and thus binds to, mannose-containing mucopolysaccharides on the surface of human buccal epithelial cells. This binding is inhibited competitively by low concentrations of mannose or

methyl-D-mannoside; washing with these sugars removes preattached bacteria. Methyl-D-mannose is not metabolizable; thus, when given to mice in their drinking water, this sugar rapidly finds its way into the urinary tract, where it significantly reduces infections caused by *E. coli*. Another example of bacterial attachment to a host cell via lectins is that of nitrogen-fixing bacteria to the root tips of legumes.

Cell-to-macromolecule interactions mediated by receptors

Among the macromolecules that influence cellular metabolism are various hormones. The autonomic nervous system affects cellular metabolism directly via signals from α-adrenergic and β-adrenergic receptors and indirectly via hormone release. In this context, the text deals with the neuroendocrine signaling that is transmitted to the cell interior by intermediation of second messengers. Two second-messenger systems

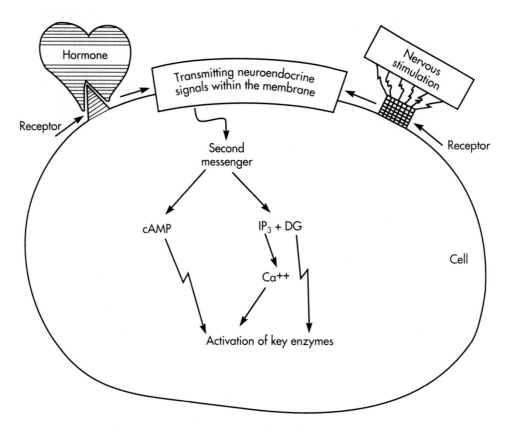

Figure 6-23. Neuroendocrine receptors on the plasma membrane.

have been reported in detail (Figure 6-23), one involving cyclic AMP, the other involving Ca^{++}, inositol trisphosphate (IP_3), and diglycerides (DG). These systems, which are not totally unrelated, are presented first. Then, some general modes of hormonal action, mediated or not by second messengers, are reviewed.

Cyclic AMP as second messenger

Hormones or neurotransmitter substances that affect cell metabolism via cyclic AMP (cAMP) are bound on the cell surface to receptors specific for those substances (Figure 6-24). This binding results in either an activation or inhibition of the enzyme adenylate cyclase, which is responsible for the formation of cAMP from ATP. Transfer of the signal from the occupied receptor on the membrane's outer face to adenylate cyclase, located on the cytoplasmic side of

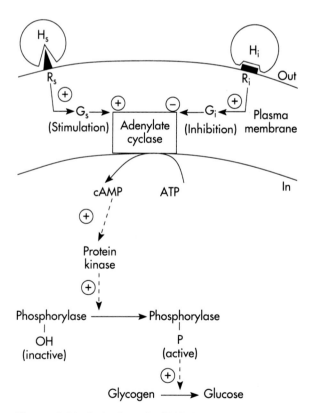

Figure 6-24. Activation of cAMP formation in liver responding to low blood sugar levels. The subscript s refers to stimulatory and i to inhibitory hormones (H), receptors (R), and G proteins that affect adenylate cyclase activity.

the membrane, occurs via G_s (stimulatory) or G_i (inhibitory) proteins, so named because their combination with GTP activates them (Figure 6-25). Activation of the G proteins is accompanied by a loss of two of the three subunits that constitute G proteins. The remaining (α_s and α_i) subunits, associated with GTP, allosterically affect adenylate cyclase activity until, because of their inherent GTP-ase activity, the associated GTP is hydrolysed. Then the stimulatory (α_s) and inhibitory (α_i) subunits dissociate from their domain on adenylate cyclase and recombine with their other subunits to reconstitute the intact G_s and G_i trimers.

Cholera toxin inactivates the GTP-ase activity of α_s, thereby blocking the inactivation of α_s and causing chronic activation of adenylate cyclase. Pertussis toxin, too, permanently activates adenylate cyclase, but does so by preventing GTP activation of α_i.

Among the numerous activators of adenylate cyclase are, glucagon, ADH, TSH, ACTH, and the β-adrenergic catecholamines. Inhibitors of adenylate cyclase include acetylcholine, somatostatin, angiotensin II, and the α_2-adrenergic catecholamines.

Some hormones that activate adenylate cyclase, HCG, TSH, LH, and FSH, have a sequence of five amino acids in common, with which they bind to gangliosides on the plasma membrane. Interestingly, this same amino acid sequence is found on the structures of the plant toxins abrin and ricin, and on cholera and diphtheria toxins, all of which have gangliosides as their membrane receptors.

The mode of action of cAMP is that it allosterically activates certain protein kinases and phosphatases. These enzymes control activation and deactivation of key enzyme activities via phosphorylation and dephosphorylation of those key enzyme proteins. A large number of these kinase enzymes are known; some are hormone-responsive, others are not. Some depend on cAMP, others on Ca^{++}-calmodulin, Ca^{++}-phospholipid, or other mediators.

The enzyme phosphodiesterase (PDE) hydrolyzes cAMP and thereby aids in the control of intracellular cAMP levels. Insulin's activation of PDE keeps cAMP levels low and, thus, antagonizes the actions of epinephrine and glucagon. Conversely, caffeine's inhibition of PDE prolongs the intracellular life of cAMP, which results in the stimulation of key enzymes that break down glycogen and fats. Since regulation of PDE activity is Ca^{++} dependent, the cAMP and Ca^{++}-dependent second-messenger systems are linked.

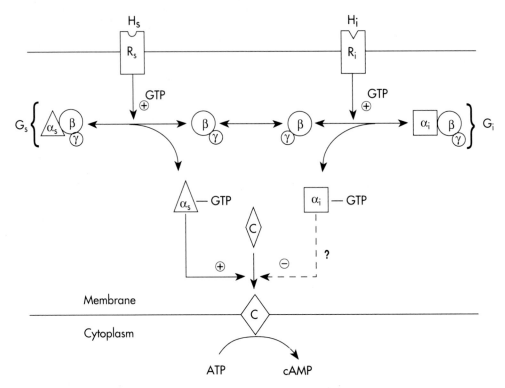

Figure 6-25. Stimulatory *(s)* and inhibitory *(i)* G proteins control cAMP formation. *Modified and reproduced with permission from Gilman AG: G proteins and dual control of adenylate cyclase, Cell 36:577-579, 1984.*

Phosphoinositol, diglyceride, and Ca^{++} as second messengers

Included among agents that stimulate cellular metabolism via this second-messenger system are the neurogenic α_1-adrenergic catecholamines and acetylcholine, and the hormones cholecystokinin, gastrin, ADH, and angiotensin II. Binding of these agents to their specific receptors on the cell membrane leads to a signal (transmitted via G protein) that activates phospholipase C within the membrane, and that enzyme activity splits the membrane lipid phosphatidylinositol-4,5-bisphosphate (PIP$_2$) into a diglyceride (DG) and inositol-1,4,5-trisphosphate (IP$_3$) (Figure 6-26). Both DG and IP$_3$ are second messengers (Figure 6-27). DG directly activates a Ca^{++}–phospholipid-dependent protein kinase. IP$_3$ effects Ca^{++} release from the endoplasmic reticulum; that Ca^{++} is bound to calmodulin and calcimedins (specific binding proteins for Ca^{++}), and it is also included in the polymeric quaternary structure of many key enzymes.

Ca^{++} binding changes the tertiary structure of these binding proteins and, consequently, those key enzyme activities (e.g., adenylate cyclase, cAMP and cGMP phosphodiesterases, glycogen synthase, pyruvate dehydrogenase, pyruvate kinase, and pyruvate carboxylase).

As the extracellular calcium concentration is thousands of times greater than the cytosolic [Ca^{++}], another mode whereby the aforementioned proteinaceous hormones increase intracellular [Ca^{++}] is by increasing Ca^{++} influx, usually via an exchange of Na$^+$ for Ca^{++}. In addition, PIP$_2$ inhibits the pump that exports intracellular Ca^{++} in exchange for H$^+$ (see Figure 6-27).

Intracellular functions of Ca^{++}, in association with various binding proteins, include the following:
- Control of key enzyme activities, either by direct attachment of Ca^{++}-calmodulin or via Ca^{++}-stimulated protein kinase or phosphatase activities.

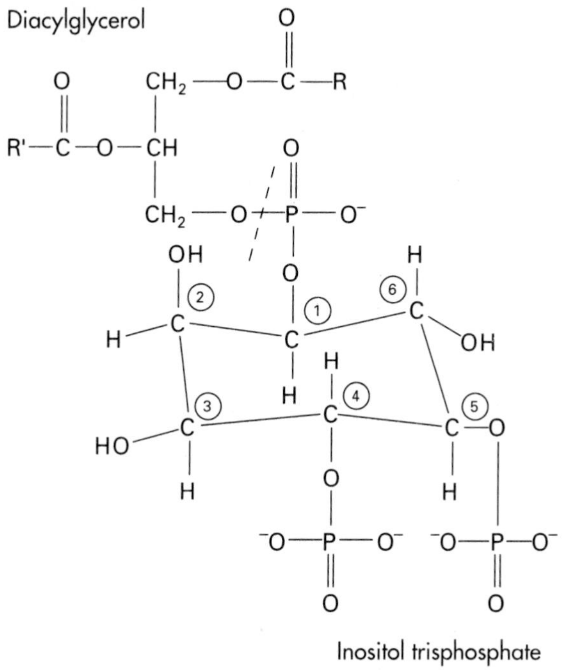

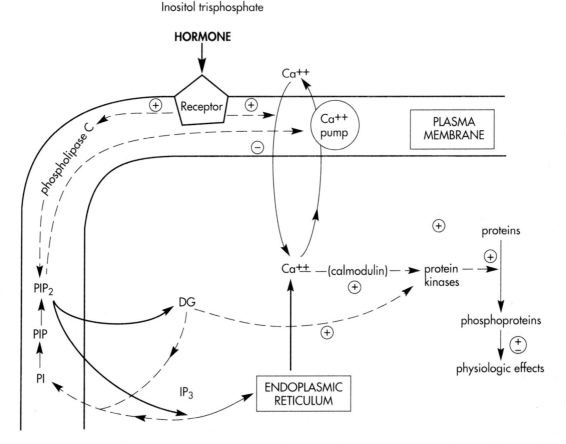

Diacylglycerol

Inositol trisphosphate

Figure 6-26. Phosphatidylinositol-4,5-bisphosphate (PIP_2). Phospholipase C, when activated, forms the second messengers diacylglycerol (DG) and inositol trisphosphate (IP_3) by hydrolyzing PIP_2 as indicated by the dotted line. [PIP, phosphatidylinositol-4-phosphate, has an OH group on carbon-5 of inositol; PI, phosphoinositol, has OH groups on both carbon-4 and carbon-5.]

HORMONE

PLASMA MEMBRANE

proteins

protein kinases

phosphoproteins

physiologic effects

ENDOPLASMIC RETICULUM

Figure 6-27. Calcium as mediator of hormonal effects on cells. Abbreviations as in previous figure.

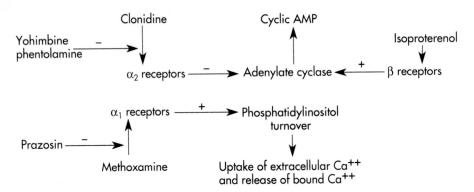

Figure 6-28. Model for regulation of cellular metabolism by catecholamines. Beta effects of catecholamines are associated with activation of adenylate cyclase, and α_2, inhibition of the cycle. In contrast, α_1 effects are mediated through separate receptors which elevate cytosol Ca^{++} and increase phosphatidylinositol turnover. Breakdown of phosphatidylinositol may be linked to the mechanism by which hormones release bound Ca^{++} and gate entry of extracellular Ca^{++}. *Reproduced with permission from Fain JN and García-Sáinz JA: Role of phosphatidylinositol turnover in α_1 and of adenylate cyclase inhibition in α_2 effects of catecholamines, Life Sci 26:1183-1194, 1980.*

- Muscle contraction.
- Cytoskeletal participation in endocytosis and secretion of endocrine and exocrine substances by exocytosis.
- Phosphorylation and dephosphorylation of nuclear proteins affecting genetic expression.

Autonomic nervous influences on the second-messenger systems

A delicate balance between activation and inhibition of the second messenger systems is provided by various adrenergic receptors (Figure 6-28). Drugs are used in research and clinical medicine to affect the activities of specific receptors.

NATURE AND ACTION OF HORMONES

Having discussed interactions of hormones with the cell surface and the roles of second messengers in conveying the hormonal message to the cell's interior, this chapter concludes with a brief survey of some general properties of hormones.

Hormone secretion and transport

Under the influence of nervous receptors that monitor the need for a given hormone and negative feedback mechanisms that control overabundance, the secretion of hormones is well controlled. Transport of hormones in the bloodstream in many cases involves a specific protein carrier (e.g., transcortin transports progesterone and corticosteroids, and thyroid hormone-binding globulin transports thyroxine) or albumin (e.g., aldosterone, testosterone). The dissociation equilibrium of bound to free hormone allows for control of the level of free (active) hormone and also prevents renal elimination of small hormone molecules. Generally, the half-lives of hormones in the circulation are short, because of urinary elimination and breakdown in tissues; especially in liver, where proteolytic enzymes degrade certain hormones (e.g., insulin and glucagon), and where other hormones are inactivated by chemical modifications, or via conjugation with glucuronic acid or glutathione prior to elimination in bile or urine.

Importance of hormone receptors

One may wonder, which is the more important: the hormone or the hormone receptor? Probably the latter, as it is possible to mimic the action of a hormone, provided the receptor is intact. Indeed, antibodies against receptor proteins may stimulate the receptor and generate hormone-like activity. Many of insulin's actions on fat cells, including down-regulation, are duplicated by stimulating the insulin receptor with antibody, spermidine, vitamin K, or wheat germ agglutinin. In contrast to the tolerance for hormone substitutes, hormone receptors are indispensable. This is apparent from the large number of inborn diseases in which a receptor is either genetically lacking (e.g., lack of ADH receptors in nephrogenic diabetes insipidus), chronically stimulated or blocked by antibodies, or has diminished hormone-binding activity (Table 6-2).

Table 6-2	Hormone receptors and diseases	
Disease	**Receptor**	**Problem**
Graves' disease (hyperthyroidism)	TSH	Antibody stimulates TSH receptor.
Acanthosis nigricans with insulin resistance	Insulin	Antibody blocks insulin binding to receptor.
Myasthenia gravis	Acetylcholine	Antibody enhances turnover of the acetylcholine receptor.
Asthma	β-Adrenergic receptor	Antibody blocks β-adrenergic binding.
Congenital nephrogenic diabetes insipidus	ADH	Receptor is deficient.
Testicular feminization syndrome	Androgen	Receptor is deficient.
Pseudohypoparathyroidism	PTH	Receptor is deficient.
Vitamin D-resistant rickets type II	Calcitriol	Receptor is deficient.
Obesity	Insulin	Hormone binding is decreased.
Diabetes mellitus type II (non–insulin-dependent diabetes mellitus [NIDDM])	Insulin	Hormone binding is decreased.

(Modified, with permission, from Murray RK, Granner DK, Mayes PA, and Rodwell VW: *Harper's Biochemistry*, ed 21, p. 471, Norwalk, Conn., 1988, Appleton & Lange.)

Classification of hormones by their mode of action

Hormones may be classified according to their mode of action and the second messenger involved. In the first instance, hormones that can enter the cell may be distinguished from those that bind to cell surface receptors and that delegate their effects to second messengers.

Glucocorticoids, after binding to cytoplasmic steroid receptors and transporting into a cell nucleus, increase the transcription of mRNA coding for key gluconeogenic enzymes. Similar modes of action have been found for other steroid hormones (sex hormones, mineralocorticoids, and dihydroxycholecalciferol) and thyroid hormones.

Numerous hormones bind to cell surface receptors and delegate their intracellular tasks to second messengers. Hormones may stimulate adenylate cyclase, and thus the production of cAMP (e.g., glucagon, antidiuretic hormone, parathyroid hormone, and β-adrenergic catecholamines), or they may inhibit cAMP production (e.g., somatostatin and α_2-adrenergic catecholamines).

Other hormones operate via the phosphoinositol/diglyceride/Ca^{++} system of second messengers (e.g., cholecystokinin, acetylcholine, and α_1-adrenergic catecholamines). The second messengers control activities of various protein kinases and phosphatases whose phosphorylation and dephosphorylation of key enzymes regulate the flow and direction of intermediary metabolism.

Finally, there are hormones for which an intracellular second messenger has not yet been found. Included in this group are various growth-promoting hormones, such as growth hormone, insulin, and nerve-, insulin-like-, platelet–derived-, epidermal-, and fibroblast- growth factors. Because of the metabolic importance of the insulin receptor, some of its features are outlined in the section that follows.

Insulin receptor

Most cells contain insulin receptors on their plasma membranes (Figure 6-29). The receptor consists of two adjacent α-subunits that are located on the outside of the membrane and are flanked by two β-subunits that span the width of the membrane and are connected to the α-subunits via disulfide bridges. Insulin is bound to the α-subunits, whereupon patching, capping, and endocytosis of insulin-receptor complexes takes place. This endocytosis is responsible for down-regulation of the number of insulin receptors in response to high insulin levels. Upon insulin binding to the receptor, the β-subunits become autophosphorylated (the receptor acts as a tyrosine kinase) and then various signals are imparted to the cell:

- Adenylate cyclase is inhibited by β-subunits.
- In fat cells, a glucose transporter (an integral membrane protein that has 12 adjacent membrane-spanning sequences) is mobilized from the Golgi to the plasma membrane.
- Various enzymes are induced, such as glucokinase in the liver, an organ where insulin does

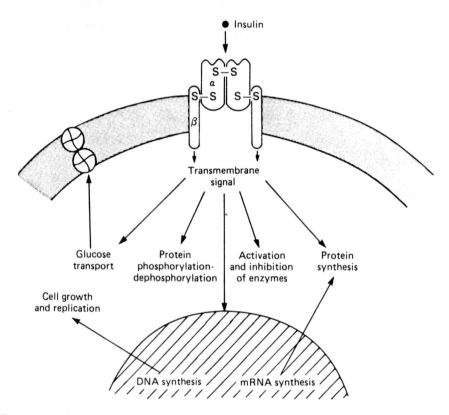

Figure 6-29. Insulin binding to its receptor generates intracellular responses. *Courtesy Dr. C. Ronald Kahn, Joslin Diabetes Center, Boston. In Murray RK et al.: Harper's Biochemistry, ed 21, Norwalk CT, 1988, Appleton and Lange.*

not promote glucose transport across the plasma membrane by directly increasing membrane permeability.

- Protein phosphorylation and dephosphorylation occur by stimulation of protein kinases (which also may activate phosphatases). A truncated list of metabolic pathways controlled by their key enzymes in this manner (by insulin) includes glycogenesis, glycogenolysis, glycolysis, gluconeogenesis, triglyceride synthesis and breakdown, and cholesterol synthesis.
- Transcriptional control by insulin induces the production of mRNA for albumin and for several key enzymes, including glucokinase, pyruvate kinase, and fatty acid synthase.

Attention has not been paid to the large area of cell-small molecule interactions mediated by receptors, which includes neurotransmission, chemotaxis of bacteria on anti-inflammatory cells, taste, phero-

mones, and CO_2-, osmo-, and glucose receptors. These topics are beyond the scope of this text.

STUDY QUESTIONS

1. *a.* List a purpose for which fluidity of plasma membranes is required.
   b. List the main membrane component responsible for fluidity.
   c. How does vitamin E protect fluidity of plasma membranes?

2. Exemplify asymmetry in plasma membrane composition.

3. List the morphologic adaptation of cell surfaces by which the rate of passive absorption is increased in liver and gut mucosal cells.

4. List factors involved in glucose transport from blood into fat cells.

5. List an important metabolic function of plasma membranes.

6. *a.* Give a function for gangliosides in cell membranes.

   b. Name a class of glycolipids on cell surfaces that function as hormone receptors.

   c. What is the cause of inborn lipidoses (e.g., Tay-Sachs disease)?

7. *a.* How do inorganic ions traverse the plasma membrane of cells?

   b. What are compounds such as valinomycin and gramicidin called collectively?

   c. Why can anesthetics enter cells so easily?

   d. List the purpose for which the pharmaceutical industry makes methyl esters (apolar) of the carboxyl groups of drugs.

   e. Give a transport-related reason for rapid phosphorylation of dietary glucose in the liver.

8. What is the name of the salient feature that regulates the brain's uptake of compounds from the bloodstream (less developed in neonates)?

9. List a membrane-related feature that causes the endocytosis of receptor-bound ligand to be impaired at 4° C.

10. *a.* What is the collective name for the subcellular attachments to the plasma membrane that aid in the signaling to and from cells?

    b. List a mineral requirement for endocytic activity of this complex.

11. List two functions of the cytoskeleton attached to plasma membranes.

12. *a.* List an example of an induced pore across a membrane.

    b. What does an ionophore (e.g., monensin) do?

13. *a.* List the microanatomical feature that bars paracellular transport of compounds across epithelial cell layers.

    b. List the lateral cell-to-cell connections that allow the exchange of small molecules.

14. Exemplify interaction between two cells mediated by cell-surface phenomena.

15. What functions have adrenergic receptors situated on the cell surface?

16. List the technical term for the small cell-surface areas where most of the low-density lipoprotein receptors reside on the plasma membrane.

17. The processes of patching and capping are involved in: (a) pinocytosis; (b) receptor-mediated transport; (c) exocytosis. (Choose one.)

18. *a.* List the subcellular site involved in allowing the receptors to escape lysosomal digestion during endocytosis.

    b. What function has CURL in the overall process of endocytosis?

    c. What is the metabolic fate of ligands contained in endosomes?

19. List the mineral + protein combination that regulates cytoskeleton intermediation in exocytosis of secretory granules.

20. *a.* List the function of the Golgi apparatus in turnover of the plasma membrane.

    b. Name the subcellular particle into which enzymes are concentrated whose carbohydrate moieties contain mannose 6-phosphate.

    c. For what important function does the Golgi utilize the presence of different lectins on various intracellular sites?

21. *a.* List the subcellular site where the ultimate preparations for the exocytosis of exocrine compounds are made.

    b. List an intracellular inorganic ion involved in exocytosis.

22. *a.* Name the kind of receptor that recognizes complex compounds by their carbohydrate structure.

    b. To which organ, and within that organ, and to which cell type is a glycoprotein targeted which has lost some of its sialic acid groups?

    c. Based on b, list a possible use of liposomes in medicine.

23. List the technique whereby a ligand is attached to an inert support in a chromatographic column, so that a receptor protein for that ligand can be selectively bound and purified on that column.

24. Indicate the mode of action by which methylmannose combats an *E. coli* infection of the urinary tract.

25. *a.* What detail (in general) is recognized by a lectin that agglutinates a certain blood group?

    b. By what surface change are senile erythrocytes recognized by reticuloendothelial cells (and thus marked for removal from the circulation)?

26. *a.* List the two well-defined second-messenger systems on cell membranes.

    b. List a connection between these two second-messenger systems.

27. *a.* List the enzyme, located on the cytoplasmic side of the plasma membrane, that responds to the combination of hormone + receptor + regulatory protein.

    b. Name the intracellular enzyme that degrades cAMP.

28. The other second-messenger system on plasma membranes has several components:

    a. Diglycerides act by stimulating which enzyme?

    b. Inositol-triphosphate acts by releasing calcium from endoplasmic reticulum, and that mineral acts in combination with a special protein. What is this protein called? This protein associates with, and activates, which key enzymes?

29. *a.* The way cAMP acts is by stimulating certain protein kinases, and this, in turn, causes the activities of some key enzymes to be covalently modified in what way?

  b. Of course, for each on-switch, there must be an opposing off-switch. List the categorical term for enzymes (also under cAMP control) that undo the work of protein kinases.

30. Knowing that epinephrine and norepinephrine are products of the nervous system, suggest two ways, via second messengers, by which nervous stimulation may affect a cell's metabolism.

31. Give the connection between the following two findings: (i) protein kinase C activates processes involved in cell division; and (ii) certain oncogenes stimulate production of diglycerides from phosphorylated phosphoinositol in cell membranes.

32. *a.* List a hormone whose membrane receptor is a ganglioside.

  b. The receptors recognized by cholera toxin, as well as by the hormones TSH, LH, and HCG, are glycoproteins. (True/False)

33. *a.* Other than rate of production, list two factors that control the functioning of a hormone.

  b. List a role of the liver in maintaining hormone balance.

34. Certain hormone-related diseases are not the result of insufficient production of the hormone but are related to _____. (Fill in the blank).

35. *a.* List the technical term for the receptor-related fact that cells become desensitized to a hormone

(e.g., insulin) or other ligands (e.g., LDL) present in high concentrations in blood.

  b. List a pathologic condition resulting from this fact.

36. Different classes of hormones.

  a. Exemplify a class of hormone that works in the nucleus.

  b. Exemplify a class of hormones that generates the second messenger, cAMP.

37. *a.* List the gland upon which thyrotropin-releasing hormone (TRH) acts.

  b. List the pancreatic hormone whose message is: "Raise the blood glucose level."

38. *a.* List a specific protein that transports thyroid hormone in blood.

  b. List two functions for such a hormone-binding protein in blood.

39. How does caffeine's inhibition of phosphodiesterase activity cause the stimulatory effects of coffee on a person?

40. To underscore the importance of hormone receptors, what are the symptoms of the following conditions?

  a. The absence of ADH receptors in the kidney.

  b. Genetically defective receptors for low-density lipoproteins (LDL).

41. *a.* List an important effect of insulin's attachment to its receptors on the plasma membranes of fat cells.

  b. Insulin affects key enzyme activities by phosphorylation and dephosphorylation of enzyme protein molecules (True/False)

  c. Insulin affects key enzyme activities by transcriptional control in the cell nucleus (True/False)

Blood: composition and function

COMPOSITION OF BLOOD PLASMA

The total blood volume increases with body weight in a nonlinear manner that is influenced by age, gender, species, adiposity, etc. In the human adult weighing 70 kg, blood volume amounts to about 8% in men and 6% in women.

When a fresh blood sample is admixed with an anticoagulant (e.g., heparin) and then centrifuged, it separates into three layers. The bottom layer consists of erythrocytes; their volume, expressed as a fraction of the total blood volume in the centrifuge tube, is the hematocrit or packed cell volume. Above the red blood cells is a thin, colorless layer (buffy coat) that contains leukocytes and platelets. The clear liquid above the packed cells is plasma. Plasma, thus, contains several soluble proteins including fibrinogen, the precursor of fibrin, a blood clotting ingredient. Allowing blood to clot before centrifugation produces serum. The yellow color of serum and plasma is due to bilirubin and carotenoids. Solutes constitute about 9% of plasma volume: proteins approximately 7%, nonprotein organic compounds approximately 1%, and inorganic salts 0.9% in humans (Table 7-1); much similarity is found in the chemical composition of blood from mature domestic animals (Table 7-2). The numerical values may vary due to physiological fluctuations (gender, age, circadian rhythm, etc.) and the laboratory methods used.

Plasma proteins can be separated by electrophoresis (Figure 7-1) into the following major fractions: albumin 52 to 68%; α_1-globulins 2.4 to 7.0%; α_2-globulins 6.1 to 10.1%; β_1-globulins 8.5 to 14.5%; γ-globulins 10 to 21%. Individual proteins are quantified using specific immunologic antibodies. The α- and β-globulins contain lipoproteins.

Functions of various plasma proteins include the following:

- Albumin transports lipids and is the major contributor to oncotic pressure because of its relative abundance. About 40% of albumin is in the circulation, while 60% is in the interstitial fluid spaces of the body. About 5% of albumin leaves the interstitial fluid each hour via lymph, then cycles through the thoracic duct, and returns to the bloodstream. Binding to albumin regulates the plasma levels, as well as the destination, of the metabolically active (unbound) forms of various substances, such as Ca^{++}, steroid hormones, and lipophilic drugs (e.g., sulfonamides, aspirin, penicillin).

- Ceruloplasmin, an α_1-globulin, binds Cu^+ or Cu^{++} and functions in the gut as a ferroxidase converting Fe^{++} to Fe^{+++} prior to incorporation of Fe^{+++} into transferrin.

- Other α_1-globulins include retinol-binding protein, thyroxine-binding globulin, sex-hormone-binding globulin, and transcortin, which transports glucocorticoids.

Table 7-1	Principal* solutes of human plasma

Solute	mg/dl
Protein, total	6.0-8.5
Nonprotein organic compounds	
Amino acids, total	60
Alanine	2.5-7.5
Glutamine (most abundant)	4.5-10.0
Carbohydrates, total	90
Fructose	6-8
Glucose (fasting)	65-110
Pentoses	2-4
Lipids, total	600
Cholesterol (free + esterified)	150-250
Fatty acids, unesterified	8-30
Phospholipids	140-225
Triglycerides	140-250
Organic acids, total	20
Acetoacetate (+ acetone)	0.3-2.0
Citric acid	1.4-3.0
Lactic acid	4-17
Wastes, total	40
Bilirubin (free + conjugated)	0.2-1.7
Creatinine	0.6-1.5
Methylhistidine	0.2
Urea	13-40
Uric acid	2.5-9.0
Electrolytes (meq/L)	
Anions, total	142-150
Bicarbonate	24-28
Chloride	96-106
Phosphate	1.6-2.5
Sulfate	0.3-1.3
Cations, total	142-158
Calcium (total)	4.2-5.3
Calcium (ionized)	2.1-2.6
Magnesium	1.5-2.5
Potassium	3.4-5.0
Sodium	135-145

Based on data from Dunagan WC and Ridner ML, eds: *Manual of medical therapeutics,* ed 26, 505-506, Boston, 1989, Little, Brown.
Smith EL, et al: *Principles of biochemistry: mammalian biochemistry,* ed 7, 4-5, New York, 1983, McGraw-Hill.
Krupp MA, et al eds: *Current medical diagnosis and treatment,* 1986, 1112-1114, Los Altos, CA, Lange.
Ganong WF: *Review of medical physiology,* ed 9, p 619, Los Altos, CA, 1979, Lange.
Schauf C, et al: *Human physiology: foundations and frontiers,* 349, 705, St Louis, 1990, Mosby–Year Book.
Murray RK, et al: *Harper's biochemistry,* ed 21, 661, 662, Norwalk, CN, 1988, Appleton & Lange.
*"Principal," meant here in a quantitative sense, allows some subjectivity. Therefore, some "minor" compounds have been included as principal waste products, whereas many qualitatively important compounds, transported in plasma, have been excluded; among those compounds are the minor entries under the listed headings and, in addition, all trace minerals, vitamins, enzymes, and hormones.

- Haptoglobins bind hemoglobin released by intravascular hemolysis. The large haptoglobin-hemoglobin complex is phagocytized in reticuloendothelial cells; iron is recycled.
- Hemopexin does not bind hemoglobin, but binds heme and transports that to the liver where iron is reutilized.
- γ-Globulins or immunoglobulins.

Turnover is approximately 25% of circulating plasma protein per day, largely via the liver and kidney. Intravenously administered albumin is taken up and lysed in tissues; amino acids are reused.

Of special importance in the turnover and resynthesis of plasma proteins is the liver, producing albumin, fibrinogen, and 80% of the plasma globulins. Hypoalbuminemia is found in hepatic cirrhosis. Lymphoid tissue and the reticuloendothelial system are sources of immunoproteins, including γ-globulin.

BLOOD CLOTTING

After injury whereby a blood vessel is damaged, blood loss must be quickly stopped. For this the body has a system of hemostasis possessing the following characteristics: (i) it is fast-acting when needed; (ii) it is not active in intact vessels; and (iii) its actions are erased after the vessel has been repaired. To meet these ends, this system of hemostasis is multifaceted. Roughly outlined, the sequence of hemostatic responses after injury is as follows (Figure 7-2). Immediate vasoconstriction occurs under neuromuscular influence. At the site of injury, blood platelets come in contact with collagen and the basement membrane, whereupon they become sticky, adhere to the collagen and to each other, forming a plug that then seals the injured vessel wall (provided the lesion or "rent" is small). It has been estimated that normal activity results in approximately 100 such rents in the vascular system per day. Platelets next release vasoconstrictive factors and a hormone that stimulates the growth of smooth muscle cells, so that damage to the vascular wall can be repaired. When tissue and platelets are damaged, a cascade of reactions is initiated that leads to blood coagulation, whereby a thrombus (blood clot) is formed consisting of a mesh of platelets with fibrin strands and trapped erythrocytes. That mesh contracts and seals off the damaged blood vessel. After tissue repair, fibrinolytic activity dissolves the clot.

In keeping with the above, the following phases of the blood clotting process will now be expanded:
- Platelet plug formation
- Vasoconstriction

Table 7-2   Ranges of some chemical constituents of blood from mature domestic animals

Constituents	Unit of measurement	Source	Horse	Cow	Sheep	Goat	Pig	Dog	Cat	Chicken
Glucose	mg/dl	P, S, WB	60-110	40-80	40-80	40-75	80-120	70-120	70-120	130-270
				80-120 (calf)	80-120 (lamb)	80-120 (kid)				
Nonprotein nitrogen	mg/dl	P, S, WB	20-40	20-40	20-38	30-44	20-45	17-38		20-35
Urea nitrogen (BUN)	mg/dl	P, S, WB	10-24	10-30	8-20	10-28	8-24	10-30	10-30	0.4-1.0
Uric acid	mg/dl	WB	0.5-1	0.1-2	0.1-2	0.3-1	0.1-2	0.1-1.5	0.2-2.5	1-2
										1-7
										(laying hen)
Creatinine	mg/dl	P, S, WB	1-2	1-2	1-2	1-2	1-2.5	1-2	0.8-2	1-2
Amino acid nitrogen	mg/dl	WB	5-7	4-8	5-8		6-8	7-8		4-10
Lactic acid	mg/dl	WB	10-16	5-20	9-12			8-20		47-56
										20-98
										(laying hen)
Cholesterol	mg/dl	P, S, WB	75-150	80-180	60-150	80-160	60-200	120-250	80-180	125-200
Bilirubin										
Direct	mg/dl	P, S, WB	-0.4	-0.3	-0.3		0-0.3	0.06-0.1	0.05-0.1	
Indirect	mg/dl	P, S, WB	0.2-5	0.1-0.5	0-0.1		0-0.3	0.01-0.5	0.15-0.3	
Total	mg/dl	P, S, WB	0.2-6	0.2-1.5	0.1-0.4		0-0.6	0.1-0.6	0.2-0.6	
Sodium	mEq/L	P, S	132-152	132-152	139-152	142-155	135-150	141-155	142-158	151-161
Potassium	mEq/L	P, S	2.5-5.0	3.9-5.8	3.9-5.4	3.5-6.7	4.4-6.7	3.7-5.8	3.4-5.4	4.6-4.7
Calcium	mEq/L	P, S	4.5-6.5	4.5-6.0	4.5-6.0	4.5-6.0	4.5-6.5	4.5-6.0	4.5-6.0	4.5-6.0
										8.5-19.5
										(laying hen)
Phosphorus	mEq/L	P, S	2-6	2-7	2-7	2-6	3-6	2-6	4-7	3-6
Magnesium	mEq/L	P, S	1.5-2.5	1.5-2.5	1.8-2.3	2-3	2-3	1.5-2.0	1.6-2.5	
Chlorine	mEq/L	P, S	99-109	97-111	95-105	99-110	94-106	100-115	117-123	119-130

P, plasma; S, serum; WB, whole blood.
Reproduced, with permission, from Swenson MJ, editor: Dukes' physiology of domestic animals, ed 10, 34, Ithaca, 1984, Cornell University Press.

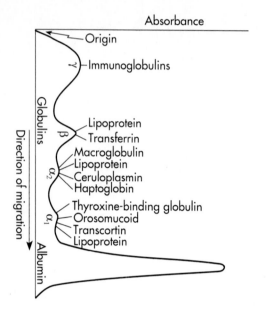

Figure 7-1. Light absorbance tracing of human serum proteins separated by electrophoresis.

- Blood clotting and fibrous organization of the blood clot
- Lysis of the blood clot

Platelets

Platelets (or thrombocytes) are nonpigmented, enucleated cell fragments derived from megakaryocytes of bone marrow (Figure 7-3). They occur in blood in concentrations of 200,000 to 400,000 per mm³. Lack of platelets (thrombocytopenia) prolongs bleeding time, and may abolish blood clotting. Causes include certain drugs, ionizing radiation, infections, anemia, and leukemia.

Platelets must be activated to participate in coagulation. This happens by adhesion of platelets to exposed subendothelial collagen, by tissue factor, or by thrombin. Activated platelets then secrete the vasoconstrictor thromboxane A_2 and ADP that activate additional platelets to bind to the adherent platelet monolayer. The result is a plug. Other factors released by activated platelets include platelet-derived growth factor (PDGF) that induces cell replication in vitro for vascular repair, and platelet factor IV, which inhibits angiogenesis and is a strong chemotactic agent for neutrophils and monocytes; this attracts anti-inflammatory cells to the site of injury.

In contrast to platelet-derived thromboxanes, prostacyclins (formed and released into blood by endothelial cells of the artery wall and also produced in the lungs) inhibit platelet aggregation. Under normal circumstances, the production of prostacyclin is sufficient to override the effect of thromboxanes so that there is no significant aggregation. However, damage to the arterial wall reduces the rate of prostacyclin synthesis and release, so that the effect of thromboxane predominates (thus causing platelet aggregation and initiation of clotting). The presence of an atherosclerotic plaque on the intima of an arterial vessel could similarly reduce the rate of production and release of prostacyclin from the arterial wall, thereby increasing the chance of thrombus formation in an otherwise undamaged artery (with possibly fatal consequences).

In addition to all of these functions, platelets are the source of blood clotting factor XIII, and they are the site of activation of clotting factors, since they provide the surface phospholipids to which these factors bind.

Vasoconstriction

Reflex vasoconstriction is caused by trauma to the vascular wall. Subsequently, there is compression of vessels by clotted blood. Activated platelets release serotonin and thromboxanes, which are powerful vasoconstrictors.

Intrinsic and extrinsic cascades of blood coagulation

Damage to a blood vessel, as caused by contact with a foreign substance, is met by an intrinsic pathway of blood clotting, whereas tissue damage evokes an extrinsic pathway of blood clot formation. Intrinsic and extrinsic cascades of hemostasis (Figure 7-4) differ in that the former exclusively requires circulating factors, whereas the latter also involves tissue factors. The final steps are the same in both pathways: prothrombin activator is produced, transforming inactive prothrombin into thrombin, which then converts fibrinogen (soluble) to fibrin (insoluble).

Circulating factors

Circulating factors are inactive until events that stimulate clotting are triggered. Then activation occurs by various mechanisms:

- A zymogen of a proteolytic enzyme is activated, the product of which, in turn, activates another zymogen by proteolytic action; ultimately, pro-

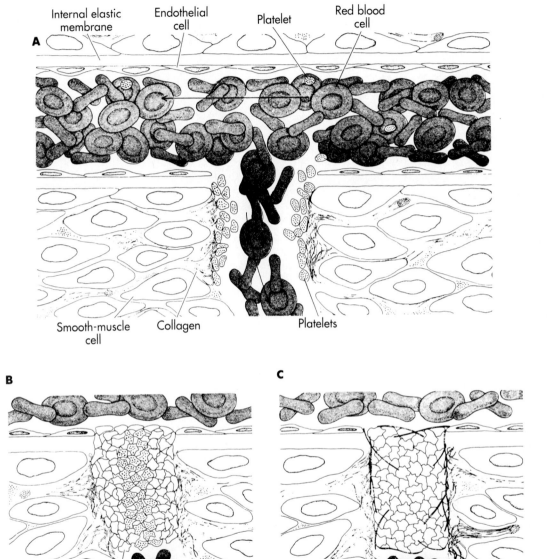

Figure 7-2. Role of platelets in hemostasis. As blood begins to flow out through a cut in the vessel wall, platelets adhere to collagen in the wall, **A.** The platelets are stimulated to secrete the contents of their granules, including ADP, and other passing platelets adhere to the first layer, building up a loose plug in the wounded channel, **B.** Changes in the platelets and contact of blood with damaged cells convert the plasma protein prothrombin into the enzyme thrombin. The thrombin in turn converts fibrinogen into fibrin strands, which reinforce the platelet plug, and it also causes platelets to pack together more closely, **C.** *Reproduced with permission from Zucker MB: The functioning of blood platelets, Sci Am 242:86-103, 1980.*

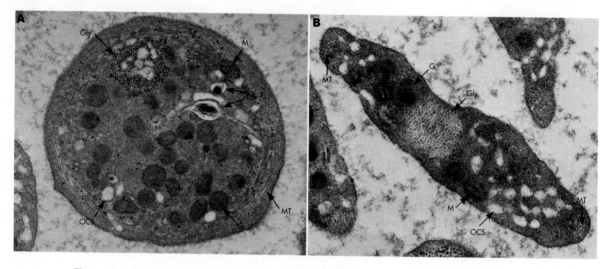

Figure 7-3. Blood platelets. Electron photomicrographs of two sections in different planes of the platelets. Microtubules *(MT)* form a rigid, disc-shaped frame around the platelet's periphery. Some of the open vesicles form a surface-connected canalicular system *(OCS)*. Numerous mitochondria *(M)* and glycogen granules *(Gly)* are present for energy provision. The dense granules *(DB)* and alpha granules *(G)* contain various substances that are secreted when platelets are stimulated and that promote the formation of platelet plugs. *Courtesy Dr. James G. White of the University of Minnesota Medical School.*

teolysis of fibrinogen yields fibrin.

- Platelets are activated.
- Proteolytic activation of some factors generates accessory factors that enhance the rates of proteolytic activation of other factors. Three kinds of accessory factors operate in these cascades: Ca^{++} ions; acidic phospholipids derived from the membrane bilayers of platelets or damaged tissues; and protein cofactors specifically required for activation of given zymogens; for example, the protein cofactor for activation of prothrombin is factor Va (see Figure 7-4).

Activated factors are designated by an "a" behind their Roman numeral. The various blood coagulation factors and their functions are listed in numerical order (Table 7-3).

Initial activation of the intrinsic pathway: contact stage

The intrinsic pathway is initiated when blood comes in contact with a foreign surface, such as a damaged vessel wall. Four factors are involved in the contact stage of clotting (see Figure 7-4): factor XII, prekallikrein, factor XI (each of which is a zymogen of a serum protease), and high–molecular-weight ki-

ninogen (HMwK), a precursor of bradykinin that also serves as an accessory factor. Bradykinin's vasodilator activity lowers blood pressure.

Factor XII becomes the protease XIIa when adsorbed to collagen or platelet membranes. Factor XIIa then converts prekallikrein to kallikrein, which in turn activates additional factor XII. This is a cyclical process called **reciprocal activation,** an autocatalytic process. Factor XIIa so produced activates factor XI, the next step in the cascade, a process that also requires HMwK as an accessory factor.

Initial activation of the extrinsic pathway

Upon tissue damage, factor VII and tissue factor (also referred to as factor III or thromboplastin) take part in the initiation of hemostasis (see Figure 7-4). Clotting is more rapid when initiated by the extrinsic rather than the intrinsic pathway.

Activation of factor X is much like prothrombin activation: Ca^{++} and phospholipid are required; the protease involved is factor VIIa, and the accessory protein is thromboplastin. Upon tissue damage, thromboplastin and phospholipids are released, enhancing the activity of factor VII, which forms small amounts of factor Xa, leading to the formation of

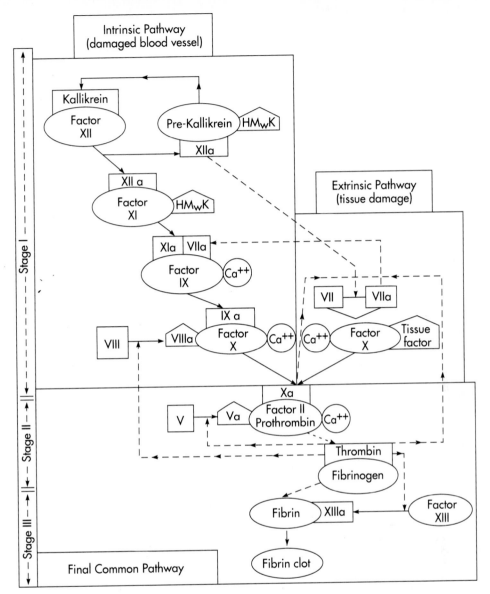

Figure 7-4. Intrinsic, extrinsic, and final common pathway of coagulation of human blood. The intrinsic pathway, initiated by damage to blood vessels in contact with foreign substances, involves components normally present in the circulation. The extrinsic pathway, activated by tissue damage, requires a tissue factor in addition to blood components. Activation of the pathways leads to the formation of prothrombin activator (Factor Xa) at the end of stage I, and then to thrombin during stage II. Thrombin cleaves fibrinogen, yielding fibrin monomers that polymerize and cross-bridge, under influence of thrombin-activated factor XIII, to form the clot (stage III). Propagation of the coagulation process occurs along the paths shown by the *solid arrows* linking clotting factors (ovals) listed by number in Table 7-3. The circulating clotting factors, which are zymogens, are converted to activated factors (indicated by the suffix 'a'; rectangles) which are proteases. Nonenzymatic protein cofactors (HMwK, VIIIa, Va, and tissue factor; pentagons), Ca^{++} *(circles)*, and in many cases a phospholipid surface are required at several stages of the cascade. *Dashed lines* indicate feedback loops whereby activated clotting factors affect other components of the cascade, as well as crossover reactions that link intrinsic and extrinsic pathways. *HMwK,* High-Molecular-weight Kininogen. *Adapted and reproduced with permission from Jackson CM and Nemerson Y: Blood coagulation, Ann Rev Biochem 49:765-811, 1980.*

Table 7-3	Human blood coagulation factors
Factor number and names*	**Function and characteristics**
I **Fibrinogen**	Soluble protein that, after proteolysis by thrombin, polymerizes to form the fibrin clot
II **Prothrombin**	Circulating zymogen transformed by factor Xa to thrombin, which converts fibrinogen to fibrin and activates factors V, VII, VIII, XIII, and XIV
III **Thromboplastin; tissue factor**	Accessory factor released from damaged tissue; Requires phospholipid for coagulation via extrinsic system
IV **Calcium ion**	Ion that bridges vitamin K–dependent clotting factors to membrane phospholipids; stabilizes fibrinogen, factor V, and other proteins; required to activate factor XIII
V **Proaccelerin**	Accessory plasma protein that, when activated by thrombin, accelerates prothrombin activation by factor Xa. Since factor Va was once called VI, currently there is no factor VI
VII **Proconvertin**	Precursor of the protease that activates factor X in the extrinsic pathway
VIII **Antihemophilic factor; von Willebrand factor**	Accessory plasma protein that, when activated, enhances factor X activation by factor IXa in the intrinsic pathway
IX **Chistmas factor**	Circulating zymogen that, when activated by factors XIa and VIIa, yields the protease that activates factor X in the intrinsic pathway
X **Stuart factor**	Circulating zymogen that, on activation by factor IXa, yields the protease that converts prothrombin to thrombin
XI **Plasma thromboplastin antecedent**	Circulating precursor of the protease that activates factor IX
XII **Hageman factor**	Circulating zymogen that, when activated by surface contact or the kallikrein system in the contact phase of the intrinsic pathway, enhances the activation of factor XI
XIII **Fibrin-stabilizing factor**	Circulating zymogen of transglutaminase that cross-links monomeric fibrin strands to form a hard clot; activated by thrombin
XIV **Protein C**	Circulating zymogen that, when activated by thrombin, yields a protease that inactivates factors V and VIII
Prekallikrein	Precursor of kallikrein that proteolytically activates factor XII in the contact stage of the intrinsic path
High–molecular-weight kininogen (HMwK)	Accessory factor for the activations of factors XI and XII; cleavage of HMwK by kallikrein yields bradykinin
Plasminogen	Circulating zymogen that, when activated by tissue activators, yields the protease plasmin that degrades fibrin after clot formation

*Names or numbers by which factors are commonly referred are printed in bold type. Modified and reproduced, with permission, from Jackson CM and Nemerson Y: Blood coagulation, *Ann Rev Biochem* 49:765-811, 1980.

some thrombin, which then converts more of factor VII to VIIa.

Amplification of initial signal

From only a very small amount of active protease (factor XIIa) formed at the initial stage of the cascade, hundreds of molecules of factor XI are formed in subsequent stages that, in turn, generate thousands of molecules of activated factor IX. An initially modest signal thus "snowballs" into a veritable "avalanche."

Concentrations of clotting factors in plasma reflect the quantities needed for triggering the next step in the cascade: concentrations of factors VII, V, II, and fibrinogen are about 0.015, 0.9, 12, and 360 mg/dl, respectively.

Retraction of the fibrin clot

Factor XIII, of platelet origin, is activated by thrombin. Factor XIIIa, being a transglutaminase, cross-links monomeric fibrin strands by connecting lysine and glutamine residues on different molecules (Figure 7-5). As a result, the fibrin clot hardens and becomes an effective seal of the damaged capillary.

Vitamin K and Ca^{++} requirements

Formation of thrombin and the active forms of factors IX and X require adequate intake of vitamin K and Ca^{++}. Vitamin K is an essential cofactor for a carboxylase, located on the lumenal side of the rough ER of liver cells, that posttranslationally carboxylates glutamyl residues in some of the newly-synthesized clotting factors. This generates γ-carbox-yglutamate (Figure 7-6), several of which are found in clusters in the vitamin K–dependent clotting factors. In human prothrombin there is a sequence of 27 amino acids, 10 of which are γ-carboxyglutamate.

Antimetabolites of vitamin K, such as dicumarol (Figure 7-7), inhibit the synthesis of the clotting factors. In dicumarol-fed animals there is simply glutamate instead of γ-carboxyglutamate. Dicumarol was first identified in spoiled sweet clover hay as the causative agent of a hemorrhagic disease in cattle. Pres-

ently it is used as rat poison; it is also used therapeutically to reduce clot-forming tendencies in individuals faced with the threat of thrombosis.

There are two adjacent carboxyl groups that form a Ca^{++}-binding site; hence, there are 10 calcium ions bound to prothrombin's 10 γ-carboxyglutamates. To demonstrate the function of Ca^{++} binding to clotting factors and the involvement of various accessory factors (phospholipids and factors Va and Xa), the conversion of prothrombin to thrombin is shown (Figure 7-8).

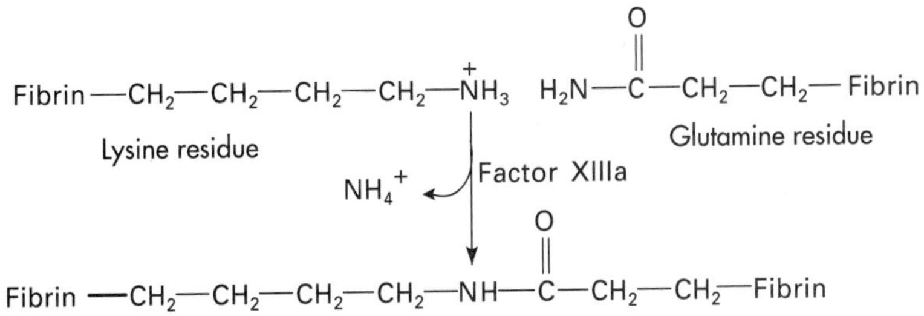

Figure 7-5. Hard clot formation by transglutaminase activity of factor XIIIa.

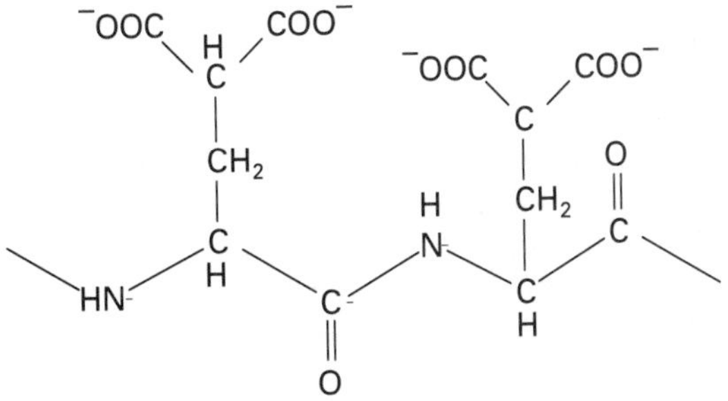

Figure 7-6. γ-Carboxyglutamate.

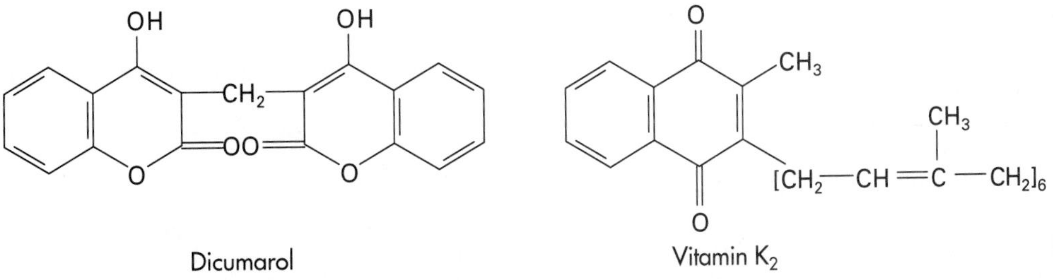

Dicumarol

Vitamin K_2

Figure 7-7. Similarity in structures of dicumarol and vitamin K.

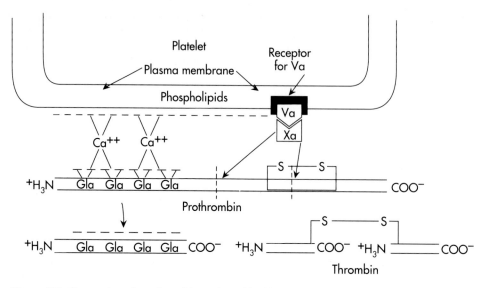

Figure 7-8. Conversion of prothrombin to thrombin. Note the involvement of accessory factors of the coagulation cascade. The many molecules of γ-carboxyglutamate *(Gla)* on prothrombin and the anionic phospholipids on the plasma membrane are linked by Ca^{++} ions; rupturing of platelets causes activation of factor V in platelets; factor Va attaches to receptors on the plasma membrane and functions in turn as a receptor that concentrates factor Xa, a protease that attacks the prothrombin peptide chain in two places to produce a molecule of active thrombin.

Control of the cascades of coagulation

Not only must the rate and extent of hemostasis in response to injury be controlled, but there must also be controls that safeguard against random clot formation.

- Concentrations of activated clotting factors (ACFs) greatly decrease by dilution in flowing blood. ACFs are only active on the relatively stagnant venous side of the microcirculation. The relative concentrations of ACFs are important (see above).
- Inhibitors to activated clotting factors exist; for example, antithrombin-III in plasma (see below). ACFs are labile and thus their time of action is limited, and are rapidly removed from the blood by the liver, in contrast to their zymogens. Especially short are the half-lives of factors VIIIa and Va. Factor Va, which is generated by thrombin, is also subsequently inactivated (lysed) by thrombin.
- Several ACFs activate or inhibit other clotting factors. Thus, thrombin activates factors V, VII, and XIII to enhance coagulation, but thrombin activation of protein C results in degradation of factors Va and VIIIa, thereby diminishing the

rate of coagulation and preventing the formation of excessive clotting, particularly outside of the immediate site of the thrombus.
- Thrombin and platelets are trapped in the fibrin mesh of a clot, so that their concentrations diminish.

Fibrinolysis

Fibrinolysis, dissolution the fibrin clot, occurs within a few days after clot formation. It serves to reopen clotted capillary vessels after tissue repair, and also to remove minor clots from terminal capillaries.

The fibrinolytic system (Figure 7-9) is composed of plasminogen, plasmin, plasminogen activators, and α_2-antiplasmin. Fibrinolysis results from activation of the plasma protein plasminogen, a zymogen of the protease plasmin, by tissue plasminogen activators. α_2-Antiplasmin is a plasma protein that specifically inhibits plasmin and aids in regulating its action.

Human plasminogen is made in the kidney. Various tissues have different plasminogen activators. A potent activator of plasminogen, made in the kidney and found in urine, is urokinase. Streptokinase, a protein from β-hemolytic streptococci, is another plasminogen activator.

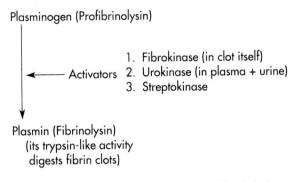

Figure 7-9. Fibrinolysis (dissolving the blood clot).

Urokinase and streptokinase are used clinically, by their application via arterial catheters, to dissolve coronary occlusions in the heart.

Anticoagulants

Anticoagulants prevent hemostasis by interfering with the enzymes or accessory factors involved in the cascade of blood coagulation. Some anticoagulants, used in vitro, remove Ca^{++} ions, which are essential in many steps of the cascade. Oxalate and fluoride bind Ca^{++} tightly, as do cation exchange resins, such as ethylenediaminetetraacetic acid (EDTA) or the more Ca^{++}-specific ethyleneglycol-bis(β-aminoethylether)-N, N'-tetraacetic acid (EGTA). Fluoride, in addition to binding Ca^{++}, stops glycolysis, which is useful if blood glucose levels are to be determined. But oxalate, fluoride, and EGTA are toxic. On the other hand, citrate, which also binds Ca^{++}, is nontoxic; thus, it permits large-scale preservation of blood for perfusion.

Heparin is an important anticoagulant in the body. It acts in conjunction with the plasma protein antithrombin-III to inhibit several of the proteases in the coagulation cascade, including factors IIa, IXa, Xa, XIIa, and kallikrein. The action of heparin is catalytic: when heparin is released from mast cells (which line the endothelium of blood vessels) or is injected, it complexes with antithrombin-III and that complex binds to, and inhibits, one of the proteases involved in coagulation. Then heparin is released from the protease–antithrombin-III complex and is ready for another round of protease inhibition. Heparin is fast-acting and is therefore used during and after surgery, and for obtaining blood plasma. Dicumarol establishes a long-term reduction of clotting tendency by inhibiting hepatic synthesis of clotting factors.

Human protein C exerts its anticoagulant activity as a zymogen of a serum protease that, upon activation, rapidly proteolyzes the activated forms of accessory proteins, especially factors Va and VIIIa.

Causes of thromboembolic conditions

A **thrombus** is defined as an abnormal clot in a blood vessel; an **embolus** is a free flowing clot that may get lodged somewhere.

When the endothelial surface of blood vessels is damaged, smooth muscle cells migrate through the internal elastic membrane and proliferate, aided by a platelet-derived growth factor; foam cells are formed, which may become infiltrated with lipids, giving rise to atherosclerotic plaques that occlude the vascular lumen. Original damage to the intima may be caused by cholesterol, carbon monoxide, cigarette smoke, fats, or epinephrine (a stress-related hormone). As discussed above, atherosclerotic lesions block the normal rate of production and release of prostacyclins from the arterial wall (natural inhibitors of platelet aggregation), thus increasing the risk of thrombus formation in an otherwise undamaged artery.

Slow blood flow caused by prolonged recumbency or occlusion may result in intravenous clotting. Under normal conditions, there is a dynamic equilibrium between clot formation and lysis. Antithrombin-III in plasma, activated by heparin, dissolves and prevents small clots. Therefore, patients with deficiency of antithrombin-III (generally inherited) have many diffuse microclots; pulmonary embolism may result. Disseminated intravascular clotting, which may be caused by bacterial endotoxins, can lead to shock.

Conditions causing excessive bleeding

Excessive bleeding occurs in the following cases:
- Vitamin K deficiency contributes to excessive bleeding, because vitamin K is needed for hepatic synthesis of prothrombin and factors V, VII, IX, and X. Inadvertent dicumarol poisoning is a rare event.
- Hepatitis or cirrhosis inhibits synthesis of clotting factors.
- Hemophilia is a hereditary deficiency of coagulation (once prevalent in European royalty). The most common cause is deficiency of factor VIII (over 85% of all cases) or factor IX. Blood transfusions may be given, but platelets from donors are easily rejected. Biosynthesized factor VIII is now available. More rarely, other coagulation factors are lacking, such as Stuart, Christmas,

or Hageman factors.

- Thrombocytopenia, having fewer than 50,000 platelets per mm³ of blood, causes internal bleeding from capillaries. This condition may result from damaging bone marrow (e.g., by irradiation, drug sensitivity, or autoimmune disorders).

THE ERYTHROCYTE

The erythrocyte, or red blood cell (RBC), functions in the transport of gases that have limited water solubility. Erythrocytes carry oxygen from the lungs to tissues and are involved in the isohydric transport of metabolic CO_2 from tissues to the lungs.

The mammalian erythrocyte is a highly specialized cell. Hemoglobin, which constitutes about one third of the cell's weight, contributes the red color and gas-carrying capacity to the erythrocyte. The lack of a nucleus, mitochondria, lysosomes, endoplasmic reticulum, and Golgi have profound metabolic consequences for the mature RBC. For instance, it cannot synthesize nucleic acids or proteins, nor can it combust fat for energy. Therefore, the erythrocyte depends on glucose as its nutrient to maintain ion pumps in its plasma membrane, cytoskeleton integrity (and therewith its cell shape), and functional hemoglobin.

Human erythrocytes have a 120-day lifetime in which they travel 175 miles through the circulation; that life span varies among domestic animal species from 65 days in pigs to 150 days in horses. As erythrocytes age, they are removed from the circulation by cells of the reticuloendothelial system, predominantly by macrophages in the spleen. Hemoglobin is degraded into its constituent protein (globin), heme, and iron. Globin is hydrolyzed, and its amino acids are reused for protein synthesis. Iron is transported to bone marrow and liver, and reutilized for heme synthesis. Heme is degraded to bilirubin and excreted in bile. To balance this erythrocyte degradation, there is a constant need for hematopoiesis, the production of erythrocytes in bone marrow.

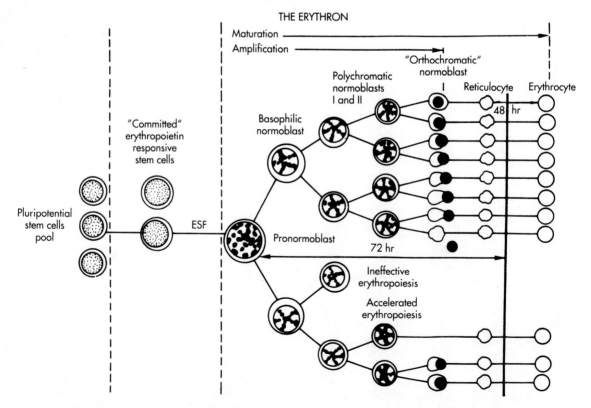

Figure 7-10. Formation of red blood cells. *Reproduced with permission from Williams WJ, Beutler E, Erslev AJ, and Rundles RW: Hematology, p 104, New York, 1977, McGraw-Hill.*

Development of erythrocytes

Several steps are involved during the maturation of precursor cells in bone marrow to circulating red blood cells (Figure 7-10).

- Stem cells are pluripotent; depending on the stimulating factor, stem cells may differentiate into erythroid (RBC), lymphoid (white blood cells), or megakaryocytic (platelets) cells.
- Erythropoietin is a hematopoietic hormone synthesized in the kidney. Its level in blood responds to a need for RBC formation, increasing greatly under conditions of hypoxemia (e.g., high altitude).
- Stimulated by erythropoietin, the stem cell forms a pronormoblast whose nucleus occupies about 80% of the cell space. After four mitotic divisions, normoblasts are formed (up to 16), and about 80% of the hemoglobin of red blood cells is produced at this stage. The normoblasts then expel their nuclei and become enucleated reticulocytes ("immature red blood cells"), which are released into the circulation and mature into erythrocytes. Maturation requires 1 to 2 days, during which the subcellular organelles decrease in size and are expelled from the cells; some reticulocyte enzymes remain in RBCs, but they are not functional.
- The capacity of hematopoiesis in an adult human is about 2.3×10^{6} cells per second. This rate of synthesis sustains a body total of about 2.3×10^{13} erythrocytes (2.5 to 3 kg). The number of reticulocytes in circulation is elevated when increased demands are made on hematopoiesis; for instance, after a hemorrhage or at high altitude.

Erythrocyte structure and composition

In humans, erythrocytes appear as biconcave disks (resembling doughnuts with their center hole not quite punched out) to increase surface area for gas exchange. Many animals have erythrocytes with a similar shape, but sizes vary greatly.

The composition of red cells (compared with that of serum) is shown in the form of Gamblegrams (Figure 7-11).

- The total number of acid-base equivalents in cells is greater than that in serum. Distribution can be predicted on the basis of Donnan equilibria when the higher intracellular protein content is taken into account.
- K^+ is the major cellular cation.

- The high 2,3-diphosphoglycerate content is specific for RBCs. It functions in the control of unloading O_2 bound to hemoglobin.
- The nonsignificant intracellular Ca^{++} level is due to a special Ca^{++}/Mg^{++} ATPase pump in the plasma membrane.

Swelling, hemolysis, and crenation of RBCs in response to medium tonicity was discussed earlier. After hemolysis, what remain are the insoluble plasma membranes and adhering proteins: "ghosts."

In addition to the Ca^{++} pump, the erythrocyte membrane has the Na^+ pump (Na^+/K^+ ATPase). Aging of the cell is accompanied by loss of functioning of both pumps, raising intracellular Na^+ and Ca^{++}, thereby inhibiting K^+-dependent enzyme activities (kinases) and decreasing stability of the cytoskeleton. The resulting cellular rigidity leads to cell destruction. Since cells no longer deform (required for passage through narrow capillaries), they get stuck and are phagocytosed by reticuloendothelial cells.

The cytoskeleton of the erythrocyte (Figure 7-12) consists of a two-dimensional net of actin and spectrin in a plane that runs parallel to the membrane. The third dimension of the cytoskeleton is provided by ankrin, which connects the two-dimensional net to

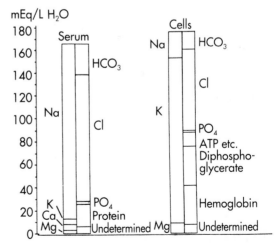

Figure 7-11. Comparing serum and erythrocyte composition. Presenting anions and cations of a fluid as bars of equal height but different composition yields Gamblegrams, named after the scientist who introduced the law of electroneutrality. *Reproduced with permission from Guest GM: Organic phosphates of the blood and mineral metabolism in diabetic acidosis, Am J Dis Child 64:401-412, 1942, American Medical Association.*

the integral membrane protein glycophorin (electrophoretically defined as band 3). The cytoskeleton determines the shape and deformability of the erythrocyte, and thereby its life span.

Blood-group antigens

Antigenic determinants (blood-group substances) are located on the cell surface of RBCs. These antigens are recognized by specific antibodies, which are thus able to agglutinate cells containing that antigen.

Fourteen human blood-group systems have been defined, comprising over 100 different blood-group antigens. All of these are genetically inherited. Knowledge of them is useful in determining familial relationship and for safety in blood transfusions.

Blood-group substances are found not only on erythrocytes but also in fluids, such as saliva, milk, gastric juice, urine, and seminal and ovarian cyst fluids.

The chemical nature of the oligosaccharide chains conjugated to membrane proteins defines blood groups A, B, AB, and O. Other such systems exist; for instance, Rh factors. The Lewis antigens (Le^a and Le^b) differ from A, B, and O antigens in that they are not synthesized in developing erythrocyte plasma membranes but are adsorbed from plasma lipoproteins onto adult cells.

The important blood group systems of domestic animal species are listed in Table 7-4. All blood-group

Table 7-4	Important blood group systems of domestic animals	
Species	**Blood group**
Dog	DEA 1.1, DEA 1.2, DEA 7
Cat	A, B
Horse	A, C, Q
Cattle	B, J
Sheep	B, R
Pigs	A, E

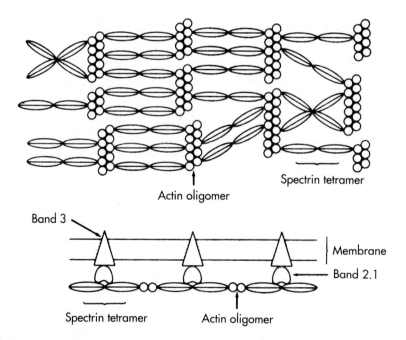

Figure 7-12. Cytoskeleton of a human erythrocyte. *Reproduced with permission from Brenner SL and Korn ED: Spectrin/actin complex isolated from sheep erythrocytes accelerates actin polymerization of simple nucleation, J Biol Chem 255:1670-1678, 1980.*

antigens described in domestic animals are inherited autosomally, and some are formed in nonerythroid tissues secreted into the blood and absorbed passively onto erythrocytes (e.g., dogs, DEA7; sheep, R; and cattle, J).

Metabolism of the erythrocyte

Those students without background in intermediary metabolism may want to skip this section and return to it after the functions, pathways, and enzymes of glycolysis (Embden-Meyerhof) and the pentose shunt have been discussed in their context of overall glucose metabolism.

The absence of mitochondria in erythrorytes implies that oxygen cannot be used to accept metabolic electrons; rather anaerobic shuttling of those electrons is needed. This rules out fats, ketones, and amino acids as sources of energy, since no anaerobic pathways for their catabolism exist. The RBC thus depends on glucose to meet its energy needs and to sustain its metabolic functions. Glucose enters erythrocytes by way of diffusion, facilitated by a specific transmembrane transporter. Glucose metabolism via glycolysis and the pentose shunt (Figure 7-13) provides energy in the form of ATP and reducing power in the forms of NADH and NADPH.

Energy produced in the erythrocyte functions for the following reasons:

- To maintain high K^+, low Na^+, and low Ca^{++} with pumps requiring ATP, so that the integrity of the cell membrane and cytoskeleton and the activities of enzymes are preserved;
- To maintain the iron of hemoglobin in the Fe^{++} oxidation state; methemoglobin, containing Fe^{+++}, is inactive as an oxygen carrier, and, thus, must be reduced; NADH and NADPH are involved here;
- To generate reduced glutathione, which has antioxidant activity; again, NADPH is involved;
- To generate 2,3-diphosphoglycerate, which controls dissociation of hemoglobin-bound oxygen in tissues.

For a steady supply of ATP via glycolysis, NAD^+ must be continuously provided to the glyceraldehyde phosphate dehydrogenase reaction (see Figure 7-13). The regeneration of NAD^+ requires that the electrons of NADH be spent. Part of it occurs by reduction of methemoglobin, and the remainder by reducing pyruvate to lactate, which is therefore the chief end product of red blood cell metabolism. Lactate is discharged into the bloodstream and converted in the

liver to glucose, so that it can continue serving RBC metabolism.

Rather than going into more detail on the common metabolic pathways of glycolysis, the text concentrates on those aspects of metabolism that are characteristic of the erythrocyte (see Figure 7-13, shaded areas).

Methemoglobin ($metHbFe^{3+}$) is constantly being formed at a slow rate by the autoxidation of hemoglobin, as is shown in the following equation. (Larger amounts of methemoglobin are formed by ingestion or inhalation of toxic substances, e.g., nitrites, tobacco smoke.)

$$HbFe^{2+} + O_2 \leftrightarrow HbFe^{2+}-O_2 \leftrightarrow metHbFe^{3+} + O_2^-$$

The O_2^- free radical is converted to H_2O_2 and O_2 by a superoxide dismutase. The formation of $metHbFe^{3+}$ is balanced by reduction back to functional $HbFe^{2+}$ under the influence of methemoglobin reductase; this enzyme uses NADH produced by glycolysis and cytochrome b_5. The toxic hydrogen peroxide formed in the autoxidation above is inactivated by reduced glutathione (GSH) under the influence of glutathione peroxidase:

$$2 \, GSH + H_2O_2 \leftrightarrow GSSG + 2 \, H_2O.$$

This vitally important enzyme contains selenium, a mineral that is essential in the diet. Catalyzed by glutathione reductase, oxidized glutathione (GSSG) is reduced back to GSH, a reaction for which the necessary electrons are obtained from the pentose shunt and shuttled by NADPH.

Formation of 2,3-diphosphoglycerate (by a mutase enzyme) competes with the formation of 3-P-glycerate (by a phosphatase enzyme) as both enzymes work on the same substrate, 1,3-diphosphoglycerate. A rise in pH favors the mutase conversion. This stands to reason, for conditions that lower O_2 tension (e.g., high altitude) tend to raise pH, thereby increasing formation of 2,3-diphosphoglycerate and favorably shifting the O_2-hemoglobin dissociation curve to the right. Conversely, a fall in pH inhibits the mutase and stimulates phosphatase.

Demise of the red blood cell

Several factors may lead to the recognition of senile erythrocytes and their removal from the circulation (in humans, about 120 days after they emerge from bone marrow). In RBCs, the key enzyme whose ac-

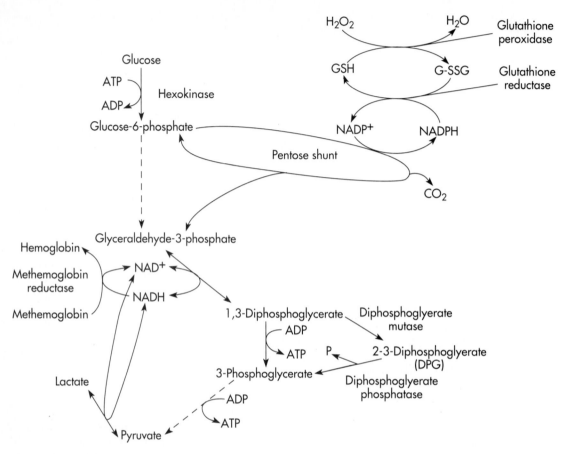

Figure 7-13. Glucose metabolism in erythrocytes. Reduction of methemoglobin, detoxification of H_2O_2, and formation of 2,3-diphosphoglycerate are highlighted.

tivity fades with age is hexokinase. A result of the senility of hexokinase is the loss of the cell's capacity to utilize glucose. Next the Na^+ and Ca^{++} ATPase pumps expire; then the cytoskeleton becomes rigid and, thus, RBCs get stuck in narrow vessels (especially the spleen and liver) and are phagocytosed by reticuloendothelial (RE) cells. Other age-related changes occur in the composition of glycoproteins and glycolipids, which attract senile RBCs to lectins on membranes of RE cells.

Hemoglobin is catabolized in the RE cells, where the protein portion, globin, is cleaved off, hydrolyzed, and exported as amino acids for reutilization in the body, while the heme portion is digested (Figure 7-14). Iron is exported (bound to transferrin in plasma) toward bone marrow (for new erythropoiesis) and other tissues (e.g., liver) for storage. Heme is oxidized

to biliverdin (a green pigment found, for instance, in bile of snakes and birds), whereby the porphyrin ring is opened up and carbon monoxide is formed (Figure 7-15). This highly toxic CO binds to hemoglobin and is expired through the lungs. Biliverdin is reduced to bilirubin and then, bound to albumin, transported to the liver. The liver takes up bilirubin by way of a specific transport system, conjugates it with glucuronic acid, and excretes it into bile (causing bile's orange color). In the gut, bacterial degradation of bilirubin produces a variety of colored and colorless tetrapyrroles (e.g., urobilin and stercobilin), small amounts of which are recycled to the liver prior to excretion in the feces and urine, contributing to their characteristic colors.

Clearing the blood of bilirubin is one of the normal liver functions. Failure of it to do so results in jaun-

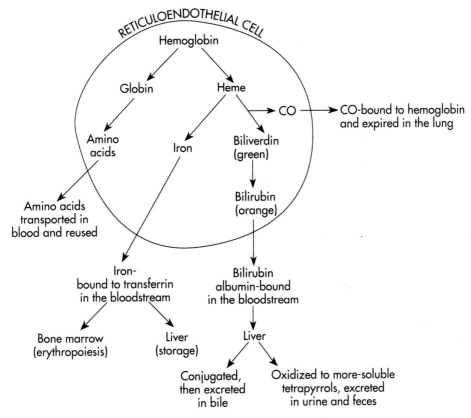

Figure 7-14. Breakdown of hemoglobin by reticuloendothelial (RE) cells; the subsequent metabolic fates of the degradation products are outlined.

dice, when a high bilirubin level in plasma imparts yellow color to skin, gums, and the white of the eyes. Such may occur under conditions of overproduction of bilirubin, for instance, in a hemolytic crisis, or when the liver doesn't function properly, as may be caused by trauma, intoxication, biliary obstruction, or hepatitis. In newborns of many species, especially in premature births, conjugation of bilirubin with glucuronic acid in the liver, and thus biliary excretion, is slow to develop. The resulting hyperbilirubinemia, neonatal jaundice, may require treatment (exposure to strong light to degrade bilirubin in blood, or blood transfusion) to avoid bilirubin accumulation in brain tissue and its dire consequences (kernicterus).

Iron metabolism

The functions of iron can be correlated best with its distribution in different body compartments. The human body contains approximately 4g of iron, of which some 65% is in the form of hemoglobin and another 10% in myoglobin, compounds involved in oxygen transport in the blood and tissues, respectively. About 20% of the iron is stored as iron-protein complexes (ferritin and hemosiderin) in tissue cells, mostly of the liver, spleen, bone marrow, and gut. Some iron is transported in plasma bound to transferrin. Several enzymes contain a porphyrin (heme) group in their structure, such as catalase, the enzyme that destroys toxic hydrogen peroxide, and the FeS- and cytochrome- or heme-containing enzymes in mitochondria that transport metabolic electrons toward oxygen in the process of oxidative phosphorylation.

To realize the amazing efficiency with which iron is conserved and reused in the body, one must take into account the continuous turnover of all iron-con-

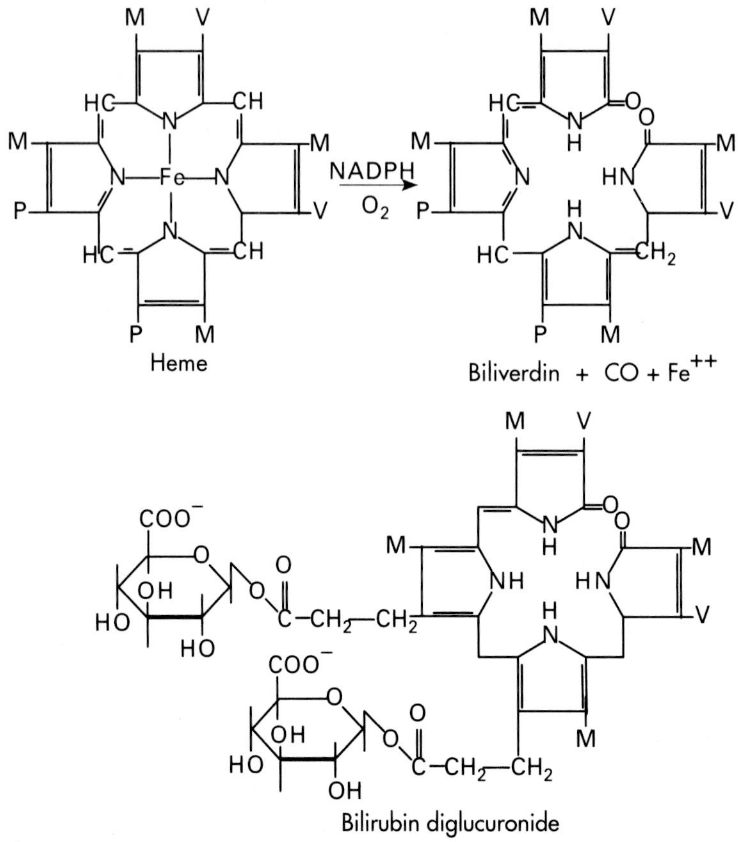

Figure 7-15. Formation of bile pigments from heme. *M,* Methyl, *P,* propionyl, *V,* vinyl groups.

taining structures and combine that with the fact that only about 1 mg of iron per day, absorbed from the gut, is sufficient to offset fecal losses of the body's total iron pool of 4g. Another consideration in iron homeostasis derives from the fact that most iron salts of organic acids are not soluble in the aqueous medium of the body. Iron must therefore be stored and made available in just the proper form and amount when and where it is needed. A synopsis of iron kinetics (Figure 7-16), whereby various iron compartments of the body interchange, requires the following explanation:

Ionized iron exists as ferrous (Fe^{++}) and ferric (Fe^{+++}) compounds. The ferric ion is the one present in the body's iron stores; the ferrous ion is the one that is absorbed from the diet, transported in blood, and used for heme synthesis.

Dietary iron comes in the forms of hemoglobin and myoglobin in meat and in nonheme compounds in fruits and vegetables. In the stomach, most iron complexes (but not heme) are digested by HCl; ferric ions are reduced to ferrous ions by ascorbic acid; and ferrous ions combine with gastroferrin, a mucopolysaccharide, which prevents the formation of insoluble iron salts at the gut's neutral pH. In the small intestines, mucosal cells elaborate transferrin, a protein that, upon binding two ferrous ions, changes its tertiary structure, and is then recognized by receptors on the gut mucosal cells and endocytosed, after which transferrin is released again. The amount of iron thus absorbed from the diet is regulated by the control over transferrin synthesis and released according to the iron needs of the body. For example, transferrin synthesis is up-regulated during growth, lactation, pregnancy, after blood loss, or at high altitude—all re-

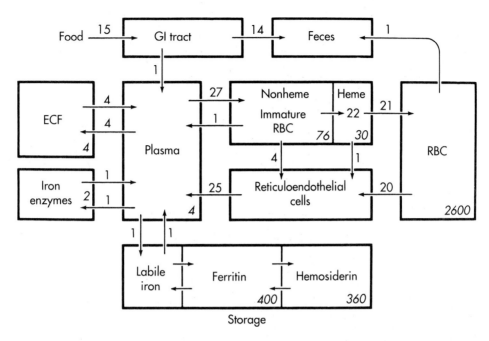

Figure 7-16. Kinetics of normal human iron metabolism. The italic numbers refer to pool sizes of compartments and transfer rates given in mg/day on the arrows. *Reproduced with permission from Pollycove M: Hemochromatosis. In Stanbury JB, Wyngaarden MB, and Fredrickson DS, editors: The metabolic basis of inherited diseases, ed 4, p 1139, New York, 1978, McGraw-Hill.*

quiring increased hemoglobin synthesis. This control mechanism by itself, though useful, is not sufficient for proper iron homeostasis: (i) since it involves protein synthesis, and is located in the gut, this control cannot respond to a rapid change in iron demand at some given site in the body; and (ii) it has no control over the uptake of heme-iron, in which transferrin is not involved. Hence, situations of over- and undersupply of iron from the diet occur. Here, a second control mechanism in the gut mucosal cell comes into play. In response to oversupply, the gut cell stores increased amounts of iron bound to ferritin and, in addition, it down-regulates the intracellular transporter that carries iron from the gut cell into the bloodstream. As gut mucosal cells are sloughed off, this store of excess iron is lost in the feces.

In the bloodstream, transferrin transports iron to cells that store or use it. Vascular endothelial cells adapt their synthesis of transferrin to the iron needs of the body. After receptor-mediated endocytosis of the Fe^{+++}-transferrin complex, transferrin is returned to the circulation. Usually, iron is first stored in the forms of ferritin and hemosiderin, proteins of homologous composition that may store up to one third of their weight in the form of ferric ions. Iron induces synthesis of the protein moiety of ferritin, apoferritin, which acts as ferroxidase, converting incoming ferrous ions to ferric ions that are stored. Stored iron is reduced by a ferrireductase to Fe^{++} in which form it is released as needed. Iron is then transported by an iron-carrying protein to mitochondria for heme synthesis as required for hemoglobin, myoglobin, cytochrome, and other compounds. Alternatively, iron may be released from a storage site (e.g., the liver or spleen) into the bloodstream for use elsewhere (e.g., hematopoiesis in bone marrow).

The major item on the iron budget is the turnover of RBCs. By and large, senescent RBCs are removed from the circulation by mononuclear phagocytes in the liver and spleen; after digestion their iron can be stored. A minor fraction (ca. 10%) of erythrocytes perishes by intravascular hemolysis after getting stuck in the microcirculation. Hemoglobin, combined with haptoglobin, and heme, bound to hemopexin, are then degraded in phagocytic cells and iron is saved.

In newborns, both hematocrit and hemoglobin concentration in erythrocytes exceed those in adults. This probably reflects up-regulation in response to low oxygen tension in the uterus. After birth the rapid destruction of excess erythrocytes and the retention of heme-iron meet iron requirements for months. This is a wise design of nature, for milk contains very little iron.

Nutritional iron requirements are difficult to estimate because of variable iron absorption in the gut. This variation depends on iron metabolism and transport in the mucosa in addition to the "availability" of dietary iron. Iron forms insoluble complexes with many organic compounds; iron may also be unavailable when diets contain high levels of inorganic phosphate. Iron from meat is readily available, since heme compounds are absorbable. Reducing agents, such as ascorbic acid, in the diet increase iron availability (see above). The recommended minimum daily intake of iron is about ten times the amount needed per day for hemoglobin synthesis. Allowances must be made for conditions that require increased hematopoiesis.

Iron deficiency is a common cause of anemia. The opposite condition, iron overload syndrome, or hemochromatosis, may be caused by an inherited dysfunction of the intestinal uptake controls, by chronic oversupply of iron supplements administered either orally or parenterally to remedy anemia, or by a hemolytic condition that leads to increased intestinal iron absorption for the purpose of compensatory erythropoiesis. Iron overload leads to an accumulation of the enlarged iron stores in the form of hemosiderin and to various clinical manifestations (e.g., skin pigmentation; pancreatic damage with diabetes ["bronze diabetes"]; cirrhosis; hepatic carcinoma; gonadal atrophy), some of which may be fatal.

Erythrocyte abnormalities

Anemia is characterized by insufficient numbers of circulating erythrocytes (low hematocrit); abnormal, nonfunctional erythrocytes; and often a below-normal hemoglobin content of erythrocytes or the presence of hemoglobin that has defective oxygen-carrying capacity caused by a genetic mutation. Anemia may be caused by blood loss, increased rate of erythrocyte destruction, or impaired erythropoiesis resulting from an enzyme or dietary deficiency.

A common feature of all forms of hereditary anemias is the production of abnormal erythrocytes that are rapidly removed from the circulation.

- Sickle cell anemia is associated with the formation of abnormal hemoglobins and abnormally shaped (sickle) RBCs, which have diminished oxygen-carrying capacities.
- Thalassemias result from diminished synthesis of one or more of the peptide chains in hemoglobin.
- Porphyrias are abnormalities of heme synthesis in which a lack of feedback inhibition causes overproduction of porphyrins, which, deposited in tissues, cause photosensitivity and discoloration of skin, bone, and teeth. Congenital porphyria (pink tooth) of cattle is the best-known of this group, although porphyria associated with photosentization has also been observed in cats and swine.
- Hemolytic anemia can be caused by a deficiency of an erythrocyte enzyme (e.g., hexokinase, pyruvate kinase, glutathione reductase), shortening the erythrocyte's lifespan by a lack of energy and reducing power.

Anemias may be accidental (e.g., hemolysis occurring in malaria or after transfusion of mismatched blood) or acquired as a result of nutritional deficiency of proteins, iron, or vitamins involved in hemoglobin synthesis, such as folic acid or cobalamine (vitamin B_{12}). Cobalamine deficiency is most commonly caused by malabsorption from the gastrointestinal tract. The stomach forms an intrinsic factor that binds cobalamine in the duodenum and targets it to receptors on mucosal cells of the ileum, which bind the complex, dissociate it, and liberate the vitamin on the serosal side. Cobalamine-deficiency anemia, or pernicious anemia, can arise from the surgical removal of the stomach (gastrectomy), parasites in the gut, or from inborn errors in the manufacturing of the intrinsic factor or the ileal receptors for it.

HEMOGLOBIN STRUCTURE AND FUNCTION; CHEMISTRY OF RESPIRATION

The structure of hemoglobin is uniquely suited for its dual functions. Hemoglobin binds oxygen in the lungs and transports it to tissues, where it unloads oxygen at a rate that adapts to the tissues' demands. As a result of metabolism, CO_2 is produced in the tissues and converted in erythrocytes to H_2CO_3, which dissociates into H^+ and HCO_3^-. The H^+ is bound to hemoglobin and carried in the bloodstream with only a minor pH shift. In the lungs, these hemoglobin functions reverse themselves: H^+ dissociates from he-

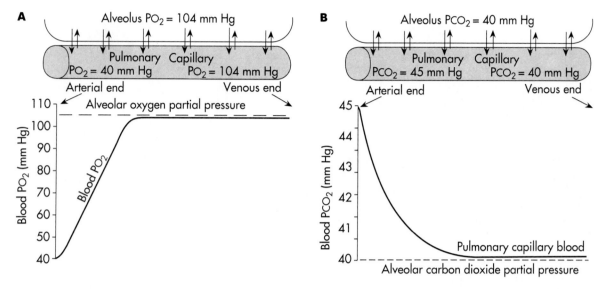

Figure 7-17. Gas exchanges in the lung. Uptake of O_2 **(A)** and release of CO_2 **(B)** require only a fraction of the vascular path length in the lung. *The graphs were constructed from data in Milhorn HT Jr and Pulley PE Jr: Theoretical study of pulmonary capillary gas exchange and venous admixture, Biophys J 8:337, 1968; reprinted with permission from Guyton AC: A textbook of medical physiology, ed 8, pp 434-435, Philadelphia, 1991, Saunders.*

moglobin and combines with HCO_3^- to form H_2CO_3, which separates into H_2O and CO_2 so that the latter can be exhaled. The loss of H^+ is accompanied by reoxygenation of hemoglobin in the lungs. Transport of oxygen and CO_2 in the blood and the exchange of these gasses in the tissues and lungs are functions of erythrocytes, and in particular hemoglobin.

Exchange of O_2 and CO_2 during respiration

In a mixture of ideal gasses, the total pressure equals the sum of the partial pressures of all components. Each gas contributes to the total pressure in proportion to its relative concentration in the mixture. Hence, about 80% of our atmospheric pressure can be attributed to nitrogen and 20% to oxygen. In alveolar air, the partial pressures of water (47 mm Hg), carbon dioxide (40 mm Hg), and nitrogen (569 mm Hg) allow 104 mm Hg for oxygen.

The partial pressure exerted by a gas trying to escape its solution is called its **tension** and is expressed as pO_2, pCO_2, etc. At equilibrium, the partial pressure of a gas equals its tension; the terms partial pressure and tension are therefore used interchangeably.

Gas exchanges in the body take place by diffusion through liquids and membranes. As O_2, CO_2, and N_2 are all highly lipid-soluble, cell membranes constitute

no barriers to their diffusion. The relative rate of diffusion then for a gas is determined by the partial-pressure gradient between two compartments for that gas and the relative size of the gas' diffusion constant. For CO_2 the diffusion coefficient (i.e., solubility coefficient [below] divided by the square root of the molecular weight) is more than 20 times that for O_2. Physiologically, this means that a small partial-pressure gradient suffices for efficient CO_2 exchange, whereas O_2 demands a much larger partial-pressure gradient. This is the exact situation in the lung, where a pCO_2 gradient of only 5 mm Hg assures rapid equilibration for CO_2. In contrast, the pO_2 gradient is 64 mm Hg (Figure 7-17). The efficiencies of O_2 and CO_2 exchange in pulmonary blood are apparent from the fact that only a fraction of the vascular path length is needed to complete gas exchange.

Hemoglobin is needed for oxygen transport in the blood

At atmospheric pressure (760 mm Hg) and at body temperature (38° C), the milliliters of gas dissolved per milliliter of plasma per atmosphere of pressure at equilibrium is called the **solubility coefficient** of that gas in plasma. As the amount of gas dissolved is pro-

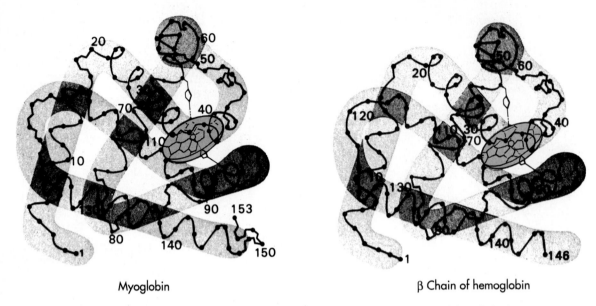

Myoglobin

β Chain of hemoglobin

Figure 7-18. Comparing the structures of myoglobin and a β-chain of hemoglobin. Only the α-carbon atoms of the amino acids are shown. Note the heme pockets where the porphyrin structures attach. *Reproduced with permission from Perutz MF: The hemoglobin molecule, Sci Am 211:64-79, 1964.*

portional to the partial pressure of that gas in the atmosphere, the volume of dissolved gas equals the product of its partial pressure and its solubility coefficient in plasma. For oxygen, the solubility coefficient in plasma equals 0.024 (compared to 0.57 for CO_2), which, multiplied by the 104 mm Hg partial pressure of oxygen available, yields a solubility of only 2.5 ml of oxygen per milliliter of plasma. This amount of physically dissolved oxygen in plasma is far below metabolic requirements. However, 15g of hemoglobin per deciliter of blood (combining with 1.34 ml of O_2 per gram) allows fully oxygenated blood to carry almost 70 times the amount of oxygen present in simple solution.

Hemoglobin and myoglobin structures

Hemoglobin transports oxygen in the bloodstream from the lungs to the tissues; inside tissue cells, myoglobin carries oxygen to subcellular sites (mitochondria; peroxisomes), where metabolic activities release electrons that must be captured by oxygen. A brief overview of some of the salient features of the structures of hemoglobin and myoglobin will aid in understanding the respiratory functions of those molecules and some genetic diseases involving abnormal hemoglobin structures.

Terminology and abbreviations used for different forms of hemoglobin are as follows:
- Hb is hemoglobin with Fe^{2+}, but uncombined with O_2; synonyms are deoxyhemoglobin, ferrohemoglobin, or reduced hemoglobin.
- HbO_2 is hemoglobin with Fe^{2+}, fully oxygenated (i.e., four O_2 per Hb); called oxyhemoglobin.
- MetHb is methemoglobin in which iron is oxidized to Fe^{3+}; it does not bind oxygen.

The protein portion of hemoglobin, globin, consists of two identical α-chains (141 amino acids each) and two identical β-chains (146 amino acids each), linked by disulfide bridges. The tertiary structures of α-chains and β-chains are remarkably similar and resemble myoglobin (Figure 7-18). Note the location of heme (Figure 7-19) in a crevice, the so-called **heme pocket.** This pocket consists of hydrophobic amino acids. The unique feature of Hb is its ability to combine reversibly with O_2 and form a stable HbO_2 complex without oxidation of Fe^{2+} to Fe^{3+}. Because of the hydrophobicity of the heme pocket, excluding water, the reaction sequence

$$HbFe^{2+} + O_2 \leftrightarrow HbFe^{2+}—O_2 \leftrightarrow HbFe^{3+} + O_2^-$$

does not proceed well all the way to the right. Consequently, the slow rates at which metHb and H_2O_2

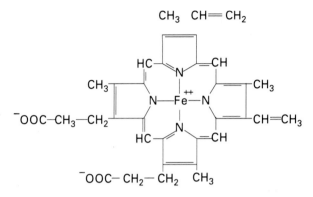

Figure 7-19. Heme or ferroporphyrin.

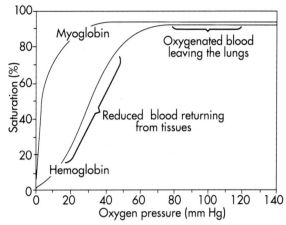

Figure 7-20. Comparing oxygenations of myoglobin and hemoglobin illustrates cooperativity and its physiologic significance.

(from O_2^-) are produced can be matched by the pace of reductive metabolism in erythrocytes.

In addition to α- and β-subunits of adult globin, in fetal blood γ-, δ-, ϵ-, and ζ-chains also exist, differing only in detail in primary structure, but having a profound effect on the oxygen-carrying characteristics of hemoglobin.

Genetic diseases relating to hemoglobin, already discussed, include sickle cell anemia and thalassemias. Presently, hundreds of abnormal globin peptide chains have been mapped. Mutations include insertion, deletion, frame shift, and extended sequences; their effects range from barely perceptible to functionally useless.

Transport of oxygen in blood

This section focuses on: (i) cooperativity in the association of O_2 and Hb, and its functional effects on oxygen loading of Hb in the lungs and unloading in tissues; and (ii) the additive allosteric effects of CO_2, H^+, and 2,3-diphosphoglycerate on the HbO_2 complex, allowing O_2 delivery at the right time and place, and at the proper rate, to myoglobin in metabolizing tissue.

Cooperative oxygen binding to hemoglobin

The kinetic observed for O_2 saturation of myoglobin with increasing pO_2 (Figure 7-20) resembles the relationship between substrate concentration and the velocity of an enzyme reaction. Since myoglobin consists of only one peptide chain and, thus, only one heme pocket to which one O_2 can bind, there can be no cooperativity in oxygen binding to myoglobin.

Hemoglobin possesses a quaternary structure, since it consists of four myoglobin-like peptide chains. Comparing the O_2-binding curves of myoglobin and hemoglobin (see Figure 7-20) illustrates cooperativity: the first O_2 molecule binds to Hb reluctantly (flat curve at low pO_2), but the attachment of the first O_2 to hemoglobin makes combination with the three additional O_2 molecules easier (curve gets steeper) until saturation is reached. Under physiological conditions, the difference in O_2 affinity between Hb and fully oxygenated HbO_2 is approximately 500-fold. Examining the two extremes of O_2 tension found in the body brings out the great physiological significance of the sigmoid shape of the O_2-Hb dissociation curve. Starting at the high pO_2 in the lungs, hemoglobin is 97% saturated (see Figure 7-20). Though in the arteries the pO_2 drops to about 80 mm Hg, hemoglobin remains virtually saturated; but then the blood enters tissues with pO_2 at or below 40 mm Hg, and there the steep portion of the curve is traversed, as hemoglobin rapidly unloads its oxygen. The pO_2 of venous blood is normally about 40 mm Hg, but during strenuous exercise it may fall to as low as 15 mm Hg. Even then, blood returning to the lungs still contains sufficient O_2 to cooperatively enhance renewed oxygenation of hemoglobin.

The unloading of oxygen in the tissues caused by the pO_2 gradient can be fine-tuned by allosteric attachments of H^+ and 2,3-diphosphoglycerate to the globin of Hb, as is examined in the following section.

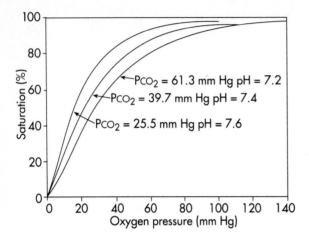

Figure 7-21. Effect of P_{CO_2} on oxygen-hemoglobin dissociation. The magnitude of the Bohr effect depends on the P_{CO_2}. *Reproduced with permission from Smith EL, Hill RL, Lehman IR, Lefkowitz RJ, Handler P, and White A: Principles of biochemistry: mammalian biochemistry, ed 7, p 116, New York, 1983, McGraw-Hill.*

Influence of CO_2 and H^+: the Bohr effect

The effect of pCO_2 on the O_2-Hb dissociation curve (Figure 7-21) is due to pH shifts caused by changing pCO_2. In erythrocytes,

$$CO_2 + H_2O \leftrightarrow H_2CO_3 \leftrightarrow H^+ + HCO_3^-$$

and, thus, the uptake of CO_2 yields H^+. The hydrogen ions engage in the equation

$$H^+ + HbO_2^- \leftrightarrow HHb + O_2$$

so that ultimately O_2 is released in response to initial CO_2 uptake (Bohr effect). This relationship is not stoichiometric: each 0.7 mol of H^+ releases 1 mol of O_2. It can also be learned from the equation that HHb is a weaker acid than is HbO_2^- (pK values are 7.71 and 6.17 respectively). The reversibility of the equation presages that reoxygenation of hemoglobin in the lungs restores the stronger acid, HbO_2^-, from which more H^+ dissociates.

The physiological significance of the Bohr effect is that O_2 unloading from HbO_2^- is finely regulated according to a tissue's metabolic need for O_2: the more metabolic activity, the more CO_2 produced, hence the more O_2 dissociation from HbO_2^- (Bohr effect) to support that high metabolic activity. In the lungs, where CO_2 is expired, lowered pCO_2 enhances O_2 binding to Hb^- (Bohr effect), and thus reoxygenation; Hb^- is saturated with O_2 at a lower pO_2.

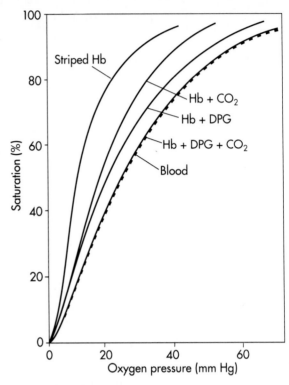

Figure 7-22. Effects of CO_2 and 2,3-diphosphoglycerate *(DPG)* on oxygen-hemoglobin dissociation are additive. The partial pressure of CO_2, when present, was 40 mm Hg; when DPG was added, its concentration was 1.2 mol of DPG per mol of hemoglobin tetramer. *Reproduced with permission from Kilmartin, JV: Interaction of haemoglobin with protons, CO_2, and 2,3-diphosphoglycerate, Br Med Bull 32:209, 1976.*

Influence of 2,3-diphosphoglycerate (DPG) on Hb-O_2 system

DPG formation in erythrocytes leads to a 4 to 5 mM concentration in the RBC—equal to the hemoglobin concentration. A tight 1:1 binding of DPG to one specific allosteric site between the two β-chains of the globin portion of Hb^- decreases hemoglobin's affinity for oxygen:

$$HbO_2^- + DPG \leftrightarrow Hb^-\!\!-\!\!DPG + O_2.$$

Therefore, at a fixed HbO_2 concentration in erythrocytes in tissues, an increasing DPG level promotes oxygen unloading from HbO_2^- (Figure 7-22). Conversely, in the lungs, increased pO_2 promotes dissociation of the Hb-DPG complex with the formation of HbO_2. The DPG effect on oxygen unloading is

| Table 7-5 | Distribution of total CO_2 in arterial and venous blood | | | |

	Arterial, mmol	Venous, mmol	Difference	
			mmol	ml
Total CO_2 in 1 L of blood	21.53	23.21	1.68	37.4
Total CO_2 in plasma of 1 L of blood (600 ml)	15.94	16.99	1.05	23.5
As dissolved CO_2	0.71	0.80	0.09	2.0
As bicarbonate ions	15.23	16.19	0.96	21.5
Total CO_2 in 400 ml of erythrocytes	5.59	6.22	0.63	14.0
As dissolved CO_2	0.34	0.39	0.05	1.1
As bicarbonate ions	4.28	4.41	0.13	2.9
As carbamino-CO_2	0.97	1.42	0.45	10.0

Reproduced, with permission, from Smith EL, Hill RL, Lehman IR, Lefkowitz RJ, Handler P, and White A: Principles of biochemistry: mammalian biochemistry, ed 7, 127, New York, 1983, McGraw-Hill.

additive to the pCO_2 (Bohr) effect (see Figure 7-22).

DPG is a sensitive control in adaptation to hypoxia: its level rises with exercise, acidemia, increases in thyroid hormones, and at high altitude; the low affinity of fetal hemoglobin for DPG compared to that of maternal hemoglobin establishes the condition for rapid oxygen unloading across the placenta (see below). Phytate, exceeding DPG in its affinity for hemoglobin, is found in the erythrocytes of birds, which unload more oxygen than human RBCs at a given pO_2. The oxygen affinity of hemoglobin in some species (e.g., cats and ungulates) does not appear to be affected by DPG.

Transport of CO_2 in blood

The relative modes of CO_2 transport, in the forms of HCO_3^-, dissolved CO_2, or as a carbamino compound bound to hemoglobin, can be assessed from the distribution of total CO_2 in plasma and erythrocytes (Table 7-5). The difference in CO_2 contents of venous and arterial blood is about 40 ml/L and, thus, each liter of blood transports about 40 ml of CO_2 from tissues to the lungs. Very little of this transported CO_2 can be carried as dissolved CO_2 (only about 8% of the total); this is advantageous, since more dissolved CO_2 would have dropped the pH markedly, whereas, in fact, only a 0.05 unit drop in pH of venous blood is observed; hence the term **isohydric CO_2 transport.** About 60% of all transported CO_2 in the blood is carried in plasma, predominantly in the form of HCO_3^- ions. Of the CO_2 transported by erythrocytes, most travels in the form of carbamino-CO_2 carrying about 25% of the total CO_2 transported in blood. It is not so much for CO_2 transport that he-

moglobin is important, but rather for oxygen transport and H$^+$ transport as HHb.

Bicarbonate

HCO_3^- is the major CO_2 compartment in plasma and the chief CO_2-transporter in blood (see Table 7-5). The formation of bicarbonate

$$CO_2 + H_2O \leftrightarrow H_2CO_3 \leftrightarrow H^+ + HCO_3^-$$

in erythrocytes is catalyzed by Zn^{++}-containing carbonic anhydrase. Subsequently, HCO_3^- leaves the erythrocyte in exchange for plasma Cl^- ions (chloride shift; see below).

Carbaminohemoglobin

CO_2 binds to the NH_2-terminals of α- and β-chains of globin

$$Hb-NH_2 + CO_2 \leftrightarrow Hb-NH-C-O^- + H^+$$

to form carbaminohemoglobin. The reaction is reversible, being determined by the pCO_2, so that in the lungs CO_2 is blown off. Furthermore, in the lungs the binding of O_2 to hemoglobin displaces CO_2, a phenomenon referred to as the **Haldane effect.**

Carbaminohemoglobin is a minor constituent of RBCs, but, because of its large arteriovenous concentration difference, it is the major CO_2-transporter of erythrocytes (see Table 7-5).

Reduced and oxygenated hemoglobin as acids

Unloading oxygen from HbO_2^- (pK 6.17) changes the tertiary structure of the protein, so that reduced Hb^- is a weaker acid (pK 7.71). Thus, oxygen un-

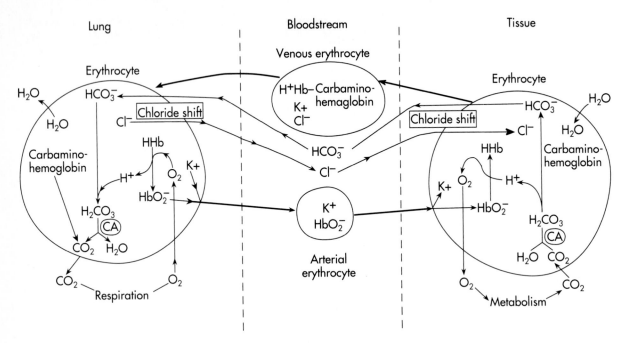

Figure 7-23. Isohydric CO_2 transport; chloride shift. In the cyclic process of CO_2 transport from tissues, via blood, to the lungs in exchange for oxygen transport from lungs to tissues, hemoglobin's oscillations between weaker acid (reduced form) and stronger acid *(HbO₂)* plays a crucial part, as does the enzyme carbonic anhydrase *(CA)*.

loading is accompanied by the acceptance of a H^+:

$$H^+ + HbO_2^- \leftrightarrow HHb + O_2.$$

In other words, if HbO_2^- would merely lose its O_2 at the site of a tissue cell, the pH would shift in alkaline direction, since reduced Hb^- is the weaker acid. However, since reduced Hb^- associates with 0.7 mol of H^+ for each mole of HbO_2^- deoxygenated, the pH remains constant. For each mole of H^+ bound to reduced Hb^- inside an RBC, 1 mol of HCO_3^- may be generated and move into plasma in exchange for Cl^-; this phenomenon is termed **Chloride shift** or Hamburger shift (named for the Dutch physiologist who discovered it, Hartog Jacob Hamburger, 1859-1924).

Isohydric CO_2 transport; chloride shift

Transport of CO_2 from tissues, via blood, to the lungs in exchange for oxygen transport from the lungs to tissues is a cyclical process (Figure 7-23). To start the cycle, it is best to consider a tissue receiving oxygen from an incoming erythrocyte carrying HbO_2. Oxygenation of the tissue is proportional to that tissue's rate of metabolism as (i) the lowered pO_2 in a tissue, reflecting the rate of oxygen consumption, determines HbO_2^- dissociation; and (ii) the CO_2 resulting from metabolism and diffusing into the RBC fine-tunes oxygen unloading via the Bohr effect. Some CO_2 is carbamino-bound to hemoglobin, but most is converted by carbonic anhydrase to $HCO_3^- + H^+$. The H^+ ions are bound to hemoglobin; hence the term isohydric CO_2 transport. It should be recalled that oxygen unloading makes hemoglobin a stronger H^+ acceptor; conversely, binding of H^+ ions to hemoglobin stimulates O_2 unloading due to the Bohr effect. H^+ binding to hemoglobin leaves one K^+ charge (formerly neutralized by HbO_2^-) to offset the HCO_3^- charge that is generated. Since the intra- and extracellular concentrations of HCO_3^- are no longer in Donnan equilibrium, HCO_3^- diffuses into plasma in exchange for Cl^- (the Chloride shift [see Figure 7-23]). Erythrocytes in venous blood, thus, are enriched with Cl^- which brings in water and causes swelling. The hematocrit in venous blood then exceeds that of arterial blood, rising from approximately 45 to 48 or 49%.

On the pulmonary side, all of the erythrocyte effects on tissue metabolism are reversed (see Figure 7-23). Diminished pCO_2 and increased pO_2 cause reoxygenation of Hb^- to HbO_2^-, whereby H^+ is liberated. Reversal of the Chloride shift moves HCO_3^- into the erythrocyte. Catalyzed by carbonic anhydrase, H^+ and HCO_3^- ions combine to form CO_2, which diffuses out of the erythrocyte and is expired. The high pO_2 also causes CO_2 release from carbaminohemoglobin (Haldane effect). Since Cl^- is replaced by HCO_3^-, and HCO_3^- is converted to osmotically inactive products, net water movement is out of the cell, thus reestablishing arterial hematocrit.

In sum, the center piece of isohydric H^+ transport is the reversible reaction $HbO_2^- + H^+ \leftrightarrow HHb + O_2$ and the conformational changes that hemoglobin undergoes as it binds and releases O_2. The net result is that O_2 is transported from the lungs to tissues in an amount sufficient to meet metabolic requirements, and that CO_2 generated in the tissues' metabolism is delivered to the lungs without an acid-base upset in RBCs, plasma, or extracellular fluid.

Myoglobin

As indicated by the oxygen dissociation curve (see Figure 7-20), myoglobin has a much higher affinity for oxygen than does hemoglobin. At a lowered pO_2 of 10 mm Hg, hemoglobin loses about 90% of its oxygen, while myoglobin is still 80% saturated. To fully place the function of myoglobin into perspective, the role of cytochrome oxidase in mitochondrial energy metabolism must be understood. In the pathway of ATP generation by oxidative phosphorylation, cytochrome oxidase combines metabolic electrons with oxygen, which it binds with an affinity that exceeds even that of myoglobin. Thus the function of myoglobin is to accept oxygen from hemoglobin at the site of a blood capillary, to shuttle that oxygen within the muscle cell, and finally to hand it over to mitochondrial cytochrome oxidase. Alternatively, the oxygen is transported to peroxisomes.

Though ubiquitous, myoglobin in mammals is abundant primarily in heart muscle. As the "go-between" in oxygen transport, it can serve as a last O_2 resort when the pO_2 drops during muscle contraction. Conversely, upon O_2 resupply, myoglobin is reoxygenated before hemoglobin.

Fetal respiration

In some species, such as sheep, cattle, goat, and man, the fetus has a different hemoglobin from that of the adult. Fetal (HbF) and adult hemoglobin (HbA) can

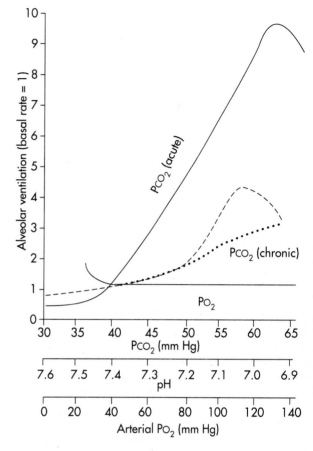

Figure 7-24. Effects of arterial Po_2, pH, and Pco_2, (both acute and chronic) on the rate of alveolar ventilation. *Modified and reproduced with permission from Guyton AC: A textbook of medical physiology, ed 8, pp 447 and 449, Philadelphia, 1991, Saunders.*

be distinguished from one another by their respective mobilities when subjected to electrophoresis, by amino-acid analysis, or by other tests.

Beside the α- and β-chains prevalent in human HbA, several other chains occur in the tetramers of hemoglobin during the development of the fetus. Prevalent is the tetramer α_2-γ_2. The disappearance of HbF after birth is rapid and provides iron for its various metabolic functions in the neonate. Proper placental O_2 transfer to the fetus is thought to be achieved because of the following:

- Fetal hemoglobin has a higher affinity for oxygen than does HbA; hence, at the pO_2-pCO_2 situation at the placenta, whereby maternal HbO_2

unloads O_2, HbF becomes more fully oxygenated; and

- Fetal hemoglobin binds 2,3-diphosphoglycerate (DPG) poorly, since uncharged serine replaces histidine in its DPG-binding site. Thus, at the same DPG level, HbA unloads O_2 while HbF is unaffected so that oxygen is directed across the placenta to the fetus.

Although nature has apparently provided HbF as a "safety factor" for oxygen exchange across the placenta, particularly in cases of maternal hypoxemia, it may not be an absolute necessity for life. In the pig and horse, for example, the hemoglobin of the fetus is indistinguishable from that of the adult, and studies have shown that human fetal blood can be replaced with maternal blood without severely compromising the potential for fetal survival.

Control of respiration by CO_2, H^+, and O_2

Increasing the hydrogen ion concentration and, much more powerfully, increasing pCO_2 stimulates the respiratory center in the brain by direct action. Contrary to this, the pO_2 has no direct action on the respiratory center, but influences respiration via chemoreceptors, located in the carotid and aortic bodies, that monitor arterial pO_2 but are more sensitive to plasma $[H^+]$ and pCO_2.

Normally, at alveolar pO_2 of 104 mm Hg, the pO_2 has no influence on alveolar ventilation (Figure 7-24). A drop in pO_2 below 60 mm Hg is required before any effect is observable, and dropping pO_2 to an extreme of 30 mm Hg raises alveolar ventilation to only 1.7 times the base rate. This can be contrasted to the feeble O_2 response to the fourfold increase in alveolar ventilation caused by lowering blood pH to 7.0 or the tenfold increase caused by increasing pCO_2 only 50% above the normal value of 40mm Hg (see Figure 7-24).

The extreme sensitivity to the pCO_2 allows respiration to respond quickly to changes in pCO_2 or pH in the blood. Increased pCO_2 (hypercapnia), or decreased pH, accompanying the condition of acidosis, raises the rate of respiration (provided the lungs are functional) so that the body gets rid of excess CO_2 and restores the value of the $[HCO_3^-]/0.03 \, pCO_2$ ratio to its normal value of about 20. Conversely, alkalosis is accompanied by hypocapnia (low blood CO_2) and, thus, leads to a hypoventilatory response. But, of course, with hypoventilation comes a lowered O_2 uptake and ultimately, the hyperventilatory response to lowered pO_2 precludes any additional lowering of respiration. (i.e., you can't kill yourself by holding your breath.) Later in the text, there is a review of the failing of lung functions as the cause of respiratory acidosis or alkalosis, and the healthy functioning of the lungs in regulating the body's acid-base balance.

STUDY QUESTIONS

1. *a.* List the functions of albumin, haptoglobin, ceruloplasmin, and transcortin.
   b. List the approximate albumin concentration in plasma.
   c. List the plasma protein absent in serum.

2. *a.* Where does the extrinsic blood clotting cascade start?
   b. List the enzyme that converts fibrinogen into fibrin.
   c. Identify the eicosanoid from the arterial wall that normally inhibits platelet aggregation.

3. When the intima of a blood vessel is damaged, there is a factor liberated that promotes the growth of smooth muscle (foam) cells. List the name and origin of that factor.

4. What substance is responsible for vasoconstrictive activity in hemostasis?

5. *a.* What are the elements that form the initial (and colorless) blood clot?
   b. List the cellular and other materials that make up a blood clot.

6. Among platelet functions is the release of thromboxane A_2 for the purpose of _____ and the release of _____ for vascular repair. (Fill in the blanks.)

7. *a.* What mineral is essential for forming a blood clot?
   b. List the vitamin that is essential for the synthesis of several clotting factors (e.g., prothrombin) and its mode of action.
   c. What antagonist to this vitamin interferes with prothrombin synthesis?
   d. Where in the body is prothrombin synthesized?

8. *a.* List the product of the mast cells that serves in vivo as an anticoagulant.
   b. How does citrate work as an anticoagulant?
   c. How does heparin-antithrombin-III complex work as anticoagulant?

9. *a.* List the function of plasmin.
   b. List the function of tissue factor.

10. *a.* For what purpose are urokinase and plasminogen produced in the kidney?
    b. For what purpose is erythroproietin produced in the kidney? List a condition that stimulates the kidney to produce more erythroproietin.

11. *a.* Why is the loss of hexokinase activity related to the life span of an RBC?
   b. Why does failure to maintain the cytoskeleton lead to the RBC's demise?
   c. Why does the loss of the Ca^{++} pump in aging RBCs lead to their demise?

12. *a.* List the kidneys' contribution to erythrocyte formation.
   b. What therapeutic measure must be taken to prevent anemia following gastrectomy?

13. *a.* What acid-base characteristic of hemoglobin is crucial for isohydric CO_2 transport?
   b. Arterial blood has a higher HCO_3^-/Cl^- ratio than does venous. (True/False)
   c. The PCV of arterial blood is higher than that of venous blood. (True/False)

14. List the toxic substance formed in the oxygenation of hemoglobin that is detoxified by glutathione-requiring enzymes in erythrocytes. List the trace mineral required for this detoxification.

15. List the metabolic pathway in the RBC that donates reducing power, so that the O_2^- radical is detoxified.

16. After hemoglobin is broken down (e.g., in the spleen):
   a. What happens to the heme moiety (breakdown product, transport in plasma, route of secretion)?
   b. What happens to the iron moiety (transport vehicle in plasma, storage protein)?

17. *a.* List two Fe storing proteins in the liver.
   b. In humans, what links vitamin C with increased availability of dietary iron?
   c. Transferrin concentration is up-regulated when diets are fed that are high in iron. (True/False)

18. In newborn animals, rapid breakdown of fetal hemoglobin:
   a. Offers a unique advantage with respect to filling the need of which mineral?
   b. Presents the danger of kernicterus, due to low glucuronyl transferase activity in liver; list the noxious compound accumulating in the blood (which in mature animals would have been excreted in bile).

19. List the avitaminosis that results from a lack of gastric intrinsic factor.

20. *a.* List three chemical forms by which metabolic CO_2 is transported from tissues to the lungs. List the chief mode of CO_2 transport in plasma.
   b. List the enzyme, located within RBCs, that catalyzes the equilibrium reactions of CO_2 with H_2O, and list its mineral requirement.

21. *a.* On a graph, draw the oxygen-hemoglobin dissociation curve obtained at a pH of 7.4. Accurately label both the ordinate and abscissa.
   b. In the same graph, draw the oxygen-hemoglobin dissociation curve obtained at a pH existing at the tissue cell level.
   c. List the advantage of the Bohr effect to a tissue cell's metabolism.
   d. List the advantage of cooperativity in oxygen-hemoglobin binding.

22. *a.* What feature in the structure of hemoglobin helps prevent the formation of methemoglobin?
   b. List the mechanism whereby erythrocytes handle the slow formation of methemoglobin.

23. Why is it that, in the pulmonary gas-exchange system, a very small partial pressure gradient suffices for CO_2 relative to O_2?

24. *a.* Diagram the exchange process of CO_2 and O_2 between tissue cells and blood; indicate all molecules, ions, and anatomical structures involved.
   b. Explain the influence that the deoxygenation of hemoglobin at the tissue cell level has on the ability of hemoglobin to bind H^+.
   c. Explain the influence that the oxygenation of hemoglobin in the pulmonary capillaries has on the ability of hemoglobin to release H^+.
   d. How does the chloride shift alter erythrocyte size in venous as compared to arterial blood?
   e. Is the normal transport of metabolic CO_2 from the tissues to the lungs a transient or permanent H^+ burden to the body?

25. List the compound that carries O_2 from hemoglobin to cytochrome oxidase in tissue cells.

26. *a.* List the advantage to a fetus of a high 2,3-diphosphoglycerate concentration in the mother's erythrocytes.
   b. Why is the production of 2,3-diphosphoglycerate in RBCs increased at high altitude?

27. Regarding the control of respiration by factors other than nervous factors:
   a. List the gas having the largest influence.
   b. What limits the hypoventilatory response of the lungs to hypocapnia?
   c. Explain how alkalosis is caused by hyperventilation.

Body fluids: volume, electrolytes, and acid-base homeostasis

This chapter focuses on the body fluids, chief electrolytes that account for osmolarity, fluid distribution and movement in body compartments, physiologic pH regulation by various organs, and, in particular, the function of the kidneys in all these. Because of their unique physiologic functions, calcium and phosphate and their homeostatic control are also examined.

BODY FLUIDS; ELECTROLYTES; KIDNEY FUNCTIONS
Water

Water, the body's chief constituent, forms an essential part of all tissue spaces in the body and perform many functions:
- Serves as a chemical reactant (e.g., hydrolysis)
- Serves as a solvent for ions and macromolecules

- Serves as a medium for transport (e.g., bloodstream, bile, urine, milk)
- Lubricates (e.g., synovial fluid)
- Absorbs shock (e.g., cerebrospinal fluid)
- Regulates body temperature by its high heat capacity and by evaporative heat loss from the lungs and skin.

Total body water volume in humans varies by less than 1% per day, despite variable water intake. More drinking leads to increased urine production (facultative water loss). But water intake in food and drink, and metabolic water formed by oxidizing H in nutrients to H_2O, must balance the sum of facultative and obligatory water losses. Obligatory losses represent evaporation in the skin and lungs, as well as fecal and urinary losses that accompany obligatory eliminations of urea, salts, and other osmotically active

Table 8-1   Daily water balance of Holstein cows eating legume hay

Water intake (L)			Water output (L)		
Source	**Nonlactating**	**Lactating**	**Source**	**Nonlactating**	**Lactating**
Drinking water	26	51	Feces	12	19
Water in food	1	2	Urine	7	11
Metabolic water	2	3	Evaporation	10	14
TOTAL	29	56	Milk	0	12
			TOTAL	29	56

Data from Leitch and Thomson, Nutr Abstr Rev 14:197, 1944.

solutes. Water turnover in resting, mature animals is about 10 to 30 ml/kg/day; as a rule, 15 ml/kg/day is the maintenance value for daily water needs. But many factors affect water turnover: species, diet, age, environment (humidity, wind, and temperature), health (fever, diarrhea, diabetes) and lactation (Table 8-1). These factors may more than double the water requirement.

Body fluid compartments

Total body water varies from 55 to 75% of body weight in domestic animals. The average value for total body water, 60% of body weight, is influenced by species, age (highest in young), gender (higher in males), and adiposity. Fat contains less than 10% water, muscle over 75%; hence the lean person has more than 70% total body water, the obese one less than 40%.

About two thirds of total body water is intracellular fluid (Table 8-2); extracellular fluid is divided into interstitial fluid, which includes lymph, cell-free intravascular fluid, which is plasma, and transcellular fluid, which includes cerebrospinal fluid, aqueous humor, synovial fluid, and, quantitatively most important, fluids of the digestive tract (Table 8-3). In an adult man, the total volume of digestive fluid secreted per day is 8.2 L (compared with a plasma volume of 3.5 L and a total extracellular fluid volume of 14 L).

Extracellular fluid may also be divided into vascular and extravascular fluids. The vascular fluid contains plasma and cells (erythrocytes, platelets, and white blood cells). Total blood volume varies with the animal species (Table 8-4), as does packed cell volume (PCV; hematocrit)—from 23% in goats to 47% in dogs.

Composition of body fluids

Fluid compartments in the body are bound by membranes, and water and respiratory gases can move freely between them. Hence when one compartment,

Table 8-2   Relative sizes of body compartments

Solids	30-50%
Intracellular fluid	30-40%
Extracellular fluid	20-25%
Interstitial fluid	14-16%
Plasma	4-5%
Transcellular fluid	1-6%

Table 8-3   Digestive secretions in humans

Secretion	ml/day
Saliva	1500
Gastric secretions	2500
Bile	500
Pancreatic juice	700
Intestinal secretions	3000
TOTAL	8200

Reproduced, with permission, from Smith EL and others: Principles of biochemistry: mammalian biochemistry, ed 7, 153, New York, 1983, McGraw-Hill.

Table 8-4   Total blood and packed cell volume (PCV) of animal species

	Volume (% of body weight)			PCV
Animal	**Total blood**	**Plasma**	**RBC**	**(%)**
Dog	8.5	4.5	4.0	47
Cat	6.7	4.7	2.0	30
Chicken	6.5	4.5	2.0	31
Cow	5.7	3.8	1.9	33
Goat	7.0	5.4	1.6	23
Pig	7.5	4.8	2.7	36
Sheep	6.5	4.5	2.0	31
Horse				
Draft	7.0	4.0	3.0	43
Thoroughbred	10.0	6.0	4.0	40
Saddle	7.7	5.2	2.5	32

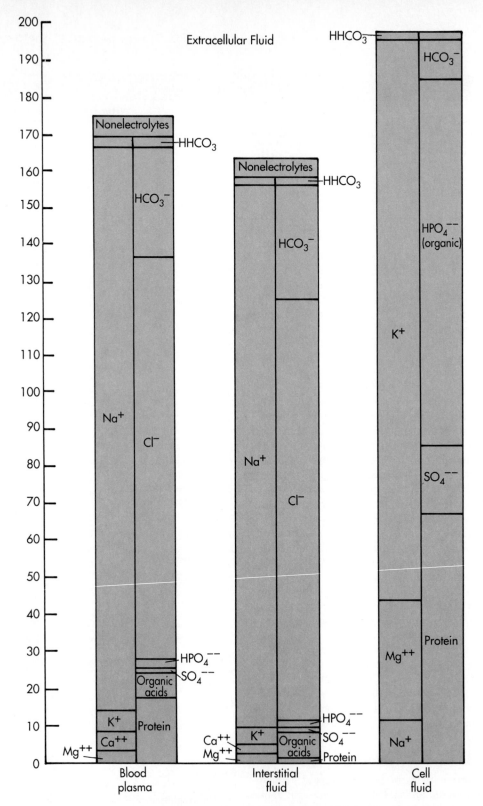

Figure 8-1. Composition of human body fluids. *Reproduced with permission from Gamble JL: Chemical anatomy, physiology, and pathology of extracellular fluid, p 5, Cambridge, 1954, Harvard University Press.*

plasma for instance, is monitored by osmoreceptors and the volume of that compartment is maintained by renal water retention or water loss, then total fluid volume is adequately controlled. Total fluid volume is primarily controlled by mineral and water retention (or loss) in the kidney, and monitored by stretch receptors and osmoreceptors. On the other hand, the distribution of fluids between compartments (and their composition) is determined by:

- Oncotic effects, since membranes are impermeable to proteins, and the various compartments differ in nature and concentrations of proteins; oncotic pressures are accentuated by satellite ions;
- Donnan equilibria, effecting uneven ion concentrations in neighboring compartments, held in equilibrium by an oppositely directed electrical gradient;
- Specific ion pumps (for Na^+, Cl^-, and Ca^{++}) requiring ATP input to maintain a steady state of nonequilibrium;
- Hydrostatic pressure (blood pressure).

With these points in mind, the composition of intracellular and interstitial fluids and plasma will be examined with the aid of Gamblegrams (Figure 8-1).

- K^+ is the principal cation in intracellular fluid; Na^+ in extracellular fluid.
- Phosphate is the primary intracellular anion, present mostly as phosphorylated organic compounds; Cl^- predominates in extracellular fluids.
- Intracellularly, the protein concentration is higher than in interstitial fluid or plasma; hence, the total electrolyte concentrations, expressed in meq/L, are also highest intracellularly.
- In the Gamblegrams, electrolyte and other solute concentrations are given in equivalents per liter (normalities). For consideration of fluid movement it is more meaningful to express these solute concentrations in osmoles per kilogram of water (osmolality). As multivalent solutes (Mg^{++} or protein) have the same osmolar effect per molecule as do monovalent ones (Na^+ or Cl^-), the intracellular osmolality equals the osmolality of interstitial fluid and is equivalent to a total osmotic pressure of 5430 mm Hg at body temperature. This equality is quite expected, since water moves freely in and out of cells. In fact, nearly all body fluids have the same osmolality. However, there is one important exception: the small difference between the osmolalities of plasma (equivalent to an osmotic

pressure of 5453 mm Hg) and interstitial fluid (5430 mm Hg). This difference of about 0.4% of the total osmotic pressure reflects the difference in oncotic pressure. This pressure difference, though small, is of vital importance in maintaining proper fluid distribution between the vascular and extravascular compartments.

- Intracellular fluid is not homogeneous. Sequestration of Ca^{++} in mitochondria and the endoplasmic reticulum, and low pH in lysosomes, are examples of uneven distributions. The composition of intracellular fluid, thus, represents a weighted average.

Interstitial fluid; lymph

The fluid remaining outside the boundaries of cell membranes is called extracellular fluid. It contains nutrients and oxygen bound for cells, and waste products destined for excretion. Extracellular fluid is in constant motion, mixed by diffusional forces in spaces between tissue cells, blood, and lymph channels. Because tissue cells live in an environment bathed by this fluid, extracellular fluid is called the **internal environment** of the body. The term homeostasis is used to mean maintenance of relatively constant (not static) conditions in the internal environment; all organs and systems of the body are involved in this process.

Microcirculation

Nutrients and cellular wastes interchange, via interstitial fluids, between tissues and blood capillaries of the microcirculation. The flow of blood in a small functional unit of the capillary bed, from arteriole to venule (Figure 8-2), pulsates through the action of sphincters. Sphincters open more frequently and for

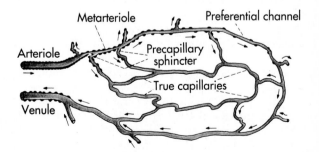

Figure 8-2. Mesenteric capillary bed. *Reproduced with permission from Zweifach BW: The character and distribution of the blood capillaries, Anatom Rec 73:475-498, 1939.*

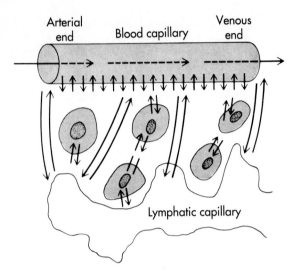

Arterial end — Blood capillary — Venous end

Lymphatic capillary

Figure 8-3. Diffusion of fluid and dissolved substances between capillary and interstitial spaces. *Reproduced with permission from Guyton AC: Textbook of medical physiology, ed 8, p 172, Philadelphia, 1991, Saunders.*

longer durations when pO_2 is low in tissues; that is, they autoregulate the flow of blood (including oxygen and nutrients) to tissues in accordance with the metabolic needs of those tissues. (This control adds to the ones discussed earlier: Bohr effect; formation of 2,3-diphosphoglycerate where and when needed; acid-base properties of oxyhemoglobin and deoxyhemoglobin; and the functionality of cooperative oxygen binding to hemoglobin.)

Various mechanisms exist for the exchange of nutrients and wastes between tissues and the microcirculation. As reviewed earlier, in the context of transport across cell membranes, intercellular clefts between endothelial cells of capillary walls allow exchange of water-solutes; pinocytosis permits exchange of any substance; fenestrae (windows) in endothelial cells function as pores; gases and lipid-solutes can move directly across capillary membranes (e.g., O_2, ethyl ether).

The presence of actin and myosin in membranes of endothelial cells causes rhythmic contractions and relaxations that pump solutes across the passage channels from the blood stream into the interstitial compartment. The result of these transport processes is a continual solute exchange that is so efficient that water and small solutes diffuse back and forth across capillaries at rates 10 to 100 times as great as the rate

at which plasma flows along capillaries (Figure 8-3).

The rate at which a solute exchanges varies inversely with the molecular diameter of the solute, suggesting a molecular sieving through pores in capillary membranes. Capillaries in most tissues allow inorganic electrolytes and small molecules (glucose, urea) to pass with relative ease while effectively blocking the passage of plasma proteins, so that oncotic gradients are formed between vascular and interstitial compartments. Different tissues derive part of their special functioning from atypical permeability of capillary membranes; for example, the extremely discriminating blood-brain barrier protects the brain; capillaries in the kidney's nephrons have properties that allow effective, yet discriminating and controllable exchange of salts and water; capillaries in the liver allow passage of blood proteins and delivery of protein-bound substances to hepatocytes.

Endothelial membranes are not perfect ultrafilters; small amounts of protein (namely albumin) enter into the interstitial fluid. Extravasated protein is channeled back to the venous side of the circulation via the lymphatics.

Lymph

Though the terms lymph and interstitial fluid are sometimes used interchangeably, it is best to reserve the term lymph for fluids contained in lymphatic ducts. The protein composition of lymph varies greatly depending on the anatomic location from which it is sampled; subcutaneous lymph has 0.25% protein, liver lymph up to 6%. Being a plasma and cellular filtrate, lymph is enriched with small proteins (albumin) rather than with the larger ones (globulins). The presence of fibrinogen and prothrombin makes lymph clot on standing. One of the vitally important functions of lymph is to carry large particulate matter, such as tissue proteins and extravasated plasma proteins, away from the interstitium and back into the blood circulation. The porosity of lymphatic capillaries enables this function. Additionally, lymph is an accessory route whereby fluids can flow from the interstitium to the blood.

The normal 24-hour lymph flow in a 70 kg human is 2-4 liters (approximately 100 ml/hr). Lymph flow is thought to be due to the following:

- Movements of skeletal muscle;
- Negative intrathoracic pressure during inspiration
- Suction effect of high velocity flow of blood in the veins in which lymphatics terminate

- Rhythmic contractions of the walls of large lymph ducts

Since lymph vessels have valves that prevent backflow (like veins), contractions of skeletal muscle push lymph toward the heart. Pulsations of arteries near lymphatics may have a similar effect. However, contractions of the walls of lymphatic ducts are important, and the rate of these contractions increases in direct proportion to the volume of lymph the vessels contain.

Agents that increase lymph flow, called lymphagogues, include a variety of compounds that increase capillary membrane permeability. In the kidneys, formation of a maximally concentrated urine depends upon an intact lymphatic circulation; removal of reabsorbed water from medullary pyramids is essential for efficient operation of the countercurrent mechanism (discussed later), and water enters the vasa recta only if an appreciable osmotic gradient is maintained between the medullary interstitium, and vasa recta blood by drainage of protein-containing interstitial fluid into renal lymphatics. Other functions of the lymphatic system (immune, phagocytic) are not the subject of this text.

Interstitial fluid; edema

The space between cells, the interstitium, comprises about 16% of a tissue. This space is filled with a gel substance consisting of collagen fibers and proteoglycan filaments. Though this gel effectively curbs the flow ("sloshing around") of fluid, diffusion of solutes occurs virtually unimpeded.

Fluid movements responsible for the distribution of fluids between vascular and interstitial space are determined by the net force that drives fluids out of arteries (net filtration pressure) or back into veins

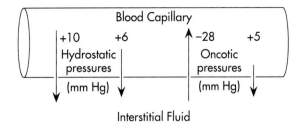

Figure 8-4. Starling forces at the capillary membrane reabsorb interstitial fluid into the bloodstream. Illustrated is a normal condition with a net reabsorption pressure of −7 mm Hg (see Chapter 5, Figure 5-3).

(net absorption pressure); that is, the algebraic sum of the four hydrostatic and osmotic pressures discussed earlier (Starling forces; Figure 8-4). Clinically important problems that arise from alterations in the normal balance between the fluids of vascular and extravascular compartments include edema and shock.

Edema, the interstitial pooling of fluid, results from abnormalities in the net hydrodynamic balance of Starling forces (Table 8-5, cases A through C):

- *Case A:* Increased capillary hydrostatic pressure may be caused, for instance, by heart failure curbing venous return, or local allergic reactions whereby histamine release relaxes blood arterioles and constricts venules, resulting in urticaria (hives).
- *Case B:* Decreased plasma oncotic pressure reflecting a lowered concentration of plasma proteins may result from improper protein nutrition, from urinary protein losses due to nephrosis, from liver disease, or from increased porosity of blood vessels allowing plasma proteins to escape (thereby raising the oncotic pressure of the in-

Table 8-5	Balance of fluid reabsorption (Starling forces) during edema				
	Hydrostatic pressure		**Oncotic pressure**		**Net fluid reabsorption pressure (mm Hg)**
Case	**Plasma (mm Hg)**	**Interstitial (mm Hg)**	**Plasma (mm Hg)**	**Interstitial (mm Hg)**	
Normal	+ 10	+ 6	− 28	+ 5	− 7
A	+ 41	− 3	− 28	+ 5	+ 15
B	+ 10	− 1	− 10	+ 8	+ 7
C	+ 10	− 10	− 28	+ 28	0

Note: Plasma hydrostatic pressure equals pressure at the venous end of a representative capillary bed in subcutaneous tissue; negativity of the interstitial fluid pressure is maintained by lymphatic pumping action; and net fluid reabsorption pressure is that drawing fluid back into the capillary at the venous end. (+) denotes pressure drawing fluid out of the capillary, and (−) denotes pressure drawing fluid back in to the capillary.

terstitium). Burning of the skin allows plasma proteins to escape from ruptured vessels and increases porosity of vessels because of pore enlargement; blisters ensue, which add to the protein loss from plasma. Other causes of increased permeability of blood vessels include bacterial toxins and allergic reactions.

- *Case C:* Increased oncotic pressure in interstitial fluid, indicating interstitial accumulation of proteins, may be caused by obstruction in the lymphatic drainage of an area such that extravasated plasma proteins accumulate. An example is the swelling that follows surgical removal of lymph nodes, as is often done in cancer cases. Filariasis is a nematode infection whereby inflammatory reactions progressively obstruct lymph-node channels with scar tissue; lymph drainage, for instance, of a leg, is totally occluded, which leads to grotesque swelling (elephantiasis) of that leg.

Shock is defined as a general failure of the circulation to adequately perfuse vital organs with blood. Shock may result from hemorrhage or increased vascular permeability, as in burns and anaphylactic reactions.

Kidney functions in control of volume and tonicity of body fluids

Volume and tonicity of body fluids are homeostatically controlled within narrow limits via the neuroendocrine system. In reaction to nervous signaling of abnormal volume or tonicity of blood, or blood pressure, various hormone-like agents are elaborated, including antidiuretic hormone, prostaglandins, atrial natriuretic factors, and products of the renin-angiotensin-aldosterone system. These agents in turn direct adaptive responses by the kidneys, as well as the thirst and salt craving mechanisms. Baroreceptors and stretch receptors monitor vascular volume, and thus (water being freely permeable across most membranes) total volume of body fluids. A constant volume, then, is maintained by appropriately varying the extent of Na^+ and Cl^- retention in the kidney in response to those nervous signals. Tonicity of the blood is monitored by osmoreceptors in the hypothalamus and is controlled by appropriately varying the extent of water retention in the kidneys. These interrelated renal functions are paradoxical: volume control is by salt regulation; tonicity control is by volume (water) regulation. Additionally, a mechanism exists for the urinary elimination of Na^+ in

reponse to elevated blood pressure under the influence of atrial natriuretic factors of cardiac origin.

Summary of metabolic kidney functions

In examining control of volume and tonicity of body fluids, the text shall highlight water, Na^+, and K^+ retention. Since the kidney is the primary organ involved, some of its major metabolic functions shall be reviewed. By producing urine, the kidney retains valuables and voids wastes and foreign chemicals, thereby controlling the composition of body fluids. As an ultimate checkpoint, the kidney has an important role in maintaining the body's acid-base balance. Endocrine functions of the kidney are quite diverse in their effects. Prostaglandins E_2 and I_2 stimulate renin release, and antagonize antidiuretic hormone (vasopressin), while they lower blood pressure and increases urine formation and electrolyte excretion. The enzyme renin, elaborated by the kidney in response to low blood pressure, leads to proteolytic activation of angiotensin II from an inactive precursor, which leads to correction of the lowered blood pressure by conserving water and electrolytes, vasoconstriction, increased salt hunger, and thirst. Another renal enzyme is responsible for converting an inactive vitamin-D derived precursor into 1,25-dihydroxycholecalciferol, which is one of the hormones in control over calcium and phosphate balance. The kidney produces several powerful vasodilators (e.g., bradykinin). Earlier, the kidney's production of erythropoietin, the hormone in control over hematopoiesis in bone marrow, and plasminogen, precursor of the fibrinolytic factor plasmin, were reviewed. The contribution of renal gluconeogenesis to the body's glucose balance will be considered later.

Functional anatomy of the kidney

Grossly, the kidney is enveloped by a tough capsule that, at the hilus, folds inward to line the sinus space (Figure 8-5). The outer layers of glandular cells, the cortex, dip down between papillae. Papillae constitute the medulla; the rays in the base portion of the conical papillae are formed by the parallel orientation of the tubules, Henle's loops, collecting ducts, and blood supply (vasa recta) of adjacent nephrons (Figure 8-6). Together, nephrons make up much of the kidney's parenchyma. Nephrons whose glomeruli are situated nearer the medulla are called **juxtamedullary nephrons;** nephrons located in the cortex are called **cortical nephrons;** their Henle's loops may not reach the medulla. Note that the collecting ducts of both

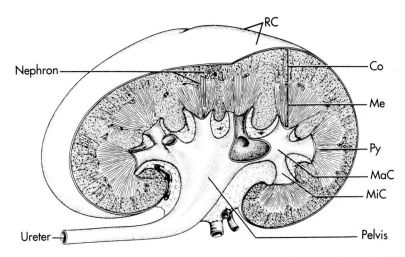

Figure 8-5. The kidney; note the nephron. The kidney is covered by a renal capsule *(RC)* composed of dense connective tissue. Kidney parenchyma is organized into an outer cortex *(Co)* and an inner medulla *(Me)* and contains more than a million functional units called nephrons. The highly coiled part of each nephron lies in the cortex while the long straight part may descend into the medulla. Each nephron drains into a collecting duct, and together they are called a uriniferous tubule. Uriniferous tubules coalesce into larger ducts and collectively form conical pyramids *(Py)*. Each pyramid and its overlying cortical tissue constitutes a lobe. There are 8-10 lobes in the human kidney, only one lobe in the kidneys of rats and other numbers in different animal species. Urine within the collecting ducts passes through openings at the papilla (apex) of the pyramid and drains into the minor calyces *(MiC)*, major calyces *(MaC)*, renal pelvis (located at the hilus), and ureter. *Reproduced with permission from Kessel RG and Kardon RH: Tissues and organs: a text-atlas of scanning electron microscopy, p 222, San Francisco, 1979, Freeman.*

kinds of nephrons traverse the medulla. The proportions of cortical to juxtamedullary nephrons vary among animal species; for example 9:1 in humans; 100:0 in beavers; and 0:100 in cats.

The nephron is the functional unit of the kidney, with respect to urine production. In human kidneys there are about 2.4 million nephrons—intermediate between the rat (30,000), the dog (80,000), the ox (8 million), and the elephant (15 million). Each nephron consists of a glomerulus, where blood is filtered, and a tubular system, where the initial filtrate is modified into urine.

Urine formed in nephrons flows through collecting ducts that merge into wider channels; then, by way of orifices at the apex of each papilla, urine flows into the renal sinus space, renal pelvis, and toward elimination via the ureter, urinary bladder, and urethra. The renal arteries coming off the aorta carry in a human at rest about 20 to 25% (renal fraction) of the cardiac output to the kidneys. This high flow rate through an organ that consitutes only 0.4% of body weight allows the kidney to control volume and com-

position of body fluids. Some 1 to 2% of the total renal blood supply flows through the vasa recta, the network of capillaries that supplies and drains medullary nephrons, and that has an important function in the formation of concentrated urine via the countercurrent mechanism.

Functioning of the nephron

Generally, one distinguishes glomerular filtration of blood, tubular secretion of metabolic waste products, and tubular reabsorption (also taking place in collecting ducts) of valuables such as water, glucose, minerals, and amino acids. Together these processes allow control over body fluid volume and composition.

Glomerular filtration

Glomerular filtration in humans produces some 180 L of filtrate per day (cf., total body water is 42 L), which may be reabsorbed for over 99.5% in the tubules. Whatever component of the filtrate that is not reabsorbed passes into the urine. An afferent ar-

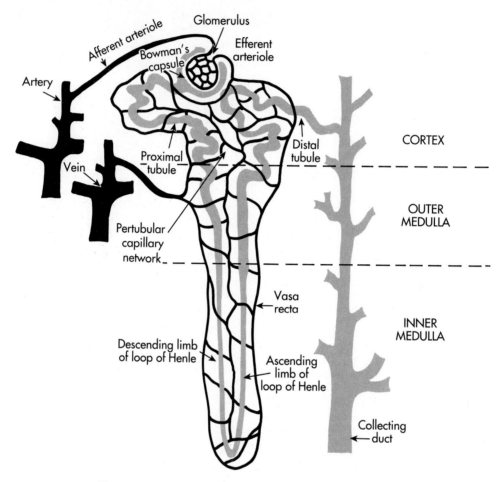

Figure 8-6. A juxtaglomerular nephron and its blood circulation.

teriole imports blood to a glomerulus, and an efferent arteriole drains the portion that has not been filtered. Enveloping the arteriolar tuft is Bowman's capsule (see Figure 8-6), where filtrate is collected and routed into the proximal tubule. Because of the magnitude of renal blood flow, both qualitative and quantitative control over glomerular filtration are of vital importance.

Qualitative control of glomerular filtration results from a series of three successive filters of decreasing pore size that stand between the bloodstream and lumen of Bowman's capsule (Figure 8-7). Small molecules can pass unimpeded, for instance, glucose and amino acids; even inulin, with a molecular weight of 5200, is filtered at the rate of water. However, blood cells and plasma proteins are not filtered. Albumin, the smallest of the main plasma proteins with a mo-

lecular weight of 68,000, is only 0.005% filtered. Hence, if a small molecular compound, such as a steroid hormone, is to avoid glomerular filtration, it must circulate in combination with a carrier protein. The pores in the glomerular filter are picked clean of obstructing proteins and debris by phagocytic (mesangial) cells.

Quantitative control of the glomerular filtration rate (GFR) results from (i) plasma oncotic pressure; (ii) glomerular blood pressure; and (iii) glomerular blood flow.

Plasma oncotic pressure is a main determinant of the net filtration pressure, the latter being the algebraic sum of the Starling forces affecting fluid distribution between arteriole and filtrate (Figure 8-8). The force driving fluid out of the arteriole and into Bowman's capsule is the arteriolar blood pressure; op-

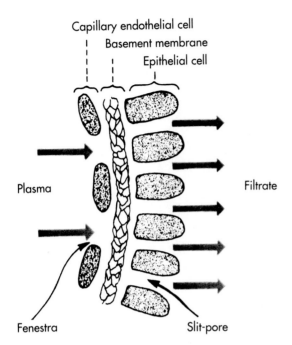

Capillary endothelial cell

Basement membrane

Epithelial cell

Plasma

Filtrate

Fenestra

Slit-pore

Figure 8-7. Filtration across the glomerular membrane. *Reproduced with permission from Guyton AC: Textbook of medical physiology, ed 8, p 290, Philadelphia, 1991, Saunders.*

posing that force, and thus directing fluid into the bloodstream, are the hydrostatic pressure in Bowman's capsule and the plasma oncotic pressure. The oncotic pressure of the filtrate in Bowman's capsule is negligible under normal conditions, since virtually no proteins are filtered. The water-conserving effect of plasma oncotic pressure is twofold: it limits GFR (by increasing as water and smaller solutes are filtered) and increases fluid reabsorption from renal tubules back into the blood (at the level of the peritubular capillaries).

Blood pressure and flow rate in the glomerulus are autoregulated, so that the GFR is relatively constant within only a few percent over a wide range (75 to 160 mm Hg) of systemic arterial blood pressure. Central in the enactment of autoregulation of GFR is the functioning of the juxtaglomerular apparatus (Figure 8-9). Where the distal tubule abuts the glomerulus, extradense tubular cells (macula densa) are in contact with granule-laden, swollen cells of afferent arterioles (juxtaglomerular cells); the granules in those cells contain renin precursor. The juxtaglomerular apparatus allows GFR to adapt to changes in systemic blood pressure, as follows.

When systemic arterial blood pressure drops, the GFR declines, resulting in enhanced time for Cl^- reabsorption in renal tubules. The macula densa senses a decreased Cl^- concentration in tubular fluid and causes dilatation of the afferent arteriole, thereby increasing glomerular blood flow and blood pressure and restoring GFR to normal. As accurate and fast as this negative feedback system may be, it constitutes only half of the autoregulatory mechanisms of GFR. The other half is regulated by the macula densa that, sensing a decreased Cl^- concentration in the tubular fluid, causes juxtaglomerular cells to release renin. Also, baroreceptors and neuroreceptors respond to lowered blood pressure by affecting renin release. The subsequent presence of angiotension II constricts efferent arterioles (which are most sensitive to angiotensin II), and that, in turn, raises the blood pressure in the glomerulus and restores GFR to normal. Thus, negative feedback mechanisms involving dilatation of afferent and constriction of efferent arterioles establishes autoregulation of GFR to such an extent that this vital process varies within only a few percent, even though systemic blood pressures may range from 75 to 160 mm Hg. The duality of the autoregulatory mechanism becomes evident when long-term effects of low arterial blood pressure on renal blood flow are considered. An acute lowering of blood pressure causes immediate dilatation of afferent arterioles and, thus, restoration toward normal renal blood flow. In a more chronic situation, the renin-angiotensin system constricts efferent arterioles, resulting in adaptation of GFR to nearly normal and a lowering of blood flow through the kidneys allowing systemic blood pressure to return to normal.

Elevated blood pressure causes increased GFR, hence less time for Cl^- reabsorption in renal tubules, a high Cl^- concentration at the macula densa, and responses of the juxtaglomerular apparatus that are opposite to those discussed above. In addition, a direct contractile response of the smooth muscle of the afferent arteriole to stretch helps to limit glomerular filtration when blood pressure is elevated.

Although autoregulation of the GFR helps to maintain fluid balance, the following four factors lead to an increased loss of body fluids:

- Increased blood pressure in glomeruli increases GFR;
- Increased blood flow through glomeruli decreases the fraction of renal blood flow that is filtered, thus the water-resorbing oncotic effect is washed out both in glomeruli and in peritubular capillaries;

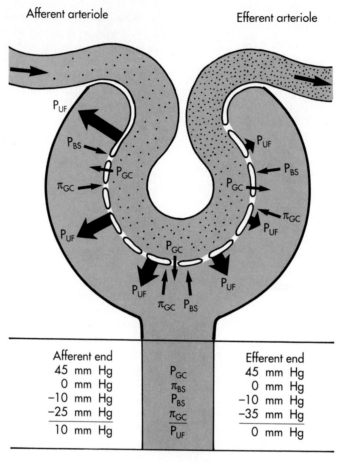

| | Afferent arteriole | | Efferent arteriole | |

Afferent end		Efferent end
45 mm Hg	P_{GC}	45 mm Hg
0 mm Hg	π_{BS}	0 mm Hg
−10 mm Hg	P_{BS}	−10 mm Hg
−25 mm Hg	π_{GC}	−35 mm Hg
10 mm Hg	P_{UF}	0 mm Hg

Figure 8-8. Starling forces controlling glomerular filtration. Net ultrafiltration pressure (P_{UF}) is the algebraic sum of hydrostatic pressures in glomerular capillary (P_{GC}) and Bowman's space (P_{BS}) and oncotic pressure in the glomerular capillary (π_{GC}). As plasma proteins are not filtered under normal conditions, the oncotic pressure in Bowman's space (π_{BS}) is zero. *Modified and reproduced with permission from Berne RM and Levy MN: Principles of physiology, p 430, St. Louis, 1990, Mosby—Year Book.*

- High rates of urine production wash out the medullary osmotic (urine concentrating) gradients of NaCl and urea (see below);
- High blood pressure in the vasa recta counters water reabsorption.

These factors combine to greatly increase urine formation in hypertensives; there may be a sevenfold increase when blood pressure goes from 100 to 200 mm Hg. Contrary to blood pressure, the rate of urine production is not regulated.

While examining factors that control GFR, discussions have progressed into various glomerular, tubular, and blood-circulatory contributions to the body's overall fluid balance. To round off that topic, the following factors are recognized:

- Sympathetic nervous stimulation and hypoxemia powerfully constrict both afferent and efferent arterioles, resulting in renal shutdown and in more blood availability systemically (e.g., exercise).
- Various hormones affect GFR: antidiuretic hormone causing water reabsorption from the distal nephron; aldosterone causing increased absorption of Na^+ and, thus, water; and prostaglandin E, produced by interstitial cells in the papillary medulla, antagonistic to antidiuretic hormone,

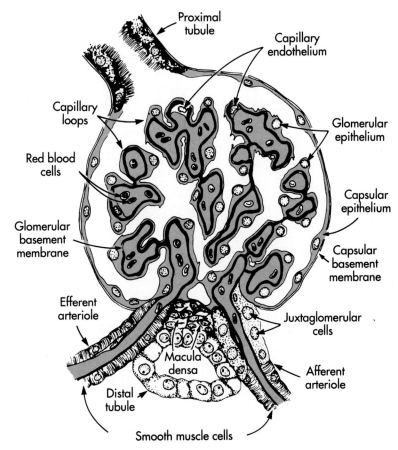

Figure 8-9. Juxtaglomerular apparatus. *Reproduced with permission from Ham AW and Cormack DH: Histology, ed 8, p 761, Philadelphia, 1979, Lippincott.*

causing water diuresis and Na^+ diuresis, as does atrial natriuretic factor (see below).

GFR is not completely balanced by tubular reabsorption of water (Table 8-6), the difference constituting an obligatory osmotic water loss. Obviously, the more particles that have to be voided in urine, the more water is lost. Thus, osmotic diuresis occurs due to high GFR of compounds that are not reabsorbed in tubules, such as urea, or injected sucrose or glucose in a diabetic.

In addition to the above listing of renal factors affecting fluid balance, a group of cardiac factors (collectively termed **atrial natriuretic factors,** or **ANF;** also called **ANP** for **atrial natriuretic peptides**) has been isolated from the atria of the heart. ANF is released in response to high blood pressure, causing the body to decrease blood pressure in various ways, such as by vasorelaxation of the afferent, but not the

Table 8-6	Glomerular imbalance	
Glomerular filtration rate (ml/min)	Rate of tubular reabsorption (ml/min)	Rate of urine output (ml/min)
50	49.8	0.2
75	74.7	0.3
100	99.5	0.5
125	124.0	1.0
150	145.0	5.0
175	163.0	12.0

Reproduced, with permission, from Guyton AC: Textbook of medical physiology, ed 7, 422, Philadelphia, 1986, Saunders.

efferent, arteriole, diuresis, and loss of sodium in urine. ANF counteracts the renin-angiotensin system by (i) decreasing thirst; (ii) inhibiting antidiuretic hormone, aldosterone, and catecholamine releases; (iii) increasing glomerular blood flow and filtration rate; and (iv) decreasing sodium and water reabsorption. Therefore, ANF intervenes in the short- and long-term control of water and electrolyte balances and of blood pressure. Clinically, the present understanding of factors that control ANF release and avail-

ability of pure ANF opens up new avenues in the therapy of hypertension.

To fully appreciate the vital importance of control over GFR, another look at Table 8-6 helps one to realize that an increased GFR from a normal value of 125 ml/min to 150 ml/min is almost, but not totally, matched by increased tubular absorption; however, increasing the rate of urine output by 4 ml/min increases urine production by a factor of five compared to normal.

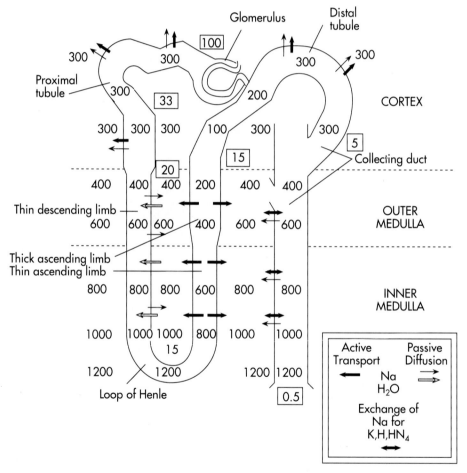

Figure 8-10. Summary of passive and active exchanges of water and ions in the juxtaglomerular nephron in the course of elaboration of hypertonic urine. Concentrations of tubular urine and peritubular fluid are given in milliosmoles per liter; large, boxed numerals, are estimated percentages of glomerular filtrate remaining in the tubule at each level. Chloride ions are actively transported in the ascending limbs of Henle's loops. The entire ascending limb of Henle's loop as well as the initial part of the distal tubule are impermeable to water, indicated by the thickened lining. *Modified and reproduced with permission from Pitts RF: Physiology of the kidney and body fluids, ed 3, p 134, Chicago, 1974, Year Book.*

Absorption and secretion in uriniferous tubules and collecting ducts

As glomerular filtrate passes from Bowman's capsule sequentially through proximal tubules, Henle's loop, distal tubules, and collecting ducts, essential substances, including water, glucose, amino acids, small proteins, and electrolytes, are reabsorbed by tubular cells and returned to the bloodstream (peritubular capillaries). Selectively, only valuables are reabsorbed; metabolic waste products are not resorbed, but voided in the urine. In addition, tubular secretion of selective waste products from the blood into the tubular lumen is an alternate means of eliminating metabolic wastes and electrolytes from the body. Thus, the nephron fulfills a dual role: it selectively removes waste products from the body, and it maintains the body's internal environment allowing for wide variations in the intake of salt and water.

A combination of microanatomical and physiological properties of tubular cells and peritubular capillaries allows the kidneys to produce dilute urine when excessive water has to be eliminated or concentrated urine when excessive water has to be conserved, and, at the same time, to rid the body of wastes by a combination of selective absorption and secretion processes in the nephrons.

The text shall follow glomerular filtrate on its way through a juxtamedullary nephron (Figure 8-10). The proximal tubules are lined with cells that have numerous mitochondria, indicative of active metabolic processes, and prominent microvillae for absorption. At this site all of the filtered glucose and amino acids, and most of the sodium and potassium, are reabsorbed by active processes, while water and anions, such as Cl^- and HCO_3^- follow passively. The descending Henle's loop traverses a huge osmotic gradient on its way down into the medulla. Its permeable tubular cells allow Na^+, Cl^-, and urea to enter the tubular fluid, and a small proportion of water to leave, so that, at the base of the papilla, the remaining tubular fluid assumes the highest osmolarity. The thin ascending Henle's loop is impermeable to water; Na^+ and Cl^- move passively into the interstitial space, whereas urea enters the tubular fluid (see Figure 8-10).

The thick ascending Henle's loop is not only impermeable to water, but also to urea; it is called the **diluting segment,** since tubular fluid is diluted to about 200 mOsm below surrounding osmolarities due to active Cl^- pumping, with Na^+, H^+, Ca^{++}, and Mg^{++} following passively. Strictly speaking, the initial portion of the distal tubule is also included in the definition of a diluting segment. The fluid is now monitored by the juxtaglomerular apparatus and continues into the distal convoluted tubule. It is important to note that this fluid has an osmolarity 200 mOsm below that of the interstitial fluid in the renal cortex and that of blood plasma. Herein lies the basis of the body's capacity to excrete hypoosmolar urine: the distal tubule and collecting duct (termed together, **distal nephron**), are impermeable to water, except in the presence of antidiuretic hormone (ADH). When ADH is absent, as in the case of hypotonic blood, the excess water is voided as hypoosmotic urine. Because the distal tubule is also impermeable to urea in the abscene of ADH (Figure 8-11), part of the tubular fluid's osmolarity resides in urea, and that allows for further reabsorption of minerals from the fluid. Approximately 10% of the filtered sodium exits the thick ascending Henle's loop and, depending on aldosterone levels, it can be reabsorbed (from 0 to 100%) from the distal tubular fluid. Also in the distal tubule, substances are actively secreted from the blood via peritubular capillaries into tubular cells and thence into intratubular fluid (e.g., H^+, K^+, and uric acid).

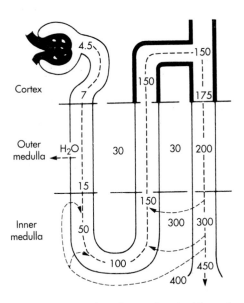

Figure 8-11. Recirculation of urea absorbed from the collecting duct. Numerical values are milliosmolalities of urea during antidiuresis caused by the presence of large amounts of antidiuretic hormone. *Reproduced with permission from Guyton AC: Textbook of medical physiology, ed 8, p 325, Philadelphia, 1991, Saunders.*

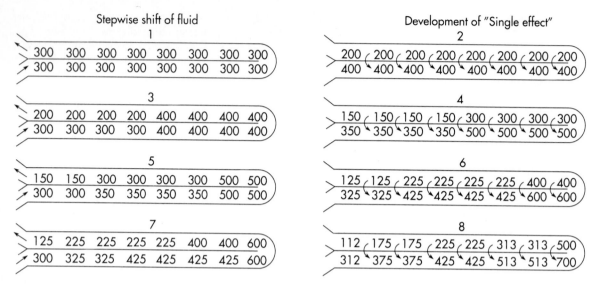

Figure 8-12. Countercurrent multiplication establishes a large osmotic gradient. The model is based on the assumption that at any level along the loop of Henle a gradient of 200 mOsm/L can be established between ascending and descending limbs by active transport of ions. *Reproduced with permission from Pitts RF: Physiology of the kidney and body fluids, ed 3, p 126, Chicago, 1974, Year Book.*

Finally, the collecting duct is permeable to water and urea, but only when ADH is present. In this case, traversing the medullary gradient pulls out the bulk of the remaining water, together with urea, by facilitated (passive) transport and solvent drag. Ammonium ions may be synthesized in ductular cells; these ions, as well as H^+ and K^+ ions, may exchange for Na^+ in tubular fluid, and this helps to control acidosis.

Osmotic gradient in the medulla

Medullary osmotic gradients of NaCl and urea are required for nephron functioning. These gradients are established and maintained by countercurrent mechanisms, that is, a countercurrent multiplication system between ascending and descending tubules and a countercurrent exchange system involving the vasa recta.

One necessary factor for countercurrent mechanisms is the parallel arrangement of tubules, ducts, and peritubular capillaries. The central feature of countercurrent multiplication is the Cl^- pump in the ascending Henle's loop. Imagine a stepwise process (Figure 8-12) in which 300 mosmolar fluid enters a loop. While stagnant, the Cl^- pump establishes 200

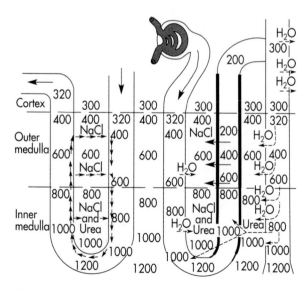

Figure 8-13. Countercurrent mechanisms for concentrating urine. Numerical values are in mOsm/L. *Modified and reproduced with permission from Guyton AC: Textbook of medical physiology, ed 8, p 310, Philadelphia, 1991, Saunders.*

Table 8-7	Concentration of urine during dehydration and medullary washout during water diuresis in dogs			
	Urine	**Cortex**	**Medulla**	**Papilla**
24 HR DEHYDRATION				
Osmolality	1725.0 ± 361.0			
Na ⎫	153.0 ± 60.0	80.8 ± 8.9	258.0 ± 18.7	320.0 ± 48.8
K ⎬ mmol/kg H_2O	162.0 ± 70.0	80.5 ± 7.9	44.5 ± 14.2	52.7 ± 5.5
NH_4 ⎪	76.2 ± 59.5	7.5 ± 0.3	14.2 ± 3.2	21.3 ± 2.3
Urea ⎭	991.0 ± 228.0	21.0 ± 4.6	532.0 ± 127.0	855.0 ± 160.0
Sum of osmolality	1771.0 ± 328.0	358.0 ± 27.5	1165.0 ± 127.0	1645.0 ± 255.0
WATER DIURESIS				
Osmolality	70.6 ± 16.6			
Na ⎫	2.8 ± 2.5	68.1 ± 5.7	134.0 ± 17.7	118.0 ± 23.1
K ⎬ mmol/kg H_2O	5.8 ± 3.7	77.2 ± 4.0	45.8 ± 5.0	48.6 ± 4.4
NH_4 ⎪	5.3 ± 2.5	7.6 ± 0.71	3.9 ± 0.51	6.8 ± 2.8
Urea ⎭	42.1 ± 16.4	10.0 ± 2.5	31.1 ± 9.9	33.4 ± 9.1
Sum of osmolality	69.9 ± 16.5	315.0 ± 13.9	401.0 ± 32.5	381.0 ± 50.7

Modified with permission, from Levitin H and others: Composition of the renal medulla during water diuresis, J Clin Invest 41:1145-51, 1962.

mosmolar differences along the way. Then fresh 300 mosmolar fluid enters and pushes the fluid forward; stagnant again, the Cl^- pump reestablishes a 200 mosmolar gradient. Multiple repetitions of this sequence produces a large gradient (Figures 8-12 and 8-13). What prevents the gradient from increasing is that materials reabsorbed from tubular fluid are carried away by the peritubular capillaries. To facilitate this process, the vasa recta has three important properties: (i) it carries 1 to 2% of the renal blood flow, which in humans translates into 12 to 24 ml/min or the entire blood volume in a matter of hours; (ii) its ascending and descending legs are adjacent; and (iii) medullary bond flow through the vasa recta is very slow (50-60 sec. for an RBC to flow from the efferent arteriole through the vasa recta and into the renal vein). Thus the vasa recta functions as a countercurrent exchanger to help maintain the medullary concentration gradient, preventing washout of solutes from the medulla. As a result, blood flowing through the vasa recta carries only a minute amount of medullary interstitial solutes away from the medulla.

The countercurrent buildup of a urea gradient in the medulla, combined with the impermeability of distal tubules and cortical collecting ducts to urea, allows urinary excretion of highly concentrated urea, the most important metabolic nitrogen waste.

The importance of the medullary gradients is further demonstrated by considering what happens in their absence. Poisoning the Cl^- pump with drugs (e.g., mercurials, furosemide) wipes out the medullary gradient and, consequently, causes severe diuresis. Drinking excessive amounts of water, inhibiting the release of ADH, causes diuresis by medullary washout (Table 8-7). Other causes of diuresis include (i) structural kidney damage (nephritis); (ii) osmotic diuresis (diabetes mellitus); (iii) poisoning glucose reabsorption (phlorizin); (iv) lack of ADH production or renal receptors for the hormone (diabetes insipidus), or inhibiting secretion of production or renal receptors for the hormone (diabetes Insipidus), or inhibiting secretion of ADH (with ethanol); (v) antagonize the actions of aldosterone or Na^+ retention (with spironolactone).

In different animal species, the kidney's capacity to concentrate urine depends on the number of nephrons present in the kidneys in relation to body size, the proportion of cortical to juxtamedullary nephrons, the magnitude of the medullary osmotic gradient, and the depth of the medulla. Large variations in maximal osmolalities of urine exist among animal species. With about 1200 mosm/L as the maximum of renal medullary osmolality, and juxtaglomerular nephrons comprising about 14% of the total, the human body (when challenged by dehydration) is able to concentrate urine to over 1200 mosm/L, which is about four times the body's plasma osmolality. At the two extremes, the beaver has about one third of a human's capacity to concentrate urine, whereas the desert rat exceeds human capacity by a factor of 4 to 5.

Na$^+$ and K$^+$ balance

In excess of 65% of Na$^+$, K$^+$, and H$_2$O of the glomerular filtrate is reabsorbed in the proximal tubules. The circular pattern of Na$^+$ entry and exit in the thin segments of Henle's loop does not make a net contribution to reabsorption. Some 25% of Na$^+$ and K$^+$ of the original filtrate accompanies the active reabsorption of Cl$^-$ in the diluting segment of the tubular system. About 10% of the filtered Na$^+$ and K$^+$ enter the distal nephron—the site of various physiologic control mechanisms.

The daily filtration of Na$^+$ is 600 g in humans, of which some 10% enters the distal nephron, an amount of Na$^+$ that equals the entire Na$^+$ content of the human body. This amount of Na$^+$ can be reabsorbed almost entirely when needed to maintain body fluid volume, in which case hardly any Na$^+$ may be voided in a day. The extent of Na$^+$ reabsorption in the distal nephron is dictated by the level of aldosterone in the blood. This hormone, acting upon the nuclei of tubular cells, enhances the synthesis of carrier proteins that function in the active exchange of Na$^+$ from tubular fluid (via tubular cells into peritubular space) for K$^+$, H$^+$, and NH$_4^+$ secreted into the tubular fluid. Aldosterone secretion, in turn, responds to various stimuli. A low Na$^+$ concentration or a low arterial blood pressure are sensed by the juxtaglomerular apparatus, giving rise to renin release, followed by angiotensin II stimulation of aldosterone release. In addition, elevated K$^+$ levels in the blood powerfully stimulate aldosterone release, since this hormone aids in K$^+$ elimination through both K$^+$ for Na$^+$ exchange in distal tubular cells, with the consequent secretion of K$^+$ into tubular fluid.

Tubular K$^+$ secretion is vitally important. As discussed earlier, maintaining a constant ratio of intra- over extracellular K$^+$ levels is a major factor in controlling the transmembrane electrical potential difference, essential for proper functioning of muscles (particularly of the heart) and the nervous system. Hence, to control the plasma K$^+$ level and avoid hyperkalemia, a system is needed that eliminates dietary K$^+$ by a mechanism, tubular K$^+$ secretion, that has a large capacity. In fact, because of its extreme sensitivity to blood K$^+$ levels, aldosterone secretion is the premier mechanism whereby blood K$^+$ levels are controlled.

Paradoxically, in contrast to K$^+$, aldosterone is of lesser importance to the regulation of blood Na$^+$ concentrations. This is because aldosterone-activated Na$^+$ reabsorption causes H$_2$O to follow osmotically, raising blood volume and pressure, thus enhancing GFR; this renders Na$^+$ reabsorption less effective, which offsets the original aldosterone effect. True, aldosterone is needed for Na$^+$ absorption in the distal nephron, but for fine control of the Na$^+$ concentration in the blood in the face of variable dietary intake, the body has the antidiuretic hormone-thirst system and the atrial natriuretic factors. When plasma Na$^+$ concentrations are elevated by approximately 1%, osmoreceptors affect antidiuretic hormone release and thirst, resulting in conservation and increased intake of water. Lowered plasma Na$^+$ concentrations, in contrast, lead to diuresis and a craving for salt. These ultrasensitive mechanisms control the plasma Na$^+$ concentration to ± 1%.

Role of the kidney in H$^+$ homeostasis

While on the topic of renal metabolic functions, the text shall overview the kidneys' contribution to H$^+$ homeostasis. Discussion of overall acid-base balance in animals will follow later.

Physiologically, the most important buffer system is the HCO$_3^-$/H$_2$CO$_3$ buffer system, since its concentration in plasma is relatively high and physiologic control mechanisms are associated with it. According to the Henderson-Hasselbalch equation,

$$pH = pK + \log \frac{[HCO_3^-]}{[H_2CO_3]} \text{ or}$$

$$pH = pK + \log \frac{[HCO_3^-]}{s \times pCO_2}$$

in which the [H$_2$CO$_3$], or [CO$_2$], is determined by the solubility of CO$_2$ in plasma (s, a physical constant), and the partial pressure of CO$_2$ (pCO$_2$), which is variable and depends on the rate of metabolism. This equation indicates that it is not the absolute concentrations of HCO$_3^-$ and CO$_2$ that are important, but rather their ratio. Given a pK value of 6.1 for the bicarbonate/carbonic acid buffer system in plasma, this ratio must equal 20:1 at a pH of 7.4. Therefore, the ratio is under physiologic control.

The lungs act upon the CO$_2$ component in the equation above and quickly respond to diminish, but never completely eliminate, the original pCO$_2$ upset. In response to acidosis, the lungs rapidly increase their rate and depth of respiration, and thereby blow off excess CO$_2$, but not the entire excess. Diminishing the elevated pCO_2 lowers the activity of CO_2 receptors, so that the hyperventilatory compensation stops short of restoring the $20:1$ ratio of $[HCO_3^-]/[CO_2]$. Conversely, decreased pCO_2 in alkalosis leads to hypoventilation, which retains CO_2; but then the lowered pO_2 is sensed by carotid body receptors and stimulates ventilation before the $20:1$ ratio is restored.

The kidneys act upon the HCO_3^- buffer component, retaining HCO_3^- by reabsorption in times of acidosis, and eliminating HCO_3^- in urine to counter alkalosis. In addition, the tubules secrete H^+ for urinary elimination as titratable acid, and secrete ammonia with which additional H^+ is voided in urine in the form of NH_4^+. Several of these renal mechanisms take days to fully respond to the conditions at hand. The value of the renal contribution to H^+ homeostasis is therefore not its rapidity, but rather its ability to completely neutralize an excess acid or alkali by restoring the HCO_3^-/CO_2 concentration ratio (and thus pH) back to normal. Following is a further examination of these renal tubular contributions to acid-base balance.

Reabsorption of filtered HCO_3^- associated with H^+ secretion. This response to changes in pH or volume of extracellular fluid is immediate (Figure 8-14, mechanism A). In humans, HCO_3^- is reclaimed to a variable extent (up to 100% if needed) in the proximal tubules, and approximately 84% of daily H^+ output is secreted by the same process. The Na^+ pump in the basolateral membrane of tubular cells drives tubular Na^+ into extracellular fluid (blood), and thereby establishes a Na^+ gradient going from tubular fluid into tubular cells. In the lumenal membrane of the tubular cell, Na^+ moves in along its electrochemical gradient in exchange for H^+.

CO_2 from the blood (extracellular fluid) diffuses into tubular cells, where it combines with H_2O in a reaction catalyzed by carbonic anhydrase. H_2CO_3, thus formed, ionizes, yielding H^+ and HCO_3^-. The H^+ moves into tubular fluid, combines there with HCO_3^- and then forms CO_2 and H_2O (catalyzed by carbonic anhydrase located in the brush border of proximal tubular cells). The HCO_3^- formed in the tubular cell accompanies Na^+ back into the bloodstream. The net result is that one HCO_3^- is reabsorbed (reclaimed) for each filtered HCO_3^- that is neutralized by H^+.

The normal serum HCO_3^- level is 24 to 28 meq/L. At this concentration, practically all of the filtered HCO_3^- is reabsorbed in the proximal tubules and returned to the plasma (Figure 8-15). When blood pH

is low (acidosis), the high pCO_2 in plasma raises the H^+ concentration in tubular cells; that, in turn, increases H^+ excretion, which stimulates reabsorption of HCO_3^- and, thus, retores the $20:1$ ratio of $[HCO_3^-]/[CO_2]$. With alkalosis, excess HCO_3^- is simply not reabsorbed and, thus, voided in alkaline urine.

Increased extracellular fluid volume enhances the glomerular filtration rate, thereby lowering Na^+ reabsorption. Consequently, as tubular HCO_3^- reabsorption is diminished, HCO_3^- is lost in urine and the body is left with an excess of H^+ ions (dilutional acidosis).

Excretion of titratable acid. In the tubular fluid, both proximal and distal, H^+ associates with $HPO_4^=$, thereby generating $H_2PO_4^-$ and freeing Na^+ for reabsorption (Figure 8-14, mechanism B). The term titratable acid refers to the amount of NaOH that must be added to a liter of urine to return its pH to 7.4.

It is important to note that, of the three renal H^+-secreting mechanisms, this phosphate mechanism is the only one that lowers the pH of urine. The value of this phosphate-acidification mechanism for H^+ secretion is that, normally, most of the HCO_3^- has already been absorbed in the proximal tubule, while still more H^+ has to be eliminated by secretion in the distal nephron. Because of a pK value of 6.8, the Henderson-Hasselbalch equation yields this tubular fluid at pH 7.4 and contains a $4:1$ ratio of $HPO_4^=/H_2PO_4^-$; that is to say, 80% of the phosphate can accept H^+. The limitation of this H^+ secretion process is the size of the H^+ gradient between tubular fluid and cells: maximally, a 1000-fold difference in H^+ concentration (3 pH units) can be maintained between tubular fluid and cells, thus limiting urinary pH to a value not less than 4.5.

Secretion of ammonium ions in urine. Secreting H^+ that has been combined with ammonia (NH_3) to form ammonium ion (NH_4^+) (Figure 8-14, mechanism C) offers a unique advantage. Ammonium ions do not acidify urine and, thus, can rid the body of excess H^+ under conditions where much of the HCO_3^- has been reabsorbed and the phosphate mechanism has topped out at pH 4.5. This mechanism uses glutamine, which is taken up from the bloodstream by both proximal and distal tubular cells. Deamidation of glutamine by glutaminase activity yields glutamate plus ammonium ion; subsequent deamination of glutamate by glutamate-dehydrogenase activity yields α-ketoglutarate, a TCA cycle intermediate, and a second ammonium ion. NH_4^+ is in equilibrium with NH_3 + H^+ in tubular cells, and since the pK of this re-

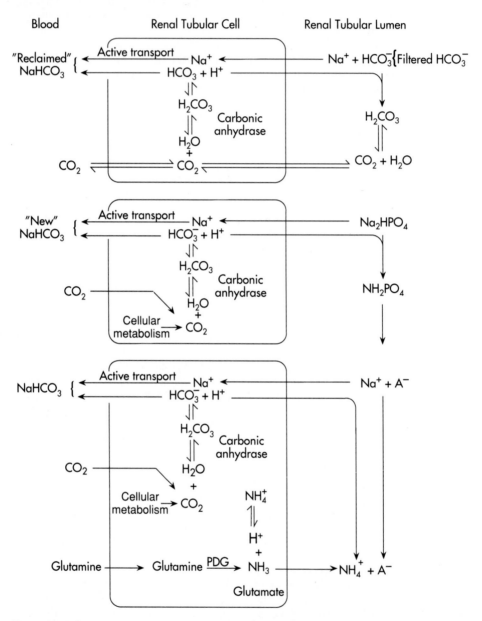

Figure 8-14. Renal tubular mechanisms for H$^+$ excretion. **A,** Reabsorption of filtered bicarbonate in association with H$^+$ secretion. **B,** Excretion of titratable acid. **C,** Secretion of ammonium ions. *PDG,* Phosphate-dependent glutaminase; *A,* anion. *Modified and reproduced with permission from Smith EL, Hill RL, Lehman IR, Lefkowitz RJ, Handler P, and White A: Principles of biochemistry: mammalian biochemistry, ed 7, p 178, New York, 1983, McGraw-Hill.*

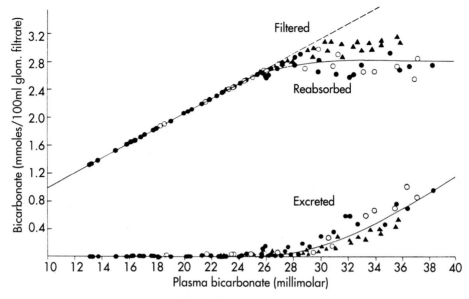

Figure 8-15. Reabsorption and excretion of bicarbonate as a function of plasma concentration in normal man. *Reproduced with permission from Pitts RF, Ayer JL, and Schiess WA: The renal regulation of acid-base balance in man. III. The reabsorption and excretion of bicarbonate, J Clin Invest 28:35-44, 1949.*

action is 9.0, the ratio of NH_4^+ to NH_3 at pH 7.0 is 100:1. However, the lipid solubility of NH_3 allows it to diffuse across tubular membranes into the tubular lumen, where it combines with secreted H^+ ions; because of their charge, NH_4^+ ions cannot be reabsorbed and, thus, pass into the urine.

Glutaminase activity in the renal tubules can be boosted to more than 10 times its normal activity under the influence of acidosis, a feature that adapts the rate of ammonia secretion to the amount of excess H^+ to be eliminated. Activation of glutaminase, thus, is a potent physiologic control over H^+ elimination. However, activation of glutaminase to these high levels requires several days, since it depends on the synthesis of new enzyme protein.

In sum, the kidneys counter alkalosis by increased HCO_3^- elimination, and acidosis by H^+ secretion, using three mechanisms: (i) combination with HCO_3^- allows complete HCO_3^- reabsorption and gets rid of H^+ in a form that does not acidify urine; (ii) combination with $HPO_4^=$ may lower the urinary pH to 4.5 as titratable acid is produced; and (iii) combination with NH_3 yields NH_4^+, which, though slow in adapting to need, offers an additional means of H^+ elimination.

The three H^+ secreting mechanisms allow the kidney tubule to reabsorb Na^+, together with osmotic water, in keeping with the renal function to control the volume of extracellular fluid in the body. H^+ secretion competes with that of K^+ in the exchange process of Na^+ reabsorption. Because of this competition, a reciprocal relationship exists, so that the presence of low K^+ concentration leads to increased H^+ secretion, while low H^+ concentration causes enhanced K^+ secretion. The following exemplify this phenomenon:

- Carbonic anhydrase inhibition by lowered H^+ generation increases urinary K^+ elimination. Na^+ reabsorption, however, is depressed, which leads to an osmotically increased urine volume; drugs that inhibit carbonic anhydrase (e.g., acetazolamide) are used as mild diuretics.
- In K^+ deficiency conditions, carbonic anhydrase-catalyzed intracellular H^+ (and thus also HCO_3^-) generation is hyperactive. The increased H^+ concentration allows Na^+ reabsorption while acidifying urine, but the augmented HCO_3^- production causes severe alkalosis. Conversely, hyperkalemia leads to alkaline urine and acidosis.

The exchange of Na^+ reabsorption for the secretion of H^+ and K^+ is under control of the adrenal mineralocorticoid aldosterone. Conditions of adrenal insufficiency (e.g., Addison's disease); feature low Na^+ and high K^+ levels in plasma. Conversely, adrenal hyperactivity (as may be caused by adrenal tumors or by pituitary- or tumor-related overproduction of ACTH, as in Cushing's disease) features hypernatremia, hypertension, hypokalemia, and alkalosis, because of abnormally elevated sodium reabsorption at the expense of increased urinary K^+ loss and urine acidification.

Clearance

To conclude the treatise of water and mineral balance and of some relevant kidney functions, the text must briefly direct the reader's attention to the quantification of these balances and organ functions and the physiologic application of the concept of clearance.

Measuring sizes of body fluid compartments

Principle; ideal case: no turnover. Generally an indicator-dilution method is used. The principle of the method is to put a known amount of indicator (e.g., a dye) in the pool for which a measurement is sought, allow time for the indicator to distribute itself evenly over the entire pool, and then measure dye concentration. Since concentration equals (amount added)/(pool volume), one finds that pool volume equals (amount added)/(concentration).

Example: To measure a dog's plasma volume, 900,000 CPM of ^{125}Iodine-labeled albumin are injected intravenously, allowing 10 minutes for mixing; then blood and plasma samples are obtained. Upon finding 2000 CPM per ml plasma, it is concluded that there are 450 ml of plasma in the dog. A problem with this simple method is that the indicator must meet various stringent criteria: They must (i) enter only the compartment to be measured (e.g., ^{125}Iodine-labeled albumin to assay plasma volume; tritium-labeled water to measure total body water); (ii) mix rapidly and evenly; (iii) not be metabolized before the concentration is measured; (iv) be nontoxic; and (v) be easily and accurately measurable.

Body pools are not stagnant. In the time it takes for the indicator to mix, turnover is already taking place because the pool is in a state of flux. Indicator disappears during mixing because of metabolism and urinary and biliary excretion. Therefore, when enough time is allowed for proper mixing, it also

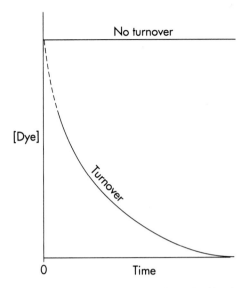

Figure 8-16. Disappearance of dye from the bloodstream.

allows for the disappearance of indicator from the pool. As a result, the indicator concentrations measured are too low, and, consequently, the estimated pool volumes too high. Clearly, one must correct for the disappearance of indicator during the time it takes to mix.

Correction for turnover. A measured relationship between dye concentration and time allows one to extrapolate and find the dye concentration at time-zero (Figure 8-16). That is the dye concentration that would have established itself initially and maintained itself if no turnover would have taken place (see Figure 8-16). Of course, the dye concentration at time-zero is the one that must be used for blood-volume estimation by the dye-dilution method.

Removal of indicator (dye) from the bloodstream, be it by liver (bile) or by kidney (urine), is a first-order process, meaning that the amount of dye removed per unit time is, at any moment, proportional to the amount of dye present at the start of that time unit. Calling dye concentration C and time t, it may be stated (for any first-order removal process): $dC/dt = -k \cdot C$. Integrating this equation from time-zero to a given point in time (t) yields:

$$\ln C_t = \ln C_0 - k \cdot t$$

and thus:

$$\log C_t = \log C_0 - k \cdot t/2.3 \qquad \text{(Eq A)}$$

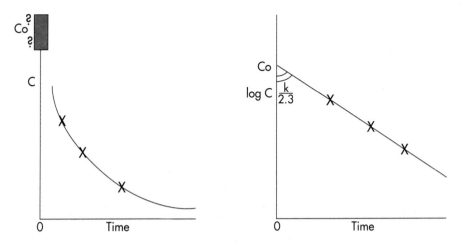

Figure 8-17. Extrapolation of the dye concentration (C) in blood to time-zero is simplified by the use of semilogarithmic graph paper.

Measuring dye concentrations at three successive times, and plotting those concentrations (C) against time on linear graph paper produces a curve (Figure 8-17) that is very difficult and inaccurate to extrapolate to time-zero. But when log C is plotted against time, a straight line is obtained (predicted by Equation A), and extrapolation to time-zero is easy and exact (see Figure 8-17).

Example: If an intravenous injection of 100 mg Evans Blue dye were given to a male dog weighing 20 kg, and dye concentrations were found of 100.53 mg/L at 10 minutes, 90.95 mg/L at 20 minutes, and 82.29 mg/L at 30 minutes, then by extrapolation it would be found that C_o = 111.11 mg/L, from which this would follow: plasma volume = 100/111.11 L, which equals 0.900 L, or about 4.5% of body weight (normal for male dogs).

In nature there are many first-order (logarithmic) processes. Those with negative slopes include dye disappearance, decay of radioactivity, light absorption, and bacterial death at a lethal temperature. First-order processes with a positive slope include bacterial growth, positive feedback, and the world's energy consumption.

Defining clearance. The aforementioned dye-disappearance curves are often referred to as **clearance curves.** These curves are determined by two parameters: the intercept with the ordinate (C_o) and the slope (k/2.3). The k value is the **fractional transfer rate.** It denotes the fraction of the pool that disappears

each minute, thus the dimension of K is minutes^{-1}. A practical expression for the slope of a logarithmic process is **half-life;** that is, the time it takes to decrease a given concentration (C_o) to half of its value (C_t). From Equation A it follows that ln (C_t/C_o) = $-k \cdot t$. Applying this to the case of one half-life, ln (½) = $-k \cdot$ half-life and, thus, half-life = (ln 2)/ k. Of course, the half-life value can also be read from the graph (see Figure 8-17).

Because k is a constant, a constant fraction of the injected dye disappears each minute. Therefore, while the dye concentration decreases with time, the fraction (though not the amount) removed each minute remains constant. It is helpful to picture that the total dye remaining, at any time, is evenly distributed over the total plasma volume, and that each minute a fraction k of that plasma volume is entirely cleared of dye. Thus, clearance is expressed as volume/time (e.g., ml/min); it is the volume (milliliters of plasma) that is totally cleared of dye per unit time (minutes). It is important to note the restricted use of the word clearance in physiology and in medicine: not an amount, but a volume is cleared over a given time. The kidneys do not clear a certain weight of glucose from plasma, but rather, they clear a certain plasma volume of glucose.

In medicine, plasma clearance of metabolites and indicators are used to quantify organ functions, pool sizes, and mineral balances.

Testing organ functions and mineral balance

Liver function tests. One of the chief functions of the liver is to clear the bloodstream of metabolic waste products. Failure of the liver to do so leads to hyperbilirubinemia (jaundice). A sensitive test for the liver's proper functioning is to follow clearance of intravenously injected dyes, such as sulfobromophthalein or indocyanine green. Within 45 minutes after injecting a standard dose of 5 mg of dye per kg of body weight, the liver should clear the blood, such that the dye concentration is below detectability.

Kidney function tests. The algebraic sum of the three renal exchange processes (Figure 8-18) represents the amount of material (dye) excreted in urine (mg/min). This equals urine flow (V_U, ml/min) times the concentration of compound X in urine (C_U, mg/ml). The sum of the three exchange processes also represents the amount of material (dye) lost from the bloodstream, which equals volume of blood totally cleared of X per unit time (V_B, ml/min) times the concentration of X in blood (C_B, mg/ml). Therefore, $V_B \times C_B = V_U \times C_U$, and thus:

$$V_B = V_U \times \frac{C_U}{C_B} \qquad \text{(Eq B)}$$

The following are notes to Equation B:

- Measuring the urinary excretion of compound X over a given period and the concentration of X in the blood (C_B) allows for the calculation of renal clearance of the blood (V_B). For example: when the average urine production over a given time amounts to 2 ml/min, and a concentration ratio of 3:1 for X in urine and blood is found, then, on the average, 6 ml of blood is cleared of X per minute.
- It is important to note that the dimension of V_B is the same as that of V_U, that is to say, ml/min.
- Different compounds have different clearances. Of course, only a certain volume of blood passes through the kidneys each minute, but 10 ml/

min may be cleared of compound X, and only 4 ml/min of compound Y.

Additional definitions used to quantify kidney functions

- Extraction ratio. Para-aminohippuric acid (PAH) passes easily through glomeruli. In addition, whatever remains in plasma after glomerular filtration reaches the tubules and is secreted there. As much as 91% of all PAH entering the renal arteries is removed in one passage through the kidneys; therefore, the extraction ratio for PAH is 91%, or 0.91. Because of the high extraction-ratio of PAH, clearance of PAH is a fair first estimate of plasma flow through the kidneys. For example, if the PAH concentration in plasma is 1 mg/100 ml, and 5.85 mg PAH/min passes into urine, then 585 ml of plasma/min are cleared of PAH, and the plasma flow through the kidneys must equal at least those 585 ml/min. Correcting for the 0.91 value of the extraction ratio, the corrected plasma flow would be (100/91) × 585 ml/min, which equals 650 ml/min. If the hematocrit were 45%, and thus the plasma volume 55% of the blood volume, then the total blood flow through both kidneys would equal (100/55) × 650 ml/min, which is 1182 ml/min.
- The filtration fraction is the ratio of glomerular filtration rate (e.g., inulin clearance) over plasma flow (e.g., PAH clearance). For example, if the glomerular filtration rate is 125 ml/min and the plasma flow 650 ml/min, then the filtration fraction is 125/650 (0.19), or 19%. This means that only 19% of the plasma presented to the kidney is actually filtered.
- Tubular load is the amount of a substance that filters through glomeruli into the tubules each minute; for example, if 125 ml of glomerular filtrate is formed per minute, and the glucose level in plasma is 100 mg/100 ml, then the tubular load of glucose is 125 mg/min. For Na^+ ions the tubular load equals 18 meq/min, and for urea, 33 mg/min.
- Tubular transport maximum is the maximal rate at which a substance can be actively reabsorbed in the tubules. The term **transport maximum** is often abbreviated as **Tm**. For glucose, Tm equals 320 mg/min, which is well above the tubular load of 125 mg/min normally encountered. Thus, at normal glucose levels in the blood, all

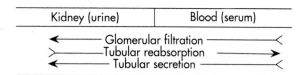

Kidney (urine)	Blood (serum)
←———— Glomerular filtration ————<	
>———— Tubular reabsorption ————→	
←———— Tubular secretion ————<	

Figure 8-18. Three exchange processes between the bloodstream and kidneys.

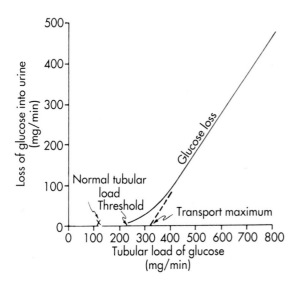

Figure 8-19. Relation of tubular glucose load to glucosuria. *Redrawn and reproduced with permission from Guyton AC: Textbook of medical physiology, ed 8, p 305, Philadelphia, 1991, Saunders.*

glucose filtered is reabsorbed and none is lost in urine. However, when the tubular load of glucose exceeds 400 mg/min, all but 320 mg/min is lost in urine. This 320 mg/min is the Tm value for glucose. Other compounds that are actively reabsorbed in tubules have different Tm values; for example, phosphate 0.1 mM/min; amino acids 1.5 mM/min; lactate 0.83 mM/min. It is important to note that there is no Tm for Na$^+$. Transport maximums are also in evidence for compounds secreted from the tubules. Some values of significance for the data in Figure 8-19 are PAH 80 mg/min and creatinine 16 mg/min.

- Threshold for substances that have a Tm: the threshold concentration of a compound in plasma is such that below that concentration all is reabsorbed, and at concentrations above it no more can be reabsorbed, and thus, all excess is eliminated in urine. In glucose, for example (see Figure 8-19), urinary loss occurs above a tubular load of 220 mg/min. The 220 mg/min threshold value of tubular load is reached (given a normal glomerular filtration rate of 125 ml/min) when plasma contains 180 mg per 100 ml; this is the threshold value for glucose concentration in plasma.

Differentiating the three renal exchange processes

For most effective treatment of renal failure, it is highly desirable to pinpoint the cause to one of the three exchange processes. Such is possible by judicious selection of test substances in clearance studies.

- Glomerular filtration rate is found by measuring inulin clearance. Inulin is a nonmetabolizable polysaccharide, which is eliminated solely by glomerular filtration (without concomitant tubular filtration or reabsorption); mannitol or iothalamate are also used.
- Renal plasma flow is indicated by clearance of PAH, since nearly 100% of the already low concentrations of PAH are removed from blood during a single passage through the kidneys by the combined processes of glomerular filtration and tubular secretion. One can correct for small amounts (ca. 9%) not removed during one passage through kidneys. Extraction ratio for PAH equals 91%; for diodrast, 85%.
- Tubular secretion is estimated from clearance of large doses of PAH under Tm conditions. A significant drop in Tm value for PAH indicates defective tubular secretion.
- Tubular reabsorption would be suspect when glucosuria is observed, while blood glucose levels were normal.

Using creatinine clearance to measure mineral balance

Complicating the clearance tests mentioned above is the fact that the concentration of compound X in blood (C$_B$) declines logarithmically, making application of Equation B cumbersome. One can solve this problem experimentally by infusing fresh X into the patient at a rate that matches renal clearance, so that C$_B$ remains constant; but this precedure would entail restraining the patient.

For these reasons, veterinarians gladly accept the help of mother nature: creatinine, a breakdown product of phosphocreatine in muscles, enters the bloodstream at the same rate at which the kidneys remove it, so no infusion is needed to maintain constant C$_B$. Creatinine is cleared almost entirely by glomerular filtration, and at a fairly constant rate; for instance in humans, plasma creatinine clearance is 95 to 105 ml/min. The constancy of creatinine clearance is used as an internal standard against which the clearances of other plasma constituents can be tested.

The disadvantage of determining the clearance of

a single substance (by using Equation B) is that blood and urine samples must be collected over a specified period of time and the volumes recorded. In most situations this is not practical. An acceptable alternative to this problem is to compute a ratio of the clearance of a substance to the clearance of creatinine, using a single collection of serum and urine:

$$\text{clearance ratio} = \frac{\text{clearance (X)}}{\text{clearance (creatinine)}}$$

The clearance ratio is most often a fraction of 1.0, but when multiplied by 100, one obtains the percent clearance ratio, which is a whole number:

$$\text{percent clearance ratio} = \frac{\text{clearance (X)}}{\text{clearance (creatinine)}} \times 100.$$

When applying the clearance formula (Equation B, with subscript S for serum):

$$\text{percent clearance ratio (X)} = \frac{\frac{C_u}{C_s} \times \text{vol}_u \ (\text{ml/min})}{\frac{\text{creat.}_u}{\text{creat.}_s} \times \text{vol}_u \ (\text{ml/min})} \times 100.$$

Simplification of that equation produces:

$$\text{percent clearance ratio (X)} = \frac{\text{creat.}_s}{\text{creat.}_u} \times \frac{C_u}{C_s} \times 100.$$

Using creatinine clearance as an internal standard cancels the impractical item, urine volume, out of the equation. Consequently, timed volumetric urine collections are not required. By determining the percent clearance ratio of a substance relative to creatinine, the actual loss of the substance from the body, through the kidneys, can be more accurately evaluated as variability caused by evaporation of the urine sample or by differences in water balance in the patient that cancel out.

It has already been pointed out that serum con-

Table 8-8	Normal percent clearance ratios in horses relative to creatinine clearance
Na$^+$	0.02-01.0%
K$^+$	15.00-65.0%
Cl$^-$	0.04-01.6%
P	0.00-00.5%

centrations of minerals (e.g., Ca^{++} and K^+) are homeostatically controlled and, thus, are unreliable as indicators of mineral balance. Therefore, the percent clearance ratio, relative to creatinine, is a convenient diagnostic tool to aid the clinician (Table 8-8).

ACID-BASE BALANCE
Importance of pH homeostasis

Maintaining pH within narrow limits around characteristic local values is vital for all body functions. Conditions that alter acid-base balance affect osmolarity and volume of body fluids, enzyme and transport processes, and, thus, metabolism and organismic functioning, as well as membrane potentials controlling nerve and muscle functions.

Normal physiologic pH is 7.4, which is the pH of most extracellular fluids. The intracellular pH averages around 7.0, depending on metabolic activity, but is much lower in certain intracellular particles (e.g., lysosomes). The 7.4 value of blood pH is midrange between 7.35 in venous blood (with its higher pCO_2), and 7.45 in arterial blood. Blood pH values significantly below the physiologic pH are referred to as acidemia, which usually accompanies a condition of acidosis; a blood pH above 7.4 defines alkalemia, a symptom of alkalosis. The blood pH range compatible with mammalian life is approximately 7.0 to 7.8.

The major effect of acidosis is depression of the central nervous system, which can be so severe (with blood pH under 7.0) that patients become disoriented, then comatose, and then die. The major effect of alkalosis is overexcitability of the nervous system, causing muscles to go into a state of tetany; tetanic convulsions may occur, and patients may die from tetany of respiratory muscles.

H$^+$ generating and depleting influences of diet
H$^+$ generating (acidifying) processes

Transport of metabolic CO_2 from tissues to lungs represents a transient H$^+$ burden because H$^+$ generation at the tissue site by the carbonic anhydrase reaction ($CO_2 + H_2O \leftrightarrow H^+ + HCO_3^-$) is offset by the same process going in reverse in the lungs, depleting H$^+$ ions. Only when some HCO_3^- is lost from the body (e.g., diarrhea) is the H$^+$ stranded, thus becoming a permanent burden.

Glucose metabolism under anaerobic conditions (heavy muscle exercise, erythrocyte metabolism) produces H$^+$ and lactate$^-$. Again, this is a transient H$^+$

burden as long as lactate$^-$ is further metabolized in the liver to either glucose or CO_2 + H_2O, since either process would use up one H^+. But if lactate$^-$ is lost in urine, as is its Na^+ or K^+ salt, a permanent H^+ burden is generated. Lactate$^-$ appears in urine at blood concentrations in excess of 50 mg/dl in most animals and prevails during heavy exercise.

Lactic acidosis in ruminants occurs when readily fermentable carbohydrates, such as grains, are overfed, from which the microbial flora in the rumen produces excessive amounts of lactic acid (including the slowly metabolizable $D(-)$ isomer) that are absorbed. Both lactic acid isomers are strong acids, and as large amounts of lactate ions are voided in urine, a H^+ burden is left that causes severe acidosis in the ruminant.

Sulfur-containing amino acids, methionine, cysteine, and cystine, are the acids that generate H^+ after a protein meal, since the neutral sulfur in them is oxidized and yields H_2SO_3. This H^+ burden is small, for even if all of the sulphur of amino acids were oxidized, it would neutralize no more than approximately 7% of the HCO_3^- formed from the α-COOH groups of amino acid catabolism.

Acetoacetic acid and β-hydroxybutyric acid, are strong acids. The liver overproduces these so-called **ketone bodies** from fats under conditions of critical carbohydrate shortage, such as during fasting, in cases of diabetes, in multiple pregnancy in sheep, and in a cow's early lactation stages. Metabolism of these acids cannot keep up with their rates of production, hence the anions are excreted in urine, leaving a large H^+ burden in the animal (ketoacidosis).

Urea synthesis from NH_4^+ ions, administered as ammoniun salts, is a H^+-generating process: $2NH_4^+$ + $CO_2 \rightarrow O = C(NH_2)_2$ (urea) + $2H^+$ + H_2O. Of course, when the NH_4^+ is first formed in the body from an amino group, it ties up H^+ ions, hence urea synthesis is not a net H^+ burden.

H$^+$-depleting (alkalinizing) processes

Metabolizable organic anions in food (e.g., lactate or citrate) alkalinize body fluids; their combustion to CO_2 + H_2O fixes one H^+ for each negative charge, thus depleting H^+. Vegetables, fruits, and leafy plant materials contain large quantities of organic acids that, upon digestion, produce HCO_3^-. Hence, typically, herbivores produce alkaline urine, carnivores do not.

Urea toxicity in ruminants occurs when urea is ingested in excess; under the influence of urease ac-

tivity in the rumen, urea yields ammonia: $O = C(NH_2)_2$ + $H_2O \rightarrow 2NH_3$ + CO_2. When more ammonia is generated than can be incorporated into the proteins of microbes, excess ammonia is absorbed and associates with H^+, forming NH_4^+. This H^+-depleting process would be offset if the liver could pick up all NH_4^+ coming from the rumen and convert it to urea, for urea synthesis generates one H^+ for each NH_4^+ used. The problem arises when hepatic urea production cannot keep pace with ruminal NH_4^+ formation. Under those conditions, NH_4^+ with fixed H^+ is lost in urine, and alkalosis ensues.

Buffering

The preceding discussion should make it clear that no acid-base homeostasis would be possible if the body did not possess buffering mechanisms that control the free H^+ and bicarbonate concentrations. The body buffers by either generating or depleting H^+, for which purpose it is equipped with chemical and physiological buffering systems. The principal chemical buffering systems of the body are: (i) bicarbonate/carbonic acid (HCO_3^-/CO_2) in extracellular fluid; (ii) phosphate ($HPO_4^=/H_2PO_4^-$) in cells and tubular fluid; (iii) proteins in tissue cells; and (iv) hemoglobin in erythrocytes.

The chemical buffers provide a fast, yet temporary, relief from acid-base challenges, but ultimately the chemical buffers must be restored to their prechallenge state and the offending acid or base permanently eliminated from the body. The latter task is accomplished by the following physiological buffering systems:

- The fast-responding, but only partly effective, reactions of the respiratory system
- The slower, but eventually completely effective, responses of the kidneys
- The exchange of H^+ ions in plasma for K^+ and Na^+ ions of tissues and bone
- The liver's removal of HCO_3^- and NH_4^+ for urea and glutamine production
- The gut's urease activity, which releases NH_4^+ from urea for use in the liver's urea cycle to neutralize additional HCO_3^-.

Permanent readjustment, however, cannot be accomplished unless the cause of the acid-base challenge has been isolated and the condition cured.

The bicarbonate/carbonic acid system (HCO_3^-/H_2CO_3) is not only a major chemical buffer, but also the system on which primary acid-base disturbances and the body's defense systems focus. The Henderson-

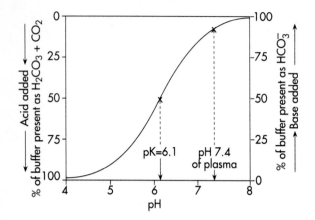

Figure 8-20. Titration curve of the bicarbonate/carbonic acid buffer system. At the pH 7.4 of plasma this system with a pK of 6.1 has little buffering capacity.

Hasselbalch equation for any buffering system

$$pH = pK + log([H^+ \text{ acceptor}]/[H^+ \text{ donor}])$$

can be applied to bicarbonate/carbonic acid (pK = 6.1):

$$pH = 6.1 + log ([HCO_3^-]/[H_2CO_3]).$$

The titration curve of the bicarbonate/carbonic acid buffer system (Figure 8-20) only has physiologic significance at around pH 7.4. Humans must live in a pH range where the chief buffer has very little capacity left to fight an alkaline challenge; a somewhat better buffering capacity (steeper slope) exists in the acidic region of liveability. Fortunately, the relatively high concentration of this buffer system in plasma provides some chemical buffering capacity, and, moreover, alkaline challenges in animals are uncommon relative to acidic ones.

H_2CO_3 (carbonic acid) and CO_2 dissolved in water are related, since $CO_2 + H_2O \leftrightarrow H_2CO_3$. The total amount of CO_2 in an aqueous medium ($H_2CO_3 + CO_2$), is proportional to the partial pressure of CO_2 (pCO$_2$) times the solubility of CO_2 in the fluid (S), $S \times pCO_2$. At body temperature, S equals 0.03 mmole/L per mm Hg of pCO$_2$. Thus, modification may be made to the Henderson-Hasselbalch equation

$$pH = 6.1 + log([HCO_3^-]/[0.03 \times pCO_2])$$

in which pCO$_2$ is expressed in mm Hg. For instance,

when we measure in arterial blood that pCO$_2$ is 40 mm Hg and [HCO$_3^-$] equals 24 meq/L, then pH = 6.1 + log [24/(0.03 × 40)], which equals 7.4.

The uniqueness of the HCO$_3^-$/CO$_2$ buffering system is significant: it is an open system, that is, it is in open contact with CO$_2$ in surrounding air. Since CO$_2$ is a major product of metabolism, there is always a large supply of potential H_2CO_3 available when required for buffering against processes that deplete H$^+$. On the other hand, since CO$_2$ is volatile, excessive H_2CO_3 generated by buffering can be expelled through the lungs into the environment. The following illustrates the advantage of the open system. In a sample of arterial blood with [HCO$_3^-$] = 24 meq/L, pCO$_2$ = 40 mm Hg, [total H_2CO_3] = 1.2 meq/L and pH = 7.4, an acid challenge gets buffered: H$^+$ + HCO$_3^-$ ↔ H_2CO_3. Now, in a closed buffering system, a drop of 4 meq/L in [H_2CO_3], bringing [H_2CO_3] down to 20 meq/L, would raise [H_2CO_3] by 4 meq/L to 5.2 meq/L, and the resulting pH would be 6.1 + log (20/5.2), which equals 6.69; it would be fatal. But in an open system, most of the H_2CO_3 formed dissociates to CO_2 plus H_2O, and reestablishes the CO_2 equilibrium value of 40 mM Hg, thus [total H_2CO_3] = 1.2 meq/L. Hence, the pH dropped to 6.1 + log (20/1.2) = 7.32; low, but survivable.

In a diagram showing the central function of the HCO$_3^-$/CO$_2$ system (Figure 8-21), HCO$_3^-$ is portrayed as the metabolic component, which is primarily affected in metabolic acid-base disturbances. The HCO$_3^-$ concentration is under the control of the kidneys, which adapt HCO$_3^-$ reabsorption to changes in pCO$_2$ caused by respiratory disorders, and by urea synthesis in the liver. These compensations tend to reestablish the 20/1 ratio of [HCO$_3^-$]/[H_2CO_3] commensurate with a pH of 7.4. The pCO$_2$ is depicted as the respiratory component, which is primarily affected in respiratory acid-base disturbances, and whose value is under control of the lungs (and respiratory center), which modify ventilation to compensate for variations in [HCO$_3^-$] caused by metabolic disorders. Buffering by other systems also affects the ratio (see Figure 8-21). Clearly, there can be only one pH value in a fluid. This truism is known as the **isohydric principle,** which states that all buffering systems actually buffer each other. Controlling one buffering system, by keeping the HCO$_3^-$/H_2CO_3 ratio constant, then controls all buffering systems and, thus, the pH of body fluids.

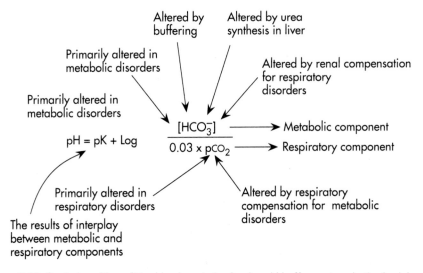

Figure 8-21. Central position of the bicarbonate/carbonic acid buffer system in the body's acid-base balance. *Modified and reproduced with permission from Schrier RW (ed): Renal and electrolyte disorders, ed 3, p 142, Boston, 1986, Little, Brown & Company.*

Respiratory regulation of acid-base balance (summary)

- Respiratory regulation acts on the pCO_2 component of the HCO_3^-/H_2CO_3 buffering system.
- pCO_2 is inversely proportional to the rate of alveolar ventilation. Doubling the rate of alveolar ventilation (to twice that of normal) causes a pH change of $+0.23$; reducing that rate to 25% of normal changes pH by 0.4. This is quite a pH range, and even larger variations in the rate of alveolar ventilation are possible.
- Two types of stimuli can either augment or diminish respiratory-center activity: humoral and neural stimuli. Humoral stimuli originate from the respiratory center, the pCO_2 of cerebrospinal fluid, or the peripheral chemoreceptors (aortic and carotid bodies). Responding to increased pCO_2, increased $[H^+]$, or decreased pO_2 in body fluids, the respiratory system acts in feedback fashion to control the rate and depth of respiration, and thereby the pH. Neural stimuli from stretch receptors in the lungs protect the lungs from overstretching by decreasing depth or tidal volume, while increasing rate of respiration; this "Hering-Breuer reflex" is not covered in this section.
- Respiratory compensation does not completely restore the pH. Gradually, as pH (and pCO_2) approach normalcy, stimulation of the respiratory center ceases. For instance, after a sudden pH drop from 7.4 to 7.0, hyperventilation restores the pH in a matter of minutes, but only to 7.2 to 7.3. Hypoventilatory compensation of alkalosis is limited by the stimulation of the respiratory center, as a consequence of the lowered pO_2 and increased pCO_2 that accompany hypoventilation.
- The buffering power of the respiratory system is one to two times as great as that of all of the chemical buffers combined.

Renal regulation of acid-base balance (summary)

- Renal regulation acts on the HCO_3^- component of the HCO_3^-/H_2CO_3 buffer system.
- Compensating for acidosis, HCO_3^- is totally reabsorbed, very little free H^+ is excreted in urine, yet somewhat more titratable acid ($H_2PO_4^-$) and NH_4^+ (H^+ induces glutaminase activity in the kidney) are excreted as a means of buffering H^+. Compensating for alkalosis, alkaline urine containing HCO_3^- is excreted.
- Renal compensation of acid-base challenge is slow (several days) but eventually complete, provided the cause of the disturbance has been isolated and the condition cured.

- HCO_3^-/Cl^- relation: with the renal elimination of H^+ in the form of ammonium ions, one Cl^- is eliminated and one HCO_3^- enters the extracellular fluid; hence, HCO_3^- substitutes for Cl^- in the extracellular fluid. Conversely, during alkalosis, when HCO_3^- passes into urine, Cl^- is reabsorbed and hyperchloremia ensues. Therefore, renal acid-base regulation also regulates the HCO_3^-/Cl^- ratio in extracellular fluid.
- Tubular reabsorption of Na^+ takes place in exchange for secretion of H^+ and K^+. Competition between H^+ and K^+ explains why a condition of hypokalemia leads to severe alkalosis, and hyperkalemia to acidosis. Because aldosterone controls Na^+ reabsorption, conditions that cause excessive aldosterone production lead to enlarged H^+ secretion in urine, and, thus, to alkalosis; conversely, depressed aldosterone production causes acidosis.

Hepatic and intestinal contributions to regulation of acid-base balance

The process of HCO_3^- elimination in the kidneys cannot cope with the rapid rate at which HCO_3^- is produced in the body from the α-carboxyl groups of amino acids. One reason the kidneys cannot excrete most of the HCO_3^- formed from amino acids catabolism is that HCO_3^- is mostly reabsorbed; another is that $CaCO_3$ is not soluble enough.

A crucial liver function in acid-base homeostasis

has been identified that remedies the problem of HCO_3^- excretion. Parenchymal liver cells may be located near the blood supply of the portal vein and hepatic artery; those periportal cells metabolize in the presence of relatively high pO_2. On the other extreme, perivenous cells located near the hepatic venous drainage have a more anaerobic metabolism. This zonation within the hepatic parenchyma is crucial for the liver's functioning in metabolism.

It is important to realize that urea formation in liver eliminates both ammonia and bicarbonate. Under normal conditions, bicarbonate formed during amino acid breakdown is in part exhaled as CO_2 by the lungs, and for the rest combined with amino groups, also derived from amino acid breakdown, to form urea in the liver's periportal cells (Figure 8-22). In perivenous liver cells, part of the amino groups combine with glutamate and leave the liver as glutamine. This hepatic glutamine and also glutamine of extrahepatic origin enter the periportal cells, where their amide group is used for urea synthesis, leaving glutamate for reuse in the perivenous cells.

During acidosis, the HCO_3^- level in plasma is lowered, so that the urea cycle's contribution to ammonium excretion is diminished. More glutamine is formed in the liver, while in kidneys the activity of glutaminase is increased; hence, increased amounts of NH_4^+ are voided in the urine of an acidotic patient (Figure 8-23).

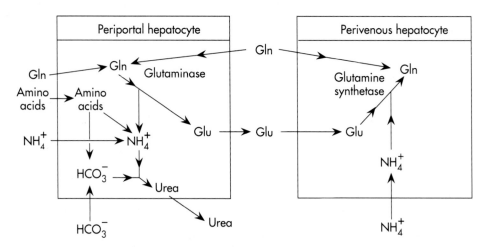

Figure 8-22. Urea formation serves for elimination of both NH_4^+ and HCO_3^-. The role of a glutamate *(Glu)*-glutamine *(Gln)* cycle between periportal and perivenous liver cells is shown. *Modified and reproduced with permission from Häussinger D: Hepatocyte heterogeneity in glutamine and ammonia metabolism and the role of an intercellular glutamine cycle during ureogenesis in perfused rat liver, Eur J Biochem, 133:269-275, 1983.*

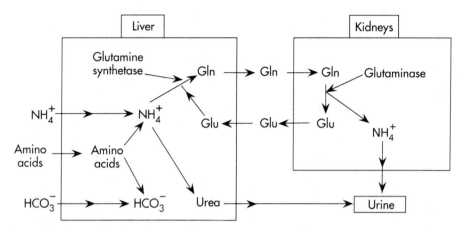

Figure 8-23. Elimination of NH_4^+ during acidosis. At low pH, the availability of HCO_3^- is limited and therefore the production of urea declines. Increased glutamine synthetase activity at low pH in the liver and stimulation of renal glutaminase during acidosis then sustain a glutamine-glutamate cycle whose function it is to eliminate NH_4^+ in urine.

Urease activity in the gut generates ammonia, which is transported to the liver via the bloodstream, where it neutralizes additional bicarbonate in the urea cycle. This contribution to acid-base balance by the gut is especially important in herbivores (e.g., ruminants), since these animals produce additional bicarbonate from organic acids in plants; their blood urea, in part, enters the saliva and, thus, is routed to the gut. In hibernating animals, this gut-liver cycling of urea is important for maintaining nitrogen balance.

Abnormalities of acid-base balance

Having dissected the homeostatic mechanisms that protect the body against changing H^+ ion concentrations, the text will now examine disturbances of acid-base balance, etiology (cause), pathogenesis (development), compensation by the body's defenses, and rationale of therapy.

Classification of primary disturbances; causes; compensation

Based on the ratio of HCO_3^- (metabolic component) over CO_2 (respiratory component), four primary acid-base disturbances can be classified: (i) primary CO_2 retention (i.e., respiratory acidosis); (ii) primary CO_2 depletion (i.e., respiratory alkalosis); (iii) primary HCO_3^- retention (i.e., metabolic alkalosis); and (iv) primary HCO_3^- depletion (i.e., metabolic acidosis).

The clinician who needs to categorize a patient is faced with two problems: (i) often, more than one kind of primary acid-base upset is present in a patient, so some of the symptoms are masked by counteracting disturbances; and (ii) symptoms are attenuated by secondary, compensatory defense mechanisms in the body, such as hyperventilation and HCO_3^- excretion. Indeed, uncompensated cases of acidosis or alkalosis are only a teaching tool. They do not exist in the live animal, since they are rapidly fatal; besides, the compensatory responses react promptly.

Before focusing on the four classes of primary acid-base disturbances, the term **respiratory** is defined as having to do with the lungs and respiratory center located in the medulla oblongata, and affecting the CO_2 component of the physiologic buffering system. The term **metabolic** then shall connote any mechanism that is nonrespiratory and affects the HCO_3^- component of the physiological buffer. The latter includes all kinds of disturbances: real metabolic ones (ketoacidosis), pathophysiologic ones (diarrhea, vomiting), nutritional ones (overindulgence in acidifying or alkalinizing substances), iatrogenic ones (physician induced), etc. Neither acidosis nor alkalosis is defined with respect to H^+; in fact, acidosis may exist in patients with alkaline plasma pH, and alkalosis at acidic plasma pH. The terms **acidemia** and **alkalemia** specifically refer to decreases or increases in blood pH, respectively.

Respiratory acidosis. The primary cause of respiratory acidosis is CO_2 retention resulting from hypoventilation. When arterial pCO_2 rises, the HCO_3^-/CO_2 ratio declines, as does pH according to the Henderson-Hasselbalch equation.

Causes include the following:
- Drugs or toxins that inhibit the respiratory center.
- Impeded CO_2 diffusion in the lung (e.g., pneumonia; emphysema; heaves in horses).
- Pneumothorax, causing one lung to collapse.
- Holding one's breath; though low pO_2 and increasing pCO_2 are sensed by carotid chemoreceptors, causing an overriding stimulus to breathe again.
- Hypoventilation of a patient on a positive-pressure anesthesia machine.

Compensation by the kidneys increases the HCO_3^-/CO_2 ratio back to normal by HCO_3^- retention and H^+ elimination in acidic urine as titratable acid and as NH_4^+. Thus, the case of compensated respiratory acidosis is characterized by increased levels of both CO_2 and HCO_3^- in plasma.

Respiratory alkalosis. The primary cause of respiratory alkalosis is CO_2 depletion due to hyperventilation. The ratio of HCO_3^-/CO_2 increases, as does pH. This condition is rarely seen in domestic animals.

Causes include the following:
- Hyperventilation of a patient on a positive-pressure anesthesia machine. (This iatrogenic cause is the most common.)
- Drugs or toxins that stimulate the respiratory center.
- Hyperventilation in states of pain, anxiety, hysteria, eclampsia in the welping bitch, early heat stroke, and NH_4^+ toxicity.
- High altitude, whereby low pO_2 causes hyperventilation.

Compensation by the kidneys decreases HCO_3^- reabsorption, produces alkaline urine containing HCO_3^- and $HPO_4^=$, and halts NH_4^+ production. Thus, the case of compensated respiratory alkalosis is characterized by decreased levels of both CO_2 and HCO_3^-.

Metabolic acidosis. The primary cause is HCO_3^- depletion, which lowers the HCO_3^-/CO_2 ratio and, thus, the pH. Primary lowering of HCO_3^- may result from buffering of acids (either ingested, injected, or formed by metabolism) or from the loss of base from body fluids. Symptoms of metabolic acidosis may include hyperventilation (compensatory), depression of the central nervous system, cardiac dysrhythmias, disorientation, and comatose conditions.

Causes include the following:
- Severe diarrhea; this constitutes a direct loss of HCO_3^- and not a loss due to buffering of acid. This is the most common cause of metabolic acidosis in animals.
- Vomition with regurgitation of upper intestinal contents; this, likewise, is a direct HCO_3^- loss.
- Renal disease (uremic acidosis), which constitutes a failure to reabsorb HCO_3^- or to excrete H^+.
- Hyperchloremia; when excess $[Cl^-]$, and thus an abnormally low level of the complementary bicarbonate anion prevails. A special case of this is dilutional acidosis due to infusion of a physiologic salt solution. Vascular volume expansion increases the glomerular filtration rate, which diminishes reabsorption of Na^+ and HCO_3^- ions.
- Hyperkalemia; when $[H^+]$ in plasma increases due to K^+ for H^+ exchange in tissue cells; also caused by diminished renal H^+ secretion when excess K^+ is excreted in exchange for reabsorbed Na^+.
- Deficient aldosterone secretion (Addison's disease); diminished Na^+ reabsorption in the kidneys is accompanied by diminished HCO_3^- reabsorption.
- Drugs or toxins that decrease carbonic anhydrase activity in the kidneys decrease HCO_3^- reabsorption.
- Overproduction of ketoacids (acetoacetic acid and β-hydroxybutyric acid) under various conditions, such as diabetes mellitus, fasting, or bovine ketosis.
- Lactic acidemia in ruminants after overfeeding grain.
- Ischemic conditions resulting in anaerobic metabolism and severe muscular exercise, both generating lactic acidemia.

Compensation by the lung in the form of hyperventilation eliminates part of the CO_2 excess, thus raising the HCO_3^-/CO_2 concentration ratio towards normal, but the CO_2-sensitive response stops short of completely compensating for the lowered HCO_3^- level. The kidneys if functional, aid in H^+ removal by increased HCO_3^- reabsorption, titratable acid secretion, and NH_4^+ generation, the latter in cooperation with the liver. The case of compensated metabolic acidosis is characterized by lowered levels of both HCO_3^- and CO_2.

Metabolic alkalosis. The primary cause is HCO_3^-

retention, which raises the HCO_3^-/CO_2 ratio and, thus, the pH. Symptoms of metabolic alkalosis may include a mild degree of hypoventilation (compensatory), and overexcitability of the nervous system, leading to tetany and, eventually, death. Given that our buffering systems are not well equipped to deal with alkali excess, it is fortunate that metabolic alkalosis is relatively uncommon.

Causes include the following:

- Vomition of gastric contents, rich in HCl. In the formation of new HCl by gastric parietal cells, HCO_3^- is returned to the bloodstream. Herbivores do not vomit; only carnivores and omnivores do.
- Hypochloremia leads to increased reabsorption of HCO_3^- in the kidneys.
- Hypokalemia leads to increased renal HCO_3^- reabsorption and more H^+ for Na^+ exchange.
- Diuretic therapy, likewise, leads to increased Cl^- loss and HCO_3^- reabsorption.
- Excessive ingestion of alkaline drugs used therapeutically to combat acidosis; such as sodium salts of bicarbonate, acetate, lactate, or citrate.
- Excessive secretion of aldosterone, causing excessive reabsorption of Na^+ and accompanying HCO_3^-.
- Ammonia toxicity in ruminants, resulting from feeding excessive amounts of nonprotein nitrogen (urea, NH_4^+).

Compensation by the lungs in the form of hypoventilation conserves CO_2 and, thus, brings the HCO_3^-/CO_2 concentration ratio closer to normal; but this respiratory compensation is limited because of potent stimulation of the respiratory drive by the increased pCO_2 and, also, by the lowered pO_2. The kidneys respond by decreasing HCO_3^- reabsorption, excreting HCO_3^- into urine, and by diminished secretion of free H^+, $H_2PO_4^-$, and NH_4^+. The case of compensated metabolic alkalosis is characterized by increased levels of both HCO_3^- and CO_2.

Summarizing compensatory mechanisms

Respiratory compensation of metabolic acidosis or alkalosis is fast and 50 to 75% effective. Renal compensation of respiratory acidosis or alkalosis takes days and can be 100% effective if the cause of the primary upset has been remedied. A concise summary chart of compensated cases of acid-base disturbances should be helpful (Table 8-9).

Table 8-9	Compensated cases of acid-base disturbances			
	pH	pCO₂	[HCO₃]	[HCO₃]/[CO₂]
ACIDOSIS				
Metabolic	down	down	down	down
Respiratory	down	up	up	down
ALKALOSIS				
Metabolic	up	up	up	up
Respiratory	up	down	down	up

Physiological basis for treatment of acid-base disturbances

Acidosis may be treated by administering alkalinizing agents, such as the sodium salts of bicarbonate, acetate, lactate, or citrate. Metabolizing the organic moieties of these salts to CO_2 plus H_2O removes H^+ ions from the body and leaves HCO_3^- stranded:

$$Na^+ \text{ lactate}^- + H_2CO_3 \rightarrow Na^+ + HCO_3^- + \text{Lactic acid}$$
$$C_3H_6O_3 \text{ (lactic acid)} + 3O_2 \rightarrow 3CO_2 + 3H_2O$$
$$\text{In sum: } Na^+ \text{ lactate}^- + H_2CO_3 + 3O_2 \rightarrow$$
$$3CO_2 + 3H_2O + Na^+ + HCO_3^-$$

These alkalinizing compounds are indicated only when the body is able to metabolize them, or else the desired therapeutic effect will not be obtained. For example, most of these compounds are poorly metabolized under hypoxic conditions, and, because of this, a more direct means of treatment, such as $NaHCO_3$, would be better when both hypoxia and acidosis are present. These compounds can be administered both parenterally and orally under most conditions.

Alkalosis may be treated with acidifying agents. Examples include (i) lysine hydrochloride, which yields HCl; (ii) NH_4Cl, from which urea is formed and HCl remains; (iii) sulfur-containing amino acids that are oxidized to strong acids; and (iv) NaCl. The latter may come as a surprise, but volume-depleted hypochloremic patients, after vomiting acidic stomach contents, would avidly reabsorb Na^+ to correct hypovolemia, with a predominance of HCO_3^- being available as accompanying anion, causing alkalosis; hence, the use of intravenous 0.9% NaCl solution in such cases, with supplementary KCl, if hypokalemia must also be corrected. Also, increased vascular volume leads to dilutional acidosis. Of course, alkalosis caused by excessive secretion of aldosterone cannot be remedied by NaCl infusion. A common clinical indication for administering urine-acidifying agents is urolithiasis (kidney stones, most commonly consisting of organic calcium salts), since calcium is kept soluble that way. However, if the stones consist of uric acid, which is formed only in primates and Dalmation dogs, urine acidification would aggravate matters, since urates are insoluble in acid media.

Clinical measurement of acid-base balance and abnormalities
Anion gap

Under normal conditions, the primary ion concentrations of plasma approximate those listed in Table 8-10. Clinically, only the cations Na^+ and K^+ are measured (together, about 148 meq/L) and the anions Cl^- and HCO_3^- (together, about 130 meq/L). The difference between these cations and anions is called the **anion gap;** its value in this example is 148 meq/L minus 130 meq/L, which equals 18 meq/L. Normal values for anion gap are 15 to 20 meq/L. The term **anion gap,** however, is something of a misnomer, since the total number of cations in plasma must equal the total number of anions.

Anion gap measurements are used to differentiate in metabolic acidosis the two causes of lowered HCO_3^- concentration in plasma, namely, HCO_3^- losses from the gut or kidneys, or net addition of endogenous or exogenous acid. It may also be useful in diagnosing hypoproteinemic metabolic alkalosis.

- When acid is added to the body, only the HCO_3^- concentration drops, while the concentrations of Cl^- and the cations remain unchanged. Hence, as illustrated in barogram C (Figure 8-24), the anion gap increases: $(144 + 4) - (105 + 15) = 28$ meq/L, which is above the normal range. Metabolic acidosis with an abnormal anion gap may result from: (i) diabetic ketoacidosis;

(ii) lactic acidosis (nutritional or ischemic); (iii) renal failure to excrete acid; or (iv) intoxication with acid-producing compounds (e.g., salicylate or ethylene glycol).
- When metabolic acidosis is caused by HCO_3^- loss from the kidneys or gut, the anion gap may remain normal (Figure 8-24, barogram B). The reason is that Na^+ accompanies the HCO_3^- lost in urine, diarrhea, or vomit. To compensate for the Na^+ loss, the kidneys increase tubular absorption of Na^+, and Cl^- goes with it. This Cl^-, added to a normal level of Cl^-, causes hyperchloremia in the presence of a normal anion gap: $(144 + 4) - (119 + 13) = 16$ meq/L. Thus, a hyperchloremic metabolic acidosis is accompanied by a normal anion gap and is diagnostic for bicarbonate loss syndromes, such as: (i) diarrhea; (ii) carbonic anhydrase inhibitors; or (iii) uremic acidosis. A dilutional acidosis caused by infusion of a physiologic salt solution also features a normal anion gap.
- When metabolic alkalosis is caused by hypoproteinemia, the anion gap may be reduced. The reason is that both HCO_3^- and Cl^- will increase in plasma in order to compensate for the lost protein anion, in effect "filling the total anion gap."

Measuring pH, [HCO_3^-], and pCO_2

Having learned about the use of anion gap in clinical diagnosis of metabolic acid-base disorders, the reader may wonder why one does not simply measure blood pH for that purpose. Measuring blood pH is in fact done; the blood sample must be kept in a closed container, since loss of CO_2 from the sample would increase the pH. It is not necessarily true, however, that acidemia accompanies metabolic acidosis; a concomitant, primary, respiratory alkalosis can cause the blood to be alkaline. Similarly, the effect on blood pH by respiratory acidosis can be offset or overwhelmed by a simultaneous metabolic alkalosis (discussed below). So blood pH is usually measured, but the pH value is not clinically interpretable unless other data are available.

Similarly, measuring plasma [HCO_3^-] is useful and common practice, but by itself it is not clinically interpretable. Increased plasma pCO_2, due to respiratory acidosis, causes a rise in the plasma HCO_3^- level, which is not the result of a metabolic alkalosis, though it could be aggravated by it. Conversely, lowering plasma pCO_2 by respiratory alkalosis decreases

Table 8-10	Electrolyte concentrations* in plasma		
Cations	**(meq/L)**	**Anions**	**(meq/L)**
Na$^+$	144.0	Cl$^-$	105.0
K$^+$	4.0	HCO$_3^-$	25.0
Ca^{++}	5.0	Phosphate	1.5
Mg^{++}	2.0	SO$_4^=$	0.5
		Organic acid	9.0
		Protein	14.0
TOTAL	155.0	TOTAL	155.0

*Typical values from within normal ranges for humans.

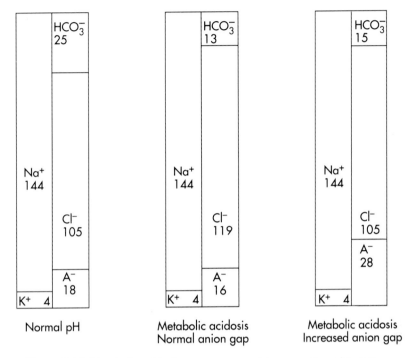

Figure 8-24. Metabolic acidosis may or may not increase the anion gap.

plasma HCO_3^-, though metabolic acidosis may not be present. Hence, to evaluate metabolic effects on blood pH, respiratory effects must be eliminated.

The pH-bicarbonate diagram

The pH-bicarbonate diagram (Figure 8-25) is used to evaluate both the type and severity of an acid-base disturbance. The diagram depicts Henderson-Hasselbalch behavior of the bicarbonate/CO_2 buffer in plasma obtained from fully oxygenated blood. Equilibrating whole blood with varying pCO_2 yields a HCO_3^- concentration versus pH relationship characterized by the more horizontal line (BD). Thus, the BD line represents the normal HCO_3^- concentration at a given blood pH. In the presence of metabolic acids, HCO_3^- is used up and, thus, a parallel line beneath BD is obtained; metabolic alkalosis, on the other hand, is indicated by the area above the BD line. Furthermore, being to the right-hand side of the normal pCO_2 (40 mm Hg) isobar (CE) indicates hypocapnia, and thus, respiratory alkalosis; pCO_2 values in excess of 40 mm Hg (hypercapnia) indicate respiratory acidosis.

The four quadrants around the "normal point" bordered by lines BD and CE each contain cases in which a combination of a metabolic and a respiratory acid-base disorder occurs. For example, a plasma sample located in the southwest quadrant indicates the combined conditions of metabolic acidosis (being below the line BD) plus respiratory acidosis (hypercapnia). The severity of a condition is gauged by the distance between a sample point and the border lines BD and CE. So, a sample point may be located close to the 40 mm Hg (normal) pCO_2 isobar, meaning either normalcy or only a mild disorder of the respiratory component, yet this sample may be far removed from the line BD, indicating a severe form of metabolic acid-base disorder. Generally, the primary disorder is the one whose effect on a blood sample causes the larger deviation from the normal pH or pO_2 border lines, while a secondary, smaller effect represents a physiologic compensation; for example, a severe metabolic alkalosis being partly compensated by a milder respiratory acidosis (increased pCO_2 caused by hypoventilation).

To exemplify compensation, one considers point P in the pH-bicarbonate diagram: apparently a rather severe metabolic acidosis prevails, yet pCO_2 is nor-

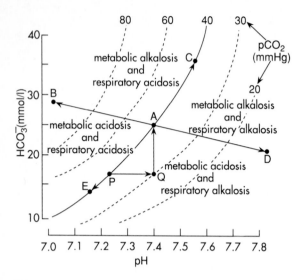

Figure 8-25. The pH-bicarbonate diagram for oxygenated human blood shows the relation between pH, [HCO_3^-], and pCO_2. The broken lines are isobars for pCO_2. Point A, the "normal point", represents average physiologic values of [HCO_3^-] about 24 mmol/L, pH about 7.4, and pCO_2 about 40 mm Hg. Other features of this diagram are explained in the text.

mal. Such an artificial condition could be established in vitro by adding acid to the plasma sample. In vivo hyperventilatory compensation would attempt to restore normal pH by blowing off excess CO_2 (moving from point P to Q); the kidneys, a bit slower to respond, would conserve HCO_3^- ions (moving from point Q up to the normal point, A). This portrayal, however, is an idealized case. In reality, neither the pH compensation nor the HCO_3^- compensation would have been 100% and, therefore, this case of primary metabolic acidosis with compensatory respiratory alkalosis yields a blood sample containing a grossly diminished level of HCO_3^- and a slightly diminished pCO_2. The pH in the blood sample remains below 7.4 until the underlying cause of the acidosis has been removed, and time has been allowed to eliminate the excess acid.

It is important to note the fallibility of blood pH as a measure of acid-base balance. A normal blood pH may result from two primary effects on pH that offset each other, such as a primary metabolic alkalosis offset by a primary respiratory acidosis. Also, an abnormal blood pH does not exclude the possibilities of metabolic or respiratory disorders, either primary or secondary; it merely indicates the presence of an overriding, pH-determining, primary metabolic or respiratory acidosis. For these reasons, a clear distinction must be made between acidosis and acidemia, and between alkalosis and alkalemia.

The Siggaard-Andersen nomogram

The Siggaard-Andersen alignment nomogram (Figure 8-26) is another aid in the differential diagnosis of the nature and severity of metabolic and respiratory acid-base upsets. Again, the pCO_2 indicates respiratory functioning, whereas metabolic effects on acid-base balance are gauged by the value of base excess (BE) in the plasma obtained from fully oxygenated blood (oxygenated hemoglobin is a stronger H^+ donor than is reduced hemoglobin). BE is defined in conjunction with buffer base (BB), which is the anion component of a buffer system. In whole blood, BB amounts to about 48 meq/L of which hemoglobin and bicarbonate each constitute about 50%. BE signifies the deviation of BB from its normal value. BE is measured as the amount of strong acid or base that must be added to a liter of oxygenated blood to attain a pH of 7.40. Hence, BE equals actual BB minus normal BB. A positive value of BE then indicates metabolic alkalosis; a negative value of BE (or base deficit) shows metabolic acidosis. The absolute value of BE reflects the severity of a metabolic acid-base disturbance. The Siggaard-Andersen nomogram is a clinical tool designed to measure BE (i.e., base excess or deficit) in a plasma sample.

The case presented in the nomogram (see Figure 8-26) shows how a measured pCO_2 of 60 mm Hg (point A), a pH of 7.08 (point B), and a hemoglobin concentration of 15 g/dl allows for the estimation of an in vitro BE in plasma of −14 meq/L (point C), an in vivo BE of −11 meq/L (point D), a [HCO_3^-] in plasma of about 17 meq/L (point E), and a total CO_2 (found practically by adding an excess of strong acid to plasma) of about 18.7 mmoles/L (point F). The elevated pCO_2 points to respiratory acidosis, and the large base deficit to metabolic acidosis. Thus, there are two primary disorders in this case.

When using the nomogram, one must realize that the buffering capacity measured in vitro differs from that of the extracellular fluid compartment of patients. The effective hemoglobin concentration is the effective buffering capacity of the hemoglobin concentration of the extracellular compartment. It amounts to about 20% of the hemoglobin concentration in the blood. Hence, the in vivo BE read from

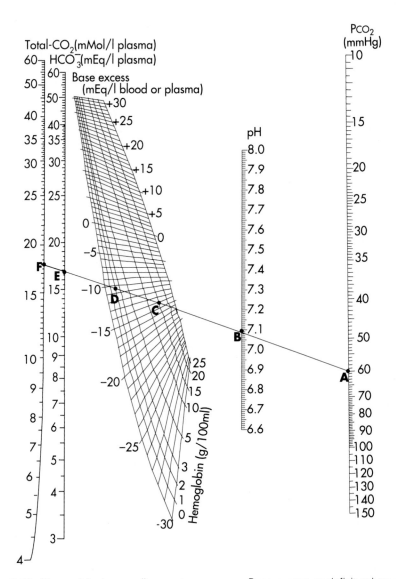

Figure 8-26. Siggaard-Andersen alignment nomogram. Base excess or deficit values are read where the middle scale is intercepted by a straight line that connects a twosome of measured values plotted on any two of the remaining four scales (see text). *Modified and reproduced with permission from Siggaard-Andersen O: Blood acid-base alignment nomogram, Scand J Clin Lab Invest 15:211-220, 1963; copyright Radiometer A/S.*

the 1, 2, or 3 g/dl hemoglobin isopleths relates to the in vitro BE on the 5, 10, or 15 g/dl isopleths, respectively. Using the in vivo value, a BE > +4 indicates metabolic alkalosis, and a BE < −4 indicates metabolic acidosis.

Here are three practical notes on the nomogram-based analysis of disturbances of the acid-base balance.

- Oxygenated (arterial) blood must be used; if only venous blood is available, corrections must be made.
- The above nomograms obtained on human blood can be used for most domestic animal species (e.g., dogs and ruminants); young pigs, however, show a positive BE of 6 to 8 meq/L, so one should

be careful using nomograms for uncharted species.

- Therapy may be based on nomogram-derived BE values. To calculate the amount (meq per whole body) of base or acid that needs to be given to remedy an acid-base disorder, one multiplies BE by 0.3 and by body weight in kilograms. The factor 0.3 comes about thusly: ⅔ of body weight is fluid, and ½ of fluid is intracellular; therefore, ⅓ of body weight is extracellular fluid.

Four clinical cases

The following guidelines are generally followed:

- pH is measured in arterial blood. In general, the pH varies in the direction similar to the primary disturbance.
- pCO_2 and BE are measured to determine the relative influences of respiratory and metabolic origin on pH.
- The results are correlated with clinical evaluation of the patient, and the primary cause(s) of the acid-base disorder is identified.

To test oneself in the use of the above concepts and nomograms, the reader should diagnose the following four cases and classify the nature and severity of the primary acid-base disturbance(s) in each case.

Case 1. A 10-year-old grade gelding with fibrinonecrotic pneumonia and pleuritis. pH 7.22; pCO_2 65 mm Hg; HCO_3^- 25.5 meq/L; and BE −3 meq/L (base deficit 3 meq/L). The lowered pH indicated acidosis. Elevated pCO_2 indicated respiratory acidosis. Base deficit indicated superimposed metabolic problem: not compensating. Kidney damage was suspected, but owners requested that a necropsy not be done when the horse died, a short time after admission.

Case 2. A 1 ½-year-old canine in for routine ovariohysterectomy. Dog induced with Suretal and then placed on gas anesthesia. The patient was apneic, so was put on controlled ventilation. Although blood gases had not been taken prior to surgery, five minutes after being put on a ventilator, an arterial blood sample was taken to determine blood gas and acid-base values of the patient. pO_2 359 mm Hg; pH 7.6; pCO_2 20 mm Hg; bicarbonate 20 meq/L; BE 0. Obviously, the problem was that the ventilator was set at a rate and pressure that overventilated the dog. Subsequent readjustment returned acid-base values to expected norms.

Case 3. A 1-week-old foal with a ruptured bladder. pH 7.31; pCO_2 31 mm Hg; HCO_3^- 14.5 meq/L; BE −10 meq/L. pH indicted primary acidosis, the low bicarbonate indicated metabolic acidosis; pCO_2 somewhat low in attempt to compensate. Foal was unable to excrete H^+ adequately and was buffered by bicarbonate.

Case 4. A 1-year-old male Labrador, dehydrated and vomiting for 2 days. pH 7.49; pCO_2 45 mm Hg; HCO_3^- 34.5 meq/L; BE 10 meq/L. Radiographs showed a spherical object obstructing the pyloric portion of the stomach. pH and bicarbonate were high, indicting metabolic alkalosis, caused by loss of HCl from the stomach; pCO_2 indicated slight hypoventilation.

FUNCTIONS AND HOMEOSTASIS OF CALCIUM, PHOSPHATE, AND MAGNESIUM

Calcium (Ca) and phosphate (P) have various vital physiological functions and constitute a significant fraction (over 3%) of mammalian body weight. The most visible form of Ca, in combination with P, is in the skeleton, which serves for support, protection, and as a metabolic reservoir, and in the teeth. Ionized Ca^{++} has an additional number of vitally important metabolic functions:

- Maintaining contractility, rhythm, and tone of myocardium;
- Maintaining normal nervous tissue irritability and transmission of nerve impulses at synapses and at neuromuscular junctions;
- Maintaning normal skeletal muscle function: myosin, the contractile protein, is a Ca-dependent ATPase;
- Maintaining normal cell membrane permeability;
- Essential for hemostasis
- Essential for milk curdling in sucklings' stomachs under the influence of rennin;
- Essential for many receptor-ligand interactions, such as glycoprotein binding to lectins;
- Essential cofactor for various enzyme systems (e.g., pancreatic lipase and amylase), some via the Ca^{++}/calmodulin interaction (e.g., glycogen synthase);
- Essential second messenger of several hormones, such as antidiuretic hormone and gastrin;
- Essential for cytoskeletal functioning in endo- and exocytosis, mediated by calmodulin.

Functions of inorganic phosphates include the structural (bones, teeth) and metabolic ones; for example, P controlling mitochondrial energy metabo-

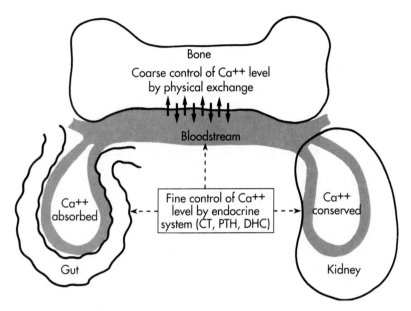

Figure 8-27. Control of the Ca^{++} level in the bloodstream. *CT,* Calcitonin; *PTH,* parathyroid hormone; *DHC,* 1,25-dihydroxycholecalciferol.

lism, P as titratable acid buffering H^{+} in urine, and pyrophosphate, inhibiting precipitation of calcium-phosphates in tissues. Functions of organic phosphates include those of phosphoproteins, phospholipids, nucleic acids, and phosphorylated intermediates in metabolism.

Considering their vital functions, it is not surprising that Ca and P homeostasis are zealously guarded. Mechanisms exist that adapt intracellular/extracellular and bone/extracellular exchange processes, urinary and fecal excretion, and intestinal absorption of Ca and P to dietary intake and to the body's need for these elements.

In this section, the text overviews: (i) the exchange processes between reservoirs (e.g., bone) and surroundings that coarse-regulate the Ca and P levels in the blood; (ii) how three hormones—parathyroid hormone (PTH), calcitonin (CT), and 1,25-dihydroxycholecalciferol (DHC)—combine their activities on the gut, kidneys, bone, and tissue cells, so as to fine-tune Ca and P levels in the blood (Figure 8-27); (iii) dietary considerations; and (iv) the conditioned and inborn disorders of Ca and P metabolism, reflecting, in part, the changing needs of the body during growth, aging, pregnancy, and lactation.

Occurrences of calcium and phosphate; bone

The adult human has 1 to 2 kg of calcium of which more than 98% is in the skeleton. Intracellular calcium (0.2 g/kg) is mostly sequestered in mitochondria and endoplasmic reticulum. In the blood, total Ca amounts to approximately 9.4 mg/dl (2.4 mmole/L), of which 41% is protein-bound (nondiffusible), 9% is complexed to bicarbonate, citrate, phosphate, lactate, etc. (diffusible), and 50% is unbound, ionized Ca^{++}. The ionized Ca^{++} (1.2 mmole/L), equilibrating between plasma and interstitial fluid, is responsible for the metabolic functions listed above. The calcium level is rigorously controlled by three hormones (PTH, calcitonin, and DHC) acting on bone, tissues, kidneys, and gut.

The same three hormones regulate the serum phosphate level (approximately 1.3 mmole/L) by regulating exchange with bone, uptake from the gut, and renal secretion. The adult human has about 1 kg of P of which 85% is in bone. As expected from the Henderson-Hasselbalch equation and a pK value of 6.8 for the dissociation of H$_2$PO$_4^-$, at pH 7.4, plasma contains a 4:1 HPO$_4^=$ to H$_2$PO$_4^-$ ratio. In order of increasing solubility, the three forms of calcium-phosphate are: Ca$_3$(PO$_4$)$_2$, CaHPO$_4$, and Ca(H$_2$PO$_4$)$_2$. At stomach pH, these salts readily dissolve; at intestinal pH, the chief calcium salts are $CaHPO_4$ and $Ca(H_2PO_4)_2$. In the body, Ca and P coexist as a supersaturated solution, prevented from crystallizing by inhibitors, such as pyrophosphate. Under conditions when pyrophosphate is hydrolyzed, calcium-phosphate precipitates out, as in bone formation and atherosclerosis. In bone, teeth, and cartilage, the main salt is hydroxyapatite, $([Ca_3(PO_4)_2]_3 \cdot Ca(OH)_2)$.

Between 90 and 95% of the organic matrix of bone consists of collagen fibers; the remainder, called **ground substance,** is composed of extracellular fluid plus proteoglycans, such as chondroitin sulfate and hyaluronic acid. A small protein of bone, called **osteocalcin,** binds strongly to hydroxyapatite, because, like the Ca^{++}-dependent blood clotting factors, it contains γ-carboxyglutamate residues, the formation of which requires vitamin K. Besides vitamin K, bone formation requires vitamin A for glycosylation of matrix proteins, vitamin C for collagen formation, and vitamin D for Ca^{++} transport.

About half of the weight and one-third of the volume of bone consists of minerals, mostly hydroxyapatite crystals, but also amorphous salts of phosphates, carbonates, fluorides, citrates, hydroxides, etc., that contain Ca^{++}, Mg^{++}, K^+, and Na^+. These amorphous salts, which are absorbed to the surface of the hydroxyapatite crystals, are of great physiologic importance, since they constitute a large and inert reservoir of exchangeable Ca^{++}, Mg^{++}, Na^+, K^+, and P that can be mobilized whenever needed; for example, to maintain serum Ca^{++} and phosphate levels; or to exchange H^+ for Na^+ and K^+ during acidosis.

The combination of collagen fibers, providing tensile strength, and hydroxyapatite, providing compressional strength, makes bone uniquely suitable for its function as the fundamental structure of the body. Bone structure represents a continual equilibrium of deposition and absorption, termed **remodeling of bone.** Osteoblasts form an organic matrix at the site where mineral deposition occurs, because of the combined effects of the loss of pyrophosphate inhibition (cleaved by alkaline phosphatase, whose level in the blood is a measure of bone-forming activity) and the affinity of collagen and osteocalcin for the minerals. Osteoclasts resorb bone by secreting acids (citric, lactic) that dissolve the minerals, and lysosomal enzymes that hydrolyze the organic bone matrix. Osteoblasts are activated by calcitonin (CT) and inhibited by parathyroid hormone (PTH); osteoclasts are activated by PTH and inhibited by CT. Provided 1,25-dihydroxycholecalciferol (DHC) is present, the antagonistic activities of PTH and CT continually, and simultaneously in the same bone, remodel each bone, thereby rejuvenating old matrices, which makes bones less brittle, and adapting skeletal form and strength to counter the degree and direction of stress applied to the bones.

Hormonal control of calcium and phosphate metabolism

In addition to their roles in bone remodeling, the forementioned hormones (PTH, CT, DHS) regulate the serum levels of Ca^{++} and inorganic phosphate homeostatically. Hormonal activities respond, by negative feedback loops, to the level of ionized Ca^{++} in serum. Then, by their effects on bone, gut, kid-

Table 8-11	Hormones that regulate calcium and phosphate metabolism		
Actions	**Parathyroid hormone**	**Calcitonin**	**1,25-Dihydroxycholecalciferol**
Serum [Ca^{2+}]	↑	↓	↑
Serum [P_i]	↓	↓	↑
Kidney	↑ Reabsorption of Ca^{2+} ↓ Reabsorption of P_i ↑ α-hydroxylase activity	↓ Reabsorption of Ca^{2+} ↓ Reabsorption of P_i	↑ Reabsorption of Ca^{2+} ↑ Reabsorption of P_i
Bone	↑ Resorption of bone	↓ Resorption of bone	Ca^{2+} mobilization from bone
Gastrointestinal tract	Indirectly causes increased absorption of Ca^{2+} and P_i by increasing production of 1,25-dihydroxycholecalciferol	No effect	↑ Absorption of Ca^{2+}, P_i

↑ = increased; ↓ = decreased.

Reproduced, with permission, from Smith EL and others: Principles of biochemistry: mammalian biochemistry, ed 7, 455, New York, 1983, McGraw-Hill.

neys, and other tissues, PTH, CT, and DHC regulate Ca and P metabolism (Table 8-11).

Parathyroid hormone

Parathyroid hormone (PTH), released in response to a lowered Ca^{++} level in serum, raises the Ca^{++} level, without simultaneously elevating the concentration of inorganic phosphate (P_i) in serum, by the following activities. In bone, PTH inhibits osteoblast-controlled synthesis of organic matrix; in addition, PTH rapidly activates existing osteoclasts, causing Ca^{++} and P_i release from bone, and, after several days, PTH activates maturation of precursor cells into mature osteoclasts and osteoblasts. Mobilization of Ca^{++} from bone is further stimulated by PTH-enhanced formation of DHC in the kidneys (discussed below). DHC activates mobilization of Ca^{++} and P_i from the bone, Ca^{++} and P_i absorption by the intestines, and Ca^{++} reabsorption in the kidney tubules. Undue accumulation of P_i in serum is prevented by PTH lowering the capacity of active phosphate reabsorption in the renal tubules, thereby causing phosphaturia. In fact, PTH is the most important control over Ca^{++} and P_i levels in serum, both in terms of magnitude and speed by which serum PTH levels respond to variations of the serum Ca^{++} level around the normal value of 9.4 mg/dl; a decrease in Ca^{++} level of only 1% can cause a 100% increase in the level of PTH. In addition, an elevated serum P_i level tends to enhance indirectly the secretion of PTH by suppressing serum Ca^{++} levels (i.e., more calcium-phosphate binding). Therefore, the phosphaturic effect of PTH elevates serum Ca^{++} indirectly by reducing extracellular calcium-phosphate binding.

The PTH effects are homeostatically regulated by antagonistic calcitonin activity, and by negative feedback on PTH secretion by DHC formed in the kidneys in response to PTH.

Calcitonin

Compared to PTH, the effects of calcitonin (CT, also called **thyrocalcitonin**) are small. Elevated serum (Ca^{++}) causes elaboration of CT from parafollicular C cells in the thyroid and, consequently, serum (Ca^{++}) is lowered by an immediate decrease in osteoclast activity, a gradual increase in osteoblast activity, and a long-term effect that prevents osteoclast formation from osteoprogenitor cells. Furthermore, CT lowers reabsorption of Ca^{++} and P_i in the renal tubules. However, CT effects are transient and small: a temporary lowering of serum Ca^{++} by CT is rapidly and effectively countered by PTH release. Besides, osteoclastic Ca^{++} release, the process stimulated by CT, is only a minor entry in the overall Ca^{++} exchange budget (discussed below).

Total thyroidectomy does not always reduce the circulating level of CT to zero. Small amounts of the hormone have also been found in cerebrospinal fluid and in the thymus, pituitary, lung, gut, liver, bladder, and other tissues. Because of this wide distribution and because PTH and DHC are far more important regulators of Ca^{++} and P_i homeostasis, thyroidectomy does not require CT replacement therapy.

1,25-Dihydroxycholecalciferol

The abbreviation DHC is used for the synonyms 1,25-dihydroxycholecalciferol and 1,25-dihydroxyvitamin D_3. DHC is a hormone that affects calcium

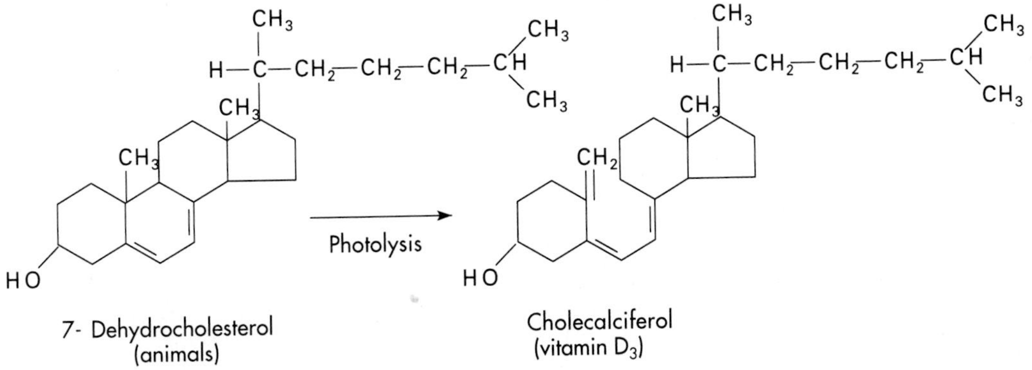

Figure 8-28. Photolysis of 7-dehydrocholesterol to cholecalciferol (vitamin D_3).

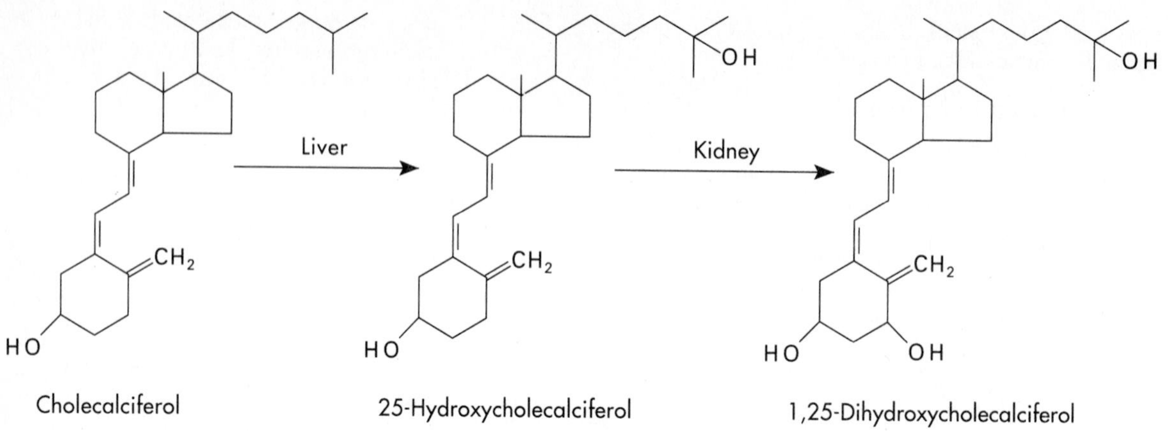

Figure 8-29. Conversion of vitamin D_3 to the hormone 1,25-dihydroxycholecalciferol (DHC).

and phosphate transport in the gut, bone, and kidneys, so as to maintain serum Ca^{++} and P_i at levels that sustain the continual mineralization of bone. The parent compound of DHC is vitamin D_3 (cholecalciferol), which is obtained either from sunlight's ultraviolet irradiation of 7-dehydrocholesterol (an intermediate of cholesterol metabolism) in the skin (Figure 8-28), or as a fat-soluble vitamin in the diet. Plants contain vitamin D_2 (ergocalciferol), a close structural analogue of vitamin D_3 and of similar potency in humans.

Vitamin D_3, as such, is biologically inactive when incubated in vitro with target tissue. In the body, to acquire hormone status, vitamin D_3 is converted to DHC in subsequent hydroxylation steps (Figure 8-29). In the liver, vitamin D_3 or D_2 is hydroxylated in a nonregulated fashion at carbon-25, and then in mitochondria of the proximal convoluted tubules of the kidneys; the hydroxylation at carbon-1 occurs, yielding the biologically active hormone DHC. These vitamins are also hydroxylated to a minor extent in bone or placenta. Additional hydroxylations (at carbon-23, carbon-24, and carbon-26) yield products that either supplement DHC activity or deactivate DHC prior to its elimination in bile.

The body's DHC activity is accurately controlled (Figure 8-30) by renal hydroxylation of 25-hydroxycholecalciferol at carbon-1. It is critical for the hydroxylation at carbon-1 that the special hydroxylase enzyme is activated by parathyroid hormone. PTH itself is elaborated in reponse to low serum Ca^{++} levels and by negative feedback loops involving

Ca^{++}, P_i, and DHC concentrations. The efficiency of this unified endocrine control system is apparent from the huge changes in plasma DHC concentration, in response to only modest variations of the Ca^{++} level around its normal level. Renal 1α-hydroxylase enzyme activity is stimulated by several other hormones (prolactin, estrogens, placental lactogen, growth hormone), and this may explain the functional adaptations of Ca and P balances to growth, lactation, and pregnancy; it also suggests a cause for bone demineralization during aging, when some of these hormone secretions decline.

DHC acts in typical steroid-hormone fashion: it enters a target cell, binds to a cytoplasmic receptor with which it then associates to chromatin in the nucleus. In gut mucosa, enhanced DNA transcription leads to the formation of three proteins—a Ca^{++}-stimulated ATPase, alkaline phosphatase, and Ca^{++}-binding protein—all related to Ca^{++} and P_i transport. Similar modes of action probably exist in kidney and bone, the other DHC target tissues. DHC promotes mineralization of bone by raising the serum levels of Ca^{++} and P_i as a result of stimulating intestinal and renal absorption of Ca^{++} and P_i, and mobilization of Ca and P to and from bones, aided by the required simultaneous presence of PTH.

Both hypocalcemia and hypophosphatemia stimulate DHC generation, resulting in increased serum levels of both Ca^{++} and P_i. When the level of Ca^{++} in serum is low and P_i is normal, the PTH response stimulates DHC formation, Ca^{++} absorption in gut and reabsorption in kidney, and the release of Ca^{++}

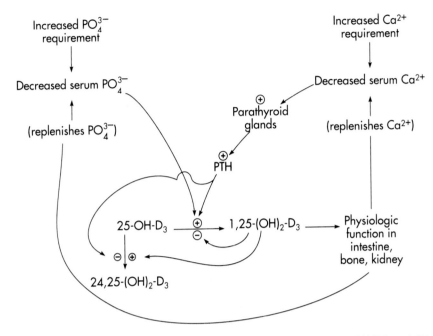

Figure 8-30. Control of the conversion of 25-hydroxycholecalciferol (25-OH-D$_3$) to 1,25-dihydroxycholecalciferol (DHC) by 1α-hydroxylase. The physiologic function of DHC is directed towards control of the serum Ca^{++} and phosphate levels. *Reproduced with permission from Martin DW Jr, Mayes PA, Rodwell VW, and Granner DK: Harper's review of biochemistry, ed 20, p 122, Los Altos, CA, 1985, Lange Medical Publications.*

from bone, so that the Ca^{++} level in the blood is normalized; but accumulation of P$_i$ simultaneously released from bone, is avoided, since P$_i$ is eliminated by phosphaturia. Conversely, when the DHC release is prompted by lowered P$_i$ level in the blood in the presence of a normal Ca^{++} concentration, the excess Ca^{++} liberated in the process of restoring the P$_i$ level is voided in urine. These examples illustrate the efficiency and quasi-independence of Ca^{++} and P$_i$ homeostasis.

Calcium and phosphate turnover; diet

Some comments are attached to the diagram depicting calcium homeostasis in adult humans (Figure 8-31).

Turnover of 1 g of Ca per day is large compared to the 900-mg Ca pool in extracellular fluid; hence, the need for three-hormone-mediated control of that Ca pool. However, the turnover of 1 g of Ca per day is small compared to the 1000-g Ca store in bone. Even the small fraction of readily exchangeable (amorphous) Ca, absorbed to hydroxyapatite in bone,

would suffice to bridge periods of low Ca intake without noticeable effects. But excessive demands on the Ca pool must be met by increased dietary intake; for instance, lactation, pregnancy, growth, or diarrhea.

Intestinal absorption of Ca occurs predominantly in the duodenum and upper jejunum by active and passive processes, both stimulated directly by DHC and indirectly by PTH, which stimulates production of DHC. A large proportion of dietary Ca is not absorbed, because it forms insoluble salts with, for instance, oxalate, phytate, and nucleic acids. Dietary phosphate, in contrast to Ca, is nearly totally absorbed by active transport, aided by DHC and, thus, indirectly by PTH. Other factors influencing intestinal absorption of Ca and P are acidity of the upper gastrointestinal tract, and the Ca/P ratio in diet. Ideally the Ca/P ratio is in the range of 1:1 to 2:1 for most animals. Increasing dietary Ca tends to limit P absorption, and vice versa. Meats are rich in P, dairy products are high in Ca.

A footnote to the kidney's role in Ca and P turnover (see Figure 8-31): of the total Ca pool, only

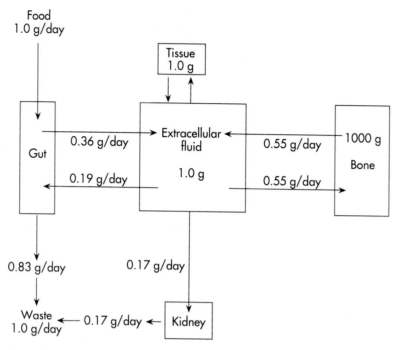

Figure 8-31. Normal calcium homeostasis in the 70-kg human. *Numerical data are from Williams textbook of endocrinology, ed 7, Wilson JD and Foster DW editors, p 1144, Philadelphia, 1985, Saunders.*

ionized Ca^{++} is filtered. Active tubular reabsorption of Ca^{++} is finely attuned to protect serum Ca^{++} homeostasis by PTH-DHC stimulating up to 100% reabsorption of Ca^{++} in times of hypocalcemia, and increasing loss of Ca^{++} in urine during hypercalcemic conditions. The P_i level in human serum is about 1 to 1.4 mmole/L, almost all of which is filtrable through the glomerulus. Serum P_i is controlled by a renal overflow system: tubular transport maximum (Tm) for active P_i reabsorption equals 0.1 mmole/min and that tubular load is reached at a serum P_i level of about 0.8 mmole/L, at which P_i starts to spill over into the urine. PTH has two direct effects relating to phosphates: bone resorption causes P_i release into plasma and PTH lowers the Tm value of active P_i reabsorption in renal tubules, thus eliminating P_i from the body by phosphaturia.

A footnote to the equilibria between extracellular fluid and bone and tissue cells (see Figure 8-31): an effective physical-chemical buffering of serum Ca^{++} and P_i levels is enacted by simple exchange (solubilization and precipitation) with bone and with Ca

sequestered in mitochondria and endoplasmic reticulum of tissue cells. About 5% of all blood, that is 1% of total extracellular fluid, flows per minute through bones, where it equilibrates with the readily exchangeable Ca and P, as well as with the Mg^{++}, Na^+, and K^+, that are absorbed in fine-crystalline and amorphous forms, so as to form a huge combined surface area. There, excess minerals are deposited, or mineral shortages in plasma replenished. On top of these gross buffering mechanisms by simple exchange, there is fine-tuning of individual Ca and P levels in serum by the three interacting endocrine controls.

Homeostasis of calcium and phosphate under normal conditions and some related disorders

The previous discussions may be summarized as follows. Under normal conditions, serum levels of Ca and P are regulated by a combination of physical-chemical exchange of serum with the bone reservoirs plus the three interacting endocrine systems controlling bone, kidney, and gut mineral metabolism. Hypocalcemia is effectively countered under the direction of PTH, which (i) prevents urinary Ca loss; (ii) stimulates absorption of Ca and P from the gut and their release from bone, while allowing excess P to be excreted in urine; and (iii) activates the production of DHC. By its effects on bone, kidneys, and gut, DHC increases serum Ca and P_i levels, so that the remineralization of bone occurs. Hypercalcemia is countered by calcitonin effects that shift the bone remodeling equilibrium toward net bone formation and by the calcitonin-directed lowering of Ca and P reabsorption in the kidneys.

The effects of deviating serum levels of Ca^{++} and P_i are diverse and serious.

- Hypocalcemia leads to increased Na^+ permeability of nerve membranes, causing increased nerve irritability, involuntary firings, muscle contractions, tetany (especially dangerous in laryngeal muscles, as such spasms obstruct respiration, thus causing death), and convulsions. Already a drop from 9.4 to 6.5 mg Ca/dl (i.e., only a 35% drop) causes these symptoms, and a drop below 50% of normal is lethal.
- Hypercalcemia depresses neuromuscular activity, affects the heart beat (lethally so, if caused by sudden intravenous Ca infusion), depresses appetite, and causes constipation by depressing contractility of the gut muscle wall. These effects appear with serum Ca levels of 12 to 15 mg/dl; above 17 mg/dl calcium-phosphate precipitates throughout the body (ectopically), including such vital places as the lung arterioles, arterial walls, and renal tubules.
- Hypophosphatemia leads to demineralization and, thus, weakening of bone; furthermore, by affecting glycolytic- and ATP-producing pathways, it causes muscle weakness, loss of leukocyte functions (thus, infections), hemolysis, and leftward-shifted oxyhemoglobin dissociation curves, because of a lack of 2,3-diphosphoglycerate.

The clinical symptoms above are visible indications of Ca or P imbalances. However, the presence of normal serum Ca and P levels does not rule out the possibility that a critical shortage exists, since these serum levels are homeostatically controlled and, thus, are the last things to change. Hence, in addition to Ca, P, and alkaline phosphatase determinations in serum, the status of Ca and P homeostasis is assessed by radiographic analysis of skeleton mineralization, and by testing renal clearances of Ca and P.

Magnesium turnover

Half the body's magnesium reserve is present in insoluble form in skeletal muscle. Most of the remainder (35%) is intracellular, being necessary for the synthesis of some protein and DNA. Magnesium is also necessary for a wide variety of enzymes' activity in intracellular metabolism. Magnesium is the second most prevalent intracellular cation (K^+ being the first), with only about 1% present in extracellular fluid. The effects of Mg^{++} on the central and peripheral nervous systems mimic those of Ca^{++}—that is, Mg^{++} enhances excitation when deficiencies exist and depresses excitation when excesses occur. The synthesis, release, and target cell effects of PTH require Mg^{++}, but excessive levels of serum Mg^{++} also inhibit the secretion of PTH and possibly its peripheral action; therefore, the optimal secretion and action of PTH depends on normal serum Mg^{++} levels.

Normal plasma Mg^{++} concentrations are about 1.5 to 2.5 meq/L. One-fourth of plasma Mg^{++} is protein bound, and that that is not is able to pass through glomeruli. Most filtered Mg^{++} is reabsorbed, reabsorption being increased by PTH. Serum Mg^{++} concentrations decrease with acute PTH deficiency resulting from parathyroidectomy.

Magnesium is by no means efficiently absorbed from the intestine and is of variable bioavailability, depending on dietary composition. Magnesium does not compete with Ca^{++} for absorption, it is not actively absorbed across the GI tract, but its absorption does depend on load (concentration gradient). Magnesium is wasted by the kidneys in acidosis, and alkaline pH's in the digestive tract impair absorption.

Neuromuscular irritability

The foregoing discussions on the effects of Na^+, K^+, Ca^{++}, P_i, Mg^{++} and H^+ on neuromuscular irritability (NI), lead us to the following generalized equation:

$$NI\alpha \frac{Na^+ \cdot K^+ \cdot P_i}{Ca^{++} \cdot Mg^{++} \cdot H^+}$$

Elevations in the serum levels of Na^+, K^+ or P_i will generally increase NI, whereas increases in the serum levels of Ca^{++}, Mg^{++} or H^+ will generally decrease NI.

Common disorders of electrolyte balance

Some common disorders are summarized below. They have been selected from a large number of conditioned and inborn abnormalities relating to Ca and P homeostasis, in order to illustrate the importance of Ca and P balances and functions.

- Eclampsia is a preparturient disorder, prevalent in bitch and sow; hypocalcemia, caused by Ca drain to the developing fetus, leads to hyperexcitability of neuromuscular system and finally to tetany.

- Milk fever, which is actually not a fever at all, occurs in dairy cows postparturiently. Low Ca and P and high Mg levels are found in serum, leading to a short period of hypersensitivity, then to paralysis, coma, and death. It should be noted that the Ca level in milk is 13 times that in plasma, and the P level some 5 to 8 times. Consequently, during lactation, there is a mineral drain from bone, via extracellular fluid, to milk causing demineralization and increased fragility of bones. This situation is further aggravated at the onset of lactation by the fact that, during the days immediately prior to and after parturition, the cow diminishes her food intake, and, thus, mineral intake. In the postparturient cow, Ca and P levels in extracellular fluid may become critically low, signifying that Ca and P mobilization from bone cannot keep up with milk letdown. Why this occurs is poorly understood, since research has shown that it cannot be attributed to either increased calcitonin or decreased PTH levels. Probably the bones of milk-fever patients are unresponsive to PTH for reasons unknown. It is not a good idea to increase dietary Ca prior to parturition, because it will lower activity of the parathyroid glands; in fact, one should feed less Ca preparturiently to stimulate PTH production. A cow with milk fever is treated by giving soluble Ca (calcium gluconate) intravenously; it should be administered slowly, for a sudden hypercalcemia can kill the cow by stopping the heart in systole.

- All-meat diet syndrome: the Ca/P ratio in meats is about 1:16, far below the desirable range of 1:1 to 2:1. This causes a secondary hyperparathyroidism, which repairs the hypocalcemia and hyperphosphatemia, but at the expense of bone demineralization.

- Hypoparathyroidism often results from careless surgical removal of the thyroid gland, together with adjacent parathyroid glands. Death from hypocalcemic tetany results, except when diets are regularly supplemented with Ca and vitamin D or its analogue, dihydrotachysterol, which is directly converted to DHC in the kidneys, bypassing the liver's control over hydroxylation at carbon-25. It should be recalled that vitamin D mimics PTH, affecting Ca^{++} and P_i resorption from bone.

- Hypervitaminosis D or vitamin D toxicity, resulting from excessive supplemetation of the diet with vitamin D, causes bone demineralization (thus, fragility) and decreased serum levels of Ca and P. A consequence is ectopic calcification in renal tubules, leading to renal failure. These effects are not caused by DHC, since the renal hydroxylase enzyme activity responsible for DHC formation is depressed under this condition. Rather, excess of the DHC precursor 25-hydroxycholecalciferol, whose formation in the liver is not as tightly controlled, is responsible.

- Hypovitaminosis D, or rickets, is seen when insufficient vitamin D is available because of poor diet and lack of sun exposure. Symptoms include decreased intestinal Ca absorption and lowered Ca resorption from bone, hypocalcemia, increased PTH levels, hypophosphatemia, phosphaturia, and impaired bone mineralization. This condition prevails in young animals in which the vitamin D requirement for bone growth is high. X-rays reveal the presence of adequate organic bone matrices, but improper mineralization of the matrices. The bones lack supporting strength, which results in bending of bones (bow-leggedness) of the young, growing animals.

- Osteomalacia occurs in adult animals and, like rickets, is a condition whereby bone is demineralized, while the matrix is not affected. The cause may be either endocrine or dietary (e.g., low Ca, low Ca/P ratio, or low vitamin D).

- Osteoporosis is the condition whereby bone matrix disappears together with a proportional amount of minerals. It can be differentiated from osteomalacia by X-ray examination. There are several etiologies for osteoporosis: (i) disuse of bone causes bone resorption, such as in aging, hibernation, or space flight; (ii) protein malnutrition; (iii) deficiencies in vitamins A, C, or K, which are needed for bone protein synthesis; (iv) pathologically elevated levels of glucocorticoids, as in Cushing's disease; bone proteins are mobilized for gluconeogenesis; (v) lack of estrogens, especially in postmenopausal women; before and during reproductive years, bone growth is accelerated by estrogen-stimulated DHC formation; (vi) hyperparathyroidism, most often due to a tumor in the gland; this condition is found mostly in females, probably because prolonged Ca drain during pregnancy and lactation overstimulates the parathyroid gland, thus predisposing to development of such tumor in later years; (vii) prostaglandin E may mediate bone resorption in certain inflammatory illnesses, such as rheumatoid arthritis and certain malignancies; inhibitors of prostaglandin synthesis, such as aspirin, prevent this condition.

• Renal rickets, or rubber jaw, is an osteomalacia caused by renal failure to reabsorb Ca. In chronic kidney disease, the damaged organ fails to produce DHC, thus losing control over Ca reabsorption in the tubules, and spilling Ca into urine. To maintain the Ca^{++} level in serum, PTH demineralizes bone, leaving the protein matrix intact; rubbery bones remain. Another renal disease leading to rickets is congenital hypophosphatemia caused by lowered P reabsorption in the tubules. This condition, vitamin-D-resistant rickets, must be treated with phosphate compounds, instead of Ca plus vitamin D.

STUDY QUESTIONS

Water balance; tonicity of body fluids

1. In each of the cases below, choose the animal that would be most likely to have the largest percentage of its body weight composed of water and briefly explain the reason for the difference.
   a. Obese animal—lean animal
   b. Cow—dog
   c. Young animal—mature animal

2. Rank in sequence of large to small: (a) intracellular fluid; (b) plasma; (c) transcellular fluid; (d) interstitial fluid; (e) extracellular fluid

3. Explain the following:
   a. Isosthenuria
   b. Diabetes insipidus
   c. Hemolysis during water intoxication in calves
   d. Osmotic diuresis
   e. Osmoreceptors

4. List the main cause for obligatory water loss in a normal human adult.

5. Which of the body fluid pools listed below would be measured by injecting radioactively labeled water intravenously and by measuring the plasma concentra-

tion of that indicator at various times thereafter: (a) extravascular; (b) intravascular; (c) total body water; or (d) plasma volume.

6. If total volume of body fluid is controlled by retention of minerals, which mineral(s) is (are) primarily retained, and what determines the distribution of body fluids between different compartments?

7. If an animal is in the physiological state of antidiuresis, it is responding to a negative water balance. (True/False)

8. List two body fluids with HCO_3^- concentrations in excess of HCO_3^- concentration in plasma.

9. List the two chief cations and the two chief anions of tissue cells.

10. Regarding the regulation of gas exchange at sites of active metabolism:
   a. List the function and control of sphincters in arterioles of the microcirculation.
   b. List the function of the Bohr effect.
   c. List a condition that prompts the RBC to synthesize 2,3-diphosphoglycerate.
   d. What is the functionality of the fact that oxyhemoglobin is a stronger acid than deoxyhemoglobin?
   e. What is the functionality of cooperative oxygen binding to hemoglobin?

11. List a function of lymphatics, related to interstitial oncotic pressure.

12. List two main solutes in peripheral interstitial fluid compartments.

13. *a.* Why would increased capillary membrane permeability, as caused by burns or allergic reactions, lead to edema?
   b. Why does occlusion of lymphatics cause edema?

14. List (or illustrate) how the endothelial cells of blood capillary walls control transport of compounds (e.g., nutrients or hormones) from the circulation to tissue cells.

15. If an animal were in the state of diuresis in the regulation of its body water balance, which of the following would be occurring:
   a. High circulating level of ADH. (True/False)
   b. High circulating level of aldosterone. (True/False)
   c. Stimulation of osmoreceptors. (True/False)
   d. Maximal permeability of the distal nephron to H_2O. (True/False)
   e. High specific gravity of urine. (True/False)

16. When using a 24-hour water deprivation test on an animal as a test of renal function, what two characteristics would one expect to find in the urine output (urine elaborated after 24 hours) from this animal if it had normal kidney function?

17. In reviewing the history of the dog with a client, the following symptoms are established: (i) excessive urination (both frequency and volume); and (ii) excessive drinking of water (polydypsia). The veterinarian finds that the urine has a low specific gravity and now wonders whether the animal is a psychogenic compulsive water drinker or perhaps is suffering from diabetes insipidus. To clinically differentiate these causes of deranged water balance, ADH is injected into the dog. Thereafter, would one expect that the dog would be able to increase its urine osmolality if:
    a. He was a psychogenic compulsive water drinker;
    b. He had Diabetes Insipidus of central origin; and/or
    c. He had nephrogenic Diabetes Insipidus?

Kidney; Na⁺ and K⁺; clearance

18. a. What percentage of the cardiac output normally goes through the kidneys?
    b. What percentage of the cardiac output flows through the vasa recta?
    c. What is a normal glomerular filtration rate in adult humans?

19. List the mechanism, controlled by the juxtaglomerular apparatus, by which glomerular filtration rate and renal blood flow are "autoregulated," and list the hormone system involved.

20. List two hormones produced by the kidneys. What are the primary functions of these hormones?

21. Which of the two types of nephrons allows an animal to maximally concentrate urine?

22. a. List two ways in which elevated plasma-oncotic pressure during dehydration diminishes water loss during the passing of blood through the kidney's nephrons.
    b. List two reasons why elevated blood pressure leads to polyuria.

23. a. Why is glucose a "threshold substance" in the kidney?
    b. List a condition under which the transport maximum for glucose in the kidneys is exceeded.

24. Sodium is more likely to be totally reabsorbed in an animal with a high or low glomerular filtration rate?

25. List the three exchange processes between blood and tubular fluid by which the nephrons control volume and composition of body fluids.

26. List the hormone elaborated to counter hyperkalemia; outline that hormone's two modes of action on the nephron, and indicate which of these modes of action allows K⁺ control independent of Na⁺ control.

27. a. List the aldosterone effect on the kidneys' tubular cells relating to serum Na⁺ levels.
    b. Why, for control over plasma sodium levels, is aldosterone not of major importance?

28. In regulating the Na⁺ balance:
    a. List the mechanism of action of antidiuretic hormone (ADH).
    b. List the mechanism of action of a cardiac hormone.

29. a. List the driving force in the nephron, whereby the osmotic gradient in the renal medulla is established.
    b. Interpret the term "diluting segment" for the part of the nephron housing that driving force.
    c. List the organic molecule important in establishing the renal medullary osmotic gradient.
    d. List the primary physiologic function of countercurrent exchange in the vasa recta.

30. What functional mechanisms are involved in concentrating urine in a normal animal?

31. If a dog is suffering from medullary washout, what renal function is impaired?

32. Explain the following clinical symptoms in a dog suffering from chronic renal failure: (a) anemia; (b) increased respiratory rate; (c) altered parathyroid hormone level in blood; (d) metabolic bone disease; (e) hyperkalemia; (f) hyperphosphatemia; (g) hypovolemia; (h) poor intestinal calcium absorption.

33. What is the clinician's number one concern related to kidney function when an animal is in shock?

34. a. List the cause of polyuria in Diabetes Mellitus.
    b. List the cause of polyuria in Diabetes Insipidus.
    c. List three causes of Diabetes Insipidus.

35. List the enzyme (and the special mineral it contains) in renal tubular cells that, under all conditions, plays a crucial role in the body's pH regulation by the kidneys.

36. a. What exactly is "titratable acid," excreted in urine?
    b. During acidosis, what is the function of increased glutaminase activity in the kidneys, and which organ is the source of the substrate for that renal enzyme?

Clearance; water balance

37. a. What renal function is specifically tested when clearance of large doses of para-aminohippurate (PAH) is measured?
    b. Which parameter is approximated by the ratio of inulin clearance to low-dose PAH clearance?

38. Despite the fact that unconjugated bilirubin is a small molecule, why is clearing the bloodstream of this compound not a renal, but rather a hepatic function.

39. A 10-kg dog with 45 mg is injected with Evans Blue resulting in: hematocrit = 45%; dye concentration in plasma after 10 minutes = 9.42 mg/dl, after 20 minutes, 8.87 mg/dl, and after 30 minutes, 8.35 mg/dl:

   a. Inthe event that the dye concentration in plasma after 10 and 20 minutes is not measured but assumed to be the same as that after 30 min (8.35 mg/dl; no turnover), what then would the calculated blood volume be?

   b. Taking the observed turnover of dye into account, find the dye concentration at time-zero (either by computing or by graphical extrapolation) and calculate the dog's blood volume.

   c. If the dog is dehydrated, would your extrapolated C_0 value be higher, lower, or equal relative to the control?

   d. If during the injection of Evans blue, the needle slips out of the vein, so that part of the injected material is extravasated, the dye dilution method would overestimate plasma volume. (True/False)

40. A dog excretes 1440 mg of creatinine in the urine per 24 hours, and the concentration of creatinine in plasma is 12.5 mg/L. Calculate the plasma clearance and give the numerical value and units in which the clearance is expressed.

41. *a.* If one wants to measure K^+ balance, why is the percent clearance ratio for K^+ relative to creatinine more reliable than simply measuring the serum K^+ level?

   b. List a nonpathological reason for the percent clearance ratio of K^+ relative to creatinine to exceed 100%.

   c. Does the percent creatinine clearance ratio of K^+ increase or decrease in a state of acidosis?

42. The advantage of expressing renal clearance of K^+ in a percent creatinine clearance ratio is that it:

   a. Makes measuring urine volume unnecessary. (True/False)

   b. Makes measuring concentration of K^+ in urine unnecessary. (True/False)

   c. Makes measurements less dependent on the dehydration status of an animal. (True/False)

43. *a.* If the percent creatinine clearance ratio of K^+ is high within its normal range, whereas at the same time that of Na^+ is low, which hormone activity is indicated?

   b. Which hormone causes the percent creatinine clearance ratio of phosphate to be high?

Acid-base balance

44. Explain the influence a H^+-producing process has on the resting membrane potential of nerve and muscle cells, and on the ability of a muscle to contract.

45. Which of the following metabolic processes are hy-drogen-ion–producing and which are hydrogen-ion–depleting? (a) ketone body production from neutral fats; (b) lactate oxidation to CO_2 and H_2O; (c) urea synthesis from ammonium ions; (d) glucose metabolism to lactic acid; (e) glucose synthesis from lactate.

46. In a dog with metabolic acidosis, the following cation and anion levels were found: Na^+ = 144 meq/L, K^+ = 4 meq/L, Cl^- = 105 meq/L, and HCO_3^- = 15 meq/L. Calculate the anion gap. What caused the elevated anion gap? Exemplify a clinical situation that leads to an increased anion gap. Give an example of another clinical situation that may lead to a decreased anion gap.

47. *a.* List the nature of the H^+ burden caused by diabetic ketosis.

   b. List the nature of the H^+ burden caused by feeding high concentrate rations to cattle.

48. *a.* What causes the "alkaline tide" in canine plasma after a meal?

   b. Why is this condition not a factor in the body's overall acid-base balance?

49. *a.* Reason as to why the renal response to alkalemia leads to hyperchloremia.

   b. Explain why hypokalemia leads to alkalosis.

   c. Explain diuresis resulting from carbonic anhydrase inhibition.

50. *a.* List two wastes removed from the body by the liver's urea production.

   b. List the liver's remedial response to alkalosis.

   c. How does intestinal urease activity help the liver to control the body's pH homeostasis?

51. Acidemia in the presence of a normal anion gap:

   a. Means that the primary cause is the loss of bicarbonate. (True/False)

   b. Is accompanied by hypochloremia. (True/False)

52. In which one of the four major categories of acid-base imbalances would a person at high altitude (low pO_2) fit?

53. *a.* Explain why infusion of NaCl into the blood leads to acidosis.

   b. Infusion of sodium lactate may be used to treat acidosis / alkalosis. (Choose one and explain why.)

54. Which of the following parameters in the blood increase in the case of compensated metabolic alkalosis: pH; CO_2; HCO_3^-?

55. A dog who has had diarrhea for several days does not eat and produces little urine of a high specific gravity.

   a. In terms of acid-base status, what important buffering compound is the patient losing from his body? What would one expect the blood pH to be compared to normal? What would one expect the compensation by the respiratory system to be? What effect has the respiratory compensation on the HCO_3^-/CO_2 ratio in the blood?

b. In relation to renal compensation to the change in acid-base status of the dog suffering from diarrhea one expects:
Increased bicarbonate in urine. (True/False)
Increased renal secretion of ammonia. (True/False)
Increased tubular fluid dibasic sodium phosphate/monobasic sodium phosphate ratio. (True/False)
Increased urinary loss of K^+. (True/False)

c. In classifying the acid-base status of this animal, which of the following correctly describes the acid-base upset: respiratory acidosis / metabolic alkalosis / metabolic acidosis / respiratory alkalosis?

56. If a Siggaard-Andersen nomogram indicates a negative value for base excess (or base deficit), and an elevated pCO_2 is measured in oxygenated blood, which two primary acid-base disturbances are then indicated?

57. You have just completed a long and difficult surgery with your patient under a positive pressure anesthesia machine. You are unsure as to whether you have used the correct ventilation rate and suspect an acid-base upset. An arterial blood sample has a pCO_2 of 20 mm Hg and a $[HCO_3^-]$ of 20 meq/L.

a. Based on the above data calculate your patient's arterial blood pH.

b. What compound could you use to treat this condition?

c. Was your ventilation rate during surgery adequate, too slow, or too fast to maintain normal acid-base status in your patient?

Calcium and phosphate; bone

58. List the daily dietary Ca requirements as a fraction of the Ca pool size in adult humans.

59. *a.* Coarse control over plasma levels of Ca and PO_4 is by which mechanical process?

b. Fine control over these plasma levels is by which three hormones?

60. What is the acute, life-threatening effect of hypocalcemia?

61. What is the intracellular role of Ca during endocytosis of low-density lipoproteins?

62. What is the connection between hypophosphatemia and decreased oxygen unloading from hemoglobin

within tissues?

63. List the primary functions of vitamins A, C, D, and K in bone formation, and indicate whether the mineral or organic matrix of bone is affected.

64. List the hormones associated with the mobilization of Ca from bone and the hormone associated with deposition of Ca in bone.

65. *a.* In an animal suffering from hypocalcemia, which hormones will be released?

b. Why are plasma phosphate levels not elevated by mobilization of bone reserves?

66. List the primary problem involved in the homeostatic maintenance of a circulating level of Ca in a cow with milk fever.

67. *a.* List the active form of vitamin D. It is activated sequentially by which body organs?

b. List the action by which this hormone affects Ca homeostasis in the kidneys, gut, and bone.

c. Decreased serum phosphate concentration activates renal hydroxylation of 25-OH-cholecalciferol. (True/False)

d. Lactation (prolactin) stimulates hydroxylation of 25-OH-D3 in position 24 of the molecule. (True/False).

68. Explain how parathyroid hormone influences Ca^{++} absorption from the small intestine.

69. *a.* How does an all-meat diet cause secondary hyperparathyroidism?

b. An all-meat diet could lead to osteomalacia. (True/False)

70. *a.* List a positive and negative nutritional consideration, related to Ca balance, that must be given to the intake of large amounts of vegetables.

b. Why is feeding increased amounts of Ca preparturiently not a good way to avoid milk fever?

71. Explain the development of "renal rickets."

72. An explanation of the etiology of milk fever involves (circle correct answer[s]): (a) low dietary Ca^{++} intake; (b) high phytate level in diet; (c) hypothyroidism; (d) unresponsiveness of bone to PTH; (e) twin calves causing excessive Ca^{++} drain; (f) hypoparathyroidism.

73. All periparturient dairy cows have a transient hypocalcemia (8 mg/dl). What is a logical reason for this dip below the normocalcemic level?

74. Indicate two conditions in a dog in which one would expect to find a lack of radiographic density of bone.

9 Gastrointestinal functions

OVERVIEW

In essence, the tissues belonging to the gastrointestinal system are the alimentary tract and the various glands that provide fluids for the chemical and physical modifications of food as needed for digestion, such as the pancreas, salivary glands, and the liver/biliary tree. These glands have in common that their exocrine secretory cells are located around spaces (acini) that are in direct connection with ducts that empty into the alimentary tract. Embryonically, these glands develop as part of the gastrointestinal structure, not different from glands that lie inside the walls of the alimentary tract.

The gastrointestinal (GI) tract starts at the mouth, where mastication (chewing) of food and admixture with saliva produces a paste that is directed via esophagus to the stomach. Digestion of stomach contents, the chyme, begins by the actions of gastric acid and enzymes. Gastric contents are directed in small boluses into the duodenum, where biliary and pancreatic ducts introduce the glandular fluids that contain HCO_3^- to neutralize stomach acid, bile salts to aid in dispersing lipids into water-soluble aggregates (micelles), and pancreatic zymogens. Most of the intestinal absorption occurs in the proximal (duodenum and jejunum) and distal (ileum) part of the small intestine. The cecum, a pouch-like structure especially developed in herbivores, harbors microflora that allow partial digestion of cellulose. The large intestines and colon modify water and salt contents before excreta reach the anus.

The gastrointestinal tract contains microflora, consisting of bacteria and protozoa, which aid in the digestion of nutrients. In ruminants, the ruminal microflora digest essentially all carbohydrates and metabolize a variable portion of proteins and lipids. In all animal species, extensive microflora are present in the large and small intestines and, to a variable extent, in the cecum.

The foremost function of the gastrointestinal system is digestion and absorption of nutrients. Though obviously located inside the body, the lumen of the gastrointestinal tract is a continuation of the outside. It is lined with epithelial cells that are constantly sloughing off, replaced with new cells with a turnover time of approximately four days. To support the digestive and absorptive functions of the epithelium and to protect from digesting its own tissues, the gut features several adaptations.

Longitudinally and transversely oriented muscle layers, responding to stimulation by the autonomic nervous system, effect mixing and analward propulsion of intestinal contents. (The topic of gastrointestinal motility is not discussed further.) Enfoldings of the luminal gut and microvilli-studded mucosal cells provide surface enlargements to maximize absorption efficiency. In open connection with the lumen of the alimentary tract are cells that produce digestive enzymes and fluids (saliva, HC1, bile, HCO_3^-, intestinal fluid), endocrine cells that elaborate numerous intestinal hormones into blood that profoundly affect intermediary metabolism, and cells whose main function is absorption. Mucus, containing mucopolysaccharides, is secreted all along the GI tract; it protects mucosal cells from attack by digestive juices and lubricates intestinal contents.

Especially important as a link between environment and the body's internal metabolism is intestinal transport of digesta from the lumen of the gut into the circulation. Specific mechanisms are present in mucosal membranes facing the lumen of the gut that actively absorb certain sugars and amino acids and facilitate transport of various nutrients, minerals, and vitamins. Other intestinal digestion products are passively absorbed. The gut is a site of stormish metabolic activity. Proteins and lipid aggregates are produced in the mucosal cells, mostly from absorbed dietary metabolites. There are two channels for transport of absorbed nutrients from the gut. Water-soluble digesta (e.g., sugars and amino acids) enter into the mesenteric blood drainage where they are directed, via portal veins, to the liver. The liver is then in a position either to remove from the bloodstream and metabolize sugars and amino acids or to let them pass unchanged toward other tissues. In contrast, lipids do not enter into the mesenteric bloodstream. Rather, lipids are packaged into large aggregates (chylomicrons and very low-density lipoproteins), which are drained from the intestines via the lymphatics. Most dietary lipids, therefore, are not directed first to the liver.

GASTROINTESTINAL HORMONES

Several criteria define gastrointestinal hormones:
- Elaboration of the hormone must be related to the intake and gastrointestinal processing of food.
- A stimulus to one part of the gastrointestinal tract must bring about a response in another, distant target; for instance, the stomach hormone gastrin has tropic effects on the distant gut.
- The effects must be independent of the central nervous system and persist after nerve connections have been cut.
- Injection of the extracted hormone must be effective.
- The effective dose of administered hormone must not exceed physiological levels.

Judged by these standards, four gastrointestinal peptides have obtained full status as hormones: gastrin, secretin, gastric inhibitory peptide (GIP), and cholecystokinin (CCK). In addition to these, many active peptides have been isolated from gastrointestinal tissues.

General properties and functions

Gastrointestinal hormones and active peptides are elaborated mostly as inactive precursors under the influence of dietary, neurogenic, or endocrine stimuli. Endocrine cells of the gastrointestinal tissues are scattered, rather than concentrated in discrete organs.

In their active form, gastrointestinal hormones and other peptides consist of only 4 to about 50 amino acids. Many of these peptides show extensive homology in their amino acid sequences. Hence, overlapping functions of these factors are to be expected and are indeed found. Each of the factors has one or more potent activities and, in addition, some lesser activities shared with other factors (Table 9-1). These

Table 9-1   Some actions of gastrointestinal hormones*

Target tissue	Action	Hormones			
		Gastrin	CCK**	Secretin	GIP***
Liver/bile	Water + HCO_3^- secretion	S	S	Ⓢ	0
	Gallbladder contraction	S	Ⓢ	S	—
Stomach	Acid secretion	Ⓢ	S	Ⓘ	I
	Pepsin secretion	S	S	Ⓢ	I
	Gastric emptying	I	I	I	I
	Gastric motility	S	S	I	I
Intestine	Intestinal motility	S	S	I	—
	Mucosal growth	Ⓢ	S	I	—
Pancreas	Pancreatic growth	S	S	S	—
	Water and HCO_3^- secretion	S	S	Ⓢ	0
	Enzyme secretion	Ⓢ	Ⓢ	S	0
	Insulin secretion	S	S	S	Ⓢ

*S: stimulates; I: inhibits; 0: no effect; —: no data available. Encircled items are effects potent enough to be of physiologic significance.
**Cholecystokinin.
***Gastric inhibitory peptide.

Table 9-2   Gastrointestinal hormones and other active peptides

Hormone/peptide	Origin	Target tissue	Major action	Secretion stimulus
Gastrin	Stomach (duodenum, jejunum)	Secretory cells and muscles of stomach; Brunner's glands	HCl, pepsin, and intestinal mucus secretion; ups gastric motility	Vagus nerve activity; peptides in stomach. HCl inhibits release
Cholecystokinin (CCK)	Duodenum; upper small intestine	Liver; gallbladder; pancreas; Brunner's glands	Gallbladder contraction; secretion of pancreatic enzymes and juice, and intestinal mucus	Fatty acids and amino acids in duodenum
Secretin	Duodenum	Pancreas; liver; secretory cells and muscles of stomach; Brunner's glands	Water, $NaHCO_3$, and intestinal mucus secretion; inhibits gastric motility; ups pepsin secretion	Food and strong acid in stomach and small intestine
Gastric inhibitory peptide (GIP)	Duodenum; upper small intestine	Pancreas; gastric mucosa and muscles; Brunner's glands	Ups glucose-mediated release of insulin; inhibits gastric secretion and motility; ups intestinal mucus secretion	Monosaccharides and fats in duodenum
Vasoactive intestinal peptide (VIP)	Duodenum		Smooth muscle relaxation; ups intestinal blood flow; ups pancreatic fluid and inhibits gastric secretion	Fats in duodenum
Bulbogastrone	Upper small intestine	Stomach	Inhibits gastric secretion and motility	Acid in duodenum
Motilin			Ups gastric and intestinal motility	
Enteroglucagon	Duodenum	Jejunum; pancreas	Inhibition of motility and secretion	Carbohydrates and fat in duodenum
Enkephalins	Small intestine	Stomach; pancreas; intestine	Ups HCl secretion; inhibits pancreatic enzyme secretion and intestinal motility	—
Somatostatin	Small intestine	Stomach; pancreas; intestines; splanchnic arterioles	Inhibits HCl and pancreatic endo- and exocrine secretions, gut motility, and splanchnic blood flow	—
Pancreatic polypeptide (PP)			Inhibits pancreatic bicarbonate and protein secretion	—
Bombesin-like immunoreactivity (BLI)			Ups gastrin and cholecystokinin release	—

activities are most diverse, since they include the following:

- Stimulation or inhibition of the secretions of digestive fluids and enzymes;
- Regulation of gut motility;
- Stimulation or inhibition of the secretion of other hormones by either endocrine or paracrine mechanisms;
- Neurotransmission in nerves of gastrointestinal tissues and in the central nervous system.

Specific hormones and peptides

To appreciate the extent to which activities of various hormones overlap, one has to look only at the tables that compare the actions of gastrointestinal hormones (Tables 9-1 and 9-2). Not all of the stimulations and inhibitions shown can be obtained with physiological concentrations of those hormones. Therefore, only some of the most potent physiological effects of the four gastrointestinal hormones have been highlighted.

- Gastrin, elaborated in response to parasympathetic stimulation (vagus nerve), to proteins in the stomach, or to stomach distension caused by the presence of foodstuffs, increases gastric HC1 secretion and gastric motility. Gastrin has numerous other activities.
- Cholecystokinin (CCK) release responds to food and HC1 coming into the duodenum. Its strongest effects are the contraction of the gallbladder, relaxation of the sphincter of Oddi, and the stimulation of pancreatic enzyme secretion. In fact, the hormone pancreozymin has been held responsible for pancreatic enzyme secretion until it was discovered that pancreozymin and CCK were the same hormone. At least five different active forms of CCK are found in tissues, ranging between 4 and 39 amino acids in length; only CCK8 and CCK12 occur in plasma. At the amino terminal of CCK33, 6 amino acids in sequence are identical to the amino terminal sequence of gastrin; hence, the many overlapping activities between those hormones.
- Secretin, the first GI hormone discovered, is also elaborated under the influence of food entering the duodenum; it responds especially to gastric HC1. Secretin strongly stimulates bicarbonate-rich fluid releases from the pancreas and liver (bile flow) with which the entering HC1 is neutralized, and the secretion of intestinal mucus for protection of the mucosa.

Table 9-3	Peptides found in gut and central nervous system

ISOLATED FROM BOTH BRAIN AND GUT

Substance P
Neurotensin
Secretin
Somatostatin
Cholecystokinin (CCK)

ISOLATED FROM EITHER BRAIN OR GUT: IMMUNOREACTIVITY FOUND IN THE OTHER ORGAN

Vasoactive intestinal peptide (VIP)
Pancreatic polypeptide (PP) and motilin
Enkephalins and endorphins
Bombesin-like immunoreactivity (BLI)
Insulin
Glucagon

Modified and reproduced, with permission, from Deveney CW and Way LW: Regulatory peptides of the gut. In Greenspan FS and Forsham PH, editors: Basic & clinical endocrinology, ed 2, 505, East Norwalk, Conn/San Mateo, Calif, 1986, Appleton & Lange.

- Gastric inhibitory peptide (GIP) is released when monosaccharides and fats enter the duodenum. Inhibition of gastrin is not nearly as potent an activity of GIP as is stimulating the pancreas to release insulin in the presence of postprandial hyperglycemia.
- Intestinal peptides that have not yet obtained full hormone status (Table 9-2) are released under the influence of gastric digesta entering the duodenum. Their functions vary from affecting gastric, hepatic, and pancreatic secretions to influencing gut motility, the release of other hormones and peptides, and splanchnic blood flow. Of special interest is the fact that many of these peptides (as well as intestinal and pancreatic hormones) have neurocrine effects as either strictly local or general neurotransmitters and neuromodulators (Table 9-3).

GASTROINTESTINAL DIGESTION AND ABSORPTION

The text examines gastrointestinal digestion and absorption of food, starting with mucus secretion, following it through the entire alimentary tract sequentially. Anatomical interludes are made where needed.

Mucus secretion

Mucus protects the alimentary tract from being digested from within by its own juices and enzymes; it also lubricates the tract's tissues and contents. Mucus is secreted from disperse mucous cells, called **goblet cells,** located along the entire alimentary tract and from complex tubular glands, such as salivary glands, glands located deep in the walls of the stomach and upper duodenum, and between intestinal villi in invaginations called **Lieberkühn's crypts.** Especially important are Brunner's glands located adjacent to the pylorus in the duodenum, where the HCl concentration is highest. Mucus secretion from these glands is under the control of the four gastrointestinal hormones (especially secretin), contact with food, and the parasympathetic nervous system. Sympathetic stimulation inhibits this mucus secretion and is thereby the most prevalent cause of stomach ulcers. Similar nervous, endocrine, and tactile influences control mucus secretions from other complex glands.

Saliva

The salivary glands (Figure 9-1) secrete a mucin-containing fluid in response to nervous stimulation; that is, cholinergic reflexes to foreign materials in the mouth, or the smell, sight, or thought of food. By its contents of water and mucin, saliva moistens and, thus, lubricates the food mass to assist swallowing.

In humans, 1 to 2 L of saliva are produced per day. The fluid is hypotonic at slow flow rates and isotonic at high rates of secretion. Saliva has a pH in the range of 6.4 to 7.0 and contains low concentrations of HCO_3^-, Na^+, and Cl^- relative to plasma, but high concentrations of K^+ and Ca^{++}. In fact, the Ca^{++} concentration in saliva may be so high that, in combination with organic materials, it can form tartar on the teeth. Saliva contains small amounts of urea, glucose, lactate, vitamins, and immunoglobulin A (IgA). Salivary transport of urea from blood to gut is especially important in herbivores, since intestinal urease liberates ammonia (which buffers rumen acid and also serves as a nitrogen source for microbial conversion of carbohydrate to protein), whose reconversion to urea in the liver neutralizes bicarbonate. Saliva also transports certain drugs out of the bloodstream (e.g., alcohol, morphine). Odiferous constituents are transported from the bloodstream into saliva, hence, for example, the odor of onions and garlic cannot be removed by mouthwash.

Enzyme activities present in saliva include carbonic anhydrase, phosphatase, lipase (which works on triglycerides of short-chain fatty acids), and an amylase, ptyalin, which initiates the digestion of starch. The latter can be experienced by chewing for

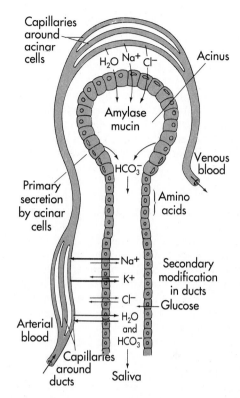

Figure 9-1. Salivary gland. *Adapted from Denny-Brown D and Robertson BG: Brain, Vol 58:256, 1935 and from Schuster MM et al.: Bull John Hopkins Hosp 116:79, 1965.*

a protracted time on bread: it tastes increasingly sweeter because of the liberation of glucose from starch.

The concentrations of Na^+ and K^+ in saliva are affected by aldosterone. Adrenocortical hyperfunction, as in Cushing's disease, causes Na^+ reabsorption in the salivary ducts in exchange for K^+, and thus, low Na^+ and high K^+ levels in saliva. Adrenocortical insufficiency, as in Addison's disease, increases the Na^+ concentration, since Na^+ is not transported out of the saliva.

Ruminant saliva differs from nonruminant saliva in having a higher concentration of Na^+, HCO_3^-, and phosphate yet a lower concentration of K^+ and Cl^-. As ruminant salivary flow increases, however, there is a reciprocal change in the phosphate and bicarbonate concentrations, keeping saliva highly buffered at all times.

In all mammalian species, facilitation of mastication and deglutition are primary functions of saliva.

This is particulary important in herbivores. For example, secretory flows as high as 50 ml/min have been recorded in a 150 kg pony during mastication, and the salivary glands of the cow secrete from 100 to 200 L/day. In the cat and dog, salivary secretion has the special function of evaporative cooling, and the parotid gland of the dog under intense parasympathetic stimulation is capable of secreting at 10 times the rate (per gm of gland) of the parotid gland in humans. Thus regulation of body heat by this means is as effective as evaporation of sweat in humans.

Gastric secretions

The gastric mucosa secretes a juice containing the following:
- Approximately 98% water;
- A pH of approximately 1.0, caused by HC1; this HC1 serves at least two functions: it kills most bacteria taken in with the diet, and it hydrolytically cleaves off a peptide from pepsinogen, and thereby converts the inactive zymogen into active pepsin, which, in turn, autocatalytically continues to activate more pepsinogen;

- The endopeptidase pepsin;
- Inorganic salts;
- Mucins, large, viscous, carbohydrate-rich glycoproteins, that serve as lubricant for and protection of stomach and intestinal surfaces;
- Intrinsic factor, a necessary carrier for facilitated absorption of vitamin B_{12} (cobalamine) in the gut;
- Small amounts of the gastric hormone, gastrin;
- A lipase that, like the salivary lipase, works on triglycerides of short-chain fatty acids.

The body and fundus of the stomach houses gastric glands that secrete HC1, pepsin, and mucus (Figure 9-2). The distal portion of the stomach, the antrum, contains the pylorus and is the site of gastrin secretion.

The following are the three cell types that line the canaliculi of gastric glands (see Figure 9-2):
- Mucous cells at the neck of the gland secrete a mucus that contains mucins;
- Parietal cells secrete HC1 and intrinsic factor;
- Chief cells secrete pepsinogen, whose activation in the lumen of the stomach by HCl produces

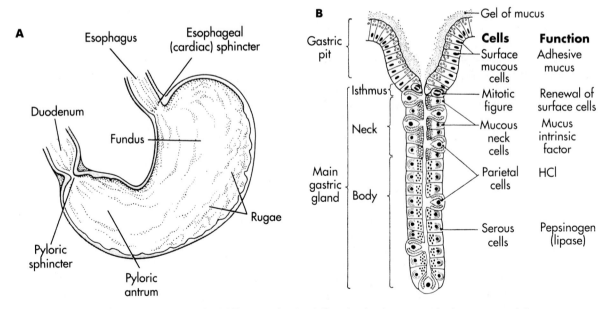

Figure 9-2. A, The stomach and **B,** a gastric gland. Gastric glands, present in the mucosa of the stomach, contain chief, parietal, and goblet cells, responsible respectively for pepsinogen, HCl, and mucus secretion. *Reproduced with permission from Passmore R and Robson JS (eds): A companion to medical studies, Vol 1, Philadelphia, 1968, Davis, p 30.13.*

the endopeptidase enzyme, pepsin.

Through active HC1 secretion at the expense of ATP (Figure 9-3), the parietal cells secrete a solution of 0.16N HC1 and 0.007M KC1. This H^+ concentration is one million times that in plasma. Carbonic anhydrase and coordinated H^+/K^+ and $C1^-$ pumps are involved. The H^+ secretion into the stomach and the coupled absorption of HCO_3^- into the bloodstream causes the postprandial rise in plasma pH, called the **alkaline tide**. This is not a permanent burden on the acid-base buffering system, because H^+ recombines with HCO_3^- in the duodenum.

Gastric secretions are regulated by the parasympathetic nervous system (vagus nerve) with acetylcholine as mediator, via intracellular Ca^{++} as second messenger. Taste, smell, or even the thought of food starts secretion. The presence of food in the stomach releases the hormone gastrin that, in turn, stimulates HC1 and pepsinogen secretions. Release of gastrin is stimulated by dietary peptides, amino acids, and the vagus nerve. Gastrin secretion is inhibited by low pH (negative feedback by HC1), and various duodenal and intestinal hormones, including secretin, somatostatin, cholecystokinin, gastric inhibitory peptide, and vasoactive intestinal peptide. Histamine, present in the gastric mucosa, is a weak stimulator of HC1 secretion.

In the stomachs of young sucklings, the enzyme rennin (rennet, not to be confused with renin, produced in the kidney [see Chapter 8]) is active. This enzyme curdles milk by using Ca ions to tie the peptide chains of the milk protein casein into a three-dimensional network of paracasein. The curdling of milk prevents it from flushing through the alimentary channel of the suckling. (Mixing milk, rennet, and $CaC1_2$ is the first step in the production of cheese.) The pH optimum for rennin activity is around 4.5. This leads to the conclusions that at pH 1.5 in adult stomachs rennin is inactive, and that the pH in the suckling's stomach is around 4.5, hence, there is no pepsin activity. Because of inactivity of pepsin, proteins in the first milk, colostrum, escape digestion in the stomach. Trypsin inhibitor in colostrum protects these proteins from attack by pancreatic endopeptidases. The result is that certain proteinaceous immune factors can be transferred from the mother, via colostrum, to the newborn suckling. (Pepsinogen is elaborated in the young stomach; when the stomach contents of a suckling are acidified with HC1 to pH 1.5, pepsin activity abounds.)

Pancreatic fluid

The pancreas produces several hormones (insulin, glucagon, somatostatin, pancreatic polypeptide) that in different ways help to regulate intermediary metabolism. For the intestinal digestion of food, however, the exocrine pancreatic functions and their regulation via intestinal hormones must be considered. The pancreatic duct empties into the duodenum in close proximity to the pylorus.

Pancreatic juice, like saliva, contains some 98% water and, in addition, inorganic salts and small amounts of proteins and other organic compounds. The pH of pancreatic juice is about 8.0 due to a high concentration of HCO_3^-. This serves to neutralize acidic stomach contents when they enter the duodenum, so an intestinal pH is maintained that allows digestive enzymes to be active. HCO_3^- contained in bile also helps in this respect. Volume and HCO_3^- content of pancreatic secretion is under control of the hormone secretin. This hormone is elaborated from the duodenum and the upper jejunum in response to gastric acid.

Secretion of digestive enzymes by the pancreas is under the control of the parasympathetic nervous sys-

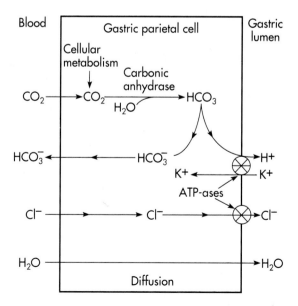

Figure 9-3. Mechanism of HCl secretion.

tem and various intestinal hormones and peptides; it is mediated by the cAMP and Ca^{++}-dependent second-messenger systems. Particularly powerful in this control is the hormone cholecystokinin, released from the duodenum and upper jejunum in response to peptides, amino acids, and long-chain fatty acids contained in the chyme leaving the stomach. Enzymes contained in the pancreatic juice primarily attack large molecular structures and start digesting them so the job can be completed further down the tract by enzymes of the small intestine.

Digestive enzymes in pancreatic juice include the following:

- Amylases, which work on starches and glycogen;
- Triglyceride lipase;
- Phospholipases;
- Cholesterol esterase;
- Ribonucleases for DNA and RNA digestion;
- Endopeptidases (trypsin, chymotrypsin, elastin) that attack proteins from within the peptide chain; and
- Carboxypeptidase, an exopeptidase specific for the carboxy terminals of peptide chains.

The endo- and exopeptidases are stored and released by zymogens. Trypsin inhibitor is contained in the cell sap of pancreatic acinar cells, and not the zymogen granules. It helps to keep trypsin in its inactive form (trypsinogen) such that the acinar cells will not be autolyzed by their own protease activity. Enterokinase, a proteolytic enzyme elaborated from the intestinal mucosa, converts trypsinogen into trypsin, which, in turn, activates all other peptidases in the intestinal lumen.

Bile

Bile is produced in the liver, where parenchymal cells secrete bile salts (needed for intestinal lipid emulsification and absorption) and metabolic waste products into bile canaliculi. The canaliculi merge into a common bile duct that empties out its contents into the duodenum near the pylorus, where chyme enters. Some species (e.g., humans, mice, dogs, cows, sheep, pigs, goats, cats, and some birds) have a gallbladder in which bile is concentrated, whereas other species do not (e.g., rats, dolphins, porpoises, whales, pocket gophers, doves, pigeons, elephants, camels, giraffes, moose, elk, deer, and horses). Bile production in the liver responds to the need to excrete waste materials from the bloodstream and to hormonal stimuli (secretin, cholecystokinin, gastrin) in response to food intake and the requirement of bile salts and bicar-

bonate for digestive purposes. One should distinguish between a bile acid-dependent fraction, which contains mixed micelles of bile salts, cholesterol, and lecithin, and a bile acid-independent fraction with a serum electrolyte-like composition. The rate of bile entry into the duodenum depends on the emptying of the gallbladder and the constriction and relaxation of the sphincter of Oddi, which is located in the bile duct near the duodenum. Both of these bile-flow determinants are controlled parasympathetically (vagus nerve) and by cholecystokinin.

A prime function of bile is that of a "sewer system" into which the liver dumps waste materials that it removes from the bloodstream. Since the pH of bile is around 7.2, bicarbonate in bile aids in the neutralization of stomach acids. Biliary bile salts and lecithin are needed for intestinal digestion (i.e., emulsification) and absorption of lipids.

Bile salts are formed in the liver from cholesterol (Figure 9-4). The formation of bile salts is under negative feedback control at the level of hydroxymethylglutaryl-CoA reductase, the key enzyme in cholesterol synthesis from acetyl-CoA, and at the level of cholesterol conversion to bile salts. The term **bile salt** is used in physiology as a functionally defined entity of great molecular diversity. Various bile acids are found in nature: cholate, deoxycholate, chenodeoxycholate, lithocholate, ursocholate (with an OH at carbon-4), etc. Furthermore, these bile acids occur, in part, conjugated to either glycine or taurine. Animal species differ in the composition of their bile salts with respect to the major bile acid, the proportion conjugated, and the glycine or taurine nature of the conjugates.

In three dimensions, the structure of bile salts is such that all of the polar groups point to one side of the plane in which the carbon-rings are situated; that orientation makes one side of the bile salt polar, the other side hydrophobic. When present above a certain concentration in a solution, bile salts can spontaneously aggregate to form micelles, or liquid crystals, in which the apolar sides interact with each other, while the polar groups interact with water (Figure 9-5). The lipid phase of micelles allows other lipids to enter, forming mixed micelles. Their propensity to form micelles, thus, makes bile salts the body's chief detergent, as micelles allow lipids to travel in an aqueous medium that is devoid of proteins. In the bloodstream or in tissue cells, proteins transport lipids via binding to apolar regions on the protein molecules; but no proteins are available to

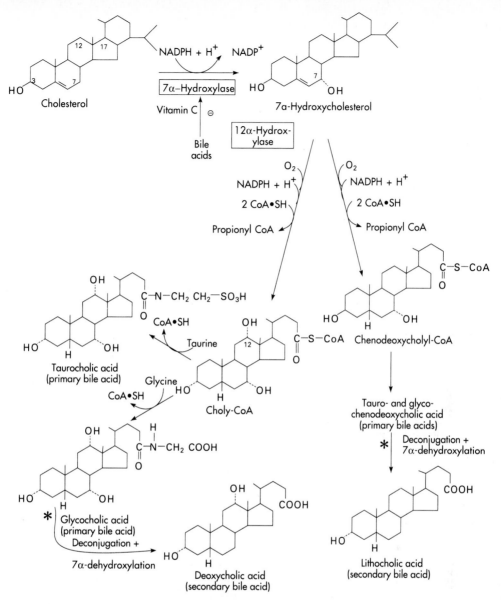

Figure 9-4. Biosynthesis and degradation of bile salts. *Catalyzed by microbial enzymes. *Reproduced with permission from Murray RK, Granner DK, Mayes PA, and Rodwell VW: Harper's biochemistry, ed 21, Norwalk, CT, 1988, Appleton & Lange, p 249.*

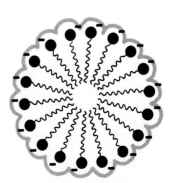

Figure 9-5. A micelle in water. Hydrophobic interactions between lipid tails and hydratation of anionic polar heads lend stability and structural order to the micelle.

carry lipids in bile or in the gastrointestinal tract. There, mixed-micelle–forming bile salts are needed. In the small intestines, bile salts carry lipid digesta to the mucosal cell surface, where lipids are absorbed and the bile salts are carried back, via the bloodstream, to the liver for another round of service (enterohepatic circulation).

Cholesterol is not only the parent compound for hepatic bile salt synthesis, but it is also excreted as such in bile. Because cholesterol is not soluble in water, it is transported in mixed-micellar form, together with bile salts and phospholipids. There are two categories of compounds in bile: those with about the same concentration as in plasma, such as inorganic salts; and those that are highly concentrated in bile, such as bilirubin (whose concentration in bile exceeds that in plasma by some thousand-fold), cholesterol, bile salts, phospholipids, and pharmaceuticals (e.g., penicillin; sulfobromophthalein). Gallbladder bile is highly concentrated and represents a precariously supersaturated solution of cholesterol and bilirubin held in balance by micelle formation. This balance can be upset, either in cases of hepatic overproduction of cholesterol or when infection or biliary obstruction leads to the formation of crystallization nuclei that, if not immediately flushed into the gut, lead to the formation of gallstones (cholelithiasis). In fact, cholesterol (literally, "solid bile") derives its name from the fact that certain types of gallstones consist predominantly of cholesterol.

Functional anatomy of the small intestine

Before reviewing the final stages of gastrointestinal digestion and intestinal absorption of nutrients, a brief overview of functional anatomy of the gut is in order. Gut motility under the direction of the autonomic nervous system produces waves of constriction and peristalsis that cause mixing and forward propulsion of intestinal contents. Surface enlargement in macro- and microanatomical form is another factor that facilitates intestinal absorption.

The illustrations of intestinal structures (Figure 9-6) show the various surface enlargements that increase absorptive efficiency, the blood vasculature and lymphatics (lacteals) that transport absorbed materials, and the tight junctions between mucosal cells that avoid paracellular invasion of intestinal contents; a mucopolysaccharide layer, or glycocalyx prevents the intestinal mucosa from digesting itself.

The gut mucosa, being an epithelial tissue, is constantly being rejuvenated. From the tips of villi, old cells slough off to be replaced by younger cells formed in the crypts of the villi and moved to the tips. The rate of mucosal turnover is controlled by the trophic action of gastrin and other intestinal hormones.

The epithelium of the small intestine secretes intestinal juice (succus entericus) consisting of viscous mucus, which is derived from goblet cells, and an enzyme-containing fluid with a composition similar to extracellular fluid that is elaborated from pits between villi, the Lieberkühn's crypts. The secretions from these crypts, amounting to approximately 1800 ml per day in humans, are immediately reabsorbed by villi, thereby creating a circular fluid pattern believed to assist in the absorption of nutrients from digested chyme.

Intestinal digestion

Digestion of nutrients, started in saliva and stomach, and continued in the duodenum, is mostly completed in the small intestines. Contrary to the pancreatic enzymes that are secreted into the lumen of the gut, intestinal enzymes are associated with the mucosal cell surface.

Proteins, after pepsin digestion in the stomach, are further broken down to peptide fragments by pancreatic endopeptidases. These fragments are attacked from both ends by pancreatic carboxypeptidase and intestinal aminopeptidase activities, so that free amino acids, a considerable amount of dipeptides, and smaller quantities of longer peptides remain to be absorbed. Pancreatic ribonucleases digest nucleic acids.

Complex carbohydrates, starches and glycogen, are digested by pancreatic amylases and various debranching enzymes before intestinal maltase, lactase, and sucrase split their corresponding disaccharides into their constituent glucose, fructose, and galactose.

Lipid digestion is complicated because of the water-insolubility of lipids. As a result of the churning action of the stomach, the motility of the intestines, and the emulsifying action of bile salts, fat is broken up into emulsion droplets that are stabilized by a coat of phospholipids. In the duodenum, pancreatic lipase attacks the emulsion droplets and breaks down the triglycerides into monoglycerides and free fatty acids, most of which are incorporated into biliary micelles. Mixed bile salt micelles carry dietary cholesterol and phospholipids, long-chain fatty acids, monoglycerides, and fat-soluble vitamins (A, D, E, and K). The mixed micelles traverse the mucopolysaccharide layer covering the gut mucosa (unstirred water layer) and deliver their lipid contents to mucosal cells. Bile salts

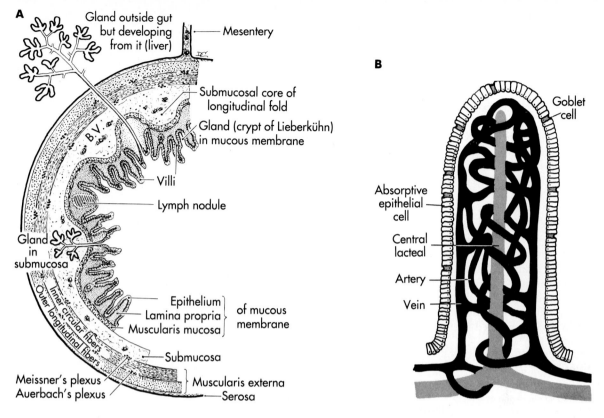

A

Gland outside gut but developing from it (liver)

Mesentery

Submucosal core of longitudinal fold

Gland (crypt of Lieberkühn) in mucous membrane

B.V.

Villi

Lymph nodule

Gland in submucosa

Inner circular fibers
Outer longitudinal fibers

Epithelium
Lamina propria
Muscularis mucosa

} of mucous membrane

Submucosa

Meissner's plexus
Auerbach's plexus

} Muscularis externa

Serosa

B

Goblet cell

Absorptive epithelial cell

Central lacteal

Artery

Vein

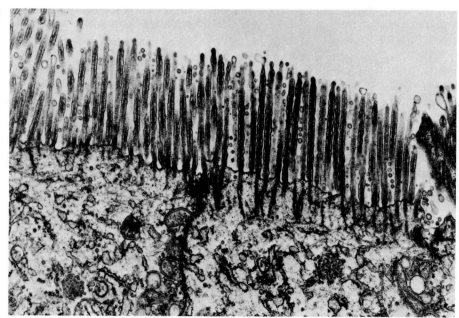

C

Figure 9-6. Anatomy of the small intestine. **A, B,** and **C** present increasing magnification. **A,** A general overview. **B,** A single villus; note absorptive cells and mucus-secreting goblet cells with their central blood circulation and lymphatics. **C,** An electron photomicrograph of neighboring ovine enterocytes; note the brush border and tight junctions between cells. *A, reproduced with permission from Ham's histology, Cormack DH (ed), ed 9, Philadelphia, 1987, Lippincott, p 492. C, courtesy Dr. Rick A. Rogers, Harvard School of Public Health.*

remain in the lumen and are absorbed in the more distal ileum. From there, absorbed bile salts are transported via the bloodstream to the liver for another round of service. The cycle from liver, via bile duct to gut, and then via bloodstream back to liver is called the **enterohepatic circulation.**

A summary of digestive processes in the gastrointestinal tract is given in Table 9-4. Further discussions on this topic are in the sections covering metabolism.

Intestinal absorption

The complex mixture of digested food and recirculating valuables of bile, pancreatic, and intestinal digestive secretions is absorbed mainly by mucosal cells of the small intestine. Practically all of the nutrient digesta are absorbed in the proximal jejunal portion of the small intestines, but bile salts and vitamin B_{12} are absorbed in the ileum. Water and electrolytes are absorbed along the entire length of the small and large intestines.

Carbohydrates and proteins are reduced to free sugars, amino acids, and very short peptides. Glucose and galactose are actively absorbed (symport with Na^+), other sugars diffuse into mucosal cells along their gradients, some aided by specific carriers. Amino acids are actively absorbed, and there is evidence for the intestinal absorption of dipeptides and somewhat longer peptides, which are then mainly converted to free amino acids inside mucosal cells. Patients with an inborn deficiency of the intestinal carrier for neutral amino acids (Hartnup disease) can satisfy their dietary tryptophan requirement by ingesting dipeptides. The absorbed sugars and amino acids that are not used for intestinal mucosal protein synthesis are transported via mesenteric and portal venous blood circulation to the liver, where their metabolic fates are determined.

Table 9-4   Summary of digestive processes

Source of secretion and stimulus for secretion	Enzyme	Method of activation and optimal conditions for activity	Substrate	End products or action
Salivary glands: secrete saliva in reflex response to presence of food in oral cavity.	Salivary amylase	Chloride ion necessary. pH 6.6-6.8.	Starch glycogen	Maltose plus 1:6 glucosides (oligosaccharides) plus maltotriose
Lingual glands.	Lingual lipase	pH range 2.0-7.5; optimal, 4.0-4.5.	Short-chain primary ester link at *sn*-3	Fatty acids plus 1,2-diacylglycerols
Stomach glands: chief cells and parietal cells secrete gastric juice in response to reflex stimulation and action of gastrin.	Pepsin A (fundus) Pepsin B (pylorus)	Pepsinogen converted to active pepsin by HCl. pH 1.0-2.0.	Protein	Peptides
	Rennin	Calcium necessary for activity. pH 4.0.	Casein of milk.	Coagulates milk.
Pancreas: presence of acid chyme from the stomach activates duodenum to produce (1) secretin, which hormonally stimulates flow of pancreatic juice; (2) cholecystokinin, which stimulates the production of enzymes.	Trypsin	Trypsinogen converted to active trypsin by enterokinase of intestine at pH 5.2-6.0. Autocatalytic at pH 7.9.	Protein peptides	Polypeptides; dipeptides
	Chymotrypsin	Secreted as chymotrypsinogen and converted to active form by trypsin. pH 8.0.	Protein peptides	Same as trypsin More coagulating power for milk
	Elastase	Secreted as proelastase and converted to active form by trypsin.	Protein peptides	Polypeptides; dipeptides

From Murray RK and others: Harper's biochemistry, ed 21, Norwalk, Conn, 1988, Appleton & Lange.

Table 9-4   Summary of digestive processes

Source of secretion and stimulus for secretion	Enzyme	Method of activation and optimal conditions for activity	Substrate	End products or action
	Carboxypeptidase	Secreted as procarboxypeptidase, activated by trypsin.	Polypeptides at the free carboxyl end of the chain	Lower peptides, free amino acids
	Pancreatic amylase	pH 7.1.	Starch glycogen	Maltose plus 1:6 glucosides (oligosaccharides) plus maltotriose
	Lipase	Activated by bile salts, phospholipids, colipase. pH 8.0.	Primary ester linkages of triacylglycerol	Fatty acids, monoacylglycerols, diacylglycerols, glycerol
	Ribonuclease	—	Ribonucleic acid	Nucleotides
	Deoxyribonuclease	—	Deoxyribonucleic acids	Nucleotides
	Cholesteryl ester hydrolase	Activated by bile salts.	Cholesteryl esters	Free cholesterol plus fatty acids
	Phospholipase A_2	Secreted as proenzyme, activated by trypsin and Ca^{2+}.	Phospholipids	Fatty acids; lysophospholipids
Liver and gallbladder: cholecystokinin, a hormone from the intestinal mucosa—and possibly also gastrin and secretin—stimulates the gallbladder and secretion of bile by the liver.	(Bile salts and alkali)	—	Fats—also neutralize acid chyme	Fatty acid-bile salt conjugates and finely emulsifies neutral fat-bile salt micelles and liposomes
Small intestine: Secretions of Brunner's glands of the duodenum and glands of Lieberkühn.	Aminopeptidase	—	Polypeptides at the free amino end of the chain	Lower peptides; free amino acids
	Dipeptidases	—	Dipeptides	Amino acids
	Sucrase	pH 5.0-7.0.	Sucrose	Fructose, glucose
	Maltase	pH 5.8-6.2.	Maltose	Glucose
	Lactase	pH 5.4-6.0.	Lactose	Glucose, galactose
	Trehalase	—	Trehalose	Glucose
	Phosphatase	pH 8.6.	Organic phosphates	Free phosphate
	Isomaltase or 1:6 glucosidase	—	1:6 glucosides	Glucose
	Polynucleotidase	—	Nucleic acid	Nucleotides
	Nucleosidases (nucleoside phosphorylases)	—	Purine or pyrimidine nucleosides	Purine or pyrimidine bases, pentose phosphate

Lipids, after digestion, present the mucosal cells with a mixture of water-soluble compounds, such as short-chained fatty acids and some of the phospholipids, and hydrophobic matter, including long-chained fatty acids, phospholipids, cholesterol, and vitamins A, D, E, and K. The water-solubles are transported via the bloodstream to the liver. The lipids are packaged and exocytosed as chylomicrons and very low-density lipoproteins into the intestinal lymphatics (lacteals) that carry them, via the thoracic lymph duct, to the left subclavian vein, where they enter the bloodstream. Thus, lipids do not travel in first instance to the liver, in contrast to water-soluble compounds absorbed in the gut. An exception to this is found in the chicken, who does not have intestinal lymphatics and routes incoming dietary lipids directly into mesenteric blood.

Water absorption is a vitally important intestinal function. In humans, about 10 L of fluid enter the gut each day. Of those 10 liters, 1.5 to 2.5 L are ingested, 1 to 1.5 L enter as saliva, 2 to 3 L are secreted by the stomach, and 1 to 2 L are secreted by the small intestine. Normally, all but about 200 ml are reabsorbed. Those 200 ml represent an obligatory water loss, osmotically associated, in part, with waste excretion, and partly for lubricating purposes. Water reabsorption from the lumen of the gut follows electrolyte reabsorption and is aided by an active sodium pump of mucosal cells that maintains a standing osmotic gradient in the lateral space between epithelial cells (cf., renal absorption of water).

Electrolytes are absorbed along gradients or accompanying, for electroneutrality, those that are actively absorbed. Inside the mucosal cell, a low Na^+ concentration is maintained by an active pump, located in the lateral membranes, that secretes Na^+ accompanied by Cl^-. In some species, such as dogs and horses, active Cl^- absorption occurs in the ileum. K^+ is for the most part passively absorbed. Intestinal absorption of Ca^{++} is an active process that requires a Ca-binding protein whose formation is controlled by 1,25-dihydroxycholecalciferol (DHC). As discussed earlier, DHC production from vitamin D_3 is stimulated by low Ca^{++} levels in the blood and the concomitant release of parathyroid hormone. Intestinal absorption of iron, exclusively in its reduced form (Fe^{++}), and adaptation to the body's need for that mineral were discussed earlier.

Malabsorption

The most prevalent disturbance due to malabsorption is diarrhea. Though the net result is a watery and often copious stool, the cause is usually related to electrolyte movements and the establishment or loss of osmotic gradients. A loosening of the tight junctions between mucosal cells, as in local tissue damage, can dispel the salt gradient between epithelial cells and, thus, diminish water absorption. The dietary intake of nonabsorbable solutes, or their formation in the gut lumen, necessitates osmotic retention of water in the stool. For example, a person lacking lactase activity cannot adequately digest lactose and, thus, develops an osmotic diarrhea as a result of drinking milk. Bacterial or viral infection (enteritis) irritates the mucosa of the distal end of the ileum and large intestine, which leads to secretion of large amounts of fluids into the lumen and increased peristalsis, so that toxins are diluted and the bacteria are removed from the body more rapidly. Cholera toxin stimulates excessive fluid secretion from the Lieberkühn's crypts in the distal ileum and colon, and, in addition, enhances the mechanism for bicarbonate-chloride exchange. This causes such a massive HCO_3^-, excretion, that it, and the immense losses of Na^+ and water that accompanies it, is often fatal. Many diseases are related to malabsorption of vitamins or minerals; for example, anemia may be caused by deficient absorption of iron, folate, or cobalamine; deficient Ca absorption may result in osteomalacia.

STUDY QUESTIONS

1. Gastric inhibitory peptide (GIP) is released in response to HCl secretion and increased motility in the antrum of the stomach. (True/False)

2. Increased parasympathetic stimulation, such as increased vagal nerve stimulation, tends to (increase / decrease / not change) gastric secretions. (Choose one.)

3. About cholecystokinin (CCK):
   a. List the CCK effect on the pancreas.
   b. List the CCK effect on the biliary system.
   c. List the CCK effect that is not related to gastrointestinal functions.

4. *a.* Name the intestinal hormones that regulate the endocrine and exocrine pancreas.
   b. What causes elaboration of these hormones?

5. List the effects that somatostatin has on the stomach, pancreas, and pituitary.

6. *a.* Name the anatomical part of the digestive tract in the horse where extensive microbial fermentation occurs.

   b. List a valuable nutritional contribution of intestinal microflora to the body's metabolism.

7. *a.* Name the channels, located within intestinal villi, into which lipids are transported after intestinal absorption.

   b. Name the microanatomical structure that prevents paracellular absorption of intestinal contents.

8. Name the circuitous route whereby bile salts are recycled and reused many times over.

9. List a function of the mucopolysaccharide layer located on the periphery of mucosal cells.

10. Why does a patient need parenteral cobalamine administration after gastrectomy (stomach removal)?

11. In a pancreatectomized dog, digestibility of starch, relative to that of maltose, is unaffected. (True/False)

12. *a.* Name the ion that establishes the standing osmotic gradient in the intercellular space of the enterocyte.

    b. Countercurrent multiplication is the mechanism whereby a standing osmotic gradient is maintained in the renal medulla and in intestinal villi. (True/False)

    c. List the active process that establishes and maintains the osmotic gradient in intestinal villi.

13. Identify primary differences between renin and rennin.

14. *a.* Name an enzyme produced by cells in the stomach (in an inactive form) that is involved in protein digestion.

    b. Name the enzyme produced in the duodenum that activates trypsinogen.

15. An initial hydrolysis product resulting from the action of pancreatic amylase on starch is (glucose / maltose / galactose). (Choose one.)

16. What are the primary structural and functional differences between micelles and chylomicrons of the digestive tract?

17. Colipase is a coenzyme involved in fat digestion that is produced by the intestinal cells. (True/False)

18. The fundamental difference in the body's routing of absorbed nutrients is that water-solubles (carbohydrates, amino acids) are transported from the gut (name the medium) to the liver, while insolubles (lipids) are transported from the gut via (name the route).

19. *a.* Small peptides can enter intestinal cells. (True/False)

    b. Large molecular weight proteins (150,000 to 900,000) can enter the intestinal cells of day-old calves intact. (True/False)

20. Elevated levels of plasma iron would tend to (increase / decrease / not change) active absorption of iron from the gastrointestinal tract. (Choose one.)

21. Name the hormone that facilitates Ca absorption in the gastrointestinal tract.

22. List a possible harm of sulphur-containing drugs administered orally to combat bacterial infections.

23. For what purposes would a rabbit practice coprophagy?

10 Introduction to metabolism

DEFINITIONS

To maintain a steady state of nonequilibrium (life), the body is in perpetual need of food, water, and oxygen intake, storage of food metabolites after a meal, parceling out these stores in times between meals, and eliminating nondigestible and metabolic waste products. The storage of intestinal digestion products of nutrients in the form of glycogen, fat, and proteins requires energy since these are anabolic processes. Combustion of fat, carbohydrate, and protein, on the other hand, goes downhill and, thus, is catabolic. The sum of anabolism and catabolism is called **metabolism.** It should be recalled that an isolated system may be anabolic (e.g., conversion of acetyl-CoA to fatty acids), but that for each anabolic process there is a catabolic one (the conversion of glucose to acetyl-CoA in the above example), which pays the energy bill and releases additional energy in the form of heat. When a large enough system is considered, all processes in nature proceed in the direction of free energy loss.

THE GLOBAL PICTURE

Homeostatic control of body composition requires the metabolic efforts of all organs and tissues, and coordination of these efforts via the nervous and endocrine control systems (Chart I). Control mechanisms exist at all levels of structural integrity, because there are organismic controls via neuroendocrine systems; organ controls, which are to some extent autonomic, such as respiration and renal functions; controls at the cell level, such as cell surface phenomena, receptors, and second messengers; and controls in subcellular organelles and cytoplasm, including cytoskeleton functions and allosteric control over key enzyme activities. Therefore, to gain an insight into the function of a metabolic process, it is imperative that the process first be considered in the overall context of the intact organism: the global picture of Chart I.

While looking at a metabolic process in the context of Chart I, one asks, What is its function? Why is that process needed, and where does it fit in the picture of the intact animal? Only after these questions have been answered, and the relevance of the process has been ascertained, can one begin to investigate how the process works and what are its enzyme and cofactor requirements (metabolic charts). Thus, physiological chemistry combines physiology (Chart I) and biochemistry (metabolic charts) and then addresses the question, How is a process controlled, so that one may be able to interpret indications that the process is deficient and, hence, devise therapeutic measures?

Before applying Chart I to any physiologic situation, three precise qualifications must be defined:
- Animal species. As there are large differences in metabolism of various species, the animal under consideration must be specified.
- Type of cell. Not all metabolic pathways occur in every cell; the cell in question must be agreed upon.
- Time of the day relative to meal intake. Throughout discussions on metabolism, the text shall distinguish three situations, each with its characteristic key word:
  Postprandial (PP)—the time immediately after a meal, characterized by storage of dietary bounty in the body's reservoirs, directed by the parasympathetic branch of the autonomic nervous system and by the hormone insulin.
  Between regular meals (BRM)—a period char-

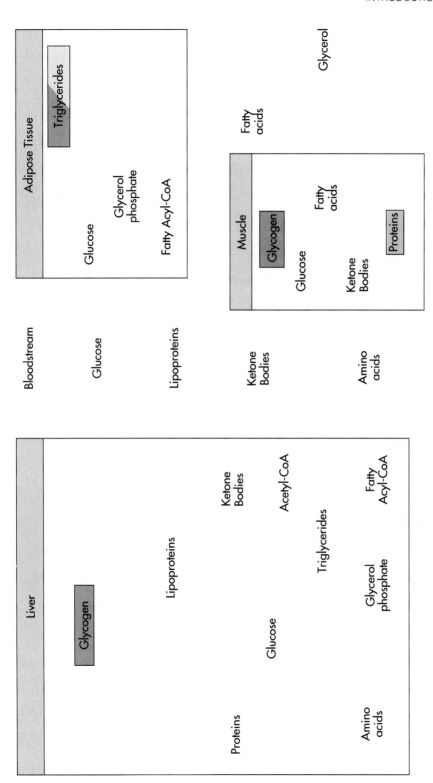

Chart I. The global picture

acterized by economy in the body's use of its stores, directed by both branches of the autonomic nervous system and by insulin antagonists, such as glucagon.

Fasting—when, due to lack of nutritionally essential factors, metabolic economy is sacrificed for the purpose of survival; directed by the sympathetic branch of the autonomic nervous system and the "panic" hormones, including epinephrine and norepinephrine.

After defining these three limits, one may discuss, for example, a pig's postprandial (PP) fat-cell metabolism. Chart I then places that fat cell within the global picture of the pig's metabolism, and may be used to demonstrate how various organs interact with the PP fat cell; for instance, the liver converts dietary sugars into fat, packages and then exports these fats as very low-density lipoproteins for deposition as triglycerides in fat cells.

METABOLIC CHARTS AND PATHWAYS

A prototype for all metabolic charts (Figure 10-1) depicts the three major body stores and energy in the four wind directions. Going down the middle, there is a "spinal" column of 6-carbon compounds (hexoses), 3-carbon compounds (glycerol, pyruvate), 2-carbon acetate, and 1-carbon CO_2. All body stores are interconnected, through that spinal column, by a multitude of pathways, some reversible, others unidirectional.

Pathways are interlocking enzyme reactions, in which the product of one step becomes the substrate of the next. The many steps that are often involved represent small free energy transitions, and, thus, allow for reversibility of a pathway. This may be likened to a staircase with many small steps; however, if one step were to be huge, a person could jump down the stairs, but would have to find an alternate route in the upstairs direction.

Considerations given a pathway in the context of a metabolic chart include qualitative controls by enzymes, vitamins, minerals, pH, and intracellular transport of substrates and products, and quantitative controls over the rate of the pathway. Among the latter are adaptive modifications of rate-limiting (key) enzyme activities by neuroendocrine, allosteric, phosphorylating and dephosphorylating, and many other influences.

Key enzymes are few in number. Adapting to variable physiological conditions, a key enzyme can either be activated or inhibited, thereby opening up or blocking the entire metabolic pathway it controls. The remainder of the metabolic pathway consists of constitutive enzyme activities present in ample amounts. Pathways are organized, in part, as multiple-enzyme complexes attached to microanatomical subcellular structures. Thus, metabolic pathways are always there and ready to go: they are part of the cell's "furniture." When their function is needed, they quickly provide their end product by activating a key enzyme that commits the starting material to traverse that pathway. Since physiological chemistry focuses on the control of metabolism, and only the key enzymes are rate-controlling, the text shall concentrate on key enzymes and not on the constitutive portions of pathways.

Key enzymes are most often found at branching points, where a pathway branches off from another. At these points, an intermediate, common to two or more pathways, is funneled specifically in the direction where needed by rate modifications of key enzyme activities.

While studying pathways of metabolism the reader should concentrate on the following:
- Name of the pathway;
- Function of the pathway in different tissues in relation to the time of meal intake;
- Place of the pathway in the global picture of the animal (Chart I);
- Place of the pathway in the general scheme of metabolism (Chart II);
- Branching point where the pathway starts;
- Rate-controlling step of the pathway;
- Name of the key (rate-controlling) enzyme;
- Cofactor and coenzyme requirements;
- Physiologic controls over the pathway.

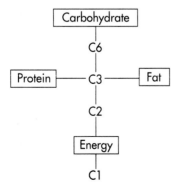

Figure 10-1. Outline of a metabolic chart.

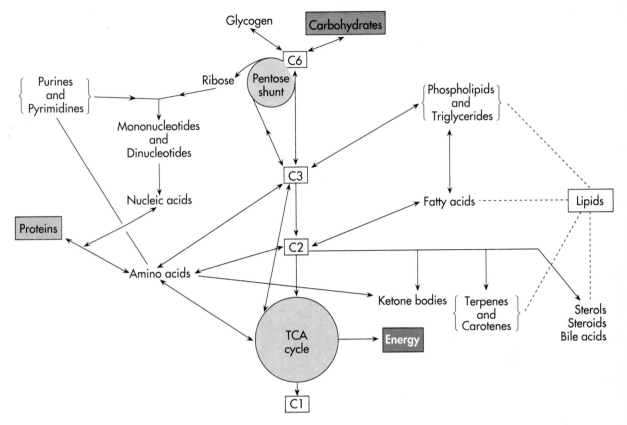

Chart II. Outline of intermediary metabolism.

OUTLINE OF INTERMEDIARY METABOLISM

Chart II conforms to the above prototype of a metabolism chart: the body's major stores and energy metabolism are located in the four wind directions, and the C6-C3-C2-C1 spinal column is clearly in evidence, as are interconnecting pathways. Chart II integrates the various pathways in a cell. The combination of Chart I and Chart II is going to be the overview for every detail encountered.

To illustrate the use of Chart I and Chart II, one may consider glycolysis. Chart II is never used as first aid. Rather, animal species (pig) is first agreed upon, as is cell type (liver), and time in relation to food intake (postprandial; PP). Then Chart I is used to find the pig's liver under PP conditions: a great deal of glucose is coming out of the gut and entering the liver. Little glucose can be stored as glycogen; the rest must be converted to fat, that is, first converted

to acetyl-CoA via glycolysis. That fat, then, is exported by the liver in the form of a lipoprotein and deposited in fat stores of adipose tissue. Now that the function of glycolysis in the PP pig's liver has been defined, Chart II may be used in a discussion of the chemistry and control of glycolysis in the context of all other metabolic pathways.

The conditions of PP and BRM metabolism may be illustrated as in Figure 10-2. It is important to note that two distinct illustrations are needed to emphasize the differences in net metabolic flow under PP and BRM conditions.

STARTING PICTURE OF METABOLISM

The caloric contents of metabolic stores in a lean man are about 85% fat, 15% protein, and 0.5% carbohydrate. These stores, of course, have functions other than their calorie count.

As the stores are replenished after a meal and grad-

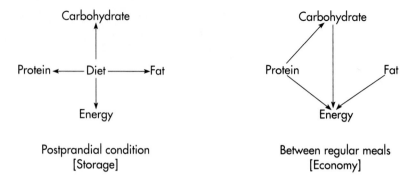

Figure 10-2. Comparing metabolic flow postprandially and between regular meals.

ually parcelled out between meals to meet bodily requirements, the ongoing metabolism reflects a state of flux. There are numerous pathways connecting the main body stores, and all of these pathways go on at tremendous speeds. Intermediates do not accumulate: they react at the same rate at which they are formed, so their concentrations are small. These metabolic pathways can be likened to small streams that are swiftly flowing. Nothing accumulates as long as all of the cofactors are there (vitamins, minerals, hormones and their receptors) and there is no inborn enzyme deficiency. But, as soon as an essential cofactor is lacking, a key reaction in a pathway can no longer proceed. Intermediates proximal to the block then accumulate, and little or nothing goes on distally from the block. It is as if a "dam" has been placed in the "river": a "lake" builds up, and it may be large. The pooling of these intermediates may become noticeable in the bloodstream and then blood analysis may give a clue as to where a metabolic block is located.

TOPICS DISCUSSED IN CHAPTERS ON METABOLISM

In the following chapters, control over metabolism is discussed in the sequence of increasing levels of structural integrity, as follows:
- Global and cellular starting pictures;
- Biological oxidation and energy metabolism;
- Pathways of carbohydrate, lipid, and nitrogen metabolism, and their controls at the subcellular level;
- Integrated cellular metabolism;
- Integrated organismic metabolism; interdependency of metabolic organ functions;
- Integrated whole-animal metabolism; related to time of food intake; neuroendocrine controls;
- Nutritional requirements (caloric, qualitative); and
- Comparative ruminant metabolism.

STUDY QUESTIONS

1. List the three items that must be precisely defined before any physiologically meaningful discussion on metabolism can begin.

2. Relating to time after food intake, three situations may be defined. List these situations and identify a term that characterizes metabolism in each situation.

3. In a well-conditioned male athlete, the body's energy stores are roughly: _____ % fats, _____ % proteins, and _____ % carbohydrates. (Fill in the blanks.)

11 Biological oxidation and energy metabolism

Bioenergetics deals with energy economy of an organism, that is to say, balancing supply and demand of energy. Supply of energy to an organism comes in the form of food (chemical energy). Metabolism converts that chemical energy, depending on demand, into other forms of energy, such as mechanical (muscle contraction), electrical (nerve and other cell membrane effects), and different chemical energy (ATP; fat and glycogen stores).

At the cellular level, energy transactions are directed by gradients. Gradients are potentials that allow energy exchange given the proper vector; for example, a current of electrons moving over a voltage difference (electrical potential), or chemicals traversing a concentration gradient (chemical potential). The combination of these two potentials is termed **electrochemical gradient.**

The problem with gradients is that spontaneous, downhill movement of vectors along their gradients wipes these gradients out; for instance, a concentration gradient disappears when compounds diffuse from the concentrated to the dilute side. Gradients must therefore be maintained at the expense of energy (e.g., Na^+, K^+, Cl^-, and Ca^{++} pumps). Spontaneous processes in nature are passive since they follow the electrochemical gradient. In contrast, for active processes, energy is required to go uphill against the electrochemical gradient.

Thus, the topic of bioenergetics holds the key to understanding the nature and mechanism of inter- and intracellular transport along or against electrochemical gradients. The topic of intermediary metabolism concerns the conversion of nutrients into proper forms of energy for maintaining those electrochemical gradients.

Electrical energy (watts) is the mathematical product of an electrial potential difference (volts) times an electron current (amperes). Electrical energy cannot be stored. It must be generated from chemical stores as needed and at the same rate that it can be used. Applied to physiology: the rates of ATP generation and utilization must match.

Chemical energy is stored as fat, protein, and glycogen. To generate electrical energy, electrons from chemical stores or from nutrients are shuttled over existing electrical potential differences. These voltage gradients are maintained in the inner mitochondrial membranes between adjacent cytochrome molecules. The necessary electrons are derived by redox reactions and shuttled by redox cofactors.

BIOLOGICAL OXIDATION
Reduction-oxidation (redox) reactions

A compound is oxidized by giving off electrons; by accepting electrons, it is reduced. The same compound under different conditions may act either as an electron donor or an electron acceptor. The following are examples of redox reactions.

Oxidized form + electrons $\leftrightarrow$ Reduced form

$$Fe^{3+} + e^- \leftrightarrow Fe^{2+} \text{ (in cytochromes)}$$
$$R—CHO \text{ (aldehyde)} + 2H^+ + 2e^- \leftrightarrow R—CH_2OH \text{ (alcohol)}$$
$$\begin{array}{l} HC—COOH \\ | \\ HC—COOH \\ \text{(succinate)} \end{array} + 2e^- \leftrightarrow \begin{array}{l} H_2C—COOH \\ | \\ H_2C—COOH \text{ (TCA cycle)} \\ \text{(fumarate)} \end{array}$$
$$\frac{1}{2}O_2 + 2H^+ + 2e^- \leftrightarrow H_2O$$
$$NAD^+ + 2H^+ + 2e^- \leftrightarrow NADH + H^+$$

The ultimate electron acceptor of mammalian metabolism is oxygen. Therein lies the link between food intake and oxygen requirement. Food is oxidized mainly inside mitochondria, where the intermediate acetyl-CoA fuels the TCA cycle. From there, electrons are shuttled by cofactors (NADH; FADH$_2$) to the intramitochondrial electron transfer chain, where voltage differences are maintained between successive redox couples (cytochromes). At the end of the chain, oxygen is ready to accept these electrons. Electrical energy is converted, in part, to chemical energy by ATP formation from ADP plus inorganic phosphate, a phosphorylation. The combined processes of electron shuttling (oxidation) and ATP formation (phosphorylation) is termed **oxidative phosphorylation.**

Enzymes and cofactors involved in redox reactions

Oxidases use oxygen as an electron and hydrogen acceptor and produce water:

$$AH_2 + \frac{1}{2}O_2 \rightarrow A + H_2O$$

Oxidases contain copper; for example, cytochrome oxidase, oxidizing the cytochrome a-a$_3$ complex at the end of the respiratory chain in mitochondria.

Oxygenases incorporate either both or one of the oxygen atoms of O$_2$ into a substrate:

$$A + O_2 \rightarrow AO_2$$

That reaction is exemplified by the oxidation of cysteine:

$$cysteine—SH \rightarrow cysteine—SO_2H$$

When only one of the oxygen atoms is used, the other forms water, using a proton and either NADH or NADPH:

$$AH + O_2 + NADPH \rightarrow AOH + H_2O + NADP^+$$

Enzymes that catalyze this type of reaction are associated with cytochromes b$_5$ and P450 that are located in the smooth endoplasmic reticulum and in mitochondria. This reaction serves several important functions. Most cells can use it to desaturate fatty acids by adding an OH-group to the molecule (which is followed by the removal of H$_2$O); for example, converting stearic to oleic acid. In the adrenal cortex the reaction contributes phenolic OH-groups to the production of steroid hormones. In the liver, these hydroxylation reactions serve to detoxify drugs (e.g., morphine). Phenobarbital is among the drugs that induce both formation and activity of enzymes and cytochrome P450 contained in the endoplasmic reticulum of the liver.

Anaerobic dehydrogenases cannot use oxygen as an electron acceptor; hence, oxidation of one substrate causes reduction of another, since electrons cannot be free:

$$AH_2 + B \rightarrow A + BH_2$$

Anaerobic dehydrogenases specifically require FAD, NAD, NADP, or GSH as cofactors to shuttle electrons; for example, the respiratory chain in mitochondria, and lactate dehydrogenase (Figure 11-1).

Aerobic dehydrogenases (Figure 11-2) oxidize a compound using molecular oxygen and produce hydrogen peroxide:

$$AH_2 + O_2 \rightarrow A + H_2O_2$$

Serving as cofactors are flavin, a yellow-colored B vitamin, and in most cases a metal (e.g., molybdenum); hence, the name metalloflavoproteins for these enzymes. Another example is the oxidative deamination of D and L amino acids.

The H$_2$O$_2$ formed is extremely toxic to the cell, and, thus, must be detoxified immediately. To that end, two different enzymes exist: (i) peroxidase, predominantly a plant enzyme (e.g., horseradish), but also found in erythrocytes, leukocytes, and milk, and (ii) catalase, the fastest-acting enzyme known, whose activity is present in all tissues, but is especially high in liver, kidneys, and bone marrow. Catalase activity is for the most part associated with small subcellular particles, **peroxisomes,** that are rich in aerobic dehydrogenase and catalase activities; apparently, these two enzymes work in tandem.

Peroxisomes

In mammals, peroxisomes are seen only in the liver and kidneys (organs with the highest catalase activ-

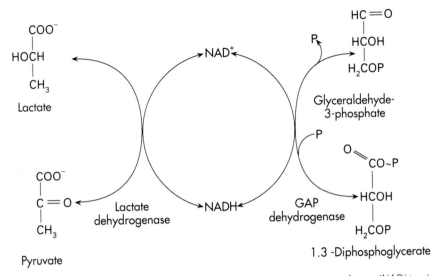

Figure 11-1. Two specific anaerobic dehydrogenases share a common cofactor *(NAD)* to shuttle electrons between two redox couples. In this case, reduction of pyruvate to lactate causes oxidation of glyceraldehyde-3-phosphate *(GAP)* to 1,3-diphosphoglycerate.

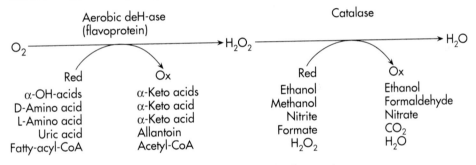

Figure 11-2. Oxidative metabolism in peroxisomes.

ities), where they occur as round particles, with a diameter of 0.5-µm, surrounded by a single membrane. Small amounts of catalase are present in all mammalian cells, associated with smaller (diameters of 0.1 to 0.2 µm) membrane-bound particles of elongated shapes, called **microperoxisomes.**

Catabolic functions

Characteristic of peroxisomes is that they contain one enzyme system, aerobic dehydrogenase, that generates H_2O_2, and another enzyme system, catalase, that breaks down the H_2O_2 (see Figure 11-2). Hydrogen peroxide is also produced outside of peroxisomes. For instance, the mitochondrial electron transfer chain contains flavoproteins and produces H_2O_2; detoxification of that H_2O_2 forms an important link between mitochondria and peroxisomes.

Another link between mitochondria and peroxisomes is fatty acid oxidation. β-Oxidation occurs not only in mitochondria, but peroxisomes, too, can β-oxidize fatty acids to acetyl-CoA (AcCoA). However, the oxidation in peroxisomes of fatty acid (and other compounds) differs from that in mitochondria in several important aspects:

- Not only are ordinary fatty acids oxidized in peroxisomes, but also (and especially) the very-long-chained fatty acids (C20, C22), as are transconfigurated fatty acids from plants.
- Peroxisomal oxidations depend on O_2 tension, unlike mitochondria in vivo, in which the O_2 tension is not rate-controlling, because of the high affinity of cytochrome oxidase for oxygen; hence, the high peroxisomal activities in the liver and kidneys.

- Peroxisomal fatty acid oxidation produces AcCoA and medium-chained fatty acids, which are exported out of the peroxisome (Figure 11-3).
- No ATP is formed in peroxisomes: heat is produced. Consequently, peroxisomal fatty acid oxidation is not under negative feedback control by high ratios of ATP/ADP, whereas mitochondrial fatty acid oxidation is. Therefore, peroxisomal fatty acid oxidation can serve as a safety valve, for it continues to oxidize fatty acids, and, thus, rids the body of an excess under conditions when high levels of fatty acids have to be coped with (e.g., during fasting or high-fat feeding). In the liver's peroxisomes, excess fatty acids can then be converted to AcCoA and medium-chained fatty acids, exported to mitochondria, and converted there to ketone bodies (which can then be transferred to plasma).
- Fatty acid oxidation (and indeed all other peroxisomal oxidation) is inducible by demand for that function, such as under conditions of feeding high-fat diets or cold stress, or administering lipid-lowering drugs (e.g., clofibrate). All of these conditions induce the peroxisomal functions, hence, over 50% of total fatty acid oxidation in the liver may be peroxisomal. Under normal conditions, peroxisomes consume some 10% of the liver's oxygen uptake, but under high-fat induction, considerably more O_2 is apportioned to peroxisomes.

- Oxidation of ethanol, methanol, etc. in peroxisomes does not involve $NAD^+/NADH$ intermediation and continues independent of metabolic influences on that redox couple (as opposed to, for instance, ethanol detoxification by alcohol dehydrogenase, which is anaerobic and does require NAD^+).

Anabolic functions

It is not correct to consider peroxisomes solely as organelles that perform oxidative catabolic functions. Peroxisomes are involved in synthetic (anabolic) functions as well (e.g., synthesis of plasmalogens [Figure 11-4]). Plasmalogens are an important class of phospholipids in all tissues; they constitute over 10% of the phospholipids in the brain and muscles. Several enzymes of the pathway of plasmalogen synthesis, and also an enzyme that contributes the necessary NADPH (isocitrate dehydrogenase), are located in peroxisomes. Also, cholic acid, a primary bile acid, is formed in peroxisomes of the liver.

Over 40 different enzyme activities have been discovered in catalase-containing microbodies (peroxisomes; glyoxysomes) in a wide variety of cells in all organisms ranking above bacteria. However, no peroxisome has been found that contains all of these enzymes. A common denominator of peroxisomes in plants and protozoa is that they contain, besides catalase, the enzymes of a glyoxylate cycle; hence, they are named glyoxysomes by some authors. The glyoxylate cycle allows plants to convert fat, via AcCoA, into carbohydrates. Such a gluconeogenic path does not occur in animals; animals cannot form glucose from fatty acids.

In view of the many vital functions of peroxisomes, it is not surprising that an inborn lack of peroxisomes (Zellweger syndrome) in human babies is fatal within one year.

Reduction potentials

As the Henderson-Hasselbalch equation for variations of the pH around the pK is dependent on the

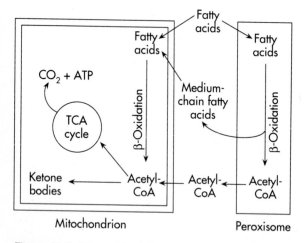

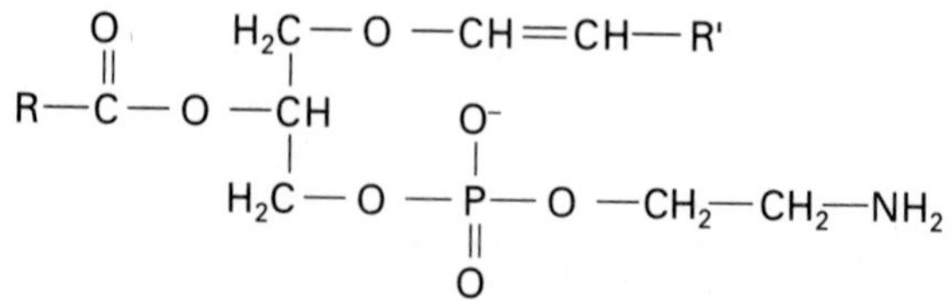

Figure 11-3. Fatty acid oxidation in peroxisomes and mitochondria.

Figure 11-4. A plasmalogen. R and R' are fatty acid chains.

logarithm of the ratio of the H^+ acceptor/donor, so is the reduction potential of a redox couple dependent on the ratio of the electron acceptor (Ox) over electron donor (Red), according to the Nernst equation:

$$E = E_0' + 0.06 \log(Ox/Red)$$

The derivation of this equation and the factor 0.06 (which is obtained under physiological conditions) were explained in Chapter 5 on Donnan equilibria. What the pH is for proton movement, the E is for electron movement. It is no wonder, then, that for maintaining constant E, redox buffers exist. In the liver, the redox couple pyruvate/lactate is the most concentrated, and thus, the most influential redox buffer. Vitamins C and E function as strong reducing agents: Vitamin C in aqueous media, and vitamin E in lipid surroundings, such as cell membranes, where they protect double bonds in unsaturated fatty acids. Redox-sensitive stains are used in histochemistry (e.g., to locate mitochondria on a tissue slide). Redox indicators are used in conjunction with enzymes, for instance, to demonstrate the presence of compounds in urine; strips impregnated with specific enzymes plus indicators to test for glucose, proteins, and ketones in the urine are available commercially.

For a 50:50 mixture of Ox/Red, the log-term in the Nernst equation equals zero and, thus, $E = E_0'$. Values for E_0 under standard conditions (30° C and pH 7.0), called **standard reduction potentials (E_0')**, are listed herein for some relevant redox couples (Table 11-1).

The following notes may be attached to the table of standard reduction potentials:

- The larger the positive value of the reduction potential, the greater the couple's affinity to accept electrons. Hence, a couple positioned above another one in the table will draw electrons away from the lower couple; in the process, the lower couple is oxidized (loses electrons), while the higher couple is reduced (gains electrons). For example, the couple oxygen/water tops the list, since it has the greatest avidity to accept electrons; hence, all other compounds can be oxidized by oxygen. For that reason, oxygen is the body's electron "sink," accepting, in the end, all metabolic electrons.

- The reduction potential table, thus, shows the direction in which redox reactions will go. In addition, from the numerical values of the reduction potentials, the extent to which the reaction will go is predictable; one can calculate the value of the equilibrium constant (K_{eq}) of a redox reaction between two couples. At equilibrium, there can be only one reduction potential (E_{eq}; Figure 11-5), and therefore, E_{eq} belonging to couple-1 must equal E_{eq} of couple-2, or applying the Nernst equation:

$$_1E_0 + \log(Ox_1/Red_1) = {_2E_0} + \log(Ox_2/Red_2)$$

Rearranging this equation yields the following:

$$_1E_0' - {_2E_0'} = \log(Ox_2/Red_2) - \log(Ox_1/Red_1)$$
$$\Delta E_0' = \log[(Ox_2/Red_2)/(Ox_1/Red_1)]$$
$$\Delta E_0' = \log[K_{eq}]$$

Table 11-1	Standard reduction potentials
Redox couple	**E_0' (volts)**
Oxygen/water	+0.82
Fe^{+++}/Fe^{++}	+0.77
Cytochrome a; Ox/Red	+0.29
Cytochrome c; Ox/Red	+0.22
Ubiquinone; Ox/Red	+0.10
Cytochrome b; Ox/Red	+0.08
Fumarate/succinate	+0.03
Methylene blue; Ox/Red	+0.01
$FAD/FADH_2$	−0.06
Oxaloacetate/Malate	−0.17
Pyruvate/lactate	−0.19
Acetoacetate/OH-butyrate	−0.27
$NAD^+/NADH$	−0.32
H^+/H_2	−0.42

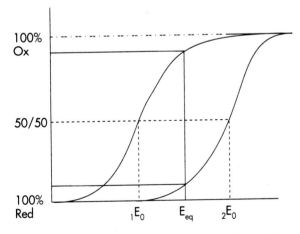

Figure 11-5. Direction and extent of a reduction-oxidation reaction. See text.

Efficiency of converting electrical into chemical energy

To estimate the available electrical energy from a redox reaction, the difference ($\Delta E_0'$) between the two redox couples involved in the reaction must be found in the table of standard reduction potentials, and then multiplied by the number of electrons (current) transferred in the reaction. (For a more accurate estimate, the ratios of Ox/Red for the two couples must be taken into account.)

Example: One wants to estimate how much electrical energy is generated when the pair of metabolic electrons shuttled by NADH traverses the entire mitochondrial sequence of cytochromes and is then captured by oxygen at the end. The standard redox potential for the oxygen couple is $+0.82$ V; for $NAD^+/NADH$ it is -0.32 V; thus the difference ($\Delta E_0'$) is 1.14 V. Since two electrons per molecule are involved, and the aim is to express the answer in Kcal (converting electron-volts to Kcal is done by multiplying by 23.062), it is in evidence that $2 \times 23.062 \times 1.14$ Kcal ($= 52.6$ Kcal) of electrical energy is generated.

These 52.6 Kcal are all of the energy liberated in mitochondria from one mole of NADH. In the process of oxidative phosphorylation, three ATP moles are formed; that is, approximately 24 Kcal of the electrical energy is trapped as ATP (ca. 46% efficiency). Energy not trapped as ATP escapes as heat. From an engineering point of view, this is called "heat loss," but for a warm-blooded (endothermic) animal, this is a source of body heat.

HIGH-ENERGY COMPOUNDS; PHOSPHORYLATION AT THE SUBSTRATE LEVEL
High-energy compounds

Upon hydrolysis, certain bonds yield extraordinary amounts of free energy: they are called **high-energy bonds.** Their energy is used to drive energy-requiring processes, such as muscle contraction, synthesis of macromolecules, and transport against gradients. For instance, while a phosphate ester yields 2 to 5 Kcal/mol when hydrolyzed, a high-energy acid-anhydride bond between phosphates in ATP yields around 8 Kcal/mol.

Examples of high-energy compounds are as follows (refer to Figure 11-6):
- 1,3-diphosphoglycerate yields 11.8 Kcal/mol converted to 3-phosphoglycerate, with 7.3 Kcal

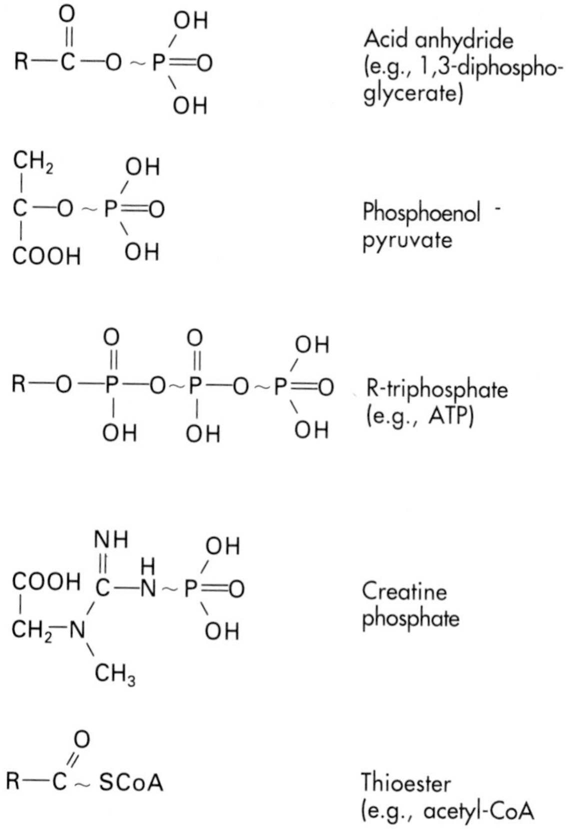

Figure 11-6. High-energy compounds.

trapped as one ATP formed at the substrate level.
- Phosphoenolpyruvate yields 14.8 Kcal/mol when converted to pyruvate, while one ATP is formed at the substrate level.
- ATP, GTP, UTP, CTP yield about 7.3 Kcal/mol when one of the two anhydride-linked phosphates is hydrolyzed. Enzymes are specific for one of these coenzymes.

Of the two high-energy bonded phosphates, most reactions split the terminal phosphate off leaving ADP; some split pyrophosphate (P ~ P) off, which is then further hydrolyzed to two phosphate molecules with energy loss as heat.
- Creatine phosphate yields 10.3 Kcal/mol. It is muscle's ready-made energy store from which ATP may be formed for contraction.
- Fatty acyl thioesters yield about 6 Kcal/mol. Examples are palmityl ~ CoA and acetyl ~ CoA.

Transfer of the acetyl unit from acetyl $\sim$ CoA yields acetate plus the needed energy for acetate to react. Coenzyme A (CoA) is a complex structure that contains the vitamin, pantothenic acid.

Phosphorylation at the substrate level

Formation of ATP by means other than oxidative phosphorylation is referred to as **substrate level phosphorylation**.

The top two high-energy compounds listed above are from the Embden-Meyerhof pathway of glycolysis. From the high free-energy values of their special bonds, it is obvious that an ATP worth approximately 8 Kcal can be amply produced.

Compared to oxidative phosphorylation (mitochondrial), phosphorylation at the substrate level (mostly cytoplasmic) is quantitatively far less important in most cells. However, in cells that must operate under conditions of low oxygen tension, (e.g., deep medullary cells in the kidneys) or that either have no mitochondria (mammalian erythrocytes) or have only few mitochondria (white muscle fiber), substrate level phosphorylation is of paramount importance.

MITOCHONDRIAL ENERGY METABOLISM
Mitochondrial structure and function

Mitochondria have an outer and an inner membrane that invaginate into the organelle and form cristae. The inner membrane consists of base pieces and knobs that point toward the inner matrix of the mitochondria. Base pieces hold elements of the electron transfer chain, including cytochrome-containing proteins; the knobs contain ATP synthase activity.

The TCA cycle, located in the mitochondrial matrix, oxidizes acetate and sends metabolic electrons to the electron transfer chain in the inner membrane. The base pieces form, anatomically and chemically a "bucket brigade" that accepts these metabolic electrons and passes them along a gradient of increasing reduction potentials from one redox couple to another, and finally to cytochrome oxidase, which donates them to oxygen, the ultimate electron acceptor. In the process of electron transfer along the chain, a proton gradient is generated by pumping H^+ into the space between the inner and outer membranes of mitochondria. This proton gradient is used to generate, by chemiosmosis, the necessary energy for phosphorylation (ATP formation) in the knobs of the inner membrane.

An intact mitochondrial structure is required for proper functioning. Damage to mitochondria, or conditions that lead to mitochondrial swelling (i.e., increasing the distance btween inner and outer membranes), leads to uncoupling of phosphorylation from oxidation, so that all electrical energy escapes as heat.

Chemical nature of oxidative phosphorylation
Energetics

An explosive energy release cannot be utilized effectively; some energy may be trapped, but most is lost. For example, the process of hydrogen fusion, by which our sun generates energy, has been duplicated explosively (H-bomb), but has not yet been "tamed." In contrast, the uranium bomb (nuclear fission) has been tamed and put to constructive use (nuclear reactors) by breaking down the energy release into smaller increments.

If the body would combust sugar by direct reaction with oxygen, it would short-circuit the electron flow. The energy explosion that would result could not be harvested and put to good use; it would escape as heat. A sugar cube can be combusted with a match to demonstrate this. Therefore, chemical pathways contain many steps, so that the small energy transitions can be harvested; also, this allows for the reversibility of pathways (cf., a staircase).

Combustion of AcCoA in the TCA cycle entails many steps. Four pairs of electrons become available in four discrete reactions (instead of one explosion), and these electrons are shuttled by various carriers to the respiratory chain (electron transfer chain).

The respiratory chain, again, consists of many reactions. If a pair of electrons were to jump straight from NADH to oxygen, about 52.6 Kcal of electrical energy would become available in one blast. Maybe, one ATP could be generated at the site of the blast, trapping less than 8 Kcal, while the remaining 45 Kcal would escape as heat. By breaking the blast up in many smaller increments, the electrons traverse as series of staggered ΔE's and produce three ATP, worth approximately 22 Kcal of chemical energy.

Chemical entities of the respiratory chain

Located within the inner matrix of the mitochondrion is the TCA cycle, where metabolic electrons are derived from nutrients. These electrons exit the TCA cycle and enter the electron transfer (respiratory) chain via two routes (Figure 11-7). The respiratory

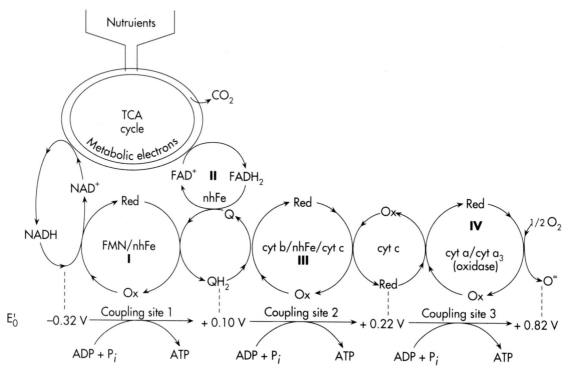

Figure 11-7. The respiratory chain transports metabolic electrons from nutrients to oxygen while the electrical energy is harvested for the production of ATP and heat.

chain consists of four protein-lipid complexes that are part of the structure of the inner mitochondrial membrane, as are the two compounds, ubiquinone (coenzyme Q, or simply Q) and cytochrome c, that move electrons from one fixed complex to another on their way to molecular oxygen (see Figure 11-7).

Three reactions of the TCA cycle release metabolic electrons in the form of NADH (niacinamide-adenine-dinucleotide); these electrons are transferred to ubiquinone by complex I, which consists of proteins that contain flavin mononucleotide (FMN) and iron in the form of ferrous sulfide (FeS), also called **nonheme iron (nhFe)** to distinguish it from iron contained in cytochromes (see Figure 11-7). NADH is thereby reoxidized to NAD^+ and is ready to accept another pair of electrons from the TCA cycle. From this it is concluded that the passing of electrons from NADH to the electron transfer chain is essential for regenerating NAD^+, and thereby for the operation of the TCA cycle.

A fourth pair of metabolic electrons escapes the TCA cycle in the succinate dehydrogenase reaction,

from where they are transferred to ubiquinone via complex II, which houses proteins associated with FAD (flavin-adenine-dinucleotide) and nhFe. Niacinamide and flavin are B vitamins that shuttle electrons. Other B vitamins function in metabolism as shuttlers, for instance, for CO_2, and amino, methyl, and ketone groups.

Ubiquinone shuttles the electrons from nhFe in complexes I and II to the chain of cytochromes, starting with complex III (see Figure 11-7). Cytochrome c conducts the electron flow from complex III to complex IV, where cytochrome oxidase finally transfers them to molecular oxygen. Cytochromes are proteins that contain a porphyrin structure at their active sites (cf., hemoglobin). Central in the porphyrin molecule is ionic iron, which can assume different valencies and, thus, shuttle electrons. Of interest, with regard to mineral requirements of animals, is the fact that the last cytochromes in the chain (a-a_3, cytochrome oxidase) contain copper in addition to iron.

Cytochrome oxidase reoxidizes the ultimate cytochrome and delivers the metabolic electrons to oxygen. In the wake of this electron transfer, all redox couples of the respiratory chain are left in their oxidized form, ready to shuttle the next pair of electrons when needed.

Phosphorylation coupled to oxidation

To form one ATP from ADP plus P_i, approximately 7.3 Kcal are needed under standard conditions. There are three so-called **coupling sites** in the respiratory chain, where a standard free energy drop in excess of 7.3 Kcal occurs (see Figure 11-7). Biochemists have tried to isolate a coupling agent that would trap these energy quanta and convey them to the site of ATP synthesis; however, such a coupling agent has never been found.

The chemiosmosis concept points to the H^+ imbalance in the equations of the TCA cycle and respiratory chain. This imbalance is resolved by moving H^+ out of the inner mitochondrial space across the inner membrane (Figure 11-8). A H^+ distribution gradient is thereby generated, which constitutes an electrochemical potential difference that is used to drive the phosphorylation reaction at the site of the coupling proteins, F_i and F_o.

Since ATP production is coupled to oxidation, oxidative phosphorylation may stop when phosphorylation cannot proceed. The sum of ADP and ATP is present in a limited amount. Therefore, when the ATP concentration is relatively high, the relative ADP level is low, and, thus, phosphorylation is inhibited. This stands to reason, because a high ATP/ADP ratio means that energy is plentiful and no more food needs to be combusted. The opposite of coupling is called **uncoupling**: detachment of phosphorylation from oxidation.

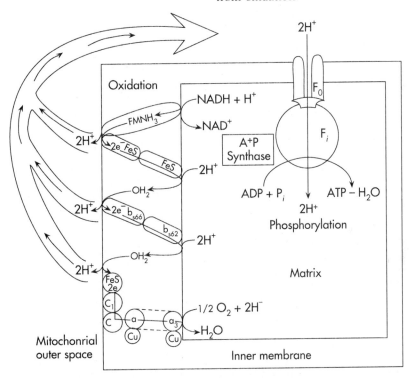

Figure 11-8. Oxidative phosphorylation by chemiosmosis. The subunits of the respiratory chain are oriented within the width of the inner mitochondrial membrane in a manner which allows translocation of H^+ ions from the matrix to the space between the two mitochondrial membranes in the process of electron transport (oxidation). H^+ ions return to the matrix via a port consisting of the membrane-spanning protein complex F_o-F_i. The H^+ gradient then is used by ATP synthase for the production of ATP from ADP and P_i (phosphorylation). *Modified and reproduced with permission from Murray RK, Granner DK, Mayes PA, and Rodwell VW: Harper's biochemistry, ed 21, Norwalk, CT, 1988, Appleton & Lange, pp 113-114.*

In order to demonstrate whether electrons enter the respiratory chain as NADH or at the level of ubiquinone, the P/O ratio can be followed; that is, the ratio of inorganic phosphate esterified to ATP per half mole of oxygen consumed. For NADH, the P/O ratio is three, since there are three ATP formed per half mole of O_2 consumed, and for QH_2 the P/O ratio equals two.

Physiologic control of oxidative phosphorylation
Autoregulation

Phosphorylation by the reaction, ADP + P_i → ATP, has a standard free-energy (G°) value listed as 7.3 Kcal/mol, as determined by the standard free energy of hydrolysis of that high-energy bond. The free energy of a compound is related to its concentration: $G = G° + RT \ln C$. It becomes increasingly tougher, logarithmically, to add more molecules to an existing concentration. (Anyone who has ever pumped a bicycle tire knows that the last pumps are the hardest.) Therefore, to add ATP to a relatively high ATP concentration takes much more energy than is needed to increase a relatively low ATP level. In fact, the necessary energy for that may not be available when electrons, traversing the electron transfer chain, jump over fixed electrical potential differences. Herein lies a basis for the autoregulation of ATP production (phosphorylation) by the ATP/ADP ratio.

Coupling of phosphorylation to oxidation is tight. Therefore, a low ratio of ATP/ADP, indicating a shortage of energy, is needed to make both phosphorylation and oxidation happen. Because of a special shuttle for ATP/ADP between cytoplasm and mitochondria, the ATP/ADP ratio in mitochondria reflects the same ratio elsewhere in the cell. So the need for energy at any place in the cell is sensed at the site of oxidative phosphorylation. The ATP/ADP pool is small and, hence, a sensitive sensor of energy need.

When energy is needed the ATP/ADP ratio is low. Phosphorylation is working and, coupled thereto, oxidation is transporting electrons from the reduced cofactors to oxygen, thereby keeping NAD^+ and FAD in oxidized forms, ready to extract electrons from the TCA cycle. The result is that more acetate, derived from food or body stores, is combusted.

When energy is plenty the ATP/ADP ratio is high. Oxidative phosphorylation is slow and, thus, NADH and $FADH_2$ are not well-reoxidized. This slows down the TCA cycle, because there are not enough cofactors to accept its metabolic electrons. Acetyl-CoA is now spared and can be used for synthetic ends; that is, to form fatty acids or ketones, depending on conditions.

Control of oxidative phosphorylation, thus, is autoregulated by the ATP/ADP ratio (i.e., the need for energy) and directs reoxidation of redox cofactors, which determine the activity of the TCA cycle and, thus, the combustion of food and body stores.

Oxygen requirement

Oxygen requirement is another element of control over oxidative phosphorylation. There are two factors involved here: the blood flow needed to transport oxygen, and the mitochondria to utilize that oxygen.

Vascularization (blood supply) differs widely among tissues. Also, ischemic conditions occur in which blood supply to tissues is impaired (e.g., atherosclerosis).

The number of mitochondria varies in different types of cells. For example, in cardiac muscle cells, there are large numbers of mitochondria, so that ATP production is sufficient to sustain the incessant muscle contractions of the heart. On the other hand, skeletal muscle cells, especially white muscle cells, contain only a few mitochondria. Consequently, during sustained exercise, the muscle's capacity to generate ATP by oxidative phosphorylation is so limited that muscles must import glucose from the bloodstream to derive ATP at the substrate level. The exercise conditioning of muscles increases both vascularization and number of mitochondria, particularly in red muscle cells.

Factors affecting oxidative phosphorylation

Unusual physiological conditions and certain drugs exist that severely impair ATP production without diminishing electron flow through the respiratory chain. Oxidation, then, continues unabatedly (in fact, it is usually increased), while phosphorylation is uncoupled from oxidation; thus, virtually all electrical energy escapes as heat. This situation may be likened unto a car engine in which the clutch has been uncoupled and then the engine is revved up; a great deal of fuel is burned but, since none of the energy is used for propulsion of the vehicle, all energy escapes as heat.

Cold stress leads to thyroxine release that specifically uncouples oxidative phosphorylation. Heat is then produced, which is necessary for temperature homeostasis. Another uncoupler of oxidative phosphorylation is dinitrophenol; when discovered, this compound promised to be an ideal drug for weight loss, since it releases dietary calories as heat, except that it was found to cause blindness in humans. Arsenic acid is chemically much like phosphoric acid, but it is biologically inactive: it cripples oxidative phosphorylation and uncouples it from oxidation.

Many agents poison oxidative phosphorylation by inactivating the respiratory chain. Examples include: barbiturates and inactivators of cytochrome oxidase, such as CO, CN, and H_2S, agents that also poison hemoglobin (a porphyrin just like cytochromes), and, thus, the oxygen supply needed for oxidative phosphorylation.

Several antibiotics cripple oxidative phosphorylation; for instance, antimycin A impairs oxidation; oligomycin and the K^+ ionophore valinomycin inhibit phosphorylation.

Place of oxidative phosphorylation in cellular metabolism

Sources of electrons for the respiratory chain

From the TCA cycle. Acetyl-CoA is a common metabolite in the catabolism of carbohydrates, proteins, and fatty acids. It fuels the TCA cycle, in the process of which the CoA splits off to be reused for the activation of the next acetate. The net reaction for the combustion of acetate via the TCA cycle is the following:

$$CH_3—COOH + 2\,O_2 \rightarrow 2\,CO_2 + 2\,H_2O$$

Both of acetate's carbon atoms are oxidized to CO_2 and its four hydrogens to H_2O. It follows from the equation, that four oxygen atoms are used; thus, four pairs of electrons are extracted from a single acetate.

The electron extractions occur in four enzyme-catalyzed steps; three of those are specific for NAD^+ (producing NADH), and one requires FAD and ubiquinone (Figure 11-9). As the levels of these cofactors are quite low, the TCA cycle immediately ceases to operate from a lack of NAD^+ and FAD if the reduced cofactors (NADH and $FADH_2$) are not immediately reoxidized. The latter takes place, imparting the electrons to the respiratory chain. Operations of the TCA cycle and the respiratory chain are, thus, tightly linked. Another such link is the cofactor ratio of ATP/ADP, discussed above.

One acetate then yields three NADH (equivalent to nine ATP) and one $FADH_2$ (converted to QH_2

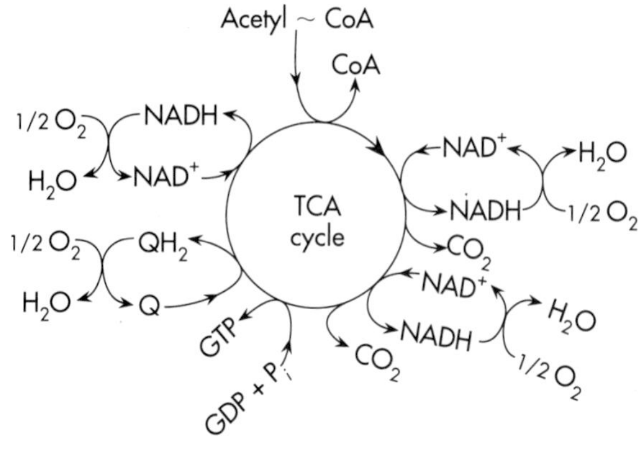

Figure 11-9. Metabolic electrons derived from the TCA cycle.

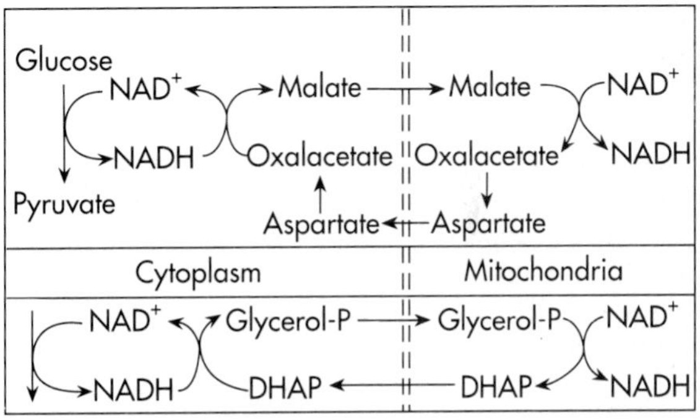

Figure 11-10. Metabolic electrons generated in the cytoplasm are shuttled into mitochondria. *DHAP*, Dihydroxyacetone phosphate.

and equivalent to two ATP); in addition, one GTP is formed at the substrate level in the TCA cycle (see Figure 11-9).

From NADH produced in the cytoplasm. Mitochondrial membranes are impermeable to NAD and NADH. So, NADH's reducing equivalent (pair of electrons), generated in the cytoplasm, is accepted by oxaloacetate and then shuttled as malate, which can cross the mitochondrial membranes (Figure 11-10). Inside the mitochondria, NADH is regenerated from malate; oxaloacetate is returned to the cytoplasm via a reversible conversion to aspartate, since the mitochondrial membranes are impermeable to oxaloacetate. Another such shuttle, used for the same purpose, involves glycerol phosphate and its oxidized product, dihydroxyacetone phosphate (DHAP; [see Figure 11-10]).

By these cyclical processes, NAD^+ is constantly regenerated in the cytoplasm, so that glycolysis of glucose to pyruvate can continue. It is important to note, though, that there are many cytoplasmic processes that utilize NADH and, thereby regenerate NAD^+, hence, shuttling to oxidative phosphorylation in mitochondria is not always needed.

Specificity of redox cofactors

In general, enzymes are absolutely specific for one redox cofactor only, be it NADH, $FADH_2$, NADPH, or GSH. Many enzyme reactions utilize NAD^+/NADH, often in catabolic reactions. NADPH, on the other hand, is not a substrate for the respiratory chain; it is usually used for anabolic purposes (e.g., biosynthesis of fatty acids or cholesterol from AcCoA). Energetically, NADH and NADPH are equivalent, each worth three ATP. In fact, many cells contain a weak enzyme activity that catalyzes this reversible reaction:

$$NAD^+ + NADPH \leftrightarrow NADH + NADP^+$$

Oxidations yield energy; reductions cost energy. Therefore, spending a NADPH on a synthetic reaction is equivalent to spending 3 ATP on that reaction. Conversely, the more reduced a compound is, the more energy it yields upon oxidation. This explains why fatty acids $(—CH_2—)_n$ are so much higher in calories than are sugars $[(—CHOH—)_n]$. A fat's $—CH_2—$ group has a molecular weight of 14 and requires 3 oxygen atoms (3 electron pairs released) to yield $CO_2 + H_2O$. In contrast, a carbohydrate's $—CHOH—$ group has a molecular weight of 30 and reacts with only 2 oxygen atoms. Hence, their metabolizable energy values are 9 and 4 Kcal/g, respectively.

Communication (shuttling) between cytoplasm and mitochondria

Mitochondria are impenetrable to most cytoplasmic compounds that do not have a special carrier system facilitating their transport across mitochondrial membranes.

- Shuttling of NADH-reducing equivalents, generated in the cytoplasm, to mitochondria was discussed above.
- The mitochondrial membranes contain a special transport system that makes them permeable to ADP and ATP. Because of this, the mitochondria sense ATP utilization and the need for energy anywhere in the cell and then adapt their rate of oxidative phosphorylation accordingly.
- A special carrier system exists that shuttles fatty acids across mitochondrial membranes, so that they can be catabolized to AcCoA and relieved of electrons via the TCA cycle. This system involves carnitine and three enzyme activities associated with the mitochondrial membranes; its mode of action and importance in control of mitochondrial fatty acid oxidation will be discussed later.
- Carbohydrates, too, are ultimately oxidized via the TCA cycle; cytoplasmic pyruvate, produced by glycolysis, permeates by carrier into mitochondria, where it is converted to AcCoA under the release of CO_2 and the formation of NADH.
- Special carriers exist for amino acids used in mitochondrial protein synthesis.
- AcCoA is generated in mitochondria from all major nutrients and body stores and is used inside mitochondria for the purposes of energy generation (TCA cycle) and ketone body production. When needed for fatty acid synthesis, which takes place in the cytoplasm of the cell, AcCoA must be shuttled out of mitochondria despite the fact that membranes bar passage of large CoA molecule. Inside mitochondria, therefore, AcCoA is converted to citrate, which exits the mitochondrion and is then reconverted to AcCoA in the cytoplasm.

In summary, although the above discrete communication channels exist, mitochondria must, in general, be considered impermeable to cytoplasmic constituents. A mitochondrion is in effect a cell within a cell.

Summary and application of oxidative phosphorylation

The above discussions of mitochondrial energy metabolism, channels of communication with the cytoplasm, and some pertinent outlines of oxidative metabolism in the cytoplasm have been summarized in Figure 11-11. Trace the following in that metabolic scheme:

- Cytoplasmic glycolysis to pyruvate with ATP formation at the substrate level. Pyruvate enters into mitochondria, where it is converted to AcCoA, ready for the TCA cycle. The reducing equivalent of cytoplasmically generated NADH is shuttled, in the form of malate or glycerol phosphate, into mitochondria and there reconverted to NADH.

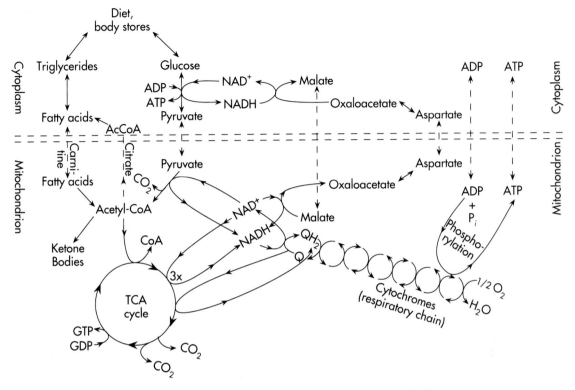

Figure 11-11. Summary of mitochondrial oxidative metabolism.

- Movement of fatty acids from the cytoplasm into mitochondria via the carnitine shuttle; breakdown (β-oxidation) of fatty acids to AcCoA, ready for the TCA cycle.
- The TCA cycle, yielding 3 NADH + 1 QH₂ + 1 GTP (at the substrate level). The redox coenzymes must be immediately reoxidized by oxidative phosphorylation, or else the TCA cycle stops for lack of electron acceptors. Therefore, oxidative phosphorylation is commonly the final oxidative pathway for carbohydrates, fats, and proteins.
- Oxidative phosphorylation reoxidizes NADH and FADH₂/QH₂ via the respiratory chain, couples phosphorylize to this oxidation, and traps approximately 50% of available electrical energy as ATP. The 50% heat loss aids in temperature regulation.
- Shuttling mechanism for ADP and ATP allows mitochondria to sense the need for energy (ratio of ATP/ADP). Since little ADP and ATP exist, this monitoring of the cell's energy needs is extremely sensitive.

- The ATP/ADP ratio is linked with the NADH/NAD⁺ ratio, for under conditions when energy is plentiful, and, thus, ATP/ADP is high, phosphorylation is inhibited and this, being coupled to oxidation, impairs the rate of reoxidation of NADH via the electron transfer chain. Consequently, NADH/NAD⁺ is high and the lack of an electron acceptor (NAD⁺) slows down TCA cycle activity, so that less food (AcCoA) is combusted. This example illustrates a general rule: metabolism is controlled by coenzymes and transport; not only oxidative metabolism, but metabolism as a whole.
- In addition to autoregulation by the need for energy, oxidative phosphorylation is controlled by the availability of oxygen and functional mitochondria; hence, the effects of exercise conditioning and ischemia on metabolism.
- The enzyme pyruvate dehydrogenase (PDH) catalyzes:

Pyruvate + NAD⁺ + CoA → AcCoA + CO₂ + NADH

This enzyme activity occurs exclusively in mitochondria. Because this step involves a tremendous release of energy, it is physiologically irreversible (see Figure 11-11). To realize the importance of the PDH reaction, one can trace the conversion of dietary glucose to fat deposits and realize that transport into mitochondria is necessary for this one step only. Since conversion of AcCoA to pyruvate is not possible, glucose cannot be formed from fat. Hence, precious protein (i.e., amino acids) must be used for the purpose of gluconeogenesis.

Alternative pathways for AcCoA exist in times when energy is plentiful. Due to a slowdown of TCA cycle activity, AcCoA tends to accumulate, but because there is precious little CoA available, alternative pathways for CoA regeneration and, thus, acetate disposal, must be followed. Consideration is given to a canine liver cell under two conditions:

- When the concentration of fatty acids is low, for instance, after a meal. As the glucose storage capacity of the body (glycogen) is limited, dietary glucose is converted to fat, as follows. Glucose in cytoplasm produces pyruvate, which enters mitochondria and generates AcCoA. The AcCoA is then transported as citrate out of mitochondria. In cytoplasm, AcCoA is regenerated and then converted to fat.

- When the concentration of fatty acids is high, for example, during fasting. High concentrations of fatty acids, mobilized from fat depots, are present in blood, and, thus, large amounts of fatty acids enter the liver, where they are converted to AcCoA in mitochondria and peroxisomes. Now that fatty acid synthesis in cytoplasm is blocked by negative feedback, AcCoA is not exported to cytoplasm. Moreover, AcCoA cannot enter the TCA cycle, since not enough NAD^+ is regenerated, nor can it go back to pyruvate (irreversible step). Hence, there is no alternative left: AcCoA is converted to ketone bodies, and a fasting ketoacidosis may develop if these ketone bodies accumulate in plasma.

The combination of the TCA cycle plus oxidative phosphorylation is present in every cell that contains mitochondria. For practical purposes, this ensemble may be likened to an electrical plug (Figure 11-12). The following notes explain the wall plug model.

- In addition to the "plug" (mitochondria), fuel and oxygen are required. Fuel comes from stores in the cytoplasm of the cell, and becomes available as AcCoA inside mitochondria. To go with the plug, an electrical outlet is drawn with AcCoA as the negative pole that releases electrons, and oxygen as the positive pole to which electrons flow.

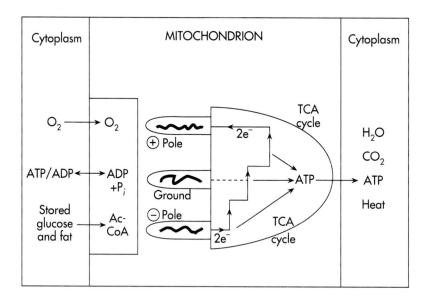

Figure 11-12. Wall plug model of oxidative phosphorylation.

- Grounding the mitochondrial energy generator with the cytoplasmic surrounding via the middle prong allows for the regulation of energy production in response to cellular ATP/ADP ratios.
- Functioning is simple: needing energy, the cell plugs its mitochondrial machinery into the socket; immediately, electrons flow from AcCoA via the electron transfer chain to oxygen, producing ATP on their way. The grounding "prong" senses when the ATP/ADP ratio is high and draws the plug out of the socket.

STUDY QUESTIONS

1. When a compound is oxidized, does it donate or accept electrons?

2. About aerobic dehydrogenase activity:
   a. List the subcellular particle in which this enzyme activity occurs.
   b. List the mineral and vitamin requirements of this enzyme activity.

3. For what purpose must catalase activity accompany the activities of flavoprotein-containing enzymes?

4. *a.* Why can peroxisomes help the liver rid the body of fatty acids under conditions (such as having "plenty of energy") when mitochondria cannot.
   b. List a synthetic function of peroxisomes.

5. List a function of cytoplasmic cytochromes in liver cells. Identify the metabolic by-product of cytochrome degradation that is normally excreted in bile.

6. List two essential nutritional factors that help protect vital structures in the body from being oxidatively destroyed.

7. Which one of the following has the highest and which one has the lowest standard reduction potential: (A) $NAD^+/NADH$; (B) Oxygen/water; (C) Cytochrome b, Ox/Red?

8. Circle the letter of the high-energy compounds only: (A) palmityl-CoA; (B) pyruvate; (C) creatinine; (D) 1,3-diphosphoglycerate.

9. Why is the conversion of phosphoenolpyruvate to pyruvate considered to be physiologically irreversible?

10. List a redox cofactor involved especially in anabolic reactions.

11. Autoregulation of oxidative phosphorylation means that the process is turned on or off by:

12. *a.* Name the pathway that converts fatty acids to AcCoA.
    b. Name the pathway that derives electrons from AcCoA.

13. *a.* List the technical term for the trapping of metabolic energy by processes other than oxidative phosphorylation.
    b. Name a pathway in which ATP is thusly produced.

14. In the chemiosmosis of mitochondrial ATP formation:
    a. Which ion is shuttled?
    b. How is uncoupling visualized in this model?

15. *a.* List two B vitamins involved in the electron transfer chain (ETC).
    b. Name two trace minerals associated with ETC function.
    c. Name a functional activity that contains the porphyrin ring.
    d. List a gas that poisons cytochrome oxidase activity (and, thus, suffocates a cell).

16. *a.* What form of energy is produced by uncouplers of oxidative phosphorylation?
    b. Name the hormone that uncouples oxidative phosphorylation during cold stress.
    c. Does the rate of nutrient oxidation (O_2 consumption) increase, decrease, or stay the same when oxidative phosphorylation is uncoupled?

17. About communication between mitochondria and cytoplasm:
    a. List a shuttler for reducing equivalents into mitochondria.
    b. Name the form in which acetate can exit mitochondria in order to serve for the purpose of cytoplasmic fatty acid synthesis.
    c. List the special carrier that allows for the transport of fatty acids into mitochondria.
    d. How can reducing equivalents generated in glycolysis by glyceraldehyde-phosphate dehydrogenase be redeemed for ATP?
    e. What features allow the mitochondrion to sense energy need elsewhere in the cell?

18. What regulates the rate of oxidative phosphorylation?
    a. In a liver cell of a healthy animal?
    b. In an exercising muscle cell?

19. List the redox cofactor ratio directly responsible for the synchronization of AcCoA combustion with electron transfer chain activity.

20. Involve rate control of oxidative phosphorylation in your reasoning to explain why high ATP/ADP ratios in cells (i.e., the situation of having "plenty of energy") lead to high $NADH/NAD^+$ ratios, and then to a slowdown of TCA cycle activity.

21. About the mammalian erythrocyte:
    a. Why can this cell not convert pyruvate to AcCoA?
    b. Given its need to keep glycolysis going, for what specific purpose must it convert pyruvate to lactate?

22. Indicate a reason why skeletal muscles, under conditions of heavy exercise, have to shift to anaerobic ATP production. Why do they not combust fatty acids?

23. List the medical term for the narrowing of afferent blood supply to a tissue. Which necessary ingredient for oxidative phosphorylation may be in short (rate-limiting) supply under this condition? What metabolic end product will this tissue produce?

24. List the enzyme whose location is responsible for the fact that mitochondria are involved in the conversion of glucose to fat after meals.

25. During fasting, when plasma–fatty-acid levels are high and, thus, the liver is burdened with the task of having to clear the plasma of those fatty acids:
    a. The fatty acids are β-oxidized in (list two subcellular organelles).
    b. Why are the AcCoA thus formed not combusted in the TCA cycle?
    c. Why is this AcCoA not used for cytoplasmic fatty acid synthesis?
    d. Therefore, this AcCoA forms which class of compounds?

26. What is the principal fate of AcCoA in the liver when the fatty acid concentration is low (e.g., after a glucose meal)?

27. By what mode does oligomycin act as an antibiotic?

28. In the wall plug model of oxidative phosphorylation (see Figure 11-12), what function has the middle (ground) prong?

Carbohydrate metabolism

REVIEW OF CARBOHYDRATE CHEMISTRY

Terminology and chemical properties of carbohydrates are briefly reviewed insofar as they are essential for understanding mammalian carbohydrate metabolism, starting with monosaccharides and progressing to complex carbohydrates.

Monosaccharides
Definitions

Monosaccharides are single chains of carbon atoms bearing multiple adjacent hydroxyl groups. One of the hydroxyl groups is oxidized to either an aldehyde or keto group, creating aldose and ketose sugars.

The general overall structure is $(HCOH)_n$, which can be written as $(C.H_2O)_n$; hence, the name carbo- (C) hydrate (H_2O).

Stereoisomers are compounds with identical composition, but different spatial configuration. Stereoisomers possess one or more asymmetric carbon atoms, that is, carbon atoms to which four different atoms or groups are attached. The simplest possible carbohydrates with an asymmetric carbon atom are those with three carbon atoms: the trioses. The convention used to name D- or L-carbohydrates is based on the orientation (right or left) of the hydroxyl group on the highest-numbered asymmetric carbon. All carbohydrates involved in mammalian physiology are of the D series; L-carbohydrates are not utilized. The reason for this is that the enzymes involved in carbohydrate metabolism recognize only D-carbohydrates.

The carbon atoms of carbohydrates are numbered beginning at the end of the chain with the most highly oxidized functional groups (e.g., aldehyde).

Classes

Trioses are three-carbon carbohydrates. Dihydroxyacetone and D-glyceraldehyde (Figure 12-1) are involved as phosphate esters in the pathway of glycolysis. Lacking an asymmetric carbon, dihydroxyacetone has no stereoisomers. D-glyceraldehyde is the isomer of importance in mammalian physiology.

Tetroses are four-carbon sugars and pentoses are five-carbon sugars. Physiologically important are the following (Figure 12-2): (i) D-erythrose, whose phosphate ester is an intermediate in the pentose shunt; (ii) D-ribose, another pentose-shunt intermediate (such as PO$_4$ ester), which is part of the structure of RNA and various nucleotides (e.g., ATP and NAD$^+$); and (iii) 2-deoxy-D-ribose, derived from D-ribose, and included in the structure of DNA.

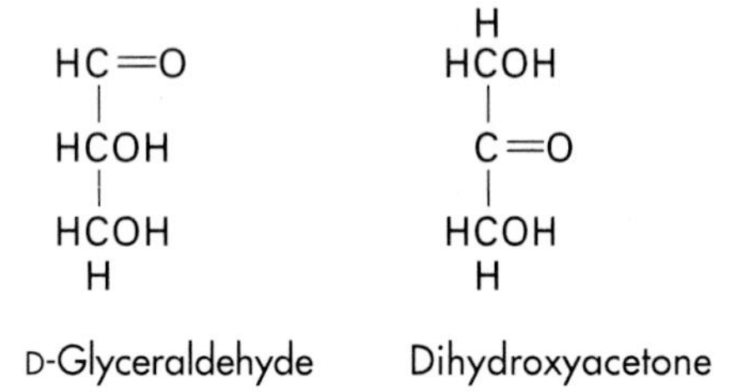

Figure 12-1. Trioses.

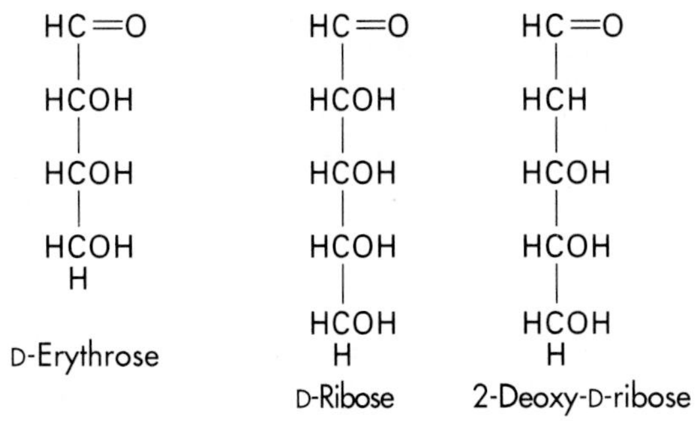

Figure 12-2. Tetroses.

Hexoses are six-carbon sugars. Since four of these carbon atoms are asymmetric, 2^4 (16) stereoisomers are possible. Of these 16, D-glucose is physiologically most important.

Glucose exists almost totally as a structure that contains a hemiacetal bond bridging carbon-1 and carbon-5. This forms a ring structure and introduces a new asymmetric carbon (carbon-1, the anomeric carbon); at the site of that carbon, stereoisomerism creates two anomers (Figure 12-3): the α-anomer of D-glucose has the OH group on carbon-1 to the right, the β-anomer has that OH group to the left. The α- and β-forms are in equilibrium with each other and with a minute proportion of glucose present in the straight-chain form.

In Haworth projection, the hemiacetal ring forms a plane with the various OH groups protruding either above or below the surface of that plane. The glucose molecule is shown in Figure 12-3 in the six-membered, or pyranose, ring form. A Haworth projection of β-D-glucose would have shown the OH group on carbon-1 above the plane of the ring.

D-fructose is a six-carbon ketose: it forms the five-membered furanose ring (Figure 12-4). D-mannose and D-galactose are epimers of D-glucose. This means that they differ in structure by approximately one carbon atom. D-mannose and D-glucose differ about carbon-2, and D-galactose and D-glucose are four-epimers. The enzymes responsible for the interconversions of these sugars are called epimerases. Epimerases require NAD(H) as a coenzyme, since the epimerization reaction proceeds via a =CO intermediate.

Reactions and derivatives

Glucose-fructose-mannose interconversion (Figure 12-5) occurs spontaneously in weakly alkaline solutions via a common enediol form. The same mechanism may be involved in the enzyme-mediated glucose-fructose interconversion that occurs in cells.

Glycosides are made up of a carbohydrate and a noncarbohydrate, or aglycone; for example, α-D-ethylglucoside is a simple glycoside (Figure 12-6). Most glycosides occur in plants and are more complex than the one depicted. Three groups of glycosides are of practical importance:

- Cyanogenic glycosides, in which the aglycone is the cyanide group. Upon eating plant materials containing this type of glycoside, animals may experience cyanide poisoning as CN$^-$ is released in the gastrointestinal tract. Cyanogenic glyco-

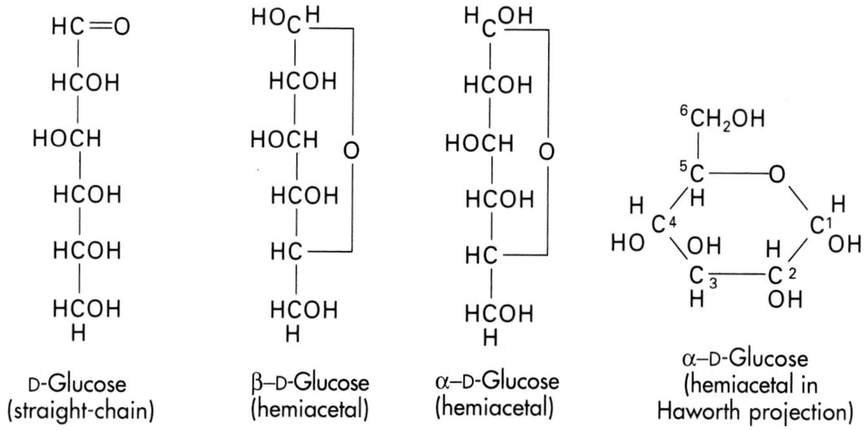

Figure 12-3. Various ways to present the structure of glucose.

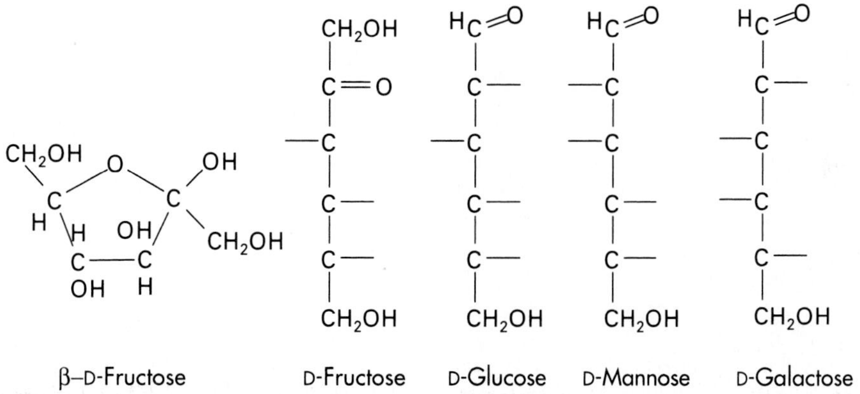

Figure 12-4. Hexoses.

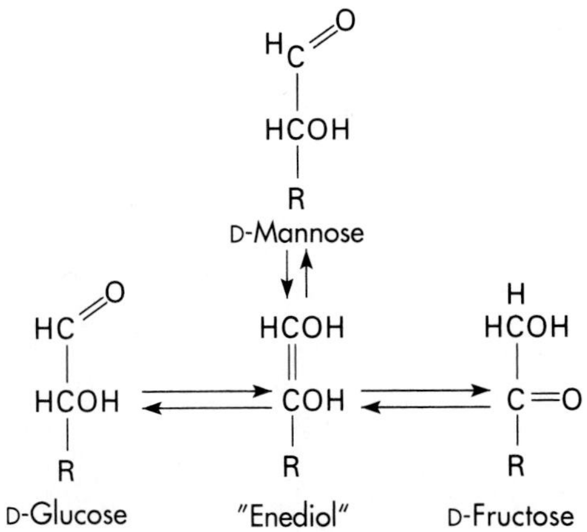

Figure 12-5. Interconversion of hexoses.

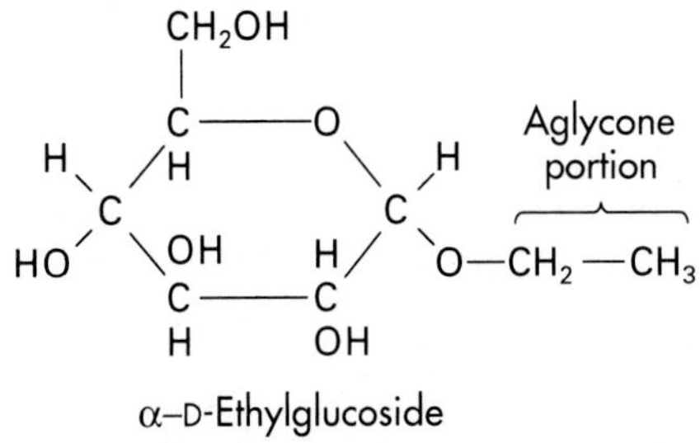

Figure 12-6. A glycoside.

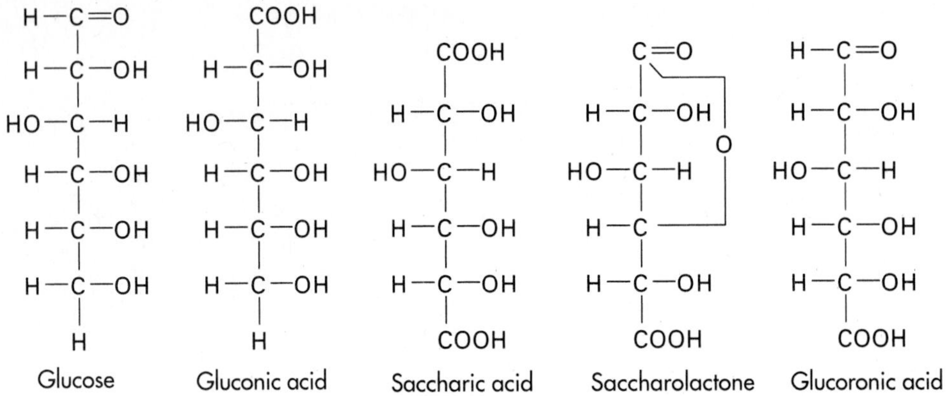

Figure 12-7. Oxidation products of glucose.

sides are present in cherry and peach leaves, stems, and pits.

- Saponins, which contain a steroid aglycone, cause inflammation and necrosis of the gastrointestinal tract as the aglycone is released. Pokeweed, for instance, contains saponins.
- Digitalis glycosides, which contain steroid aglycones. These compounds, though of great value in the treatment of congestive heart failure, can also cause poisoning in animals. The foxglove plant is a rich source.

Oxidation of hexoses at carbon-1 to a —COOH group yields acids that bear the -onic suffix; for example, gluconic acid is derived from glucose in the pentose shunt (Figure 12-7). Oxidation at carbon-6 of hexoses to carboxylic groups yields uronic acid derivatives; for instance, glucuronic acid, derived from glucose in the liver, is used to prepare various metabolic wastes and noxious compounds for transport in bile.

Disaccharides

Two monosaccharides linked by a glycosidic bond constitute a disaccharide. There are many possible combinations between two hexoses: carbon-1, carbon-2, carbon-3, carbon-4, or carbon-6 of one of the hexoses may be linked to carbon-1, carbon-2, carbon-3, carbon-4, or carbon-6 of the other for a total of 25 possible combinations. This is only half of the possibilities; in addition there are α- and β-glycosidic linkages depending on whether the bridge spans under (α) or above (β) the plane of the hexose rings. The distinction between α- and β-linkages is of great metabolic importance, because digestive enzymes are specific for either α- or β-linked saccharides.

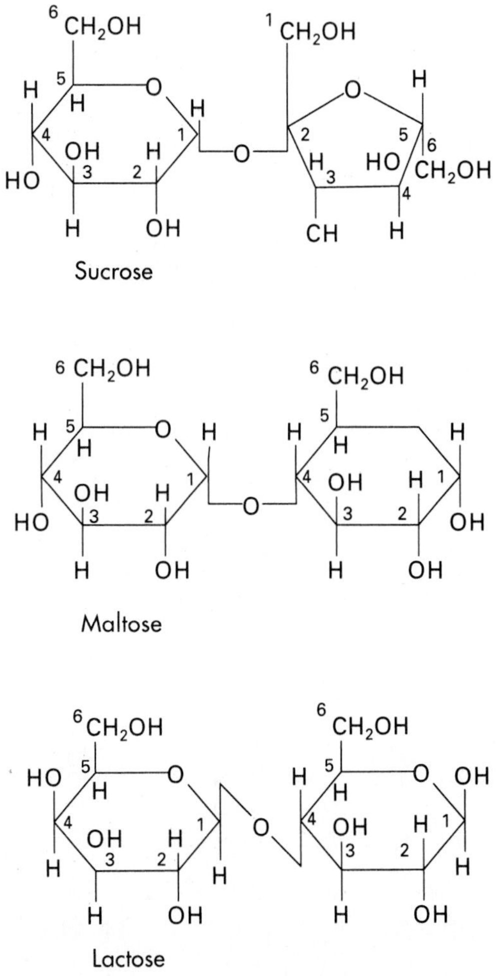

Figure 12-8. Disaccharides.

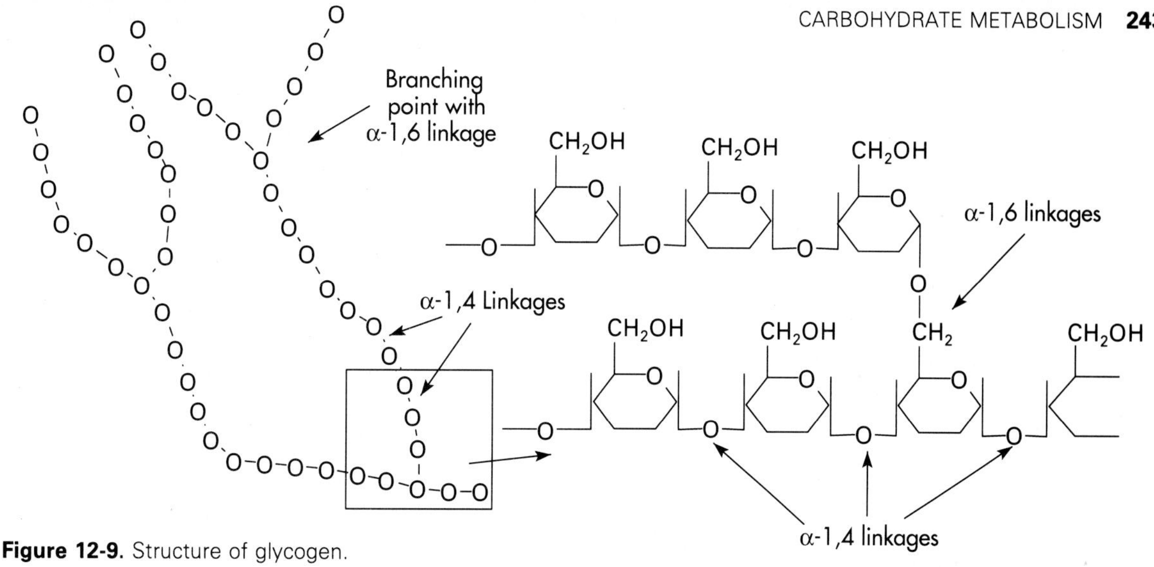

Figure 12-9. Structure of glycogen.

Some disaccharides of physiological importance are as follows (Figure 12-8):
- Sucrose, household sugar, consists of an α-D-glucose whose carbon-1 is linked via an α-glycosidic bond to carbon-2 of β-D-fructose.
- Maltose, formed by intestinal digestion of starch, consists of two α-1,4 linked α-D-glucose molecules.
- Lactose, milk sugar, is composed of β-D-galactose whose carbon-1 is β-glycosidically linked to carbon-4 of β-D-glucose.

Polysaccharides

If two hexoses can combine in 50 different ways, one can imagine the complexity of a polysaccharide structure consisting of hexoses, in which an additional complication is that a single hexose may engage in glycosidic linkages to adjacent hexoses at the site of one, two, or even three of its carbons. The latter case gives rise to branched structures.

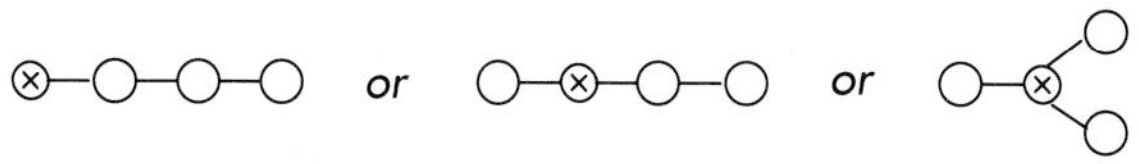

Finally, a great variety of monosaccharides and derivatives are present in the polysaccharide structures found in biological materials. Polysaccharides are macromolecules with molecular weights that may exceed one million (>1000kDa).

To relate to biological functioning, the sequence and three-dimensional structure in which the various monosaccharides are arranged in their straight or branched chains is important. Moreover, it is im-

portant to know whether or not polysaccharides are present as glycoproteins or glycolipids.

Three physiologically important polysaccharides that consist entirely of glucose are reviewed:
- Glycogen, the form in which animal tissues store glucose, has a basic structure that consists of α-1,4 linked D-glucose molecules. Once in every 11 to 18 linkages a branching point occurs via an α-1,6 linkage, which yields a tree-like structure (Figure 12-9). The molecular weight of glycogen ranges from one to over four million.
- Starch, the glucose store of plants, contains 15 to 20% amylose and 80 to 85% amylopectin. While both of these polysaccharides consist totally of a α-D-glucose, amylose is nonbranched and amylopectin contains about one α-1,6 branch per 30 α-1,4 linkages.
- Cellulose consists of nonbranched β-1,4 linked glucose units (Figure 12-10). Due to that β-linkage, cellulose is nondigestible by enzymes of mammalian origin. Cellulose, containing over 50% of the carbon in plant material, is the most abundant organic compound in the world.

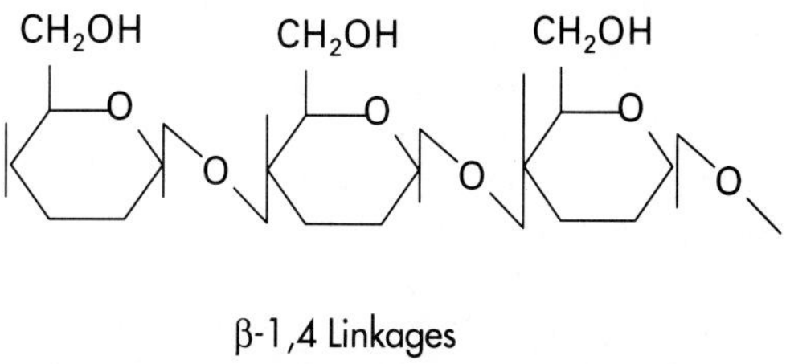

β-1,4 Linkages

Figure 12-10. Portion of the cellulose structure.

Carbohydrate portion of macromolecular structures

Too often one thinks of carbohydrates solely as readily metabolizable fuel. However, carbohydrates and their derivatives are also parts of more-permanent body constituents, usually in the form of macromolecular complexes. In these macromolecular complexes, carbohydrates are linked in either straight or branched chains consisting of the following:

- Ordinary hexoses, such as glucose, mannose, and galactose;
- Deoxysugars, such as deoxyribose in DNA; and fucose (6-deoxygalactose) in various glycoproteins, including those of blood group substances;
- Sulfated sugars, as in heparin;
- Hexosamines (amino sugars), such as glucosamine, mannosamine, galactosamine, and the N-acetyl derivatives of those hexosamines. Of interest is sialic acid, found at the end of sugar chains, imparting anionic charges (Figure 12-11).

The combinations of carbohydrates with proteins (glycoproteins) and with lipids (glycolipids) serve various key functions in cells.

- Mucopolysaccharides exist in mucous secretions and serve as a protective layer, covering, for example, the surface of the intestinal mucosa.
- Chytin, the hard protective exoskeleton of insects, consists of long strands of N-acetylglucosamine connected by the undigestible β-linkage.
- Plasma proteins and cell proteins are mostly glycoproteins. Among the various functions of the carbohydrate moieties of glycoproteins is that their recognition by carbohydrate-specific receptors (lectins) gives direction to intra- and extracellular transport.

- Several proteinaceous hormones are glycoproteins (or glycopeptides), for instance luteinizing hormone (LH) and human chorionic gonadotropin (hCG).
- Many enzymes are glycoproteins.
- Glycoproteins and glycolipids on cell membranes perform a multitude of vital functions that have already been discussed (e.g., receptors, cell adhesion, blood groups).

CARBOHYDRATE FUNCTIONS AND MAJOR PATHWAYS

Sectioning the field of metabolism into carbohydrate metabolism, lipid metabolism, protein metabolism, etc., is done for teaching purposes primarily; it has less significance in the intact organism where these primary nutrient groups are rapidly and easily interconverted. Therefore, close attention must be paid to integrate carbohydrate metabolism into the complex of overall metabolism. The importance of placing all aspects of metabolism first in relation to the intact animal (see Chart I, Chapter 10) and then in the context of overall metabolism (see Chart II, Chapter 10) before going into further detailed discussions cannot be overstated.

Dietary carbohydrates and their metabolic destination
Gastrointestinal digestion and absorption

Digestion by gastrointestinal enzymes presents mucosal cells with a mixture of monosaccharides. Intestinal uptake of glucose and galactose is by active transport, which makes it independent of sugar concentrations in the gut and blood. On the other hand, fructose, mannose, and the pentoses are passively, and thus less efficiently, transported.

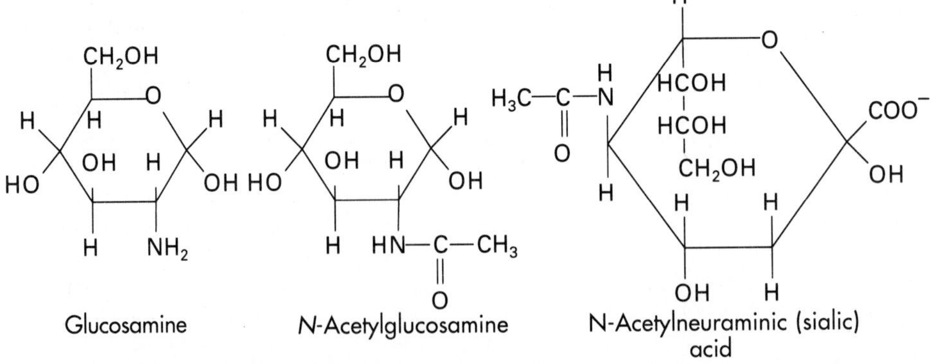

Figure 12-11. Aminosugars.

Postabsorptive destination of dietary carbohydrates

Absorbed dietary sugars are carried via the portal vein to the liver, where the following alternatives are decided.

- To allow enough glucose to exit via the hepatic vein to maintain a level of blood glucose within its normal postprandial range;
- To convert galactose, mannose, and fructose to glucose;
- To replenish the limited glycogen stores with the incoming glut of dietary glucose;
- To combust glucose to obtain energy for the many postprandial functions of the liver; and
- To convert the remainder of the dietary glucose bonanza to fat; then export that fat in the form of lipoproteins into the bloodstream from where the fat can be removed for deposition in adipose tissue.

This abridged list of liver options on the disposal of dietary carbohydrates establishes a need to consider pathways of carbohydrate metabolism and their physiologic control.

Overview of metabolic functions and pathways of carbohydrate metabolism
Metabolic functions of carbohydrates

- Glucose oxidation is a primary nutrient source of energy in nervous tissue, and nearly the sole source in erythrocytes, retina, deep medullary cells of the kidneys, and the germinal epithelium of the gonads.
- Fat deposition in triglyceride stores requires a supply of glycerol phosphate with which to esterify fatty acids. Fat cells derive their glycerol largely from glucose.
- Pentose components of nucleic acids are formed, in part, from glucose.
- In the liver, glucose metabolism yields glucuronic acid and glucosamines, required for synthesis of certain macromolecules and for detoxification of wastes.
- Glucose is needed for fetal development and for milk sugar synthesis in the dam during lactation.

Glucose stores

Despite the aforementioned vital functions of glucose, the body stores are limited. For example, a 70-kg man has approximately 100 g of glucose stored as liver glycogen, 250 g as muscle glycogen, 25 g as adipose tissue glycogen, and 10 g of free glucose in the extracellular fluid compartments. Under normal conditions, muscle and adipose tissue glycogen are of little use for general metabolism, since these tissues cannot contribute glucose to the general circulation (no glucose-6-phosphatase), and blood glucose contributes nothing since its level is maintained constant. This leaves 100 g of liver glycogen, the equivalent of approximately three potatoes or seven slices of bread, as the body's main glucose reserve that can be exported to the circulation.

In light of these limited stores of ready-made glucose, it is not surprising that, under conditions other than those immediately after a meal, glucose utilization is reserved mostly for the aforementioned vital functions. In addition, with increasing time after dinner, glucose synthesis from noncarbohydrate sources, predominantly proteins, gains steadily in importance. The delicate balance between glucose intake and utilization forms a focal point in the discussion of intermediary metabolism.

Names and functions of major pathways of carbohydrate metabolism

Chart III places carbohydrate metabolism's major pathways in the overall metabolic scheme in which carbohydrate, protein, lipid stores, and energy metabolism are interrelated.

The glycolysis (Embden-Meyerhof) pathway provides for the conversion of glucose to pyruvate and the production of NADH and of ATP at the substrate level. In cells that possess mitochondria, pyruvate is mostly oxidized, via AcCoA formation, in the tricarboxylic acid (TCA) cycle. In tissues lacking mitochondria (or oxygen), pyruvate is converted to lactate and exported out of the cell.

The citric acid cycle (TCA cycle or Krebs cycle) is the common oxidative pathway for AcCoA derived from carbohydrates (via pyruvate), proteins (via amino acids), and fats (via β-oxidation). Electrons derived by the TCA cycle from acetate are shuttled by NADH and $FADH_2$ to the adjacent mitochondrial pathway of oxidative phosphorylation for ATP generation.

Glycogenesis is the synthesis of glycogen from glucose, glucose metabolites, or metabolic precursors of glucose. **Glycogenolysis** is the breakdown of glycogen to glucose. Only in liver and kidney is free glucose formed and made available to the entire body via the bloodstream. In other tissues, such as muscle and adipose tissue, the stored glycogen cannot deliver glucose to the bloodstream, because the glucose-phosphates formed cannot be dephosphorylated (i.e., these tissues lack the enzyme glucose-6-phosphatase).

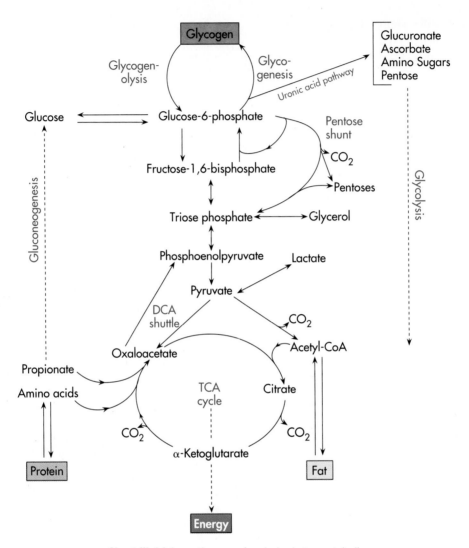

Chart III. Major pathways of carbohydrate metabolism.

The hexose monophosphate shunt (pentose shunt or pentose phosphate pathway) is a cytoplasmic pathway that oxidizes glucose to CO_2 and H_2O. In addition, it is the generator for NADPH and pentoses (ribose).

Gluconeogenesis is the synthesis of glucose from noncarbohydrate precursors (mainly amino acids, glycerol and, in ruminants, propionate). This process reverses the reactions of glycolysis and must negotiate the irreversible (energy requiring) reactions of glycolysis via alternate routes, e.g., the dicarboxylic acid (DCA) shuttle.

The uronic acid pathway in the liver functions by providing glucuronic acid with which metabolic wastes and toxic substances are conjugated in preparation for their biliary elimination, ascorbate (primates lack this particular uronic acid pathway function and have to take vitamin C in their diet), and part of the carbohydrate moieties of glycoproteins and glycolipids.

MAJOR PATHWAYS INVOLVING HEXOSES

Chart IV details the top of Charts II and III, and, thus, shows the main metabolic routes for hexoses: interconversion of various hexoses, glycogen synthesis

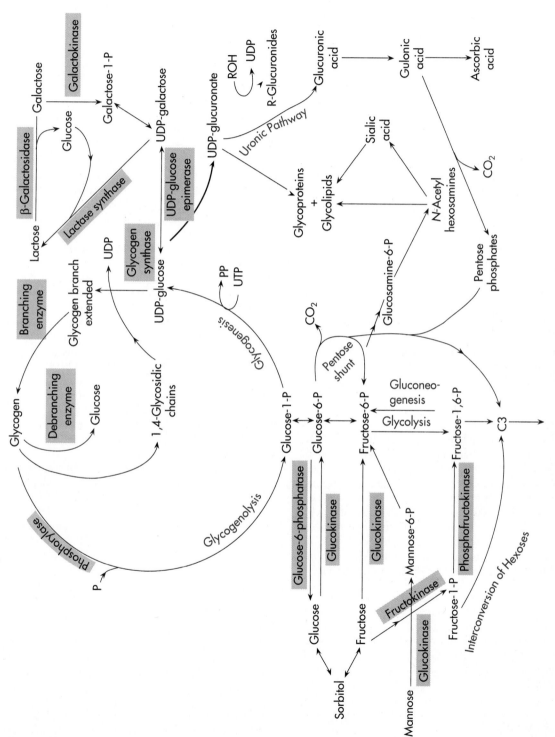

Chart IV. Main pathways at the hexose level.

and breakdown, glycolysis and gluconeogenesis, the uronic pathway, and the formation and catabolism of milk sugar. Glucose 6-phosphate, located in the center, will be the starting point for all discussions pertaining to this chart.

Hexokinase; glucokinase; specific kinases

Glucose metabolism starts with a phosphorylation that also serves to keep glucose in the cell, since the charged phosphate group precludes diffusion of glucose back out of the cell. G-6-P, thus formed, is a substrate from which multiple pathways branch out.

Enzymes that catalyze glucose phosphorylation, glucokinase and hexokinase, require energy input (ATP). Other necessary cofactors for these kinase activities are Mg^{++} and K^+; hence, the high intracellular concentrations of these cations. Kinase steps are highly exergonic and, thus, irreversible.

Hexokinase

Hexokinase is present in all cells in low concentrations (small V_m). The low K_m for hexokinase ($10^{-5}M$) means that the enzyme is working at maximal velocity at very low glucose concentrations. But the enzyme is powerfully inhibited by its product, G-6-P. Hence, when G-6-P is not rapidly used up, that is to say, no longer needed by the cell, hexokinase activity stops. This enzyme is not inducible.

Glucokinase

Glucokinase is a liver enzyme. It has a high K_m ($10^{-2}M$) meaning that high concentrations of glucose can be phosphorylated before V_m is reached. The enzyme is inducible, so that enzyme activation (and enzyme synthesis) meet the acute (and chronic) needs for more glucokinase activity. Glucokinase activity is not induced in the livers of adult ruminants, because not enough glucose escapes degradation by the ruminal flora. Unlike hexokinase, glucokinase is not inhibited by its product, G-6-P, yet its activity is stimulated by insulin.

Specific kinases

Hexokinase and glucokinase phosphorylate not only glucose, but also fructose and mannose to their -6-P derivatives. In addition, there are kinases that phosphorylate carbon-1, namely, fructokinase, phosphofructokinase, and galactokinase. The importance of these specific kinases, initiating alternate pathways for the various hexoses, is apparent under conditions when the glucose pathways are obstructed; for ex-

ample, in diabetes, fructose can be readily metabolized, while glucose cannot.

Glucose 6-phosphatase

Glucose 6-phosphatase (G-6-P-ase) catalyzes the breakdown of G-6-P to free glucose and P_i. The enzyme is present in the liver, kidneys, and gut. In the gut, it is probably involved in the transport of glucose from the lumen into the bloodstream. In the liver and kidneys, G-6-P-ase is a key enzyme in regulating the blood sugar level.

Hepatic G-6-P-ase activity is inhibited by insulin; hence, when glucose levels in the blood are high and, thus, insulin is released by the pancreas, G-6-P-ase activity is inhibited while glucokinase activity is stimulated. This makes sense, since there would be no point in adding more free glucose to an already high blood glucose level. When blood glucose levels drop, and insulin levels decline, G-6-P-ase becomes active and supplies glucose to the bloodstream. Of course, in diabetes mellitus, where high blood sugar levels are present because of an insulin deficiency, unbridled G-6-P-ase activity aggravates the condition. Consequently, the level of G-6-P is chronically low, and this in turn leads to impaired glycogenesis.

The significance of the absence of G-6-P-ase from muscle cells is that muscle glycogen cannot contribute directly to the blood glucose level. Instead, the muscle uses its hexose resources exclusively for its own purposes, albeit that anaerobic glycolysis in muscles produces lactate that can be converted by the liver to blood glucose.

G-6-P-ase activity is part of a multienzyme complex located on the luminal side of the endoplasmic reticulum (Figure 12-12). Besides hydrolyzing G-6-P, the enzyme can also hydrolyze pyrophosphate (PP) and carbamoyl phosphate (CP). It can also transfer the phosphate groups of PP or CP onto glucose, thereby generating G-6-P, but the latter is usually of minor physiologic importance in the intact system. Specific translocases shuttle substrates and products across the endoplasmic reticular membrane. (See Figure 12-12: T1, T2, and T3.) Insulin deficiency or administration of glucagon increases activity of the catalytic unit relative to translocase activity. In contrast, glucocoricoids stimulate G-6-P hydrolysis by increasing translocase activities rather than the catalytic unit. Glycogen storage disease Type I, caused by deficient G-6-P-ase activity, may have various etiologies, relating to impairment of either the catalytic unit of the enzyme or one of the translocases.

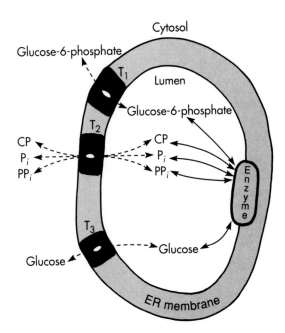

Figure 12-12. The glucose-6-phosphatase system of the endoplasmic reticulum in liver. The catalytic unit (enzyme) is located on the lumenal side of the endoplasmic reticulum *(ER)* membrane. Transport of substrates and products is via translocase units *(T₁, T₂,* and *T₃). CP,* Carbamoyl phosphate. *Reproduced with permission from Arion WJ, Lange AJ, Walls HE, and Ballas LM: Evidence for the participation of independent translocases for phosphate and glucose-6-phosphate in the microsomal glucose-6-phosphatase system, J Biol Chem 255:10396-10406, 1980.*

Hexose monophosphates

Since G-6-P, G-1-P, and F-6-P are at approximately the same energy level and readily interconvertible by reversible enzyme reactions, the text shall consider them as one pool, a hexose monophosphate pool.

Branching points

It is necessary to consider the following compounds as important branching points (see Chart IV): F-6-P, G-6-P, and UDP-glucose. It is from these points that various pathways diverge. These compounds are, thus, the direct substrates of competing enzymes. Rate-controlling (key) enzyme activities for diverging pathways are found at these branching points.

Glycogen metabolism

The body's capacity to store carbohydrate is limited: in a 70-kg human, the liver may contain 6% glycogen

by wet weight postprandially, or approximately 100 g total; muscle contains less than 1% glycogen, or roughly 250 g total; adipose tissue contains about 25 g total; add to that 100 mg glucose per 100 ml of extracellular fluid, or approximately 10 g total, to arrive at a combined total of some 385 g of stored carbohydrates. The caloric equivalent of carbohydrates being 4 Kcal/g, the human body's store totals only 1540 Kcal. Of that amount, the largest part, contained in muscle, is used by the muscle itself for contraction. Glucose in the blood cannot be depleted without fatal consequences. Hence, only glycogen stored in the liver is available directly for maintaining the blood sugar level and performing the many vital carbohydrate functions in different parts of the body.

This leads to three conclusions:
- For meeting daily energy needs, the body uses fat stores, since the total calories in the sugar stores would not last through even a single day.
- The ready-made carbohydrate stores are too small to even meet daily carbohydrate needs; therefore, gluconeogenesis is of vital importance to assist glycogenolysis in the production of glucose.
- The main sites for glycogen synthesis are muscle and liver; but in the utilization of glycogen these tissues differ; hence, different hormonal control mechanisms must be used for glycogen metabolism in these tissues.

Glycogenesis; glycogen synthase

G-1-P is converted to UDP-glucose; pyrophosphate is liberated and split by pyrophosphatase, a ubiquitous enzyme, into two phosphate groups. (See Chart IV.) Hence, the conversion of G-1-P to UDP-glucose costs the equivalent of 2 ATP and is irreversible.

At the UDP-glucose branching point, decisions must be made as to whether there are needs for the functions of the uronic pathway or milk sugar production, or can the body afford to store the glucose unit in the form of glycogen.

Glycogen synthase is the committing and rate-limiting step of glycogenesis. Being a key enzyme, its activity can be inhibited by phosphorylation of the enzyme, or activated by dephosphorylation. Postprandial conditions activate glycogen synthase activity in various ways. The parasympathetic nervous system has a direct effect via the triphosphoinositol-mediated Ca^{++}/calmodulin messenger system, and an indirect effect via nervous stimulation of insulin release from the pancreas. Insulin, the hormone that promotes storage of dietary bounty, stimulates glycogen synthase by causing dephosphorylation of the enzyme; an additional effect of insulin on glycogenesis is the inhibition of G-6-Pase activity. This makes G-6-P available, which serves not only as the indirect substrate, but also as an allosteric feed-forward activator of glycogen synthase activity. When activated, glycogen synthase tags individual glucose units on to the outer branches of the glycogen tree, or to protein-bound "glycogen primer" molecules, while UDP is liberated. When the α-1,4-linked branches have grown to lengths of 6 to 11 glucose units, a branching enzyme transfers groups of 6 or more glucose units and attaches these short chains with an α-1,6-linkage to an annex branch (Figure 12-13).

Glycogenolysis; phosphorylase

Phosphorylase splits single glucose units, in the form of G-1-P from the outer branches of glycogen

by cleaving 1,4-glycosidic bonds with the aid of inorganic phosphoric acid. (See Chart IV.) When phosphorolysis has left four glucose molecules in a chain, then a transferase enzyme transfers a group of three glucoses, after which a debranching enzyme removes the 1,6-bonded glucose hydrolytically, thereby forming free, nonphosphorylated glucose (Figure 12-14).

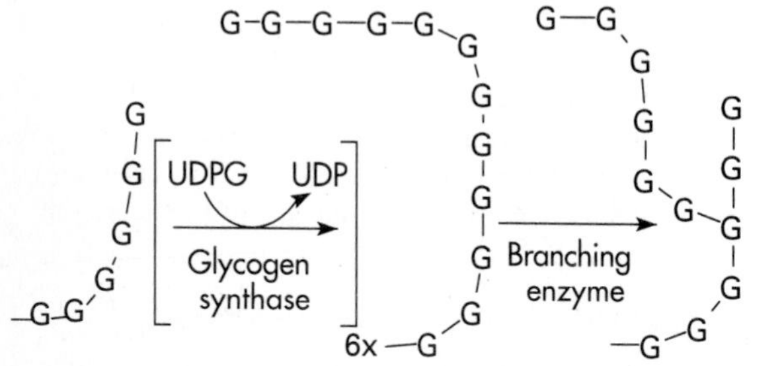

Neuroendocrine control over glycogen synthase and phosphorylase by phosphorylation and dephosphorylation of enzyme molecules

Glycogen synthase and phosphorylase are key enzymes whose activities must be carefully controlled. Obviously, during glycogenesis, the enzymes responsible for glycogen degradation must be inactive; and vice versa, when phosphorylase activity is needed, glycogen synthase must be inhibited. Therefore, to enable the enzymes to switch from dormancy to activity, an active and an inactive form exists for glycogen synthase and phosphorylase; and to avoid simultaneous occurrence of these antagonistic enzyme activities, the same mechanism that activates one inactivates the other. In their phosphorylated forms, glycogen synthase is inactive, phosphorylase active; in their dephosphorylated (OH-) forms, glycogen synthase is active but phosphorylase is not.

What then are the conditions that lead to phosphorylation or dephosphorylation of enzyme molecules? The autonomic nervous system has a direct effect on phosphorylation of the key enzymes. The parasympathetic branch stimulates dephosphorylation and, thus, activation of glycogenesis; in addition, it prompts insulin release from the pancreas. The

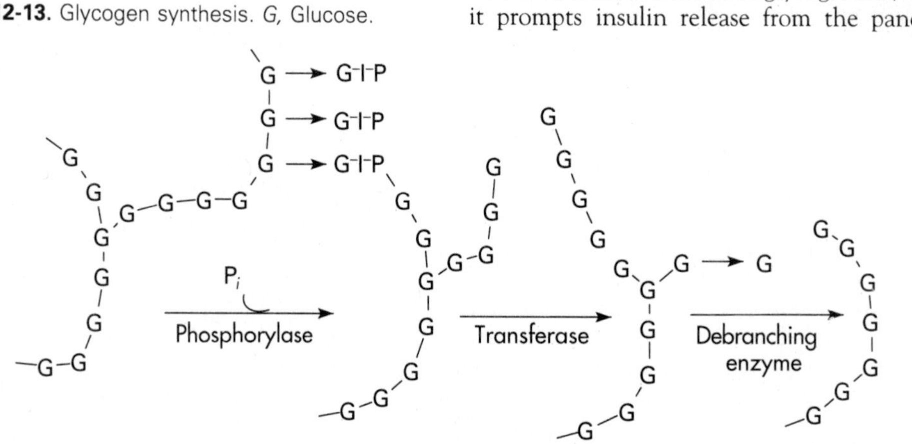

Figure 12-13. Glycogen synthesis. *G*, Glucose.

Figure 12-14. Glycogen degradation, *G*, Glucose; *P*, phosphoric acid; *G-1-P*, glucose-1-phosphate.

sympathetic branch activates glycogenolysis, and causes elaboration of glucagon, epinephrine and norepinephrine. A discussion of endocrine influences may be centered around control of cAMP-dependent protein kinase activity (Figure 12-15). After a meal, the concentration of cAMP in the cell is low, because adenylate cyclase is inactive and, in addition, insulin stimulates phosphodiesterase activity that degrades cAMP. Consequently, cAMP-dependent protein kinase is inactive and allows glycogen synthase and phosphorylase to be in their dephosphorylated (OH) forms. Also, inactive glycogen synthase is activated by dephosphorylation under the influence of synthase phosphatase. Postprandially, therefore, glycogen synthesis is stimulated and glycogenolysis inhibited. But after the bounty of the meal has been anabolized, and insulin and G-6-P levels have dropped, glycogenesis is no longer stimulated. Demands are then made upon the liver glycogen store for maintenance of the blood

sugar level in the time between meals. Under hormonal influence (glucagon; catecholamines) the hepatic cAMP level increases, and activation of cAMP-dependent protein kinase causes phosphorylation of glycogen synthase and phosphorylase, resulting in mobilization of stored glycogen by inhibition of glycogenesis and activation of glycogenolysis.

In the processes of glycogen synthesis and breakdown, the first examples are found (many will follow) of key enzymes whose active forms can be either the phosphorylated or the dephosphorylated enzyme. In general, key enzymes in pathways that produce blood glucose (glycogenolysis, gluconeogenesis) are activated by phosphorylation, whereas pathways that consume glucose (glycolysis, fatty acid synthesis) are inhibited by it. For instance, in the liver, glucagon enhances enzyme phosphorylation, whereas insulin inhibits it.

The chemical identities of glycogen synthase and

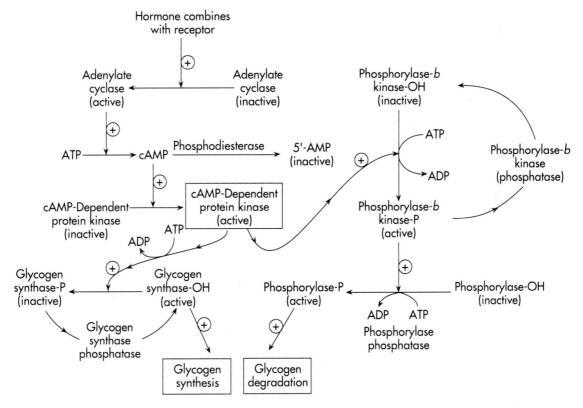

Figure 12-15. Hormonal control over glycogen metabolism. Note that phosphorylation, via cAMP-dependent protein kinase, inhibits glycogenesis while stimulating glycogenolysis; dephosphorylation activates glycogenesis while inhibiting glycogenolysis.

phosphorylase in muscle differ from those in the liver, even though they perform the same functions and show great similarity in their activations by phosphorylation and dephosphorylation. The liver has a specific glucagon receptor allowing the organ to control the blood sugar level by utilizing its glycogen store; muscle lacks this glucagon receptor. Both tissues respond to epinephrine and norepinephrine, and, thus, under stress conditions that lead to elaboration of these hormones, muscle glycogen is mobilized. Another functionally important feature of muscle phosphorylase is that its activation is coordinated with muscle contraction.

Glycogen storage diseases (glycogenoses)

Glycogen storage diseases are characterized by glycogen accumulation in the liver, kidneys, and muscles, caused by the deficiency of one of the enzyme activities needed for glycogen utilization. For instance, lack of muscle phosphorylase (McArdle's disease) causes glycogen accumulation in muscles; muscles are enlarged but cannot exercise; however, liver phosphorylase is unaffected. In Type I glycogen storage disease (von Gierke's disease), G-6-P-ase activity or one of the translocases is lacking in the liver, kidneys, and intestines. Glycogen accumulates in the tissues of these organs, but blood glucose levels are critically low and hyperlipidemia and ketosis occur. Hormones, elaborated in response to the critically low blood glucose level, prompt increased rates of gluconeogenesis, generating a great deal of G-6-P. Because of the defective G-6-P-ase activity, the bulk of this G-6-P is available for glycogenesis, stimulated via the feed-activation of glycogen synthase. Other glycogen storage diseases feature a lack of branching or debranching enzymes or of phosphorylase activities.

UDP-glucose as a branching point

Besides being the substrate for glycogen synthase, UDP-glucose holds the keys to two additional pathways, namely, the uronic acid pathway and the formation or degradation of milk sugar, lactose. (See Chart IV.)

Uronic acid pathway

This pathway starts with the oxidation of UDP-glucose to UDP-glucuronate. (At pH 7.4, most acids are dissociated; hence, the interchangeable use of the name of the acid and its anion: e.g., ascorbic acid and ascorbate.) The liver and, to a lesser extent, the kidneys use UDP-glucuronate for conjugation reactions with toxic substances, which these organs remove from the bloodstream. In Chart IV, conjugation to ROH with liberation of UDP and formation of R-glucuronides is portrayed. R may stand for bilirubin, a natural breakdown product of hemoglobin and cytochromes, for certain drugs, or for steroid hormones, whose inactivation by conjugation is as important as their elaboration in the maintenance of hormonal balance. All of these compounds are removed from the blood by the liver (and kidneys), conjugated, and eliminated in bile or urine.

Alternatively, UDP-glucuronate may be hydrolyzed and, via glucuronate and gulonate, converted to ascorbate. In species that lack the enzyme activity responsible for conversion of gulonate to ascorbate, such as primates and the guinea pig, ascorbate is a vitamin (Vitamin C) that must be included in the diet. Gulonate can also be decarboxylated and then phosphorylated to pentose phosphates, which then can be used for synthesis of nucleotides and nucleic acids. (See Chart IV.)

Of great importance is the formation of carbohydrate-protein complexes (glycosaminoglycans, mucopolysaccharides, glycoproteins) via the uronic pathway, starting from UDP-glucose and from F-6-P. (See Chart IV.)

Glycosaminoglycans are macromolecular carbohydrate complexes, attached to protein, that consist of repeating disaccharide units formed from a uronic acid (glucuronate or iduronate) linked to N-acetyl-galactosamine or N-acetyl-glucosamine. The amino sugar is in many cases sulfated. Some examples of glycosaminoglycans and their disaccharide units include the following:

- Chondroitin sulfate (glucuronate + N-acetyl-glucosamine sulfate);
- Dermatan sulfate (iduronate + N-acetyl-galactosamine sulfate); and
- Hyaluronic acid (glucuronate + N-acetyl-glucosamine).

These complexes occur in various body structures: cartilage, bone, skin, umbilical cord, heart valves, arterial walls, cornea, and tendons. Hyaluronic acid also occurs in synovial fluid and vitreous humor; it serves to lubricate the joints and to hold water in interstitial spaces.

Heparin's repeating disaccharide unit consists of glucuronate (or iduronate) and sulfated glucosamine or N-acetyl-glucosamine. Heparin is produced and stored in mast cells and is known for its anticoagulant and lipid-clearing activities.

In summary, the uronic pathway has four major synthetic functions: (i) synthesis of the sugar moieties of various classes of glycoproteins; (ii) production of glucuronate for conjugation; (iii) ascorbate production; and (iv) service as a minor route for the formation of pentose phosphate. Rate-control of the uronic acid pathway is by demand for its products. Since conjugation processes go on even under conditions of severe carbohydrate shortage (hypoglycemic coma), it appears that the uronic path has a high priority in the utilization of carbohydrates.

Conversion of UDP-glucose to lactose

UDP-glucose is converted, via an epimerase reaction in mammary tissue, to UDP-galactose, which combines with a glucose molecule to form lactose. Lactose formation is energetically preferred over glycogen formation; hence, production of lactose in adequate amounts will occur as long as the mother is milked out properly. Immediately upon weaning the suckling, lactose production stops because of product inhibition.

It is of interest to speculate on the presence of lactose rather than glucose in milk. One possible reason for the use of an "unusual sugar" is that glucose metabolism in the mammary gland can be directed toward the synthesis of a specific sugar for milk. However, this reasoning would lead one to predict the presence of a simple sugar like galactose rather than lactose. The significance of a disaccharide in place of a monosaccharide may lie in the effective halving of the osmotic concentration (for a given energy content), for lactose is a major contributor to the osmotic pressure of milk.

Digestion of lactose

When milk sugar is digested by intestinal lactase, it yields glucose and galactose. Galactose, whose intestinal absorption efficiency exceeds that of glucose, is converted in the liver to galactose 1-phosphate by a specific galactokinase. Galactose 1-phosphate is then converted to UDP-galactose, which is subsequently epimerased to UDP-glucose and then converted to glycogen. (See Chart IV.)

An inborn metabolic disease (galactosemia) constitutes a lack of the enzyme activity that converts galactose 1-phosphate to UDP-galactose; this leads to accumulation of galactose in the blood and galactosuria after dietary intake of milk products. A possible complication of galactosemia is the formation of cataracts in the eye lens, an osmotic effect of the accumulation of galactitol formed by reduction of galactose. Therefore, in galactosemic patients, the intake of galactose must be curtailed. This can be done without risking a shortage of galactose in the body because, even in galactosemic patients, UDP-glucose can still be converted to UDP-galactose, so that plenty of endogenously synthesized galactose is available for synthesis of the numerous vital compounds that contain galactose, such as glycoproteins, glycosaminoglycans, and glycolipids.

Fructose metabolism

Fructose is found in high concentrations in semen. It is synthesized from glucose via sorbitol. (See Chart IV.)

Cells geared to metabolize fructose have various alternative pathways: conversion to F-6-P is probably of minor importance, because the affinities of hexokinase and glucokinase for fructose are low compared to their affinities for glucose. But very active in the liver is the enzyme fructokinase, which converts fructose to F-1-P. The latter can be converted to Embden-Meyerhof (E-M) glycolysis intermediates by two different routes: either phosphofructokinase converts the F-1-P to F-1,6-bisphosphate, or else, a special enzyme, fructoaldolase, splits the F-1-P into triose intermediates of the E-M path.

The advantage of multiple pathways is that fructose can escape a defect in one pathway (e.g., defective glucokinase can be bypassed by taking an alternative path). The beneficial effects of fructose feeding to diabetics derive from the fact that fructokinase, unlike glucokinase, is not affected by lack of insulin.

Though fructose is intestinally absorbed only half as efficiently as glucose, it is important because diets may contain substantial amounts of fructose in the form of table sugar. Essentially all dietary fructose is converted to glucose and glucose metabolites in the gut and liver. After removal of the liver, the carbohydrate demands of animals cannot be met by feeding fructose as the sole carbohydrate.

Not all tissues metabolize fructose to the same degree. The small intestines in humans, but not in rats, convert a large part of dietary fructose into glucose. The liver metabolizes fructose faster than glucose, probably because fructose bypasses the rate-limiting enzyme reactions of glucokinase and phosphofructo-kinase; hence, fructose is referred to as **rapid fuel.** Muscle and brain tissues use fructose only after its conversion into glucose by the liver. Adipose tissue in vitro metabolizes fructose about as well as it does glucose.

Mannose

Dietary mannose can be metabolized by glucokinase and an isomerase to F-6-P. (See Chart IV.) Since mannose is passively absorbed in the intestine, diet is an insignificant source of mannose. N-acetyl-man-nosamine, needed for the production of sialic acids and glycoproteins, can be synthesized from F-6-P.

The pathways in the top triangle of Chart II have now been detailed. Later this information shall be integrated with lipid and protein metabolism, and put together functionally. To be able to do that, the reader must condense the material discussed thus far, so that the more critical concepts can be recalled when needed.

Once again, one must review the functions and limitations of the body's carbohydrate stores. It is necessary to consider the functions of the various pathways, and neuroendocrine activation or inactivation of key enzyme activities that control the directions in which pathways go. One must establish a functional mental picture of the branching points for F-6-P, G-6-P, and UDP-glucose in Chart II and name the key enzymes involved in pathways that compete for substrate at the branching points.

GLYCOLYSIS; EMBDEN-MEYERHOF PATHWAY
Functions of glycolysis

- Since carbohydrate storage capacity in the form of glycogen is limited, glycogen stores are soon replenished in the period immediately following a meal so that excess glucose is stored as fat. The conversion of glucose to fat in the liver and fat cells entails Embden-Meyerhof (E-M) glycolysis of glucose.
- For production of glycerol phosphate used by fat cells in triglyceride synthesis, glucose is catabolized.
- In periods between meals, the utmost economy is observed in spending glucose. To meet energy demands, most tissues combust fats and ketone bodies via the TCA cycle. But since there are "leaks" in the TCA cycle via which cycle intermediates leak

into other pathways, a little bit of glucose or of glucogenic intermediates is needed to resupply cycle intermediates. Thus, some glucose may be catabolized via the E-M pathway to "grease" the TCA cycle "machinery," enabling it to combust fats and ketones to meet the energy demands of most tissues.
- There are some tissues that feed themselves under normal conditions exclusively with glucose, such as retinal tissue and red blood cells.
- Cells that have to function under reduced oxygen tension cannot use their mitochondrial energy-generating machinery and, thus, are limited to cytoplasmic ATP formation by the anaerobic fermentation of glucose. Examples include deep medullary cells in the kidneys and skeletal muscle cells during severe exercise.

Overview of the Embden-Meyerhof pathway

Following the phosphorylation of glucose to G-6-P, and an internal rearrangement to F-6-P, the key enzyme, phosphofructokinase (PFK), transfers a high-energy phosphate from ATP to F-6-P to form fructose-1,6-bisphosphate (Chart V). The latter is cleaved into two triose phosphates, which are oxidized by NAD^+ and then rearranged to produce pyruvate. Depending on the availability of mitochondria and oxygen, pyruvate is then oxidized in the TCA cycle or reduced to lactate and exported out of the cell.

The energy yield per molecule of glucose converted to pyruvate is 4 ATP + 2 NADH. However, since 2 ATP are initially invested to phosphorylate glucose and F-6-P, the net energy yield is 2 ATP + 2 NADH (together worth about 8 ATP) when pyruvate is produced. If lactate is the end product, the 2 NADH are used to reduce pyruvate, hence, 2 ATP are the total net yield of anaerobic fermentation.

To examine E-M glycolysis, one starts by applying Chart I, the global picture, to the postprandial situation in a dog. In the liver cell, the arrow from glucose to AcCoA indicates E-M glycolysis. The aforementioned functions of the pathway should be apparent. Now glycolysis is located in the context of overall metabolism outlined in Chart II and further detailed in Chart V. It is important to concentrate on the irreversible (committing) steps, as well as the key enzymes and cofactors. It is also important to note how the carbohydrate pathways are interwoven with lipid, protein, and energy metabolism. The use of Chart V will be helpful when studying the following notes.

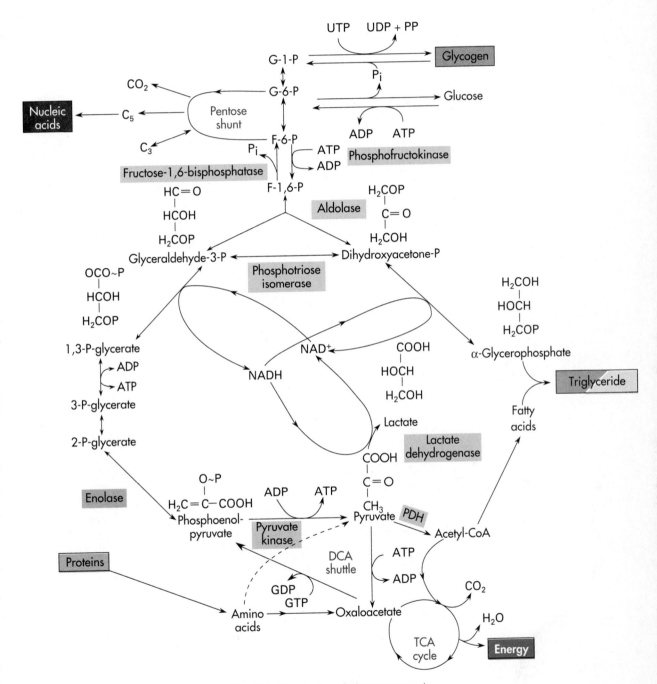

Chart V. Glycolysis and gluconeogenesis.

Embden-Meyerhof glycolysis and its controls

Two glycolytic pathways for glucose 6-phosphate

One catabolic pathway for G-6-P is named after its co-discoverers: the Embden-Meyerhof pathway of glycolysis. The English word "enzyme" derives from the Greek "en zume," which means "in yeast" where cellular enzyme activity was first demonstrated. Later, glycolysis was found in virtually every cell.

The alternate oxidative pathway for G-6-P, the hexose monophosphate shunt by which energy is ob-tained from G-6-P, is especially useful for cells that do not have the TCA cycle (e.g., erythrocytes); it is found in most cells, and is also used for purposes other than energy production (discussed below).

Phosphofructokinase reaction

Function. Glycolysis via the E-M pathway starts with an irreversible (committing) step in which the key enzyme phosphofructokinase (PFK) pulls F-6-P out of the hexose monophosphate pool and converts it to fructose-1,6-bisphosphate. As is common for kinase reactions, ATP, Mg^{++}, and K^+ are required for optimal PFK activity.

$$\text{Fructose-6-phosphate} \underset{\underset{\text{ATP} \quad \text{ADP}}{\xrightarrow{\hspace{2cm}} \text{Phosphofructokinase}}}{\overset{\overset{P_i}{\xleftarrow{\hspace{2cm}} \text{Fructose-1,6-bisphosphatase}}}{}} \text{Fructose-1,6-bisphosphate}$$

In the liver, PFK's low concentration makes it rate-limiting for glycolysis. The rate of glycolysis is con-trolled right at the branching point, where a portion of the hexose monophosphate pool is to be committed to degradation. Because of glucose economy between regular meals, it is to be expected that PFK activity will remain inhibited unless a demand for energy is signaled in the form of ADP and AMP, the products of ATP after its energy has been spent. Postprandially, a unique activator of PFK, fructose-2,6-bisphosphate, enables conversion of dietary glucose to fat. Control of PFK activity by both of these factors are considered in the following passages.

Control of PFK activity by AMP, ADP, ATP, and citrate. AMP and ADP are allosteric activators of phosphofructokinase (PFK), whose activity adapts to the signal "demand for energy," so that energy can be provided via glycolysis.

Fine control over the adaptation of PFK activity to the cell's need for energy is mediated by the enzyme adenylate kinase, present in most tissues, catalyzing:

$$\text{ATP} + \text{AMP} \leftrightarrow 2 \text{ ADP}$$

At equilibrium, the concentration of ATP is ap-proximately 50 times that of AMP. Consequently, spending only a small proportion of the ATP produces (via ADP) a large percentage increase in the AMP concentration. This fact, combined with allosteric PFK activation by AMP, makes PFK activity ex-tremely sensitive to even the smallest changes in a cell's energy status, so that the amount of precious carbohydrate spent on glycolysis is accurately con-trolled.

On the other hand, ATP and citrate powerfully inhibit PFK. Breakdown of fat yields high levels of ATP and citrate. Under this condition, energy is plentiful and PFK inhibition spares glucose from gly-colytic breakdown.

Control over glycolysis and gluconeogenesis by fructose-2,6-bisphosphate. Postprandially in the liver, dietary glucose must refill the glycogen stores; since these stores are small, most incoming glucose is converted to fat. The latter conversion requires glycolysis. There is a problem in that the rate-con-trolling enzyme activity of glycolysis, PFK, is allos-terically depressed by ATP and citrate, compounds whose levels are elevated in this high-glucose state. Fructose-2,6-bisphosphate now relieves inhibition of PFK by ATP and citrate as it substantially lowers the K_m for F-6-P.

Fructose-2,6-bisphosphate (F-2,6-P_2) is a potent stimulator of PFK and an inhibitor of fructose-1,6-bisphosphatase (F-1,6-P_2-ase). Thus, it stimulates gly-colysis and inhibits gluconeogenesis. F-2,6-P_2 is formed from F-6-P in the liver by a specific 6-phos-phofructo-2-kinase, and converted back to F-6-P by a specific F-2,6-P_2-ase. These two enzymes activities occur on a single protein with two active sites. The functionality of this arrangement is that phosphory-lation of the enzyme protein activates one of the enzyme activities, while it concomitantly inactivates the enzyme activity of the other site, and vice versa for dephosphorylation. Phosphorylation of that protein activates F-2,6-P$_2$-ase activity (Figure 12-16: site 1), and the resulting lowering of the F-2,6-P$_2$ concentration decreases glycolysis and facilitates gluconeogenesis. In contrast, hydrolytic loss of phosphate from the protein activates 6-phosphofructo-2-kinase enzyme activity (See Figure 12-16: site 2), thereby generating F-2,6-P$_2$ and stimulating PFK activity and, thus, glycolysis. Clearly, then, phosphorylation and dephosphorylation of the protein carrying the two opposing enzyme activities is that which controls the level of F-2,6-P$_2$ and, thus, the delicate balance between glycolysis and gluconeogenesis. This phosphorylation requires the activity of either cAMP-dependent protein kinase or phosphorylase kinase, whereas the dephosphorylation is catalyzed by a protein phosphatase.

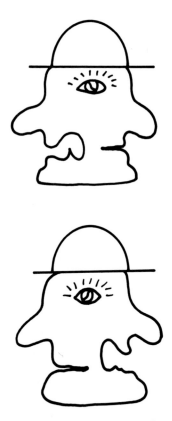

Figure 12-16. A dual-function enzyme; when in the phosphorylated (P) form, fructose-2,6-bisphosphate is hydrolyzed to fructose-6-phosphate at site 1. When the enzyme is in the dephosphorylated (OH) form, its site 2 is active and phosphorylates fructose-6 phosphate to fructose-2,6-bisphosphate.

Formation and breakdown of F-2,6-P$_2$ assists hepatic control of carbohydrate metabolism, alternating glycolysis and gluconeogenesis for the general good of the body. Generation of F-2,6-P$_2$ is positively correlated to the rate of glycolysis and negatively correlated to gluconeogenesis. It has been observed that during fasting the concentration of F-2,6-P$_2$ in the liver decreases to 10% of normal, but overcompensates to 250% of normal by feeding high-carbohydrate diets. Administering gluconeogenic precursors, such as alanine, lactate, glycerol, or fructose (broken down to C3), powerfully lowers F-2,6-P$_2$ production in the liver to enable gluconeogenesis. F-2,6-P$_2$ is an intracellular signal in the liver cell after a meal, indicating that glucose is abundant. In this respect, its action is opposite to that of cAMP, which is a hunger signal, indicating a glucose shortage and, thus, a need for gluconeogenesis.

Hormonal control over PFK via F-2,6-P$_2$ is different in the liver and extrahepatic cells. In the liver, glucagon, epinephrine, diabetes (insulin deficiency), and starvation all raise the concentration of cAMP. Protein kinases that increase activities of phosphorylase, F-1,6-P$_2$-ase, and F-2,6-P$_2$-ase are activated, thereby inhibiting glycolysis and stimulating gluconeogenesis. In fact, glucagon's action in lowering F-2,6-P$_2$ levels in the liver, and hence inhibiting glycolysis, is an essential requirement for net gluconeogenesis. Insulin counteracts glucagon and epinephrine by dephosphorylating the two-enzyme protein, thereby increasing formation of F-2,6-P$_2$ and enhancing glycolysis. However, while insulin deficiency or fasting lowers the level of F-2,6-P$_2$ in the liver, no such drop has been observed in skeletal muscle. In perfused hind-limb muscles of rats, not only insulin but also (and in contrast to liver) epinephrine elevated the F-2,6-P$_2$ concentration and stimulated glycolysis. In perfused heart muscles, epinephrine increased glycolysis but did not elevate the level of F-2,6-P$_2$.

The production of F-2,6-P$_2$ in glycogen-rich hepatocytes is increased by α-sympathetic nervous activation (electrical or by agonists), but only when glucagon is absent. In the presence of glucagon, these α-sympathetic stimulations of glycolysis are prevented, since inhibited formation of F-2,6-P$_2$ stimulates gluconeogenesis.

Perinatal change in the level of F-2,6-P$_2$ correlates well with profound changes in fetal and postnatal carbohydrate metabolism. Three days before term, when hepatic glycogen synthesis is initiated, the concentration of F-2,6-P$_2$ is at a minimum; two hours after birth, it increases rapidly, as does glycogen mobilization. Neonatal hypoglycemia reflects the high rate of glucose utilization for the purpose of heat production.

It should not be concluded from the above that all control over PFK activity revolves around F-2,6-P_2. To the contrary, in many tissues, and also in the liver under conditions other than postprandial conditions, the activity of PFK is controlled not by F-2,6-P_2, but by the level of AMP; for example, electrical stimulation of the hind limb causes muscle contractions and a huge increase in lactate production, but the level of F-2,6-P_2 is low; also under ischemic conditions, control over PKF is by AMP.

Fructose-1,6-bisphosphatase reaction

Just as glycolysis is regulated by PFK, so is gluconeogenesis controlled by the reverse step: the F-1,6-P_2-ase reaction. Tissues that lack this enzyme activity cannot generate glucose by gluconeogenesis. F-1,6-P-ase activity is absent from adipose tissue, from heart muscle, and from smooth muscle. On the other hand, the enyzme is active in striated muscle, kidneys, and liver. Since the liver is geared toward production of glucose by gluconeogenesis (to maintain the blood glucose level), the level of F-1,6-P_2-ase is higher than that of PFK.

Futile cycles

If both opposing enzymes, PFK and F-1,6-P_2-ase, were allowed a free rein constantly, one would witness a futile cycle whose only achievement would be that it converted ATP to ADP + P_i and heat. Therefore, the rates of opposing key enzymes must be controlled, so that a gain in one's activity is accompanied by a loss in the other's activity. Stimulators of PFK, such as ADP and AMP, inhibit F-1,6-P-ase, and inhibitors of PFK (e.g., ATP) stimulate F-1,6-P-ase. Other than by ATP, hydrolytic activity of F-1,6-P-ase is stimulated by fasting, glucocorticoids, and by fructose feeding.

Despite these considerations, three futile cycles exist in carbohydrate metabolism:
- Glucokinase vs. G-6-P-ase;
- PFK vs. F-1,6-P-ase; and
- Pyruvate kinase vs. the DCA shuttle.

Futile cycles may serve various functions. One is to generate body heat. A second is to allow better quantitative control over the direction of a net flow of intermediates; for instance, when the ratio of glycolysis/gluconeogenesis goes from 95:5 to 90:10, gluconeogenesis doubles with little loss in glycolysis (Figure 12-17). Such fine control would not be possible in an all or no enzyme activation/inhibition system. A third function is to regenerate ADP, so that ATP-producing pathways may continue; for example, conversion of glucose to fat aided by a futile cycle of triglyceride formation and breakdown in fat cells.

Aldolase reaction

This step is a reversible conversion between F-1,6-P_2 and two triose phosphates, glyceraldehyde phosphate (GAP) and dihydroxyacetone phosphate

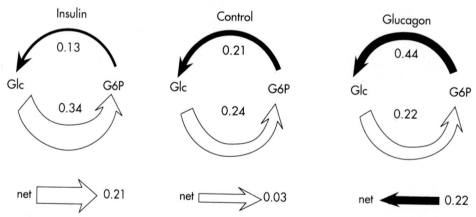

Figure 12-17. Hormonal control over a futile cycle. Total and net flux through the glucose/glucose-6-phosphate *(Glc/G6P)* cycle in cultured rat hepatocytes are expressed in µmol/min per g wet weight. Note the antagonistic effects of insulin and glucagon. *Reproduced with permission from Christ B, Probst I, and Jungermann K: Antagonistic regulation of the glucose/glucose-6-phosphate cycle by insulin and glucagon in cultured hepatocytes, Biochem J, 238:185-191, 1986.*

(DHAP). These two triose phosphates are readily interconvertible. Thus, when GAP is used in the subsequent glycolytic pathway, DHAP may be converted to yield additional GAP.

Metabolic fates of triose phosphates

DHAP can be reduced by a NADH-requiring reaction to yield glycerol phosphate, a necessary ingredient in the formation of triglycerides and phospholipids. For cells, such as adipose tissue, that lack the enzyme glycerokinase and, thus, cannot obtain glycerol phosphate by means of phosphorylating free glycerol, synthesis of glycerol phosphate via glycolysis up to DHAP is a must. Here is one important link between glucose uptake and triglyceride formation in adipose tissue.

GAP is the direct precursor for subsequent glycolysis. In the remainder of the E-M pathway, GAP gets oxidized. This is where the initial energy investment is harvested. For thus far, the hexose has been "primed" by tagging on two phosphates at the expense of ATP. But in the triose end of glycolysis, from each triose two ATP are harvested at the substrate level and one NADH (equivalent to three ATP) is produced.

Glyceraldehyde phosphate oxidation to 1,3-diphosphoglycerate

Under the influence of GAP dehydrogenase, a pair of hydrogen atoms, including a pair of electrons, is taken from GAP, so that the phosphorylated aldehyde is oxidized to a phosphorylated glyceric acid. NADH is formed and an inorganic phosphate is incorporated. The net reaction can be written as follows:

$$\text{Glyceraldehyde phosphate} \xrightleftharpoons[\; P_i \;]{NAD^+ \quad NADH} \text{1,3-Diphosphoglycerate}$$

Glyceraldehyde phosphate dehydrogenase

In muscle and other extrahepatic tissues, oxidation of GAP is rate-limiting for glycolysis, because of low enzyme concentration.

Triose end of glycolysis

In the conversion of 1,3-diphosphoglycerate to 3-phosphoglycerate, an ATP is formed at the substrate level. Then the P shifts from the 3-carbon to the 2-carbon of glycerate, after which enolase catalyzes the loss of water and formation of phosphoenolpyruvate

(PEP). Enolase activity is inhibited by fluoride ions (F^-). Since F^- also complexes Ca^{++}, the addition of fluoride to a blood sample serves at once as an antiphysiologically coagulant and as a block against glycolysis; such is necessary if one wants to measure plasma glucose levels.

Glycolysis leading up to the formation of PEP is physiologically reversible, albeit that different enzymes may be involved in forward and backward reactions. (See Chart V.) But the difference in free energy between PEP and pyruvate is in excess of 12 Kcal, which makes the free energy jump of the pyruvate kinase reaction too big to be traversed in the opposite direction under physiologic conditions, since one ATP can contribute only 7 to 8 Kcal worth of free energy to a reaction. Part of the 12 Kcal is trapped in the formation of an ATP at the substrate level.

The irreversibility of the PEP-to-pyruvate conversion by pyruvate kinase has large implications for the process of gluconeogenesis from pyruvate or lactate. In order to bring pyruvate up to the free energy level of PEP, two ATP are needed. At the expense of one ATP, pyruvate is carboxylated to become oxaloacetate, and at the expense of a second ATP equivalent (in the form of GTP), oxaloacetate is decarboxylated and phosphorylated to PEP, from where it is converted to glucose via reverse glycolysis. This two-step conversion of pyruvate via oxaloacetate to PEP, called the **dicarboxylic acid shuttle** will be discussed in the context of gluconeogenesis.

It is critically important that the conversion of PEP to pyruvate, that is the activity of pyruvate kinase (PK), be well controlled. Glucose formation from amino acids (via PEP) can occur only when the energetically preferred conversion of PEP to pyruvate is blocked; that is, when PK activity is inhibited (Figure 12-18). Alanine allosterically inhibits pyruvate kinase activity. In addition, pyruvate kinase activity is controlled by protein kinase and phosphatase enzymes:

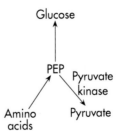

Figure 12-18. For gluconeogenesis from amino acids, the pyruvate kinase reaction must be inhibited.

phospho-PK is inactive and dephospho-PK is active. PK activity is augmented under conditions that stimulate glycolysis (insulin) and by feed-forward activation by $F-1,6-P_2$, while it is inhibited when glycolysis is not required and gluconeogenesis must take place (glucagon).

Energetics of glycolysis

Reducing equivalents (NADH) generated in the cytoplasm can be transported into mitochondria and "cashed in" for 3 ATP. But the NADH formed from GAP does not necessarily have to be reoxidized via the mitochondrial process. NADH generated in the cytoplasm can partake directly in reducing reactions, such as the cytoplasmic reduction of DHAP to glycerol phosphate. (See Chart V.) Either way, an NADH may be counted as the equivalent of 3 ATP. As all conversions of C3 compounds following the aldolase step have to be multiplied by two to relate back to the degradation of 1 hexose molecule, it follows that—after investing 2 ATP early in glycolysis from glucose—10 ATP equivalents are obtained from GAP to pyruvate, making a net 8 mol of ATP produced for 1 mol of glucose converted to pyruvate.

Metabolism of pyruvate

The metabolic fate of pyruvate formed by glycolysis depends on oxygen availability and on a tissue's machinery to utilize available oxygen; that is, the number of mitochondria, vascularization, etc. Muscle fibers vary greatly in their numbers of mitochondria. During vigorous muscular exercise, the muscle has to produce great amounts of energy, which are needed for muscular contraction. Under such a condition, the muscle's demand for oxygen may exceed the rate at which oxygen is supplied by the bloodstream and the rate at which the small numbers of mitochondria can utilize it. The muscle is then said to have incurred an oxygen debt. How the muscle can keep up its energy supply during anaerobic and aerobic conditions will now be examined.

Under aerobic conditions. When oxygen is available, pyruvate, formed via glycolysis in the cytoplasm, enters the mitochondrion, where it is completely oxidized to CO_2 and water via the TCA cycle. In this process, 15 ATP are produced from 1 pyruvate, or 30 ATP from the 2 pyruvates derived from 1 hexose molecule. One should compare this to the net formation of only 8 ATP in the pathway from hexose to pyruvate. Hence, a total of 38 ATP are produced

from 1 hexose molecule. But this process requires oxygen for a least two reasons: (i) to accept the electrons taken from pyruvate during oxidation in the TCA cycle and use them for oxidative phosphorylation; and (ii) to reoxidize the NADH generated in the cytoplasm at the GAP dehydrogenase step, for without continuous supply of NAD^+, glycolysis would soon cease and the muscle would run out of energy.

Under anaerobic conditions. Under anaerobic conditions, NADH is reoxidized to NAD^+ by losing its two metabolic electrons to pyruvate. This process, catalyzed by lactate dehydrogenase (LDH), converts pyruvate to lactate. (See Chart V.) In muscle, under anaerobic conditions, lactate is a metabolic end product. To become metabolizable, it would have to convert back to pyruvate, which cannot happen under anaerobic conditions. Instead, most of the muscle's lactate goes via the bloodstream to the liver, where gluconeogenesis converts it to glucose that can then be taken up from the blood by the exercising muscle and glycolyzed back to lactate (Cori cycle; see below). The conversion of pyruvate to lactate in order to generate NAD^+ is energetically costly. Above, it was calculated that 6 of the 8 ATP equivalents derived from glucose in its glycolysis to pyruvate were derived from the formation of NADH at the GAP dehydrogenase step. At this point, those 6 ATP equivalents are sacrificed, bringing the net total efficiency of anaerobic glycolysis down to 2 ATP per hexose molecule, compared with 38 ATP under aerobic conditions. But as low-yielding as anaerobic glycolysis may be, it does allow completion of muscular activity.

Cori cycle. ATP is required for muscular contraction. The muscle stores energy in the form of phosphocreatine and as glycogen. During contraction, ATP is formed from ADP plus phosphocreatine, and when phosphocreatine is depleted, glycogenolysis and subsequent glycolysis produce more ATP. During exercise, as noted above, pyruvate and increasingly larger proportions of lactate are formed in muscle. Small proportions of pyruvate and lactate are metabolized via the muscle's TCA cycle or excreted in urine. By far, most of the lactate/pyruvate pool is released as lactate into the bloodstream, converted by hepatic gluconeogenesis to blood glucose, and taken up again by muscle. That glucose-lactate cycle is called the **Cori cycle** (Figure 12-19). The net reaction of the Cori cycle is that the liver invests ATP during gluconeogenesis from lactate, and the muscle extracts that ATP energy during glycolysis. The ex-

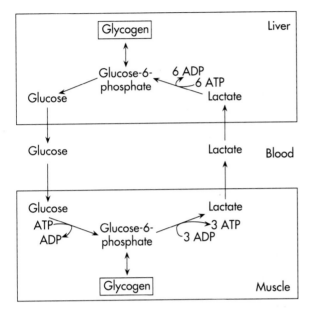

Figure 12-19. Cori cycle. Maintaining anaerobic glycolysis in exercising muscle requires assistance from the liver.

ercising muscle uses the liver's mitochondria. It is important to note that the Cori cycle does not spend any of the body's small glucose reserve; whatever glucose it uses it regenerates.

Pasteur effect

Pasteur noted that glycolysis is linked to respiration, that is, oxygen consumption. The rate of glycolysis—glucose disappearance and lactate appearance—is lower under aerobic conditions than anaerobically. Another way to state the effect is that admission of oxygen to a glycolyzing system spares glucose.

Explanations for the Pasteur effect include the following:

- Aerobically, pyruvate is combusted via the TCA cycle, so that from 1 glucose molecule 38 ATP are produced. But anaerobically, with lactate as the end product of glycolysis, only 2 ATP are produced from 1 glucose molecule. Comparing these two conditions, one can understand that the energy needs of a cell can be met aerobically by glycolysis of fewer glucose molecules than is the case under anaerobic conditions.
- The rate-controlling enzyme phosphofructokinase, and thus glycolysis, is not inhibited when the ATP concentration is low because of a shortage of oxygen.

The inverse of the Pasteur effect is named after Crabtree: hexose feeding causes a drop in oxygen consumption.

It is important to recall: under anaerobic conditions, no oxygen is available to accept electrons from the TCA cycle. Hence, fats and ketones cannot be used as food, and glucose is the only food left.

The conversion of glucose (or G-6-P) to pyruvate is referred to as the E-M pathway of glycolysis. The other glucose-catabolizing pathway, namely, the hexose monophosphate (pentose) shunt will now be examined, after which the text shall return to examination of the pyruvate/lactate pool.

PENTOSE SHUNT

The hexosemonophosphate shunt is present in most cells, where it constitutes an alternate route for the combustion of G-6-P. Being located in the cytoplasm of cells, the oxidative capacity of the pentose shunt is of special importance to cells, such as erythrocytes, that lack mitochondria. The synonym pentose shunt derives from the fact that this pathway produces ribose (and thus indirectly deoxyribose) for the synthesis of nucleic acids and nucleotides. Another function of the pentose shunt is the generation of reducing equivalents in the form of NADPH, which is essential for fat storage, sterol synthesis, and other vital cell functions.

Biochemical overview

The pentose shunt branches from G-6-P (Chart VI). It involves the oxidation of carbon-1 of G-6-P to a carboxyl group, with G-6-P-dehydrogenase as a key enzyme, and uses $NADP^+$ to accept electrons. This is the rate-controlling step of the oxidative portion of the pentose shunt. The next step oxidizes the carbon-3 to a keto group, producing another NADPH. After a decarboxylation step (in which carbon-1 is split off as CO_2), the nonoxidative part of the pentose shunt begins, in which heptose-, hexose-, pentose-, tetrose-, and triosephosphates interreact. The transketolase steps require thiamin pyrophosphate (TPP) as a cofactor; thiamin is vitamin B_1.

Reaction equations of the pentose shunt

Oxidative reaction:

$$3 \text{ G-6-P} + 6 \text{ NADP}^+ \rightarrow$$
$$3 \text{ Ribulose-5-P} + 6 \text{ NADPH} + 3 \text{ CO}_2$$

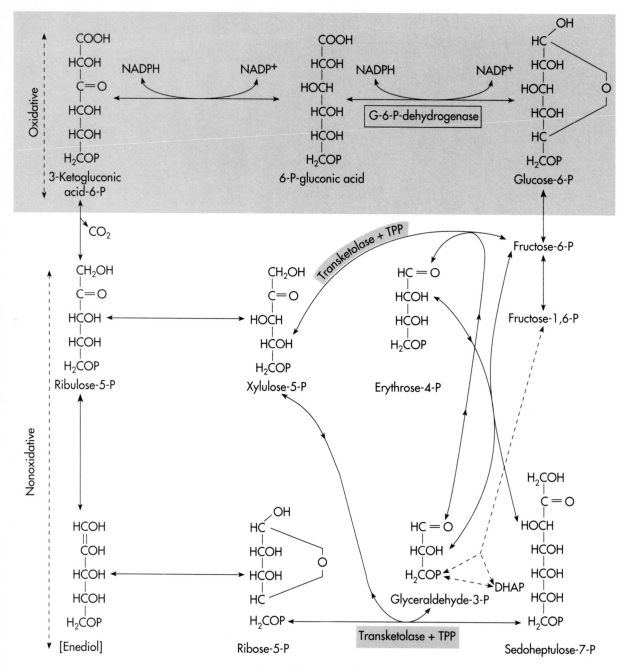

Chart VI. Pentose shunt.

Nonoxidative reaction (GAP stands for glyceraldehyde phosphate):

3 Ribulose-5-P ↔ 2 Xylulose-5-P + Ribose-5-P

Ribose-5P + Xylulose-5-P ↔
Sedoheptulose-7-P + GAP

Sedoheptulose-7-P + GAP ↔
Fructose-6-P + Erythrose-4-P

Erythrose-4-P + Xylulose-5-P ↔
Fructose-6-P + GAP

In these equations, the products of one step are the reactants of the next step. Hence, by adding reactions, all intermediates cancel out, so that the net sum can be stated as follows:

3 G-6-P + 6 NADP$^+$ →
3 CO_2 + 2 F-6-P + GAP + 6 NADPH

Since F-6-P and G-6-P both belong to the hexosemonophosphate pool, and two GAP can form one G-6-P, the pentose shunt can also be summarized as follows:

Glucose-6-P + 12 NADP$^+$ →
6 CO_2 + 12 NADPH + P$_i$

Products of the pentose shunt

Except for the decarboxylation step, all reactions of the pentose shunt are reversible (even the rate-limiting step). In cells that contain fructose-1,6-bisphosphatase, the pentose shunt can form a closed loop. Traversing the loop six times completely oxidizes 1 glucose molecule and produces 6 CO_2, together with 12 NADPH, which are equivalent to 36 ATP. This can be compared with the 38 ATP produced when G-6-P is oxidized via the E-M pathway and the TCA cycle.

GAP produced via the pentose shunt can be used for glycerol phosphate formation or E-M glycolysis. GAP can also be used to produce pentoses via reversal of the nonoxidative part of the pentose shunt. The latter is of major importance in tissues (e.g., skeletal muscle) that lack the oxidative portion of the pentose shunt and thus, cannot form pentoses directly from G-6-P.

Rate control over the pentose shunt

The rate at which the pentose shunt operates depends on metabolic pull. The cell may need pentoses for nucleic acid and nucleotide syntheses, or NADPH for fat or steroid synthesis. The activity of the oxidative part of the pentose shunt is stimulated by insulin. This probably reflects an increased demand for NADPH. Allosterically, the activity of G-6-P-dehydrogenase is inhibited by galactose. In the lens of the eye, metabolism depends a great deal on proper functioning of the pentose shunt. Cataracts develop during galactosemia from an accumulation of galactitol, formed by reduction of galactose.

Cofactors of the pentose shunt

B vitamins are shuttlers. Thiamin (vitamin B_1) in the form of TPP and as cofactor of transketolases (see Chart VI), shuttles ketocompounds from one molecule to another. Nicotinamide (the N of NAD and NADP) shuttles hydrogen atoms, including their electrons.

The vast majority of biological redox reactions requires NAD(H), but certain enzymes, for instance in fatty acid and steroid syntheses, have an absolute requirement for NADPH and do not take NADH as a substitute. The rate at which an NADPH-producing pathway (such as the pentose shunt) operates is dictated by the demand for NADPH in the cell. Pentose shunt activity is, thus, synchronized with fatty acid synthesis by two circumstances: (i) the absolute specificity of NADP(H)-producing and NADP(H)-utilizing enzyme reactions; and (ii) the scarcity of NADP(H), which necessitates that the rates of utilization and production of NADPH must match exactly. Though the reducing equivalent of NADPH can be transferred to NAD$^+$ and thence cashed in for ATP, NADPH should be considered primarily as a cofactor used in synthetic reactions.

Functions of the pentose shunt

Complete combustion of glucose for energy is found in nearly all cells, but is especially important in erythrocytes, which lack the TCA cycle. Note that in the pentose shunt CO_2 is produced, which is not the case in the E-M pathway of glycolysis from glucose to pyruvate.

The pentose shunt is one of the three major sources for the production of NADPH (the other two pathways for NADPH production branch off from TCA cycle intermediates). NADPH, in turn, is required for cytoplasmic lipid synthesis.

Synthesis of pentoses is another essential function of the pentose shunt. Ribose is a constituent of ATP, NAD(P), and other nucleotides, and of RNA; deoxyribose of DNA is derived from ribose. Intestinal absorption of ribose is too limited to meet demands; hence, the importance of the pentose shunt in this respect. In the liver, pentoses can also be derived via the uronic pathway.

Production of ribose via the pentose shunt can occur either oxidatively (from G-6-P) or nonoxidatively (from GAP) by reversal of the nonoxidative part of the pathway. In muscle, where G-6-P-dehydrogenase activity is lacking, oxidative pentose shunt activity is very low and the nonoxidative part of the shunt is the main route for ribose synthesis. In other tissues, the oxidative part of the shunt produces ribose.

Pentose shunts in different tissues

Competition between the E-M pathway and the pentose shunt for catabolism of G-6-P in various tissues is studied by labeling glucose with radioactive carbon (^{14}C). The CO_2 produced via the shunt is derived from carbon-1 of glucose (see Chart VI), whereas CO_2 produced via the E-M pathway and the subsequent TCA cycle is derived from all six carbon atoms of glucose. Thus, comparing for a given tissue, the production rates of radioactive CO_2 from specifically carbon-1 labeled glucose (glucose-1-^{14}C) with the $^{14}CO_2$ production from glucose-6-^{14}C yields an estimate of the proportion to which G-6-P is catabolized by the two pathways.

These proportions are different for various tissues, and vary a great deal depending on physiological conditions, especially during the time after a meal. Most tissues can catabolize G-6-P by both pathways, but muscle, deficient in G-6-P-dehydrogenase activity, lacks the oxidative pentose shunt. Activity of the pentose shunt is especially high in adipose tissue, which requires NADPH for fatty acid synthesis. High pentose shunt activity is found in endocrine tissues, which need NADPH for synthesis of cholesterol and steroid hormones, or use ribose for nucleic acids involved in the production of proteinaceous hormones. In the mammary gland, pentose shunt activity is very high during lactation for the production of milk fats and proteins, but absent in the nonlactating state.

The pathway discussed above has only been found in fat cells; hence, it is referred to as the **F-type.** A different pathway, the **L-type,** is found in liver and other tissues. Functionally, the two pathways are identical. Chemically, the L-type distinguishes itself by the presence of an eight-carbon sugar phosphate, and by the involvement of 1,7-bisphosphorylated sedoheptulose. There is evidence that fructose-2,6-bisphosphate (the regulator of glycolysis) also controls the flow of intermediates through the pentose shunt, at the level of sedoheptulose-7-phosphate to sedoheptulose-1,7-bisphosphate conversion.

Metabolic considerations

After a meal, liver and adipose tissue convert glucose to fat. G-6-P is an all-inclusive "kit" for the "assembly" of fatty acids:

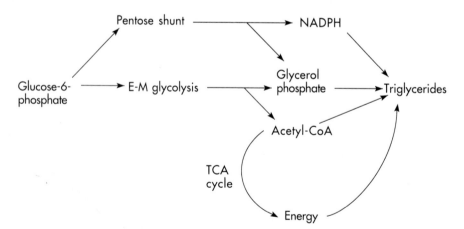

At this point, it is beneficial to summarize the pentose shunt for easy recall: functions of the shunt; where in the cell it is found; rate-controlling step, enzyme, cofactors; rate-control of the shunt; in which tissues the shunt is particularly active and why; on which points in the mainstream of carbohydrate metabolism the shunt touches; determine whether the shunt is the only pathway for NADPH production; rating of the energy-economy of glucose catabolism via the shunt.

Having dealt with highlights of the upper portion of Chart II, the text returns to the lactate/pyruvate pool and considers its aerobic fate. To this end, the discussion shall leave the realm of cytoplasm and enter into that of mitochondrial metabolism.

OXIDATIVE DECARBOXYLATION OF PYRUVATE

Under anaerobic conditions, pyruvate is converted to lactate, so that NAD^+ is regenerated for continued operation of glycolysis and ATP formation in the cytoplasm. Under aerobic conditions, pyruvate may enter mitochondria, where pyruvate dehydrogenase activity converts it to AcCoA and CO_2. Because this reaction entails both an oxidation (NADH is formed) and a decarboxylation (CO_2 is produced), it is an oxidative decarboxylation. Because of its pivotal place in metabolism (see Charts II, V, and VII), this step warrants careful attention.

Pyruvate as a branching point

- By transamination, pyruvate becomes alanine, which can be incorporated into proteins.
- Via the DCA shuttle, pyruvate can be carboxylated to become oxaloacetate, from where further conversion to PEP and reversal of the E-M pathway lead to production of glucose.
- Pyruvate can be oxidatively decarboxylated to become AcCoA, after which further conversion to either fatty acids or, via the TCA cycle, to CO_2, H_2O, and energy can occur. The text shall consider the latter pathway.

All pathways discussed thus far are present in the cytoplasm of the cell, but the conversion of pyruvate to AcCoA occurs only in mitochondria. Another mitochondrial process is the TCA cycle, funneling electrons into the pathway of oxidative phosphorylation. Hence, for its combustion via the TCA cycle, AcCoA does not have to leave the mitochondrion. However, the main pathway for fatty acid synthesis from AcCoA is located in the cytoplasm of the cell. Therefore, when glucose is converted to fats, pyruvate formed via E-M glycolysis has first to be transported into mitochondria, and the AcCoA formed there (by oxidative decarboxylation of pyruvate) has to be exported back into the cytoplasm (discussed below).

Mechanism of the pyruvate dehydrogenase step

The step under discussion is the C3 to C2 conversion of Chart II. In fact, this is a multistep conversion, catalyzed by a multienzyme complex, collectively called **pyruvate dehydrogenase.** Five different enzyme activities are included in the pyruvate dehydrogenase

NET: Pyruvate + NAD⁺ CoA ⟶ Acetyl~CoA + NADH + CO₂

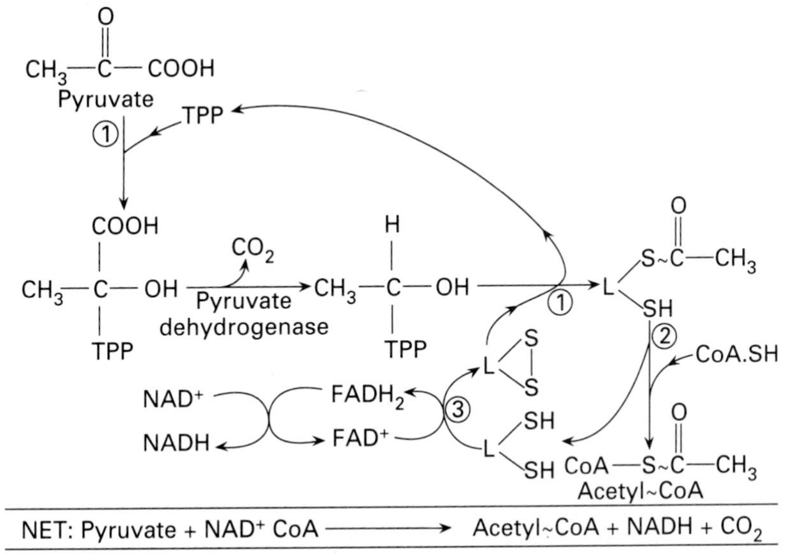

Figure 12-20. The pyruvate dehydrogenase (PDH) reaction. The PDH complex employs three enzyme activities in the oxidative decarboxylation of pyruvate. *1*, Pyruvate dehydrogenase; *2*, dihydrolipoyl transacetylase; *3*, dihydrolipoyl dehydrogenase. Two additional enzyme activities are involved in the rate control of the PDH reaction (Fig. 12-21). *TPP*, Thiamin pyrophosphate; *L*, lipoic acid.

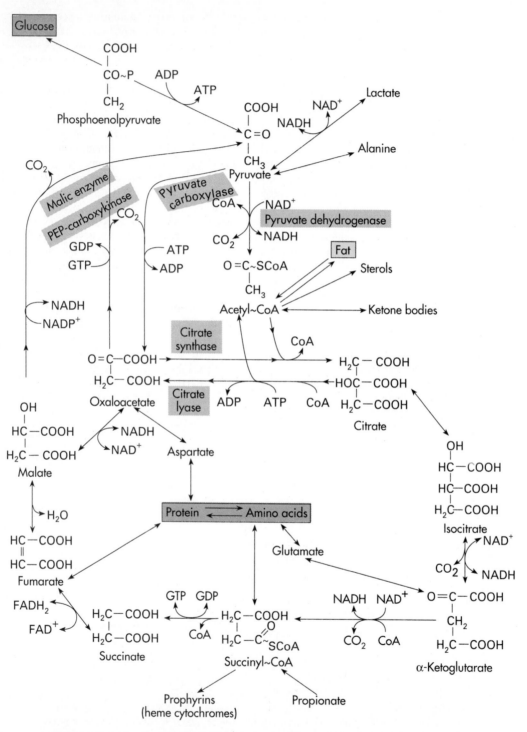

Chart VII. The tricarboxylic acid acid (TCA) cycle and dicarboxylicacid (DCA) shuttle.

complex. Two of these, involved in phosphorylative and dephosphorylative rate control, are discussed below. The others are indicated by numbers in the illustration (Figure 12-20). Pyruvate dehydrogenase activity (enzyme #1) links thiamin pyrophosphate (TPP) to pyruvate, then decarboxylates pyruvate, ties the ethanal that is formed to the oxidized form of lipoic acid, which becomes reduced while acetate is formed. Next, the enzyme (#2) dihydrolipoyl transacetylase combines the acetyl group with coenzyme A and sets the reduced form of lipoic acid free, to be reoxidized by dihydrolipoyl dehydrogenase (enzyme #3). Thus, the oxidized form of lipoic acid is regenerated for a new round of action, while the electrons are transferred from lipoic acid to flavin, then to NAD⁺, and ultimately to the electron transfer chain.

No less than five B vitamins are involved in their regular roles as shuttlers: thiamin, lipoic acid, flavin, niacin, and pantothenic acid, the latter a component of coenzyme A. The pyruvate dehydrogenase reaction is not unique: in the TCA cycle, the oxidative decarboxylation of α-ketoglutarate to succinyl-CoA follows the identical reaction mechanism.

In addition to NADH formation, the enormous free-energy drop from pyruvate to acetate is further harvested by bringing acetate to a higher free-energy level by forming ACoA. AcCoA, containing the energy required for uphill reactions, is an important branching point (Chart VII) for the following:

- Fatty acid synthesis
- Sterol synthesis
- Ketone body synthesis
- Entry into TCA cycle by condensation with oxaloacetate, forming citrate
- Various acetylation reactions (e.g., acetylcholine)

The huge free-energy drop between pyruvate and AcCoA means that the reaction is physiologically irreversible. Therefore, AcCoA cannot go back to glucose, and, thus, fatty acids (as they are catabolized to AcCoA) cannot form glucose. For gluconeogenesis, amino acids, glycerol, lactate, and propionate (ruminants) are used.

Rate control of pyruvate dehydrogenase activity

Included in the multienzyme complex are two enzymes that control the activity of the pyruvate dehydrogenase step (Figure 12-21): (i) a protein kinase that phosphorylates the enzyme protein, thereby decreasing its enzymic activity; and (ii) a phosphatase

that dephosphorylates and thereby stimulates enzyme activity. High ratios of ATP/ADP, NADH/NAD⁺, or AcCoA/CoA stimulate protein kinase and, thus, impair pyruvate dehydrogenase activity. These high ratios are present under conditions when energy is plentiful (e.g., during fat oxidation). Glucose degradation via pyruvate is then blocked. In keeping with its role of converting glucose to fat postprandially, insulin stimulates pyruvate dehydrogenase activity; fasting inhibits it which spares glucose.

THE TRICARBOXYLIC ACID CYCLE

The terms tricarboxylic acid (TCA) cycle, citric acid cycle, and Krebs cycle are synonyms.

The TCA cycle, in concert with oxidative phosphorylation, is the major pathway of intracellular respiration in aerobic organisms. Inside mitochondria, AcCoA is derived from: (i) pyruvate; (ii) fatty acids; (iii) amino acids; or (iv) ketone bodies. The AcCoA is oxidized by TCA cycle enzymes, some of which are freely dispersed in the mitochondrial matrix, whereas others (notably the redox steps) are attached to the

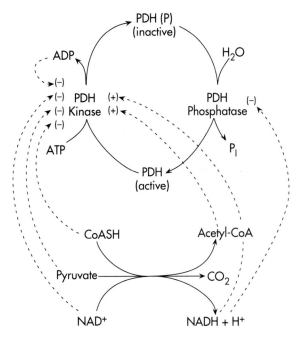

Figure 12-21. Rate control over the pyruvate dehydrogenase (PDH) reaction. PDH is inactivated by phosphorylation under influence of the products of the reaction; the substrates of the reaction prevent the active form of the enzyme from being phosphorylated.

inner surface of the inner mitochondrial membrane, hence, in close contact with enzymes associated with oxidative phosphorylation.

But the TCA cycle is more than a common channel for the ultimate oxidation of carbohydrates, lipids, and proteins. Its intermediates and enzymes also serve a variety of anabolic purposes, such as gluconeogenesis (from lactate, amino acids, and propionate), lipogenesis, and synthesis of nucleotides, and hemoglobin.

With Chart VII as a guide, the text shall move in a clockwise direction around the cycle and highlight its major metabolic significance and control.

The TCA cycle and its controls
Citrate-condensing enzyme (citrate synthase)

This is a key step that commits AcCoA to complete oxidation. AcCoA condenses with oxaloacetate to form citrate, a tricarboxylic acid. Because this reaction involves the splitting of the high-energy bond between acetate and CoA, the step is irreversible under physiological conditions. The reverse reaction (see Chart VII) by **citrate lyase,** also called **citrate cleavage enzyme,** requires the energy of an ATP to form AcCoA.

It would appear that citrate is a symmetric molecule, but the condensation of acetate to oxaloacetate (OxAc) is asymmetric. The two molecules of CO_2 released later in the same passage through the TCA cycle are derived from the original OxAc, and, thus, the carbons of the acetate molecule that are condensed last become part of the OxAc regenerated at the end of the passage through the TCA cycle. This can be demonstrated with the use of labeled acetate.

Elevated concentrations of ATP (i.e., high ATP/ADP ratio) in mitochondria inhibit citrate synthase activity by raising the K_m of this enzyme for AcCoA. Decreasing amounts of AcCoA then go through the cycle. This control is advantageous, because when energy is needed (ATP level is low) citrate synthase activity is high, so that energy may be obtained from fat via AcCoA combustion in the TCA cycle. Conversely, when less energy is needed (ATP level is high) citrate synthase is inhibited, so AcCoA is spared from combustion. Consequently, the AcCoA level (i.e., the ratio of AcCoA/CoA) increases, and that in turn: (i) inhibits pyruvate dehydrogenase, thus sparing glucose; (ii) allosterically stimulates pyruvate carboxylase activity (see Chart VII), which promotes gluconeogenesis via pyruvate under the proper conditions; (iii) may promote fatty acid synthesis; and (iv) may lead to increased production of ketones under conditions adverse to glucose and fatty acid synthesis. Such high ATP/ADP (and, hence, AcCoA/CoA) ratios usually come about by fat oxidation in periods between meals or during fasting. The sparing of glucose and increased gluconeogenesis are then needed.

Conversion of citrate to α-ketoglutarate

Citrate and isocitrate are in a reversible equilibrium. Under influence of the enzyme isocitrate dehydrogenase (ICD), isocitrate loses a CO_2 and a pair of electrons in its conversion to α-ketoglutarate. Mitochondrial isocitrate dehydrogenase requires NAD^+ to accept electrons from isocitrate. But in the cytoplasm of cells, many enzyme activities similar to the ones of the TCA cycle are found, including an ICD. Cytoplasmic ICD requires $NADP^+$ for its activity and, thus, produces the synthetic redox cofactor NADPH. This NADPH source, compared to the other two major sources (HMP shunt and malic enzyme [discussed below]), may add significance because of a putative interchange between NADPH and NADH via cytoplasmic and mitochondrial ICD activities (Figure 12-22).

It is important to note that α-ketoglutarate is interconvertible (by transamination; discussed below) with the amino acid glutamate. The amino acids ornithine, proline, histidine, and glutamine, which all yield glutamate in their degradative pathways, as well as glutamate itself, are, thus, all potential TCA cycle intermediates. Conversely, transformation of α-ketoglutarate to glutamate constitutes a drain (or leak) of TCA cycle intermediates.

Conversion of α-ketoglutarate to succinyl-CoA

Succinyl-CoA is formed when α-ketoglutarate loses CO_2 and a pair of electrons in an oxidative decarboxylation reaction analogous to the pyruvate dehydrogenase step. This step is irreversible under physiological conditions.

At this point in the TCA cycle, it has been shown that two carbon atoms in the form of AcCoA entered the cycle, and that two carbon atoms were lost from the cycle in the form of CO_2. Hence, in the cycle from oxaloacetate to succinyl-CoA, there is no net gain of carbon atoms. AcCoA being unable to go back to pyruvate, and being completely combusted in the TCA cycle, can never be converted to glucose.

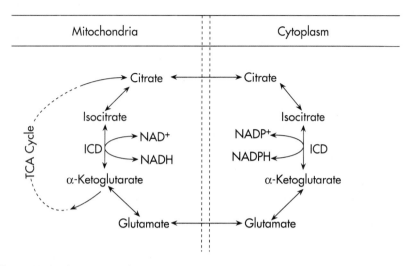

Figure 12-22. Interconversion of reducing equivalents. *ICD,* Isocitrate dehydrogenase.

Hence, fatty acids, whose intermediate oxidative breakdown product is AcCoA, cannot contribute to gluconeogenesis; but amino acids, whose breakdown products are TCA cycle intermediates, are the main ingredients for gluconeogenesis.

Succinyl-CoA as a branching point

The high-energy bond of succinyl-CoA allows it to engage in synthetic reactions or substrate phosphorylation.

- The combination of succinyl-CoA with glycine is the pacemaker in the synthesis of porphyrins (e.g., heme and cytochromes) in mitochondria. Biosynthesis of porphyrins constitutes a constant drain of succinyl-CoA away from the TCA cycle.
- Several amino acids (methionine, isoleucine, and valine) are converted to succinyl-CoA, as is propionic acid. These amino acids and propionate, entering the cycle at the intermediate stage of succinyl-CoA, are all gluconeogenic precursors via further TCA cycling to oxaloacetate, then to PEP and on to glucose. (See Chart VII.)
- In the TCA cycle, succinyl-CoA is hydrolyzed, whereby part of the free-energy release associated with the liberation of free CoA is trapped in the formation of one GTP from GDP at the substrate level.

It may be significant that the key enzyme in gluconeogenesis, PEP-carboxykinase, requires GTP when converting oxaloacetate to PEP. (See Chart VII.) Hence, glucogenic amino acids that enter the TCA cycle at the stages of either α-ketoglutarate or at succinyl-CoA, and propionate, traverse the step from succinyl-CoA to succinate, and thereby generate the GTP required to boost them over the PEP-carboxykinase step on their way to becoming glucose.

Other important metabolic requirements for GTP include: (i) activation of fatty acids, the first step in the combustion of fatty acids for energy; (ii) various steps in protein synthesis; and (iii) regulation of transmembrane and intracellular signaling to make cellular metabolism responsive to neuroendocrine stimuli.

Oxidation of succinate to fumarate

This step involves FAD. Unlike NAD, which can be isolated as a free compound, FAD is attached to the enzyme succinate dehydrogenase, where it transmits electrons taken from succinate to ubiquinone; from there, only two ATP are produced in the pathway of oxidative phosphorylation. The glucogenic amino acids phenylalanine and tyrosine enter the TCA cycle at the stage of fumarate.

Conversion of fumarate to malate

By saturating the double bond in its structure with water, fumarate is converted to malate. The importance of malate outside the TCA cycle is summarized in the following:

- Mitochondrial membranes are permeable to malate, so that malate can shuttle reducing equivalents of NADH from cytoplasm into mitochondria; NADH itself cannot permeate mitochondrial membranes.

- In the cytoplasm, malate can be converted to pyruvate by oxidative decarboxylation under the influence of malic enzyme, which produces NADPH in the process. (See Chart VII.) Besides the pentose shunt and the cytoplasmic isocitrate dehydrogenase reaction, malic enzyme is the third major source of NADPH.
- Malate is an effective precursor for the cytoplasmic synthesis of fatty acids (See Chart VII): via its conversion to pyruvate it produces both AcCoA and NADPH. Of course, depending on conditions, malate also serves as a precursor for gluconeogenesis.

Oxaloacetate: formation and branching point

Oxidation of malate produces oxaloacetate and NADH, and with that the TCA cycle is closed. By transamination, oxaloacetate is in reversible equilibrium with the amino acid aspartate. The oxaloacetate/aspartate pool is an important branching point, as can be seen from Chart VII.

- Oxaloacetate itself cannot cross mitochondrial membranes, but, via reversible conversions to either malate or aspartate, cytoplasmic and mitochondrial oxaloacetate/aspartate and oxaloacetate/malate are single pools that serve both cell compartments.
- As a gluconeogenic precursor, oxaloacetate may be formed from amino acids, lactate, or propionate via either the pyruvate carboxylase or malate dehydrogenase steps, or by deamination of aspartate. PEP-carboxykinase then converts oxaloacetate to PEP on its way to forming glucose.
- The use of aspartate for protein synthesis is another drain on TCA intermediates.
- Aspartate is the "building stone" of pyrimidine bases (uracil, thymine, cytosine), which are components of nucleotides and nucleic acids.
- The involvement of oxaloacetate in the TCA cycle is not considered to be a drain on the oxaloacetate/aspartate pool, since the TCA cycle does not use it up.

Leaks in the TCA cycle and replenishment

Thus far in the exploration of the TCA cycle, the text has encountered several branching points along which TCA intermediates leak away. Obviously, these intermediates must be replenished or else the TCA cycle would dry up. In listing leaks and replenishing processes, various catabolic and anabolic functions of the TCA cycle can be summarized and the central position of the cycle in metabolism ascertained (Figure 12-23; see Chart VII).

Leaks in the TCA cycle.

- Citrate is permeable across mitochondrial membranes, and, hence, it may leave mitochondria. In the cytoplasm, under the influence of citrate lyase, it may be split into oxaloacetate and AcCoA, with the latter used for cytoplasmic fatty acid synthesis.
- Likewise, aspartate, malate, glutamate, and α-ketoglutarate are permeable and may be used for various cytoplasmic functions.
- Pyruvate, α-ketoglutarate, and oxaloacetate can be transaminated to their corresponding amino acids (alanine, glutamate, and aspartate, respectively; discussed below) and then incorporated into proteins.
- Oxaloacetate can engage the PEP-carboxykinase step on the way to gluconeogenesis.
- Malate is siphoned off to provide NADPH via the malic enzyme reaction, converting it to pyruvate.
- Succinyl-CoA leaks out of the cycle to form porphyrins, such as heme for hemoglobin and the cytochromes for electron transport.
- The oxaloacetate/aspartate pool is constantly tapped for the synthesis of pyrimidines (uracil, cytosine, thymine) that are part of the structures of nucleotides and nucleic acids.

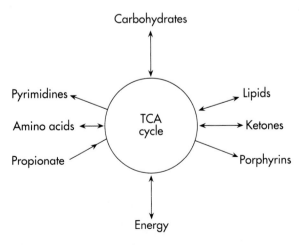

Figure 12-23. Leaks and replenishment of TCA cycle intermediates.

Replenishment of TCA intermediates. Because of all the anabolic involvements for which TCA cycle intermediates leak away, cycle activity would soon become deficient (so that not enough AcCoA could be oxidized) if there were no processes whereby TCA intermediates are replenished.

- One of the functions of glucose is to replenish the TCA cycle machinery, so that AcCoA (derived from fat) can be completely oxidized. Pyruvate, formed from glucose via E-M glycolysis, can be carboxylated by pyruvate carboxylase to replenish oxaloacetate. The saying goes that "fats are burned in a carbohydrate flame."
- Proteins yield amino acids that can be converted to TCA intermediates by transdeamination and, thus, serve the purpose of gluconeogenesis.
- Propionate is a source for replenishment through gluconeogenesis, since it is metabolized to succinyl-CoA. Though not of importance in the diet of monogastric animals, it is of the utmost importance for ruminants who rely on gluconeogenesis from propionate, amino acids, glycerol, and lactate for their glucose supply. Propionate conversion to succinyl-CoA requires the B vitamins, biotin and cobalamine (Figure 12-24).

At this point, it is helpful to consider the two B vitamins involved in propionate's conversion to succinyl-CoA, biotin and cobalamine. It is important to remember that B vitamins function as shuttlers.

Biotin shuttles CO_2. In combination with the metal manganese (Mn) it plays a part in the CO_2-shuttling reactions catalyzed by carboxylases. Examples are: AcCoA carboxylase, converting AcCoA to malonyl-CoA; pyruvate carboxylase, lengthening the C3 substrate pyruvate to the C4 product oxaloacetate;

and propionyl-CoA carboxylase (see Figure 12-24) tagging a carboxyl-group onto the middle carbon of its substrate to form methylmalonyl-CoA. Biotin is formed, usually in adequate amounts, by the bacterial flora in the gut, but oral antibiotics may create biotin-deficiency. In young animals, extra demands on biotin, which is needed for growth, are met by feeding a biotin-supplemented diet. Biotin forms an inactive complex with the egg-white protein avidin; avidin is denatured by boiling the eggs. Raw eggs should therefore not be fed to young animals, since biotin would remain bound to avidin in the GI tract.

Cobalamine (vitamin B_{12}) shuttles methyl groups. Examples are: the conversion of methylmalonyl-CoA to succinyl-CoA (as shown) and the formation of heme. Cobalamine is a large molecule containing the metal cobalt. This vitamin is also formed by the intestinal flora and, in addition, it is derived from the diet. Absorption of cobalamine from the gut requires a transport-facilitation factor, called **intrinsic factor,** which is produced in the stomach. After gastrectomy, a patient must receive vitamin B_{12} intravenously. A patient whose stomach genetically lacks the capability to make intrinsic factor exhibits a hemoglobin deficiency, called **pernicious anemia.** After intestinal absorption, cobalamine is transported in blood by a special carrying protein, transcobalamine, and stored in the liver. Because liver and red meats are prime sources of vitamin B_{12}, vegetarians have difficulties obtaining sufficient amounts of the vitamin from their diet. Ruminants derive B vitamins through microbial synthesis.

Energetics of the TCA cycle

Pyruvate combustion in mitochondria via pyruvate dehydrogenase and the TCA cycle yields five reducing

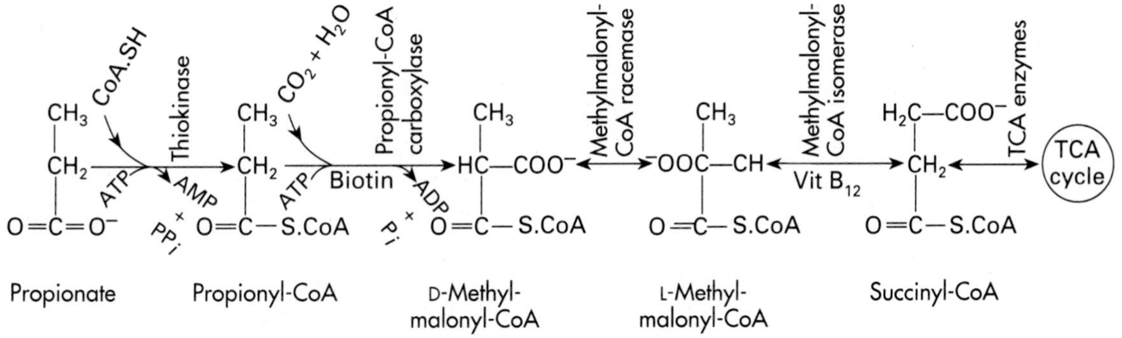

Figure 12-24. Conversion of propionate to succinyl-CoA.

equivalents of which four are carried by NAD^+ and one by FAD/ubiquinone. The net reaction is as follows:

$$C_3H_4O_3 \text{ (pyruvate)} + 5 \text{ O} \rightarrow 3 \text{ CO}_2 + 2 \text{ H}_2O$$

As a result of that complete combustion, 14 ATP can be produced by oxidative phosphorylation, in addition to 1 ATP equivalent (GTP) produced at the substrate level. Considering that 1 mol of glucose yields 2 mol of pyruvate, the mitochondrial portion of glucose combustion yields 30 ATP equivalents, as compared to 8 ATP equivalents for the cytoplasmic portion. With 1 mol of glucose approximating 686 Kcal worth of energy, and 1 ATP high-energy phosphate bond being equal to about 7.6 Kcal, it follows that approximately 42% of the energy of glucose is captured in the form of ATP during complete combustion.

The remainder of the energy of glucose escapes as heat, which aids in the regulation of body temperature. Of course, eventually, all energy of glucose is released as heat after the ATP is used up from serving its multipurpose.

Conversions of amino acids to TCA intermediates

Instead of referring to later discussions of amino acid metabolism, the text shall now consider processes whereby amino acids lose their amino groups on their way to becoming TCA intermediates.

Transamination

By transamination, amino acids are in reversible equilibrium with their corresponding α-ketoacids in a manner whereby one amino acid (e.g., glutamate) loses its amino group (and, thus, becomes α-ketoglutarate), while that amino group is transferred by pyridoxamine (vitamin B_6) to an α-ketoacid (e.g., pyruvate), which is thereby converted to the corresponding amino acid (alanine). This example describes the glutamate-pyruvate transaminase (GPT) reaction (Figure 12-25).

By the same mechanism, transamination between aspartate-oxaloacetate and α-ketoglutarate-glutamate is catalyzed by glutamate-oxaloacetate transaminase (GOT). Generally, all nonessential amino acids are in equilibrium with their α-ketoacids via transamination. The B vitamin pyridoxamine shuttles-NH_2 groups; another function of this vitamin is to shuttle CO_2 in the decarboxylations of amino acids to primary amines (e.g, tyrosine decarboxylation to tyramine).

The same transaminases in serum have an S as prefix and are called SGPT and SGOT; they are assayed for diagnostic purposes. Normally, the serum levels of these enyzmes are quite low, since GPT and GOT are predominantly intracellular enzymes. But

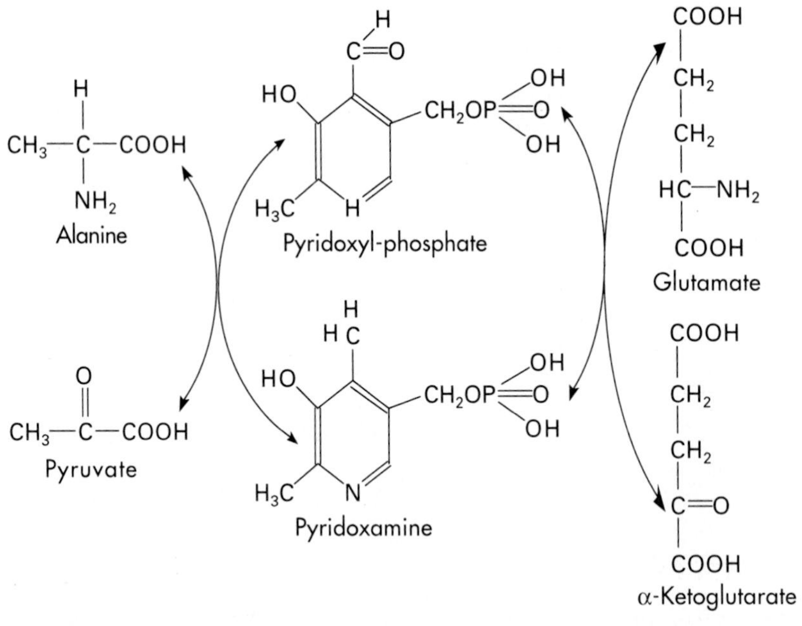

Figure 12-25. The glutamate-pyruvate transaminase reaction.

after tissue damage, the enzymes are liberated into serum. In addition to specific isozymes of LDH (see Chapter 4), corroborative evidence for a myocardial infarction may be obtained by observing elevated levels of SGOT, because the heart muscle is richer in GOT than in GPT. On the other hand, in acute liver disease, the level of GPT in serum may be elevated more than that of GOT. It should be emphasized, however, that GOT/GPT ratios of various tissues differ among animal species.

For the net conversion of amino acids to carbohydrate intermediates, transamination is not enough, since one amino acid is gained for each one lost. Transamination, then, serves only to supply a particular amino acid needed (e.g., for protein synthesis) at the expense of another amino acid. For the net conversion to a carbohydrate intermediate, an amino acid must not merely exchange, but rather get rid of the amino group.

Oxidative deamination

Straight oxidative deamination removes the α-amino group and produces the corresponding α-ketoacid and NH_3, which is detoxified in the liver's urea cycle. Quantitatively, though, this reaction is less important in animals, since the necessary enzymes for this process are present in few tissues and then only in low activities. Also, few amino acids are substrates for this reaction.

Transdeamination

For the net conversion of amino acids to carbohydrates and TCA intermediates, there are two specific transaminases present in most animal tissues: alanine transaminase and glutamate transaminase (Figure 12-26). These enzymes, with the help of pyridoxamine, reversibly transfer amino groups from almost any amino acid to pyruvate (forming alanine) and to α-ketoglutarate (forming glutamate). Since alanine is also a substrate for glutamate transaminase, all amino groups derived from different amino acids can be concentrated in glutamate. Glutamate, in turn, can be

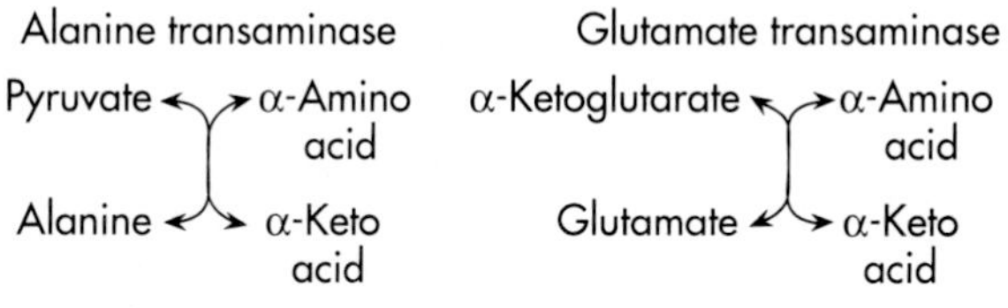

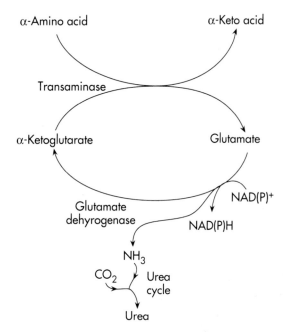

Figure 12-27. Transdeamination of α-amino acids.

oxidatively deaminated by glutamate dehydrogenase; the NH_3 formed is converted to urea in the liver (Figure 12-27).

By these mechanisms, all nonessential, and some essential, amino acids can be converted to their corresponding α-ketoacids. Most of these ketoacids are in equilibrium with TCA cycle intermediates or with pyruvate, and are therefore glucogenic. Some amino acids yield AcCoA and ketoacids, and, thus, are ketogenic (Figure 12-28). Glucogenic amino acids predominate in the composition of dietary proteins.

Citrate lyase

When sugar is converted to fat, the two cytoplasmic processes, that is, glycolysis to pyruvate and fatty acid synthesis from AcCoA, are separated by one mitochondrial step (conversion of pyruvate to AcCoA) and the transport of AcCoA from mitochondria to cytoplasm. In that transport, citrate serves as carrier, and AcCoA is liberated from citrate by citrate lyase (or cytrate cleavage enzyme) in the cytoplasm (Figure 12-29).

- The combination of mitochondrial citrate synthase and cytoplasmic citrate lyase works as a pump that shuttles AcCoA from mitochondria to cytoplasm. The pump is fueled by ATP, which is needed in the citrate cleavage process to es-

Alanine transaminase

Pyruvate ⇄ α-Amino acid

Alanine ⇄ α-Keto acid

Glutamate transaminase

α-Ketoglutarate ⇄ α-Amino acid

Glutamate ⇄ α-Keto acid

Figure 12-26. General transamination reactions. Not shown here is the involvement of pyridoxamine.

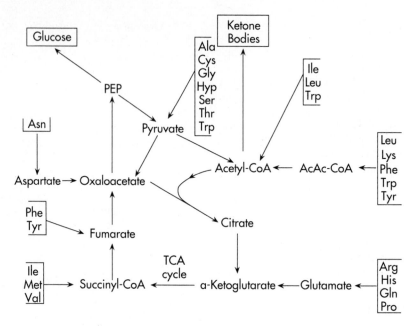

Figure 12-28. Glucogenic and ketogenic amino acids.

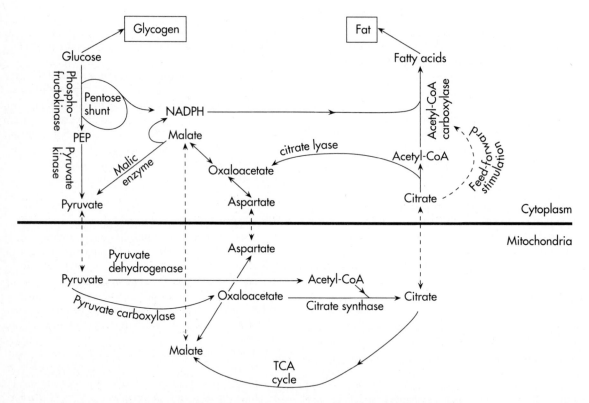

Figure 12-29. Role of citrate lyase in the conversion of glucose to fat.

tablish the high-energy bond between acetate and CoA.

- Ruminants obtain acetate from the rumen and activate that to AcCoA in the cytoplasm. Therefore, adult ruminants do not need the AcCoA shuttle, and citrate lyase activity is low in their livers.
- The illustration in Figure 12-29 brings out three key roles of citrate: (i) shuttler of acetate; (ii) feed-forward activator of fatty acid synthesis by stimulating AcCoA carboxylase; and (iii) NADPH source for fatty acid synthesis via isocitrate dehydrogenase and via malic enzyme.
- It is important to appreciate the pivotal function of citrate lyase for the purpose of lipid synthesis.

GLUCONEOGENESIS; DICARBOXYLIC ACID SHUTTLE
Functions and precursors of gluconeogenesis
Functions of gluconeogenesis

Since glycogen storage capacity is limited, the need for gluconeogenesis arises soon after a meal, because of the various metabolic functions for which glucose is indispensable. In concert with glycogenolysis, gluconeogenesis assists in maintaining a reasonably constant blood sugar level. Between regular meals, humans derive 75% of their glucose needs from glycogenolysis and 25% from gluconeogenesis, predominantly in the liver and renal cortex.

Gluconeogenesis removes lactate from the bloodstream. Lactate arises in resting human subjects from glycolysis under anaerobic conditions; that is, in erythrocytes, white blood cells, kidney medulla, and testis. Lactate also derives from muscle during exercise, and the liver converts lactate back to glucose via the Cori cycle.

Gluconeogenesis also removes glycerol from the bloodstream. In adipose tissue, the synthesis and breakdown of triglycerides (fat stores) is a continuous process. In the breakdown of triglycerides, free glycerol is formed. Adipose tissue lacks the enzyme glycerokinase, which in other tissues converts glycerol to glycerol phosphate, so that it can serve again for the synthesis of triglycerides. Therefore, glycerol is a waste product of adipose tissue metabolism that is allowed to diffuse into the bloodstream, from where tissues that contain glycerokinase, such as the liver and kidneys, remove and phosphorylate it. Then, depending on the need for glucose and on the availability of other glucogenic precursors, glycerol phosphate is used either for synthesis of triglycerides and phospholipids (and released into the blood in the form

of lipoproteins by the liver), or it is used for synthesis of glucose. One can trace this course of events in Chart I.

Gluconeogenesis in different tissues

Most tissues are theoretically capable of gluconeogenesis, but erythrocytes, adipocytes, heart, and smooth muscle are not, (since these tissues lack fructose-1,6-bisphosphatase activity). The liver and kidneys, especially, exhibit abundant gluconeogenesis, because the presence of G-6-P-ase activity allows these organs to produce free glucose for export into the bloodstream. Studies on hepatectomized animals have assigned a great value to the kidney's role in glucose homeostasis.

Gluconeogenic precursors

The following compounds serve as endogenous substrates for hepatic and renal glucose production via gluconeogenesis:

- Amino acids have a variety of vital synthetic functions and are, therefore, used conservatively for gluconeogenesis. During their conversion to carbohydrate, their amino groups are irretrievably lost (excreted as urea). The utmost economy in expenditure of essential amino acids for gluconeogenesis is observed in order to save them as much as possible for protein synthesis. The majority of the amino acids form TCA intermediates and pyruvate, and are therefore glucogenic; other amino acids form AcCoA and, thus, are ketogenic. Especially important for gluconeogenesis are alanine in the liver and glutamine in the kidneys. It has been estimated that the contribution of the indispensible or semi-indispensible glucogenic amino acids to ruminant glucogenesis is about 5 to 7% of glucose produced in both the fed and fasted states.
- Lactate serves the purpose of gluconeogenesis in tissues with adequate oxidative metabolism, such as the liver and kidneys. Lactate is also readily oxidized in cardiac muscle, which is rich in mitochondria and rarely becomes hypoxic. A good source of glucose during exercise is lactate, and during concentrated carbohydrate feeding (where rumen lactate concentrations are greatly increased), L-lactate may be one of the major hepatic gluconeogenic precursors.
- Glycerol, the waste product of lipolysis in fat cells, is converted to glucose in tissues that contain glycerokinase activity; in particular, the liver and kidneys.
- Propionate, a volatile fatty acid produced by mi-

croflora of the rumen and those of the cecum (horses), is a major gluconeogenic source of glucose and glycogen. The percentage of glucose formed from propionate varies with diet, from a maximum of about 70% under heavy grain feeding in ruminants, to virtually none during starvation. Acetate and butyrate, the other major volatile fatty acids produced by gut microflora, and free fatty acids, generated from lipolysis, do not contribute to net synthesis of glucose.

Fructose-1,6-bisphosphatase

The pathway of gluconeogenesis is essentially a reversal of the E-M pathway of glycolysis. But there are four irreversible steps in the latter pathway that have to be circumnavigated in gluconeogenesis (see Charts V and VII):

- Conversion of PEP to pyruvate by pyruvate kinase.
- Conversion of pyruvate to AcCoA by pyruvate dehydrogenase.
- Conversion of fructose-6-phosphate to fructose-1,6-bisphosphate by phosphofructokinase.
- Conversion of glucose to glucose-6-phosphate by hexokinase.

The first two of these obstacles are circumvented by the dicarboxylic acid shuttle, the third one by pacemaking enzyme activity, fructose-1,6-bisphosphatase, and the fourth one by glucose-6-phosphatase.

Fructose-1,6-bisphosphatase (F-1,6-P_2-ase) is an inducible, key enzyme in gluconeogenesis. Factors and conditions that stimulate the dicarboxylic acid (DCA) shuttle, such as high ATP levels, also stimulate the F-1,6-P_2-ase reaction. Practically, thus, the gluconeogenic activities of the DCA shuttle and F-1,6-P_2-ase are synchronized. The DCA shuttle and F-1,6-P_2-ase are simultaneously stimulated by glucagon and glucocorticoids that are secreted in response to low blood sugar levels, and inhibited by insulin. The balance between glycolysis and gluconeogenesis is controlled at the level of hexose-phosphates by the fact that F-2,6-P_2 is both the allosteric activator of phosphofructokinase (i.e., glycolysis) and the inhibitor of F-1,6-P_2-ase (i.e., gluconeogenesis).

As F-1,6-P_2 stimulates conversion of PEP to pyruvate by feed-forward activation of pyruvate kinase, lowering the F-1,6-P_2 level will direct PEP, formed via the DCA shuttle, in the direction of gluconeogenesis. Such lowering may be due to: (i) stimulated F-1,6-P_2-ase activity by ATP and glucocorticoids or glucagon; or (ii) inhibited phosphofructokinase activity by high ATP or citrate levels.

F-1,6-P_2-ase is also, in another sense, the key to gluconeogenesis: some tissues have it, others do not. It is abundantly present in the liver and kidney and has been demonstrated in striated muscle tissue. On the other hand, erythrocytes, adipose tissue, and smooth muscle do not contain F-1,6-P_2-ase activity. Since only liver and kidney tissues contain glucose-6-phosphatase activity, only these organs can contribute glucose to the circulation via gluconeogenesis.

Dicarboxylic acid shuttle

The pathway from pyruvate to oxaloacetate and then on to PEP is called the **dicarboxylic acid** or **DCA shuttle.** (See Chart VII.) It allows pyruvate and compounds that can be converted to pyruvate, such as lactate and various amino acids, to be metabolized to PEP without having to traverse the irreversible step from PEP to pyruvate in the wrong direction. The free-energy drop from PEP to pyruvate is so large that two ATP equivalents would be needed to boost pyruvate back up to the energy level of PEP, which is accomplished through the DCA shuttle.

Pyruvate carboxylase

Pyruvate carboxylase tags a CO_2 on to pyruvate, so that oxaloacetate is formed. To drive the reaction energetically, one ATP is needed. Furthermore, the B vitamin biotin is involved as a shuttler for CO_2 obtained from bicarbonate. As expected, this reaction and, thus, gluconeogenesis is impaired in biotin-deficient animals. The mineral manganese is required for pyruvate carboxylase activity. Pyruvate carboxylase activity is especially high in the liver and kidneys, the main sites of gluconeogenesis.

Pyruvate carboxylase is a mitochondrial enzyme. By producing oxaloacetate, it replenishes TCA cycle intermediates and opens up the way for gluconeogenesis from pyruvate and compounds that are converted to pyruvate, such as lactate and various amino acids. For its activity, a high level of AcCoA (or better, a high AcCoA/CoA ratio) inside mitochondria is required. AcCoA serves as an allosteric activator of pyruvate carboxylase activity, even though AcCoA itself does not partake in the reaction.

Activation of the pyruvate carboxylase step by AcCoA is that which links energy metabolism to gluconeogenesis (Figure 12-30). The level of AcCoA starts to rise when fatty acids are broken down to fill a demand for energy, and this rise in AcCoA causes pyruvate carboxylase to replenish the TCA cycle, so that AcCoA can be combusted. But when the nec-

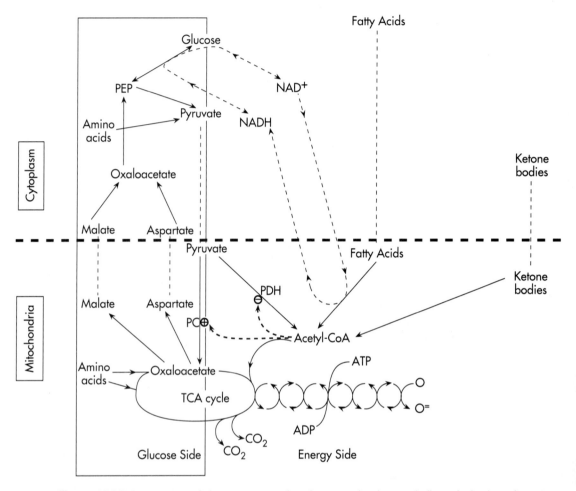

Figure 12-30. Importance of the pyruvate carboxylase reaction in metabolism. Activation of pyruvate carboxylase by acetyl-CoA links energy metabolism with gluconeogenesis. *PC,* Pyruvate carboxylase; *PDH,* pyruvate dehydrogenase.

essary energy has been supplied, ATP/ADP and NADH/NAD$^+$ ratios rise to the point where they inhibit TCA cycle activity. Consequently, the AcCoA/CoA ratio increases, causing inhibition of pyruvate dehydrogenase (PDH) and stimulation of pyruvate carboxylase (PC) activity, so that high levels of oxaloacetate are established for gluconeogenesis via the PEP-carboxykinase step. The latter situation occurs in periods between meals, when fatty acids are combusted for energy, and gluconeogenesis supplies needed glucose.

PEP-carboxykinase

Conversion of oxaloacetate to phosphoenolpyruvate (PEP) is catalyzed by PEP-carboxykinase, which requires the energy of either GTP or ITP to drive the reaction in the uphill direction of PEP. This reaction is the focal point of gluconeogenesis, because all gluconeogenic pathways, either via pyruvate or TCA cycle intermediates, merge at oxaloacetate. (See Chart VII.)

The activity of PEP-carboxykinase responds to the intracellular level of cAMP. Thus, glucagon has a direct positive effect on the enzyme's activity. Glucocorticoids, by themselves, do not influence PEP-carboxykinase activity directly, but they do amplify glucagon stimulation. In the liver, epinephrine activates the enzyme, as do thyroid hormones and α-adrenergic stimulators. As expected, insulin decreases PEP-carboxykinase activity; after all, insulin acts to lower glucose levels, not to stimulate gluconeogenesis.

For the PEP-carboxykinase reaction to take place, the level of oxaloacetate must be high. Hence, pyruvate carboxylase must be active and this requires allosteric activation by AcCoA. AcCoA levels become elevated at times (e.g., between meals) when fat oxidation provides the body's energy. Also at these times, gluconeogenesis becomes increasingly more important. High levels of AcCoA then stimulate pyruvate carboxylase activity directly and PEP-carboxykinase activity indirectly (via elevated oxaloacetate concentrations), so that the DCA shuttle is ready to go when gluconeogenesis is called for.

Another way to look at oxaloacetate as the branching point of the TCA cycle and PEP-carboxykinase (gluconeogenesis) is that when ATP levels are low, citrate synthase has the lower K_m for oxaloacetate, thus directing oxaloacetate preferentially into the TCA cycle. Higher ATP levels decrease the affinity of citrate synthase for oxaloacetate and, thus, open up the pathway of gluconeogenesis.

PEP-carboxykinase is in the cytoplasm of the cell, but this has only a minor effect on interrelationships between the mitochondrial TCA cycle and cytoplasmic gluconeogenesis (with oxaloacetate in the branching point position.) Mitochondrial and cytoplasmic oxaloacetate readily exchange via reversible conversion to either malate or aspartate to which mitochondrial membranes are permeable.

For fat storage, adipose tissue requires a constant source of glycerol phosphate, since the tissue lacks glycerokinase. One such source is glucose, which is taken from the bloodstream and converted via dihydroxyacetone phosphate to glycerol phosphate. (See Chart V.) During fasting, when glucose is in short supply, adipose tissue removes increased amounts of lactate and amino acids (alanine) from the bloodstream. It is significant that the activity of PEP-carboxykinase in adipocytes is greatly increased during fasting; by this route, glycerol phosphate is generated.

REGULATION OF CARBOHYDRATE METABOLISM

Because of the numerous metabolic functions of glucose and its derivatives, and furthermore, since there are so many metabolic pathways that either lead to the formation of carbohydrates or that compete for carbohydrate utilization, there must be a well-balanced and adaptable control over carbohydrate metabolism. Such control needs to be centrally located, so that all aspects of carbohydrate metabolism, no matter where they occur in the body, are simultaneously taken into account. The central medium in which changes in the rates of production and utilization of glucose (no matter where they occur) are reflected is the bloodstream. Fluctuations in the blood glucose level are sensed by nervous receptors, which then transmit nervous signals to endocrine glands, which, in turn, secrete the appropriate hormones that direct pathways to counter blood sugar fluctuations. Such control over pathways is, of course, exerted at the location of rate-controlling steps.

Thus far, the text has concentrated on metabolism at the cellular level. However, nervous-endocrine control over metabolism involves not just single cells, but rather the interplay of various tissues and organs: an organism. It is now necessary to examine first lipid and protein metabolism at the cellular level, then the peculiarities of different tissues and organs, and ultimately the organismic functioning of the sum of all tissues before a more comprehensive outline of the nervous-endocrine control over metabolism can be meaningful. Meanwhile, though, a few notes on the regulation of carbohydrate metabolism are in order; in the process, some salient features of previous discussions are summarized.

Functions of glucose and its derivatives

- Nutrition (energy) for nervous tissue and red blood cells, white blood cells, retina, testis, and other tissues that lack either mitochondria or an adequate oxygen supply via the bloodstream (e.g., heavily exercising muscle).
- Storage as glycogen in various tissues to bridge periods between meals. This is especially important in the liver (blood glucose) and muscles.
- Serving as the source for glycerol phosphate needed for storage of fat as triglycerides in adipose tissue. Triglycerides supply glycerol for gluconeogenesis in periods between meals and during fasting.
- Serving to replenish TCA cycle intermediates (to grease the TCA machine), so that fats and ketone bodies can be combusted for energy purposes.
- Fueling the pentose shunt, which provides NADPH for synthetic processes (fatty acids; steroids) and ribose for the synthesis of nucleotides and nucleic acids.
- Serving in the liver, via the uronic acid pathway, to conjugate toxic compounds, so that these compounds can be excreted in bile; to provide

hexoses and hexosamines for the synthesis of glycoproteins and glycolipids; and to produce ascorbic acid (vitamin C) only in animals that lack this function of the uronic acid pathway, such as primates and guinea pigs.
- Producing lactose (milk sugar).
- Providing, together with other sugars that are interconvertible with glucose, the carbohydrate moiety of glycoproteins and glycolipids.
- Serving, via sorbitol (see Chart IV), as a source for fructose, which serves in the motility of sperm.
- Serving in the gut to support uptake and subsequent transport of dietary lipids, by providing the glycerol phosphate needed for intestinal esterification of lipids.

Need for carbohydrate supply
Dietary carbohydrates

Without dietary carbohydrates, lipid metabolism would be severely compromised, as can be seen from the list of carbohydrate functions. Also, protein metabolism, and, thus, the nitrogen balance, would suffer because increased demands for gluconeogenesis would deaminate amino acids with consequences that are eventually fatal. In short, since all carbohydrates (except vitamin C) can be synthesized in the body, there are no essential carbohydrates that have to be taken in with the diet, in contrast to fatty and amino acids, some of which the body cannot synthesize and, hence, are essential. But inclusion of carbohydrates in the diet is crucial for proper metabolic balance and for the highest feeding efficiency.

The ability of an animal to utilize dietary glucose may be determined by measuring its glucose tolerance (Figure 12-31). This relates the blood glucose concentration with the time after administering a test dose of glucose. When a normal animal is fasted and glucose is then given either orally or parenterally, the blood glucose level will temporarily increase and then return to normal fasting levels. Responsible for the return of blood glucose to normal levels is an increased concentration of insulin caused by stimulation of the pancreatic β cells by hyperglycemia. Insulin enhances facilitated transport of glucose into tissue cells and metabolic conversions leading to storage in the form of glycogen and triglycerides. In fact, the insulin response is large enough to cause a temporary hypoglycemia (see Figure 12-31), which may cause dizziness and even loss of consciousness. This situation then corrects itself by the release of glucagon and catecholamines. The glucose tolerance test is used clin-

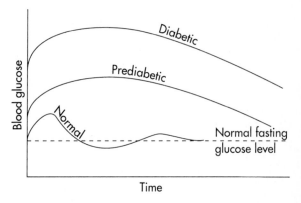

Figure 12-31. Glucose tolerance curves.

ically to aid in the diagnosis of diabetes mellitus. The disability to utilize glucose is demonstrated by an excessive and long-lasting hyperglycemia in response to a glucose challenge, a decreased glucose tolerance. In humans, having a normal blood glucose level but decreased glucose tolerance is characteristic of a latent form of pancreatic insufficiency, which later in life may develop into diabetes. Hence, the term **prediabetic.**

Gluconeogenesis

The body's carbohydrate storage capacity is very limited. The liver of a 70-kg adult human can store approximately 100 g of glucose in the form of glycogen. Regular meals restock this store, so that in periods between meals it supplies about 75% of the blood glucose. Between regular meals, thus, gluconeogenesis supplies 25% of the body's blood glucose, but that proportion increases to nearly 100% after a fast of over one day, which suffices to deplete hepatic glycogen. The relevance of gluconeogenesis in humans during starvation is that a constant glucose supply is of vital importance, as the following account will exemplify (Table 12-1).

In human subjects, the brain combusts glucose, and glucose is catabolized to lactate in anaerobic tissues, such as red blood cells, white blood cells, kidney medulla, retina, and testis. During exercise, muscle is added to this list.

The anaerobic tissues require approximately 40 g of glucose per day. Since these tissues cannot derive energy from any other source, this demand for glucose must be met even during prolonged starvation. Lactate produced by these tissues is converted back to

Table 12-1 Importance of gluconeogenesis in humans during starvation

	Glucose required per day		Glucose produced per day	
Early stage	Anaerobic tissues	40 g	Lactate (via Cori cycle)	40 g
	Brain	120 g	Glycerol (from adipose tissue)	20 g
		TOTAL = 160 g	Muscle protein (via Ala + Gln)	100 g
			TOTAL =	160 g
Later stage	Anaerobic tissues	40 g	Lactate (via Cori cycle)	40 g
	Brain	35 g	Glycerol (from adipose tissue)	> 20 g
		TOTAL = 75 g	Muscle protein (mostly Gln)	< 15 g
			TOTAL =	75 g

After the liver's glycogen stores have been exhausted, the brain's adaptation to the utilization of ketone bodies spares muscle protein.
Ala = Alanine; Gln = Glutamine

glucose in the liver at the expense of fatty acids for energy (the Cori cycle).

In early stages of starvation, the brain uses about 120 g of glucose per day. Once liver glycogen stores are depleted, this glucose must be provided by gluconeogenesis. Glycerol, released by adipose tissue, can support synthesis of about 20 g of glucose per day. The remaining 100 g must then come from amino acids derived from protein breakdown in muscle tissue. Measuring arterial-venous differences in muscles during starvation shows that 60% of the amino acids are released as alanine and glutamine, formed in the muscle from other amino acids. As starvation proceeds, the glucose requirement of the brain decreases to approximately 35 g per day, because ketone bodies are oxidized in preference to glucose by certain areas of the brain. Because of this, protein degradation in muscles needs only to supply roughly 15 g of the required glucose after prolonged starvation, and this conserves muscle protein. The decreased rate of gluconeogenesis from amino acids during prolonged starvation reflects mainly a decreased rate of hepatic gluconeogenesis from alanine. Consequently, as starvation proceeds, the relative importance of the liver as a site of gluconeogenesis decreases, while that of the kidney cortex, which uses glutamine, increases.

The following are two notes relating to the above:

• Gluconeogenesis from either glycerol or amino acids represents a net gain of carbohydrates for the body. In contrast, gluconeogenesis from lactate is merely a recycling (the Cori cycle) of carbohydrate.

• The ruminant liver is in a continual state of gluconeogenesis, whether being fed or fasted, since no glucose as such is derived from the digestive tract. Demands for glucose are increased during exercise, pregnancy, and lactation.

Control over carbohydrate metabolism by the autonomic nervous system

Metabolic functions of the autonomic nervous system

Functions of the autonomic nervous system (ANS) deal with emergency situations, repair mechanisms, and maintaining a constant internal environment (i.e., homeostasis). The ANS therefore is the center of neuroendocrine control over organ function.

The nervous pathway that connects detection of an environmental signal by a receptor to an organ or muscle for corrective action is called the **reflex arc.** For the ANS, a reflex arc consists of a receptor that is connected via an afferent nervous pathway to the hypothalamus, and from there via an efferent nerve (vagus nerve for parasympathetic and splanchnic nerve for sympathetic nervous system) to target organs, such as the liver, pancreas, gut, and adrenals.

Divisions of the ANS are the sympathetic and parasympathetic nervous systems.

• The sympathetic nervous system is associated with the "fight or flight mechanism." To this end, the liver makes glucose available, as glycogenolysis and gluconeogenesis are activated by direct nervous stimulation of key enzymes (phosphorylase, G-6-P-ase, and PEP-carboxykinase) and inhibition of pyruvate kinase. Lipolysis is stimulated by the activation of triglyceride lipase to provide needed energy. Thus, the overall effects of sympathetic nervous stimulation on metabolism are catabolic.

• The parasympathetic nervous system is associated with the postprandial "vegetative" situation and has, therefore, an anabolic effect on metabolism; for example, glycogen synthase activity and fat storage are stimulated under the influence of insulin.

Transmitter substances and second messengers of the ANS differ and allow differentiation of various receptors and ANS innervations. Adrenergic receptors are specific for epinephrine and norepinephrine and belong to the sympathetic branch. Cholinergic receptors are cholinesterase-specific and belong to the parasympathetic branch. Peptidergic receptors are sensitive to neurogenic peptides (e.g., bombesin, vasoactive intestinal peptide, cholecystokinin, and somatostatin) that travel via axonal transport. Specific activators and blocking agents exist whose actions help define subclasses within the above main classes of receptors. To exemplify the use of these agents: isoproterenol stimulates β-adrenergic receptors, while propanolol is used as a β blocker; when about 50% of a sympathetic effect on a target cell still prevails in the presence of propanolol, then peptidergic receptors must be involved. These receptors, called α_2 receptors, are defined by their inhibition of adenylate cyclase activity; clonidine stimulates α_2 receptors; the drugs yohambine and phentolamine negate clonidine's effect and are used to verify that an effect was mediated by α_2 receptors.

The various transmitter substances, when bound to their specific receptors, involve all three major second messenger systems (Figure 12-32):

- β-Adrenergics work via cAMP and protein kinases.
- α-Adrenergics work via IP_3 and Ca^{++} release from ER.
- Neurogenic peptides allow uptake of extracellular Ca^{++} and involve calmodulin.

ANS effects on metabolism are fast (mere seconds) and, because of the opposing sympathetic and parasympathetic branches, ANS effects are reversible.

Glucose homeostasis via the autonomic nervous system

Glucose receptors are present in the mouth, gut, liver (portal vein), and hypothalamus. These receptors sense deviations from the normal glucose concentration and send, via afferents, messages to the hypothalamus, which interprets them as either "too much" or "not enough glucose."

The hypothalamus is divided into ventromedial and lateral nuclei, among others.

- From ventromedial nuclei, sympathetic efferents (splanchnic nerve branches) go to target cells, such as liver, pancreas, adrenal, fat, gut, and heart tissue cells.
- From lateral nuclei, parasympathetic efferents

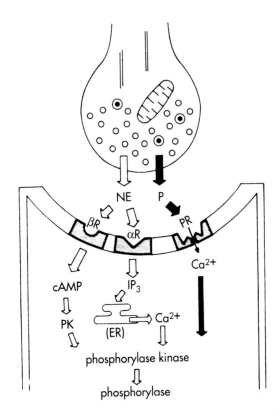

Figure 12-32. Second messenger systems of receptors of the autonomic nervous system. Postulated mechanism by which norepinephrine *(NE)* and a putative neuropeptide *(P)*, released simultaneously from sympathetic nerve terminals, lead to phosphorylase activation in a liver cell. *αR,* α-Adrenergic receptor; *βR,* β-adrenergic receptor; *PR,* putative peptide receptor; *IP,* inositol-1,4,5-triphosphate; *cAMP,* cyclic 3',5'-AMP; *PK,* protein kinase; *ER,* endoplasmic reticulum. *Reproduced with permission from Shimazu T: Neuronal regulation of hepatic glucose metabolism in mammals, Diabetes/Metabol Rev 3:185-206, 1987.*

(branches of the vagus nerve) go to target cells.

ANS effects on carbohydrate metabolism are outlined in Figure 12-32.

The lateral hypothalamus contains the feeding center, and the ventromedial section the satiety center. The effect of these antagonistic centra is that glucose glut inhibits food intake, while glucose shortage activates feeding.

Parasympathetic effects promote storage of glucose by effecting insulin release from the pancreas and activating glycogen synthase in the liver (Figure 12-33). Sympathetic effects counter a drop in blood glu-

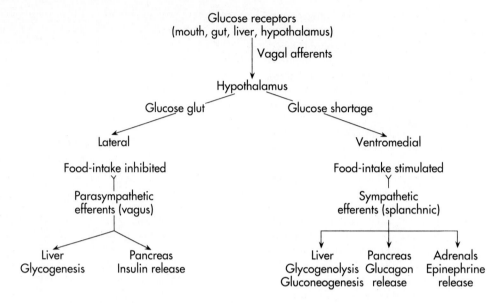

Figure 12-33. Control of glucose metabolism by the autonomic nervous system.

cose level by stimulating the key hepatic enzymes for glycogenolysis (phosphorylase) and gluconeogenesis (PEP-carboxykinase), and by effecting releases of pancreatic glucagon and adrenal epinephrine.

ANS stimulation releases epinephrine from adrenals, and glucagon and insulin from pancreas, all with strong effects on liver metabolism. This creates a problem if one wants to establish the fact that key liver enzymes are activated directly, that is, without intermediation of these hormones. As ANS efferents adhere in their effector organs to the vascular endothelium, the ANS in the isolated perfused liver may be electrically stimulated at the site of an isolated blood vessel. By this method, direct ANS effects on key hepatic enzyme activities have been demonstrated (Figure 12-34).

Endocrine influences on carbohydrate metabolism

The bloodstream is the central medium in which the balance between glucose supply and demand for the entire organism is reflected. Various tissues and organs can make adjustments in their glucose utilization, such that they take up more glucose when the blood glucose level is high and then economize on glucose when blood sugar drops. Examples of this are numerous.

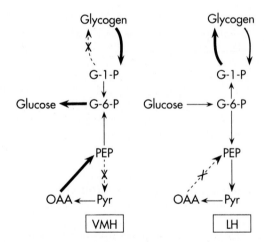

Figure 12-34. Reciprocal influences if the ventromedial *(VMH)* and lateral hypothalamus *(LH)* on carbohydrate metabolism in the liver. Broad arrows show steps stimulated and crosses denote steps inhibited. *G-1-P,* Glucose-1-phosphate; *G-6-P,* glucose-6-phosphate; *PEP,* phosphoenolpyruvate; *Pyr,* pyruvate; *OAA,* oxaloacetate. Reproduced, with permission, from Shimazu T: Neuronal regulation of hepatic glucose metabolism in mammals, Diabetes/Metabol Rev 3:185-206, 1987.

- The liver contributes glucose to the bloodstream, by glycogenolysis and gluconeogenesis, when the blood sugar level is low-to-normal, but takes glucose from the bloodstream, via glycogenesis and conversion to fats, when the blood sugar level is elevated.
- At low-to-normal blood sugar levels, muscle tissue feeds itself with fats and ketones from the blood, but at higher blood sugar levels, a shift toward uptake and metabolism of glucose, aided by insulin, is observed.
- The kidneys can serve as a blood glucose emergency valve when the tubular load exceeds the transport maximum for tubular reabsorption; in humans, this happens at a normal glomerular filtration rate when the concentration of blood glucose exceeds 180 mg glucose per 100 ml plasma, the same concentration as the Km for glucokinase in liver tissue.
- The brain shifts toward ketone body utilization during fasting.

As useful as these adaptations in the metabolism and functioning of various tissues are, they would by themselves be too insensitive, and too slow to avoid large and possibly detrimental changes in carbohydrate stores. Adaptations must be centrally organized and finely adapted to small fluctuations in blood sugar level by the neuroendocrine control system.

Hormones that affect carbohydrate metabolism are secreted either directly or indirectly in response to even small variations in the blood sugar level. However, the blood glucose level in the blood is not the only factor that causes the release of these hormones: fatty acids, ketone bodies, amino acids, and especially the presence of another hormone in the blood may influence the secretion of a given hormone. And this is understandable, for the same hormones that influence carbohydrate metabolism also modify lipid and protein metabolism.

For each hormone that influences metabolism in one direction, there is an antagonistic hormone that affects metabolism in the opposite direction. Hormones that activate the committing step in a metabolic pathway work in an inhibitory fashion on the key enzyme of an antagonistic pathway; for instance, insulin stimulates phosphofructokinase while inhibiting F-1,6-P$_2$ activity. In general, conditions that favor secretion of a given hormone are inhibitory to the release of antagonistic hormones. Also, the action of one hormone causes activation or inhibition of other hormones.

The text shall now consider the influence of various hormones on carbohydrate metabolism, limiting the discussion to the so-called **metabolic hormones.** It should be kept in mind, though, that numerous other hormones, whose primary functions are nonmetabolic, also affect carbohydrate metabolism, such as antidiuretic hormone and sex hormones.

Insulin

Insulin is secreted by the pancreas in response to high blood sugar levels, certain amino acids and intestinal hormones, parasympathetic nervous system activation and β-adrenergic agonists. Its mission is to store sugars, fats, and amino acids derived from the diet in their appropriate metabolic stores, that is, glycogen, triglyceride, and protein. Insulin also enhances uptake of K$^+$, derived from the diet, into muscle, erythrocytes, liver, and bone. Insulin promotes glucose transport into extrahepatic tissues (e.g., muscle and adipose tissue) and these tissues then shift their metabolisms to increased glucose utilization. In the liver, glucose uptake is not controlled by insulin, but insulin does affect hepatic glucose metabolism by counteracting the effects of glucagon. The activity of glucokinase is enhanced and that of G-6-P-ase inhibited, leading to increased production of G-6-P, which stimulates deposition of blood glucose in the form of glycogen (Figure 12-35).

Fat synthesis is stimulated by insulin, since the glycogen stores are rapidly filled and additional dietary glucose has to be stored as fat. Therefore, insulin stimulates: (i) all key enzymes required to convert G-6-P to AcCoA (phosphofructokinase, pyruvate kinase, pyruvate dehydrogenase, and citrate lyase); (ii) all three NADPH-generating systems (G-6-P-dehydrogenase of the pentose shunt, malic enzyme, and cytoplasmic isocitrate dehydrogenase); and (iii) AcCoA carboxylase, the key enzyme for fatty acid synthesis from AcCoA. The glycerol moiety of triglycerides is an important carbohydrate reserve for periods between meals.

Glucagon

Glucagon is the pancreatic antagonist of insulin: it is secreted in response to a lowering of the blood sugar level, exercise, stress, and β-adrenergic agonists (more so than insulin). Its function is to restore the blood glucose level back to normal and to control the economic use of the body's resources between regular meals. Glucagon acts chiefly on the liver, where the bloodstream carries it from the pancreas. It stimulates adenylate cyclase, and the second messenger cAMP

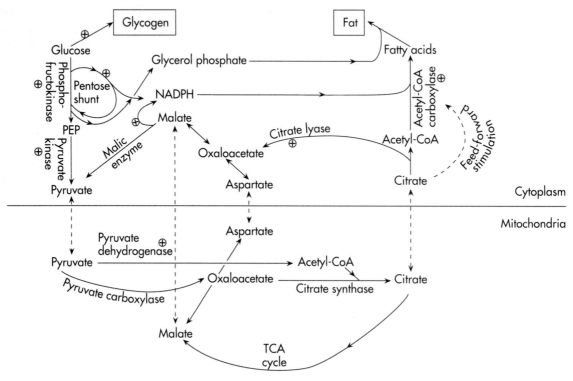

Figure 12-35. Effects of insulin on carbohydrate metabolism. Important direct stimulations are marked.

then activates phosphorylase (i.e., glycogenolysis). Since G-6-P-ase is also activated, free glucose is formed from glycogen and excreted into the blood-stream. Glucagon has no effect on muscle phosphorylase, so liver glycogen can be mobilized without simultaneously depleting muscle glycogen. In addition to its glycogenolytic action, glucagon stimulates generation of glucose by inducing key enzymes of hepatic glucoeneogenesis, by enhancing hepatic uptake of alanine (the chief amino acid exported from muscle) from the blood, and by supporting pyruvate transport from cytoplasm into mitochondria (Figure 12-36). Energy for gluconeogenesis, and metabolism in general, is provided by glucagon's stimulation of lipolysis. Fatty acids are β-oxidized to AcCoA and this promotes gluconeogenesis by (i) generating reducing equivalents in the form of NADH; and (ii) stimulating pyruvate carboxylase activity, thereby raising the concentration of oxaloacetate. Glucagon may in-

crease muscle uptake and catabolism of circulating fatty acids; however, it functions mainly at the level of the liver. Few effects of glucagon on muscle tissue have been described.

It is important to note that the metabolic chart, depicting the situation in the liver between regular meals, is divided into an energy side and a glucose side. It shows that energy is obtained from fat combustion, while the glucose balance is maintained at the expense of the protein stores. The two connections between the energy and glucose sides are (i) the formation and use of reducing equivalents (NADH/ NAD$^+$); and (ii) the formation of AcCoA from fat inhibiting pyruvate dehydrogenase (which spares glucose), while allosterically stimulating pyruvate carboxylase and, thus, gluconeogenesis (Figure 12-37).

To fully appreciate the antagonistic actions of insulin and glucagon, the respective schemes should be compared.

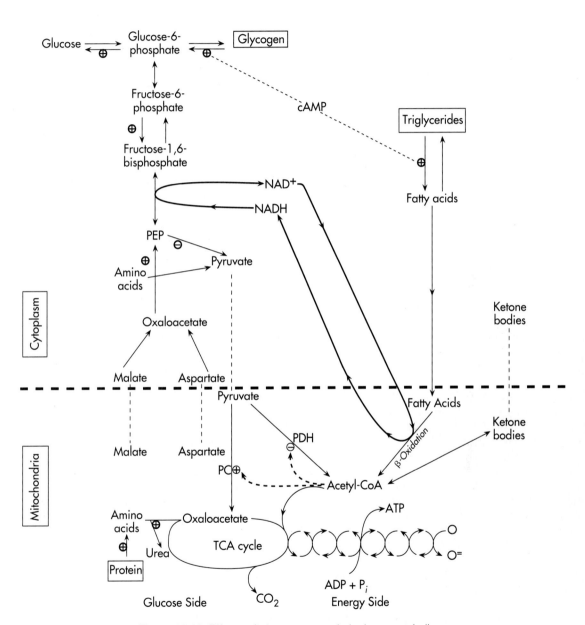

Figure 12-36. Effects of glucagon on carbohydrate metabolism.

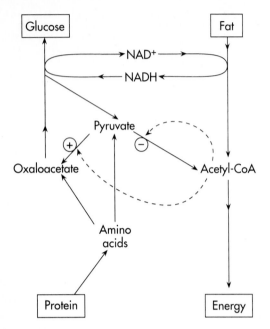

Figure 12-37. Two sides of metabolism and their connections.

Adrenocorticotropic hormone

Adrenocorticotropic hormone (ACTH) is one of the hormones secreted by the anterior pituitary in response to stress and hypoglycemia. Relating to carbohydrate metabolism, the most important function of ACTH to be considered is that it stimulates the release of glucocorticoid hormones from the adrenal cortex, namely cortisol.

Glucocorticoids

Glucocorticoids are steroid hormones secreted by the adrenal cortex in response to ACTH; their function is to restore a lowered blood glucose level back to normal. Glucocorticoids affect cellular metabolism by enhancing transcription of DNA-encoding key enzymes, such as phosphorylase, G-6-P-ase, F-1,6-P_2-ase, and PEP-carboxykinase; their mode of action is therefore slow, compared to that of glucagon, but enduring. Metabolic effects of glucocorticoids result from (i) stimulating lipolysis in adipose tissue; (ii) decreasing glucose uptake and increasing proteolysis and amino acid release in extrahepatic tissues; (iii) stimulating gluconeogenesis in the liver by increasing the synthesis of inducible enzymes; and (iv) increasing urea cycle (arginase) activity, needed to detoxify ammonia liberated in the conversion of amino acids

to glucose. Glucocorticoids have a "permissive" role; by themselves, glucocorticoids only slightly alter the rate of hepatic gluconeogenesis, but they are required for maximal glucagon stimulation of glucose production. Thus, glucocorticoids are insulin antagonists.

Epinephrine

Epinephrine (adrenaline) is secreted by the medulla of the adrenal gland in response to signals from the sympathetic nervous system. Stress, fright, cold, anxiety, nervousness, and hypoglycemia are conditions leading to a sympathetic nervous response. The function of epinephrine under these conditions is to provide the individual with quick energy. This energy, of course, has to come from combustion of glycogen and fat. But fatty acid combustion requires that the TCA machine in all cells be replenished with intermediates, for which purpose the liver has to provide glucose when glycogen stores are depleted.

Epinephrine stimulates lipolysis, glycogenolysis, and gluconeogenesis by both cAMP-dependent and Ca^{++}/calmodulin-dependent mechanisms. In adipose tissue, a cAMP-induced increase in triglyceride lipase activity causes fatty acid release, providing free fatty acids as a nutrient to muscles and, at the same time, promoting gluconeogenesis in the liver. (See Figure 12-36.) In muscle, epinephrine activates phosphorylase, so that glycogen is degraded and lactate exported. Stimulation of hepatic gluconeogenesis by epinephrine is primarily mediated by a large increase in the mobilization of lactate and alanine from extrasplanchnic tissues (as witnessed, for instance, by a dramatic increase in Cori cycle activity after pharmacological epinephrine infusion). To support the rapid release of glucose from the liver, the activities of key enzymes involved in glycogenolysis and gluconeogenesis are activated: phosphorylase, G-6-P-ase, F-1,6-P_2-ase, pyruvate carboxylase, and PEP-carboxykinase.

More often than not, elaboration of one hormone affects various other hormones. These endocrine interrelationships complicate the task of assigning specific metabolic actions to specific hormones. Case in point: epinephrine inhibits insulin and increases glucagon release, in addition to having effects on numerous other hormones.

Thyroid hormones

Thyroxine (tetraiodothyronine) and triiodothyronine affect metabolism in a concentration-dependent manner. In low concentrations, thyroid hormones are protein-anabolic, in high concentrations catabolic. Triiodothyronine is the faster acting of the two hormones. Cold stress releases large amounts of the thyroid hormones; their function is to produce heat. To this end, they uncouple oxidative phosphorylation, so that energy produced by nutrient oxidation is released as heat, instead of being partly trapped in the form of ATP. To compensate for increased rates of nutrient oxidation, food intake must increase or else the patient will lose weight rapidly. Similar effects are produced by either injecting animals with high doses of thyroid hormones or by administering drugs that stimulate the thyroid to overactivity.

The effects of thyroid hormones on key enzymes are mediated by interaction with DNA in the nucleus. Thyroid hormones stimulate hepatic gluconeogenesis from alanine and lactate in the following manners: (i) pyruvate kinase, and, thus, glycolysis, is inhibited; (ii) β-adrenergic receptor synthesis is stimulated, thereby potentiating the actions of catecholamines (iii) by lowering the activity of phosphodiesterase, the level of cAMP is raised, and this in turn may also explain why thyroid hormones potentiate the actions of glucagon and the catecholamines; (iv) by stimulating hepatic uptake of alanine, the substrate concentration for gluconeogenesis is increased. Hypothyroidism reverses all of these effects.

Growth hormone

Growth hormone (somatotropin) promotes growth by stimulating both the transport of amino acids into cells and DNA and RNA syntheses. In carbohydrate metabolism, the growth hormone has diabetogenic properties, since its action antagonizes that of insulin. In the liver, the growth hormone increases glycogenolysis and gluconeogenesis from amino acids. These effects lead to elevated blood glucose levels and, thus, to stimulation of insulin production. In muscle, growth hormone impairs glucose uptake and glycolysis; fatty acids are used for energy, because of the lipolytic action of growth hormone.

Control of growth hormone secretion from the pituitary is by two hypothalamic peptides: growth hormone releasing factor and growth hormone release-inhibiting factor. The latter factor, also called **somatostatin,** is produced not only in the hypothalamus, but also in the stomach and in D cells of the islets of Langerhans in the pancreas. Somatostatin serves as: (i) a paracrine factor, inhibiting both insulin and glucagon release; (ii) an inhibitor of growth hormone release; (iii) an agent that diminishes Ca^{++} uptake by cells, thereby suppressing the effects of growth hormone; (iv) a neurotransmitter in the brain; (v) an inhibitor of gastric emptying, gastric acid production, and gut motility by which flux of nutrients in the gut is regulated. The latter function is finetuned to need by the fact that a major stimulus for the elaboration of somatostatin into the portal blood is the presence of high levels of glucose or amino acids.

In the liver, the growth hormone stimulates the production of somatomedins (sulfation factors). These promote growth, since they bind to insulin receptors on cells, where they exhibit insulin-like activity, including down-regulation of insulin receptors; therefore, they are potentially diabetogenic.

Control over pathways

Metabolic charts show that carbohydrate metabolism can be considered as the metabolic "backbone" to which lipid and protein metabolisms are attached. All metabolic pathways are normally in a state of balance, and challenges are met by shifting directions of pathways. Such shifts are brought about by modifying the rate-controlling steps.

Metabolism never stops: pathways go either one way or the other, but they do not stand still. Thus, conditions that activate glycogen synthase inhibit phosphorylase; fructokinase is inhibited by conditions that activate $F-1,6-P_2$; high levels of AcCoA inhibit the oxidative decarboxylation of pyruvate, but they activate pyruvate's anabolic route of entry into the TCA cycle as oxaloacetate.

Whether a pathway goes in the forward or reverse direction is, to a large extent, determined by the presence of allosteric factors, the levels of which, in turn, may be controlled by hormones. These factors regulate the activities of rate-controlling enzymes in metabolic pathways by feed-forward and negative feed-back controls. Allosteric factors determine not only the direction of a given pathway; they also interrelate different pathways, so that, for instance, carbohydrate and fat metabolism become integrated. Examples of the synchronization of different pathways are: (i) uptake and glycolysis of glucose by adipose tissue and the rate of triglyceride synthesis; (ii) uptake and phosphorylation of glucose in the liver (glucokinase) and glycogen synthase activation; and (iii) provision of energy by fatty acid oxidation, establishing high levels of ATP and citrate, which then inhibit phosphofructokinase, so that glucose is spared from going through the destructive E-M pathway of glycolysis, and gluconeogenesis can take place.

Especially important in meshing the gears of various pathways are the cofactors, not so much their concentrations (for they do not fluctuate much), but their ratios: AMP/ATP, NADH/NAD$^+$, etc. Examples are (i) the activity of phosphofructokinase as it is affected, via adenylate kinase, by AMP/ATP; (ii) pentose shunt activity that provides NADPH, which is then used for lipid synthesis; and (iii) TCA cycle activity tied to oxidative phosphorylation by production and utilization of NADH.

Phosphorylation/dephosphorylation is a powerful means whereby the activities of key enzymes are synchronized. In general, phosphorylation activates processes that generate free glucose (glycogenolysis and gluconeogenesis), whereas dephosphorylation activates key enzymes involved in storage of glucose, either as glycogen or fat. For example, when insulin lowers the level of cAMP (by stimulating phosphodiesterase activity), it inactivates cAMP-dependent protein kinases, so that glycogen synthesis can occur; insulin activity facilitates conversion of glucose to fat by keeping all key enzymes dephosphorylated and, thus, active (e.g., phosphofructokinase (via stimulated F-2,6-P$_2$ formation); pyruvate kinase; pyruvate dehydrogenase; citrate lyase; and AcCoA carboxylase).

Paradoxes

Evidence, based largely on radiolabeled compounds, indicates that a proportion of glycogen deposited in the postprandial state is not derived directly from glucose, but rather indirectly after part of the glucose has been converted in the liver and extrahepatically to pyruvate/lactate, and the latter has regenerated G-6-P via gluconeogenesis in the liver. This finding, reported by several groups of researchers and contested by others, implies that in the liver gluconeogenesis would proceed postprandially and that at the same time glycolysis would go on to support conversion of glucose to fat. The most cogent explanation for this paradox is zonation in the liver: there are large differences in enzyme activities of periportal (zone 1) and perivenous (zone 3) liver cells. In acid-base balance discussions, the text has already taken note of zonation (i.e., ureagenesis in zone 1 during metabolic alkalosis; glutamine synthesis in zone 3 during metabolic acidosis). In carbohydrate metabolism, zonation could explain the simultaneous occurrence of opposing pathways in the liver (i.e., gluconeogenesis in zone 1; glycolysis in zone 3).

Another paradox surrounds pyruvate kinase activity in the liver. Despite increased pyruvate kinase activity, allowing glucose conversion to lactate, gluconeogenesis thrives via the DCA shuttle. One might ask, Why is it that PEP produced via the DCA shuttle does not all leak away toward pyruvate, as energetics would predict? Again, compartmentation in the liver may be the answer. These, and other controversial findings, suggest that much is still lacking in the overall understanding of carbohydrate metabolism.

So numerous are the interrelations between carbohydrate, lipid, and protein metabolism, that it would be misleading for this text to continually separate them. In looking upon metabolism from the carbohydrate point of view, many of the main aspects of lipid and protein metabolism have already been covered. Discussion shall now proceed in subsequent chapters to explore lipid and protein metabolism at the cellular level.

STUDY QUESTIONS

1. Regarding carbohydrate chemistry:
   a. Why are only D-sugars found in animals?
   b. List two common epimers of D-glucose.
   c. Name a nine-carbon, anionic amino-sugar in glycoproteins.
   d. Name a deoxysugar found in glycoproteins (e.g., blood group substances).
   e. Name a source of cyanogenic glycosides.
   f. List a glycoside that contains a steroid aglycone.
   g. List the monosaccharides that make up "milk sugar."
   h. How are the three α-D-glucose units linked at the site of a branching point in glycogen?

2. a. List the vital function of carbohydrates that is related to hypoglycemic coma.
   b. List two types of cells that derive their energy chiefly from blood glucose.
   c. List the main class of dietary ingredients that would not be intestinally absorbed if glucose were lacking in the diet.

3. Dietary glucose, entering the liver in large amounts after a meal, must be immediately disposed of. Some can be combusted for energy, but by far most of it is stored in two forms, namely _____. To that end, the "hormone of plenty," namely _____, activates three key enzymes that are active at the hexose level, namely _____. (Fill in the blanks.)

4. What is the homeostatic significance of having a Km for hepatic glucokinase equivalent to the glucose concentration at which receptors in renal proximal

tubular cells become saturated, thereby allowing glucose to appear in urine?

5. Roughly, how much glycogen does the human liver store? If calorically insignificant, what makes the glycogen stores so important?

6. Explain why muscle glycogen cannot contribute directly to blood glucose, but can do so indirectly.

7. *a.* Explain the functionality of the fact that glucagon does not activate muscle phosphorylase.
   b. List a hormone that enhances glycogenolysis in muscle.

8. *a.* List two hormones that activate G-6-P-ase. Explain the functionality of this control.
   b. Give the collective term and one etiology for disorders in which liver and/or tissues are crammed with glycogen, while hypoglycemia may prevail.

9. Given the hormonal response to hypoglycemia and G-6-P-ase deficiency as the cause of a glycogen storage disease, explain the loss of control over glycogen deposition in the liver.

10. List the general modification in key enzyme structures responsible for the fact that hormonal stimulation of glycogenolysis simultaneously inhibits glycogenesis. Name these key enzymes.

11. *a.* How does glucagon (too large to traverse cell membranes) stimulate glycogenolysis?
    b. List an ensemble of mineral and protein involved in cAMP-independent stimulation of protein kinase activity.
    c. Given that thyroid hormones inhibit phosphodiesterase, what effect do these hormones have on glycogenolysis?

12. *a.* List the compound where glycogenesis branches away from lactose formation.
    b. List the polysaccharide that is an intermediate in the conversion of galactose to glucose.

13. *a.* List the clinical symptom resulting from intestinal lactase deficiency.
    b. List the clinical symptom of galactosemia.

14. Why is fructose referred to as a "rapid fuel"?

15. *a.* How is the uronic acid pathway involved in hepatic maintenance of the body's endocrine balance?
    b. List a uronic acid pathway function in dogs that is lacking in primates.
    c. In newborn animals (and humans), the low activity of glucuronyl transferase in the liver is manifested by what?
    d. Does severe carbohydrate shortage stop all functioning of the uronic acid pathway?

16. What important function has E-M glycolysis in the liver right after a meal? In adipose tissue? In muscle?

17. In the times between meals when the liver has to supply blood glucose, the glucose is obtained via two routes, namely _____. To this end, glucagon, by means of the cofactor _____, activates three key enzymes that are active at the hexose level, namely _____. (Fill in the blanks.)

18. List the cofactor that, in the liver, conveys the signal, "need for energy," and whose level is amplified by adenylate kinase, so as to stimulate / inhibit (choose one) glycolysis.

19. *a.* For what purpose must the postprandial liver overcome the inhibition of glycolysis caused by high energy levels in the cell?
    b. What allosteric activator of phosphofructokinase helps the postprandial liver overcome this inhibition?

20. *a.* A factor that stimulates the kinase activity that phosphorylates F-6-P in the 2-position inhibits glycolysis. (True/False)
    b. Anoxia activates glycolysis. (True/False)
    c. Citrate activates glycolysis. (True/False)
    d. Glucagon decreases the level of $F\text{-}2,6\text{-}P_2$. (True/False)

21. *a.* The activities of phosphofructokinase and pyruvate kinase are linked via feed-forward activation by which compound?
    b. What is another control mechanism that synchronizes activation of these two rate-controlling steps of E-M glycolysis?

22. *a.* Why must the pyruvate kinase step be stimulated postprandially and inhibited between meals in a liver cell?
    b. List the hormones responsible for these regulatory effects and their modes of action on pyruvate kinase.

23. List the pathway needed to traverse the pyruvate kinase step in the opposite direction, so that gluconeogenesis from lactate or alanine can occur. List the function of allosteric inhibition of pyruvate kinase activity by alanine.

24. Other than as an anticoagulant, why would one add fluoride to a blood sample?

25. Name the route whereby the liver converts the end product of glycolysis in a heavily exercising muscle back to the original nutrient of that muscle.

26. List the cofactor responsible for the fact that anoxia in exercising muscle cells leads to the production of lactate.

27. The presence of oxygen drastically increases the amount of glucose that must be catabolized to meet the cell's energy need. (True/False)

28. *a.* Considering the chief nutrient of erythrocytes, and their lack of mitochondria, what is the most

important metabolic end product that the mammalian red blood cell returns to the bloodstream?

b. List the pathway, other than E-M glycolysis, by which red blood cells derive energy from glucose.

29. As fat cells lack glycerokinase activity, by which pathway must they obtain the glycerol phosphate needed for postprandial fat deposition?

30. a. What links the rate of the pentose shunt to fat synthesis in adipose tissue after a meal?

b. What function has the pentose shunt in endocrine cells that contain an abundance of rough ER?

31. List two B vitamins involved in both the nonoxidative part of the pentose shunt and the pyruvate dehydrogenase reaction.

32. a. Why can muscles not generate NADPH via the pentose shunt?

b. List a function of the HMP shunt in muscles.

33. Why do pyruvate and lactate levels in the blood rise during thiamin deficiency?

34. List a condition (list cell type and time in relation to meal intake) whereby glycolysis and pyruvate dehydrogenase activity are high despite the fact that "plenty of energy" is available.

35. List two cofactor-related functions of malate in the cytoplasm.

36. Indicate leaks in the TCA cycle for the production of RNA bases and porphyrins.

37. a. Name the class of enzymes requiring biotin as a cofactor.

b. List the special mineral required for biotin-mediated reactions.

c. List two major pathways under the control of these enzymes.

d. Give a cause of biotin deficiency.

38. a. Name the trace mineral that must be fed to a cow so that her liver can convert propionate, produced in the rumen, to glucose.

b. What disease results from a lack of intrinsic factor?

39. a. What does a high ATP/ADP ratio mean to a cell?

b. How does the effect of this high ATP/ADP ratio on oxidative phosphorylation impede TCA cycle activity?

40. List the adipose tissue's important nonnitrogenous source for net glucose synthesis in the liver between meals.

41. Why can fatty acids not replenish TCA cycle intermediates?

42. List a purpose for, and a vitamin requirement of, the measurement of SGOT/SGPT ratios in plasma.

43. a. By which route is an amino acid converted to a TCA cycle (gluconeogenic) intermediate?

b. List the enzyme involved in getting rid of the amino moiety of amino acids in their conversion to glucogenic intermediates.

c. Identify two ways for the liver to metabolize NH_3, either entering from intestines or produced endogenously?

d. The brain exports NH_3 as _____. This is especially important in the brain, since NH_3 is very toxic to the central nervous system. (Fill in the blank.)

44. Sometimes it is better to have more than one good reason for doing something. Case in point: fat combustion spares glucose because:

a. High ATP/ADP ratios inhibit phosphofructokinase. (True/False)

b. High citrate levels activate $F-1,6-P_2$-ase.

c. High AcCoA levels inhibit pyruvate dehydrogenase.

d. Lactate dehydrogenase becomes activated.

e. High ATP lowers the K_m of citrate synthase for AcCoA.

45. For gluconeogenesis from alanine or lactate, what allosteric effect links the rate of fat oxidation with activity of the DCA shuttle?

46. For what purpose is phosphoenolpyruvate formation via the DCA shuttle stimulated in adipose tissue during fasting?

47. Regardless of whether amino acids are converted to pyruvate or to TCA intermediates, in their gluconeogenic pathway they are all converted to the TCA cycle intermediate _____, which can exchange between mitochondria and cytoplasm after conversion to _____. (Fill in the blanks.)

48. Citrate is an important metabolite for various reasons.

a. It shuttles _____ out of mitochondria. (Fill in the blank.)

b. It stimulates the production of _____ by feedforward activation. (Fill in the blank.)

c. It stimulates / inhibits (choose one) gluconeogenesis at the hexose-phosphate level.

49. a. List the enzyme that must be activated to transport "building stones" for fatty acid synthesis out of mitochondria.

b. List the hormone that activates this enzyme.

50. What criticism must one level against the statement that, in the postprandial liver, AcCoA generated by β-oxidation of fatty acids is shuttled out of mitochondria by the citrate lyase pump?

51. Indicate three sources of NADPH and list two uses for it.

52. *a.* Why is the lactate (produced by erythrocytes and the subsequent Cori cycle) not a source for net glucose synthesis?

  b. Why is glycerol a better precursor for net gluconeogenesis?

53. *a.* Can the muscle, at rest oxidize fatty acids? Ketone bodies?

  b. Is glucose the only energy source for the heavily exercising muscle, or can the muscle oxidize fatty acids?

54. *a.* Exemplify a futile cycle.

  b. What is the net reaction of a futile cycle?

  c. Give two physiologic advantages of a futile cycle.

55. Choose whether lactate or pyruvate is the better precursor for hepatic gluconeogenesis.

56. About meshing gears (synchronizing) of pathways, explain why:

  a. In an exercising muscle, the activity of GAP dehydrogenase is geared to lactic dehydrogenase activity.

  b. In adipose tissue after dinner, glucose uptake must accompany fat deposition.

  c. In the liver after dinner, pentose shunt activity parallels fat formation.

57. In times of glucose scarcity, what adaptation does brain metabolism make to spare muscle protein?

58. When a portal glucose receptor in the liver monitors a glucose glut:

  a. Will the appropriate autonomic nervous response be evoked via sympathetic or parasympathetic efferent signaling?

  b. List the efferent nerve that tells the pancreas what to do, and list what the pancreas then does.

  c. List a direct nervous effect on a liver enzyme.

59. This entire question deals with neuroendocrine effects mediated by the autonomic nervous system (ANS) in response to hypoglycemia.

  a. Where are afferent signals from glucose receptors processed?

  b. List the transmitter substance of adrenergic sympathetic nervous activity.

  c. List two major glucose-producing pathways (and one key enzyme in each one) in the liver and a lipolytic key enzyme in adipose tissue that are directly stimulated by that adrenergic sympathetic nervous activity.

  d. The sympathetic division of the ANS stimulates release of which pancreatic and which adrenal hormone?

  e. Hypothalamic elaboration of ACTH-RH leads to: (i) which hormone release from the anterior pituitary, and which, ultimately, from the adrenals? (ii) which remedial metabolic effects in the liver?

60. Why, when all adrenergic ANS receptors are blocked with drugs, are ANS effects on cells still in evidence?

61. *a.* List a synonym of epinephrine, and explain its function of simultaneously stimulating phosphorylase and triglyceride lipase; list the intracellular second messenger involved.

  b. In what direction and by which mechanism would a sudden epinephrine release influence blood glucose?

  c. For what purpose would glutamate dehydrogenase activity and the urea cycle be increased in the liver after epinephrine administration?

62. *a.* Outline two effects of glucocorticoids that promote gluconeogenesis.

  b. Explain why stimulation of gluconeogenesis and protein breakdown occur simultaneously under glucocorticoid stimulation.

  c. For what purpose do glucocorticoids stimulate arginase activity?

63. *a.* List an intestinal hormone that regulates the rate at which the stomach empties and, thus, the rate at which glucose is released from the gastrointestinal tract.

  b. Why do somatomedins act in an insulin-like fashion?

64. Circle the enzyme that makes each statement true.

  a. Insulin stimulates: PEP-carboxykinase; phosphorylase kinase; F-2,6-P_2-ase; F-1,6-P_2-ase; citrate lyase; malic enzyme.

  b. Glucagon stimulates: Pyruvate carboxylase; pyruvate dehydrogenase; pyruvate kinase; adenylate cyclase; phosphodiesterase.

65. What is the significance of the fact that glucagon activates the "A" system for alanine transport into the liver?

66. Why, in liver, are glucagon's effects more immediate than glucocorticoids' effects? Why is glucagon secreted into the circulation faster than glucocorticoids?

67. Explain why, due to its actions on carbohydrate metabolism, growth hormone is sometimes called "diabetogenic factor."

68. What are the reactions of an animal when its blood glucose level drops below a critical level?

69. *a.* Why would overweight middle-aged people be prevalent among prediabetics?

  b. What causes glucosuria in diabetes mellitus? Think of other causes for glucosuria.

70. In the time between regular meals:

  a. List the purpose served by protein and fat stores.

  b. List the connection whereby fat oxidation inhibits glycolysis.

13 Lipid metabolism

LIPID STRUCTURES AND FUNCTIONS
Definitions and functions

Lipids are insoluble in water but soluble in solvents such as ether and benzene. Functions of lipids are varied:

- Structural elements in cell membranes (fluid mosaic model), in myelin, and in the form of fat pads;
- Storage for energy (triglycerides in fat cells);
- Certain vitamins are lipids (A, D, E, and K);
- Certain hormones are lipids (sex hormones, glucocorticoids, aldosterone, prostaglandins).

Other functions of lipids are implicit from the discussions that follow. Familiarity with terminology and chemical properties of some major lipid classes is essential for understanding lipid metabolism.

Classification

Single lipids and conjugated lipids may be differentiated. Among single lipids are the short, medium, and long-chain fatty acids, fatty acid esters with glycerol (mono-, di-, and triglycerides), ordinarily referred to as fats and oils, waxes (esters of fatty acids with larger-sized alcohols), and sterols and steroids and their esters. Among conjugated lipids are phospholipids, glycolipids, sulfolipids, and lipoproteins.

One should not be too rigorous in classifying lipids as being water-insoluble, mainly because such a thing as "insoluble" does not exist; it is always a matter of degree. Short-chain, volatile fatty acids (C2-C4), such as acetate, propionate, and butyrate (important fermentation products of ruminal metabolism), are quite soluble in water, as are ketone bodies (acetoacetic acid and β-hydroxybutyric acid), but the larger the fatty acid, the less soluble it is in water. Some lipids, such as phospholipids and fatty acids, carry charges on their molecules. Uncharged lipids are generally called **neutral lipids** (e.g., fats and cholesterol).

Saturated fatty acids

The carbon chain of fatty acids consists of —CH_2— groups and is terminated on one end by a —CH_3 and on the other end by a —COOH (carboxyl) group. The carbon atom carrying the —COOH group is called the **α-carbon,** and the adjacent one the **β-carbon.** These terms surface, for instance, in α-ketoacids and β-oxidation of fatty acids. The ultimate carbon at the other end is called the **omega-carbon** (after the last letter of the Greek alphabet) or **n-carbon.** At neutral pH, the —COOH group is fully dissociated (—COO^-), giving the fatty acid a polar "head." As long as the polar head constitutes a large proportion of the fatty acid molecule, the compound is water-soluble. Saturated fatty acids are referred to by their total number of carbon atoms: thus, C18 is stearic acid, C16 is palmitic acid, C4 is butyric acid, C3 is propionic acid, and C2 is acetic acid. Because of their dissociation at physiological pH, fatty acids are often referred to by their anionic names: stearate, palmitate, etc.

Note that most fatty acids, saturated and unsaturated, have an even number of carbon atoms; this is because biosynthesis of fatty acids generally starts with acetate (2 carbons) and proceeds by tagging more acetates on.

Unsaturated fatty acids

Unsaturated fatty acids contain —C = C— double bonds. Adding a double bond to a linear, saturated fatty acid promotes twisting of the molecule. Thus, unsaturated fatty acids occupy more space and therefore are less tightly packed in biological membranes. Their loose structure in biological systems also imparts a lower melting point to unsaturated fatty acids compared with the more tightly packed, linear saturated fatty acids. Thus, desaturation of structural membrane fatty acids (i.e., addition to double bonds) is associated with lowering the melting point (making them oils at room temperature), and increasing membrane fluidity.

Oleic acid, a monounsaturated fatty acid, is one of the main lipids stored as triglycerides in the adipose tissue of most animal species; in ruminants, however, stearic acid predominates, making for harder fat. Oleic acid is formed from stearic acid by desaturating the bond between carbon atoms 9 and 10 in the middle of the chain (Figure 13-1).

Mammalian enzyme systems cannot desaturate fatty acids between carbon-1 (the omega- or n-carbon) and carbon-9. Therefore, polyunsaturated fatty acids (see Figure 13-1) with double bonds in that region are obtained from the diet. Linoleic acid is the principal fatty acid in oil obtained from plant seeds, such as corn or safflower oil. Since its ultimate double bond is at carbon-6, linoleic acid is the parent of a family of n-6 polyunsaturated fatty acids. Subsequent elongation and desaturation of linoleic acid at sites beyond carbon-9 yields arachidonic acid. Chloroplasts of plants contain an enzyme that desaturates linoleic acid at carbon-3, giving rise to linolenic acid, the parent of an n-3 family of polyunsaturated fatty acids. Elongations and desaturations beyond carbon-9 yield a C20 fatty acid with five double bonds (eicosapentaenoic acid) and a C22 fatty acid with six double bonds (docosahexaenoic acid). Though present in green leaves, certain vegetable oils (especially soy oil), and milk, eicosapentaenoic acid and docosahexaenoic acid are particularly concentrated in oils from fish and other marine animals, since they are synthesized by phytoplankton at the base of the marine food chain.

Because arrangements at the two sides of double bonds are all in cis-configuration, polyunsaturated fatty acids have a crescent shape. This explains why cholesterol is almost exclusively esterified to polyunsaturated fatty acids: the crescent shape provides a great deal of overlap, thus stabilizing lipid-lipid interaction between sterol and fatty acid. The other preferential binding site for polyunsaturated fatty acids, especially arachidonic acid, is the β-position of phospholipids (e.g., lecithin) in cell membranes and lipoproteins. Later, when discussing cholesterol transport from tissues to liver, the text shall elaborate on a crucial enzyme activity that transfers the polyunsaturated fatty acid from lecithin to cholesterol.

Polyunsaturated fatty acids have many functions

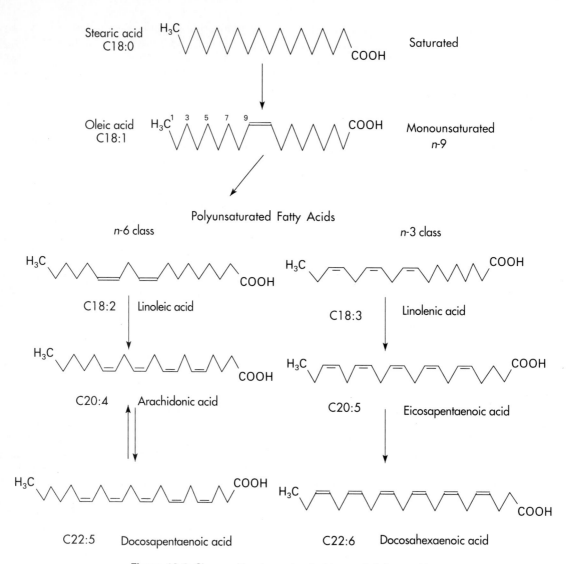

Figure 13-1. Classes of polyunsaturated (essential) fatty acids.

that are of vital importance. Because the body has difficulty synthesizing them, they must be included in the diet; hence, they are called **essential fatty acids (EFA),** namely, linoleic, linolenic, and arachidonic acid. Dietary EFA deficiency leads to retarded growth, reproductive failure, and changes in many organs including the skin, liver, and kidneys. Many of these, and other effects, are mediated by prostaglandins and leukotrienes, which are derived from arachidonic acid. Recently, the high concentration of docosahexaenoic acid in the phospholipids of the cerebral cortex, retina, testis, and sperm have led to defining

involvements of the n-3 family of EFA in various brain, optical, and reproductive functions. The n-3 fatty acids are now regarded as essential nutrients with their own specific functions, distinct from those of the n-6 EFA.

The essentiality of the longer-chained EFA is hard to prove, since animals, in general, can derive their n-6 and n-3 families from the parent compounds, linoleic acid and linolenic acid. The cat may be the only animal who lacks the desaturase enzyme activity that desaturates fatty acids at carbon-6; therefore, cats must be fed the longer-chain EFA, such as are found in fish. Young infants also have a limited capacity to metabolize the parent EFA into the longer-chained ones, and must be fed docosahexaenoic acid for brain and eye development. To this end, lactating mothers must increase docosahexaenoic acid in their milk by eating fish, and baby formula diets should contain docosahexaenoic acid and arachidonate.

Although ruminant animals normally receive a diet low in lipid, most incoming dietary saturated fatty acids pass unchanged through the rumen to be subsequently incorporated into animal tissues; however, dietary unsaturated fatty acids are subjected to hydrogenation by rumen microbes before passing into the intestine. In addition, microbes of the rumen carry out extensive lipolysis of dietary triglyceride; therefore, the small intestine receives mainly saturated, free fatty acids of dietary origin, rather than triglyceride and unsaturated fatty acids. One might ask the question then, "How does the ruminant animal derive its essential fatty acids?" Essential fatty acids for ruminant animals are derived from digestion of microbes in the small intestine and absorption of microbial lipid (i.e., recycled dietary carbohydrate).

Another dietary consideration for nonruminant animals is the ratio of linoleate (n-6) over linolenate (n-3), since those two EFA compete for the same desaturase and elongase enzymes. Hence, a 50 to 100 fold excess of linoleate (as in corn, safflower, sunflower, or peanut oil) can severely depress the body's synthesis of the n-3 family; soy oil is better balanced. Fish provides all necessary n-3 EFA at the lowest caloric intake. A striking example of the importance of this (n-6)/(n-3) ratio is that diets high in fat from vegetable and nonaquatic animal sources [rich in linoleate (n-6) and saturated fatty acids, deficient in n-3 EFA] lead to insulin resistance (non–insulin-dependent diabetes). A likely explanation for this is that n-3 EFA are potent inhibitors of lipoprotein production in the liver. When n-3 EFA are lacking, there is no inhibition of hepatic production of very low-density lipoproteins; peripheral tissues are then nourished by triglycerides contained in these lipoproteins, so that glucose is not removed from the bloodstream. The resulting high insulin levels lead to down-regulation of insulin receptors. Replacement of only 6% of the linoleate with long-chain n-3 EFA from fish oil prevents the development of insulin resistance, probably as a result of "fuel switching" with reduced fatty acid and increased glucose utilization in peripheral tissues.

Epidemiologic studies on Eskimos and on people in coastal villages (fisherpersons), compared to inland-dwelling farmers, have shown a correlation between increased fish consumption and decreased levels of blood cholesterol and mortality from coronary artery disease and strokes. Subsequent physiologic studies of the antiatherogenic property of fish oil have revealed a multitude of possibly beneficial EFA effects, including the following:

- EFA lower triglyceride, cholesterol, and apoprotein B production in the liver, and, thus, the secretion of hepatic, very low-density lipoproteins. This lowers serum cholesterol levels, as does an increased rate of cholesterol conversion to bile salts and excretion of the latter in feces under the influence of fish oil.

- In the process of hemostasis, platelets convert arachidonate to thromboxane A_2, which constricts arterioles and causes platelets to aggregate, so as to form a blood clot. The n-3 EFA of fish oil compete with arachidonate, and by inhibiting thromboxane A_2 production they work toward vasodilation and less platelet aggregation.

- Additional effects of n-3 EFA by which they decrease the viscosity of blood include increased deformability of erythrocytes, which improves oxygen supply to tissues under ischemic conditions, and increased fibrinolysis.

- Fish oils may suppress intimal smooth-muscle proliferation by decreasing the production of endothelial-cell–derived growth factors.

Adverse effects of supplementing diets with EFA are the increased conversion of polyunsaturated fatty acids to lipid peroxides and the toxic effects (cancer; aging of cells) associated with the latter. A possible increase of the requirements of vitamins E and C as antioxidants may be associated with EFA supplementation of diets.

Prostaglandins, thromboxanes, and leukotrienes

These three classes of compounds, collectively called the eicosanoids, are derived from arachidonic acid (Figure 13-2). The latter occurs predominantly in cell membranes, on the β-carbon (or A_2 position) of glycerol in lecithins and phosphatidylinositols. Certain agonists stimulate phospholipase A_2 activity, thus liberating arachidonate. Agonists have specific target cells: for example, thrombin for endothelial cells and platelets; bradykinin for renal tubular cells. Once released, arachidonate activates both cyclo-oxygenase and lipoxygenase enzymes; which of the three classes (and which specific compound) is produced depends on the cell's need.

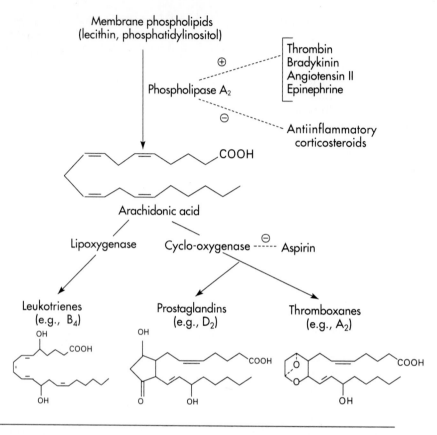

Figure 13-2. Formation of leukotrienes, prostaglandins, and thromboxanes from arachidonic acid.

The amount of arachidonate initially released provides the greatest push. Hence, the antiinflammatory potency of glucocorticoids, since they activate synthesis of a protein that inhibits phospholipase A_2 activity in cell membranes and, thus, inhibit formation of compounds derived from all three classes involved in inflammatory reactions. In contrast, aspirin specifically inhibits cyclo-oxygenase activity, but allows synthesis of leukotrienes; hence, aspirin inhibits blood clotting (mediated by prostaglandins and thromboxanes), but has no effect to ameliorate asthma (leukotriene effects).

Prostaglandins are active as hormone-like agents in lowering blood pressure, controlling microcirculation in tissues, stimulating smooth-muscle organs, and functioning in reproduction. Their pharmaceutical uses are being actively pursued.

Thromboxanes differ from prostaglandins in having a six-membered ring (instead of the five-carbon ring) that contains one oxygen atom in the ring structure and one bound between two of the ring's carbons. Produced by platelets in the process of hemostasis, thromboxane A_2 counteracts the main prostaglandin (i.e., PGI_2 or prostacyclin produced by the endothelial cells of the vascular system in that it promotes vasoconstriction and platelet aggregation.

Leukotrienes are elaborated by macrophages and leukocytes under immunologic and other stimulation. Leukotrienes are involved in many diseases with inflammatory and immune hypersensitivity reactions; for instance, they constrict bronchial airway musculature (hundreds of times more potently than does histamine), and they cause swelling and blisters by increasing vascular permeability. The slow-reacting substance of anaphylaxis (SRS-A) is a mixture of leukotrienes.

Sterols and steroids

A specificly conjugated ring structure is typical of this class of compounds (Figure 13-3). Apparently, small differences in molecular structure make for enormous differences in the functions of the various steroids. Cholesterol is the parent compound of the steroid family. Therefore, a brief discussion of cholesterol is in order.

Cholesterol is needed for the production of bile salts (for function in intestinal lipid absorption), ste-

roid hormones (sex hormones, glucocorticoids, and mineralocorticoids), cell membranes of animals (not plants), myelin, and lipoproteins (involved in lipid transport).

Cholesterol is present in every animal cell and, hence, it is taken in with the diet by carnivores and omnivores. Herbivores do not consume cholesterol in their diet, yet cholesterol is present in their tissue cells and milk: evidently cholesterol is synthesized in adequate amounts in the body.

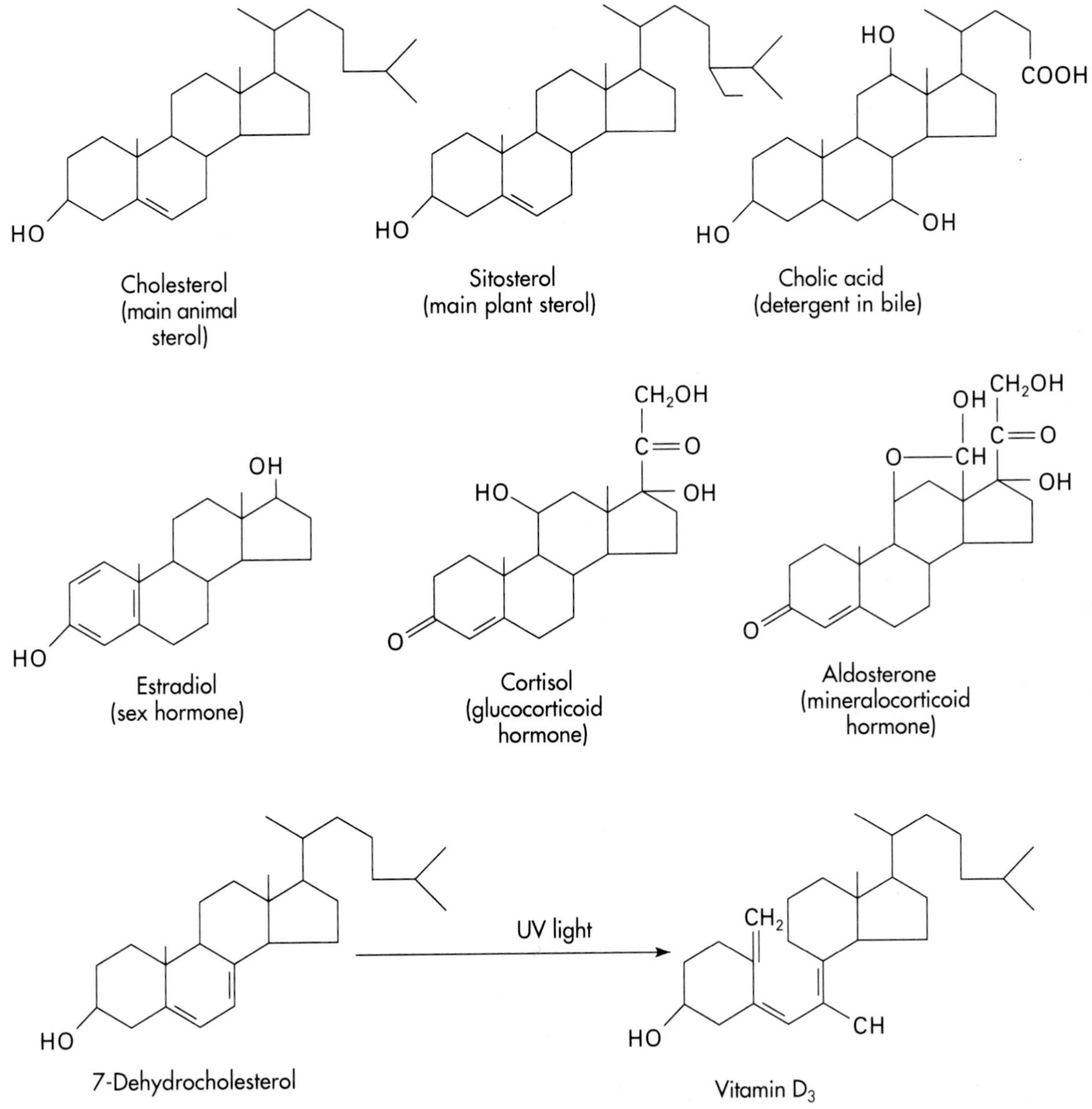

Cholesterol
(main animal sterol)

Sitosterol
(main plant sterol)

Cholic acid
(detergent in bile)

Estradiol
(sex hormone)

Cortisol
(glucocorticoid hormone)

Aldosterone
(mineralocorticoid hormone)

7-Dehydrocholesterol

UV light

Vitamin D_3

Figure 13-3. Diverse functions of steroids.

Cholesterol biosynthesis (Figure 13-4) takes place in the cytoplasm; the building block, AcCoA, which is formed in mitochondria from pyruvate or from fatty acid oxidation, must first be shuttled into the cytoplasm via the citrate lyase pathway. From three AcCoA molecules one hydroxymethylglutaryl-CoA (HMG-CoA) is produced. Then follows the rate-controlling step for the synthesis of cholesterol (or dolichol), namely, NADPH-requiring reduction of HMG-CoA to mevalonic acid under the influence of HMG-CoA reductase. The activity of HMG-CoA reductase is modulated according to the need for cholesterol synthesis. The enzyme is under allosteric (negative feedback) control by cholesterol and bile acids. In addition, its activity is regulated, in tandem with triglyceride lipase and AcCoA carboxylase, by adenosine monophosphate-activated protein kinase: phosphorylation inhibits HMG-CoA reductase activity. The HMG-CoA reductase step and subsequent conversions of the hydrophobic isoprene derivatives, via squalene, to cholesterol and steroids occurs in the membranes of the smooth endoplasmic reticulum.

Cholesterol has only one polar group, the phenolic OH-group, and hence, it is practically insoluble in water (and even less so when the OH-group is esterified to a fatty acid). Essential fatty acids esterify to cholesterol, since their crescent shapes allow lipid-lipid interaction. Under extreme conditions cholesterol precipitates in bile, where it is most concentrated, and gallstones are formed. This, in fact, is the origin of the word cholesterol (Greek "chole" means bile, "stereos" means solid).

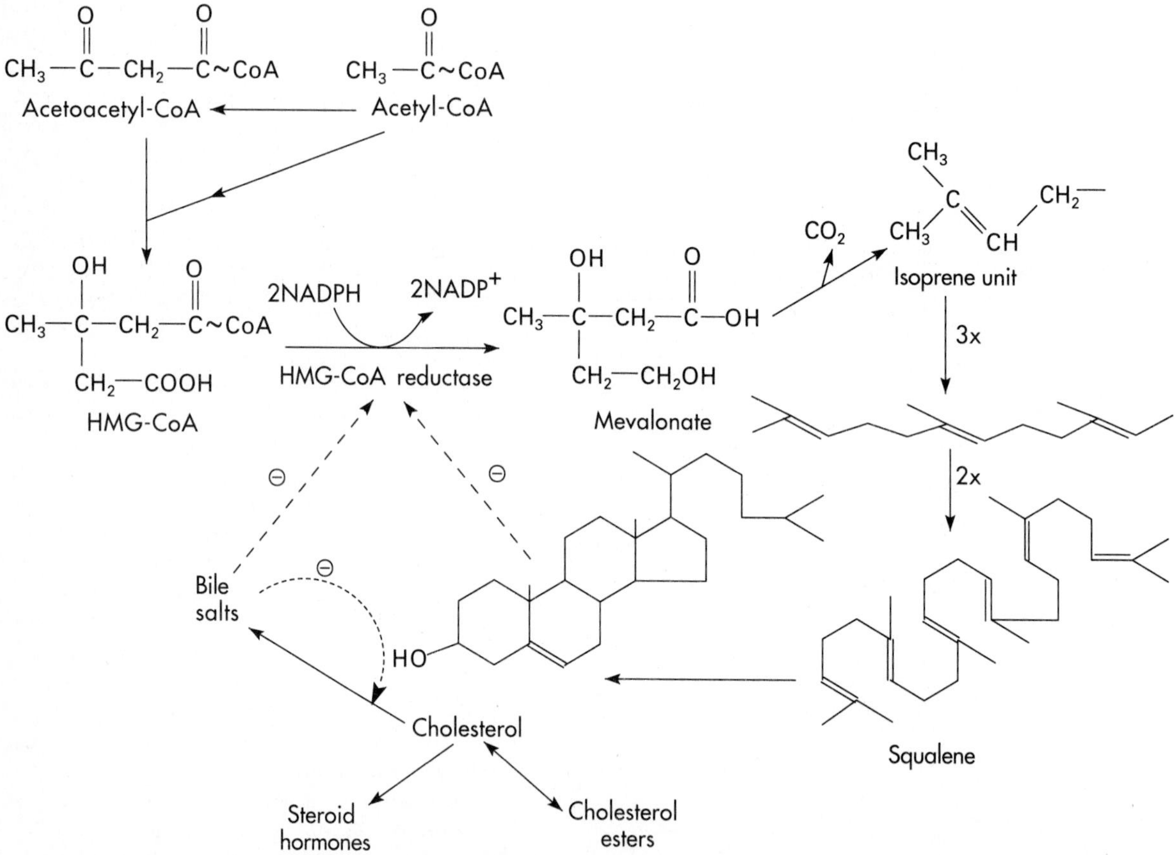

Figure 13-4. Cholesterol and steroid biosynthesis. *HMG,* Hydroxymethylglutaryl-CoA. Note the rate-controlling step, HMG-CoA reductase requires NADPH and is under negative feedback control by cholesterol and bile salts *(broken arrows).*

In three dimensions, the conjugated ring structure of cholesterol looks like an arrangement of can openers (Figure 13-5). In this way, the planar structure of the molecule becomes apparent, and it is easy to visualize how multiple cholesterol molecules can stack up to form a sheathlike structure, as in myelin.

Although cholesterol can be synthesized by all tissues of the body, synthesis in the liver, intestinal tract, and skin contributes to 97% of total cholesterol synthesis. Dietary cholesterol is normally less than half of total body cholesterol synthesis per day, and the amount of cholesterol used in steroid hormone synthesis is only 10% of that used in bile acid synthesis. Although bile acid synthesis and excretion by the liver is a major drain on the body's cholesterol pool, biliary cholesterol excretion is also a major route for cholesterol elimination. As an average over a 24-hour period, about 75% of the cholesterol normally present in the small intestine is that derived from bile.

Most cells that are capable of cholesterol biosynthesis produce just enough sterol for their own use. Exceptions are as follows: (i) during myelinization, Schwann cells in the peripheral nervous system produce huge amounts of cholesterol as an important constituent of myelin sheaths; (ii) small intestines produce large amounts of sterols for lipoprotein (chylomicron) formation; and (iii) cholesterogenesis in the liver serves the purposes of bile salt and lipoprotein production.

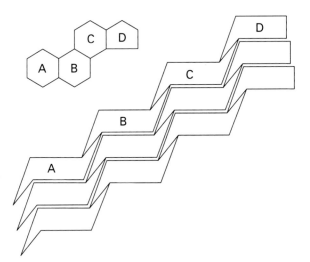

Figure 13-5. Two- and three-dimensional representation of the conjugated ring system of cholesterol.

As indicated above, the main catabolic route for cholesterol is its excretion in bile, mostly after being converted to bile salts, but also as free sterol. Conversion of cholesterol to steroid hormones requires NADPH, and this explains the high pentose-shunt activity during steroidogenesis in the adrenals and ovaries. Vitamin C also plays a role in the formation of phenolic —OH groups during steroidogenesis; after ACTH stimulation, the level of ascorbate in the adrenal cortex drops while corticosteroids are generated.

There is cholesterol homeostasis in the body: levels of the sterol in the blood and tissues are held constant. This means that the more cholesterol obtained from the diet, the less the body synthesizes, and vice versa. The average American diet contains about 0.6 g of cholesterol per day. Because cholesterol turnover amounts to roughly 2.4 g/dl, the body's rate of endogenous production is about 1.8 g/dl; that is, threefold that which is eaten. Cutting down on dietary intake, therefore, only slightly affects the body's cholesterol pool. One can, however, overindulge in foods that are rich in cholesterol (eggs, brain, lobster) to an extent that meets, or exceeds, the daily cholesterol needs. Under such conditions, endogenous synthesis does not cease completely, so that even more cholesterol is added and the pool size increases, giving rise to elevated blood and tissue cholesterol levels. The human body will protect itself by lowering the efficiency of intestinal cholesterol absorption and by negative feedback on the rate-controlling enzyme, HMG-CoA reductase.

An important aspect of cholesterol metabolism is the transport of this lipid in the form of lipoproteins. Later, under this heading, the text discusses the transport of dietary cholesterol from the gut to the liver, the distribution and redistribution of cholesterol from cells that have an excess to cells that need it, and the route of cholesterol elimination from cells to the liver to bile. The text discusses inborn and conditioned abnormalities related to lipoprotein metabolism that give rise to the formation of atherosclerotic lesions in blood vessels, which cause heart attacks and strokes.

The main plant sterol, sitosterol, differs from cholesterol in having one additional ethyl group attached to the side chain. As this extra ethyl group sticks out of the plane of the molecule, it forms a barb that blocks its passage across the membranes of the intestinal mucosa; hence, sitosterol is poorly absorbed from the diet. In fact, by forming mixed crystals with cholesterol in the gut, plant sterols impair absorption of

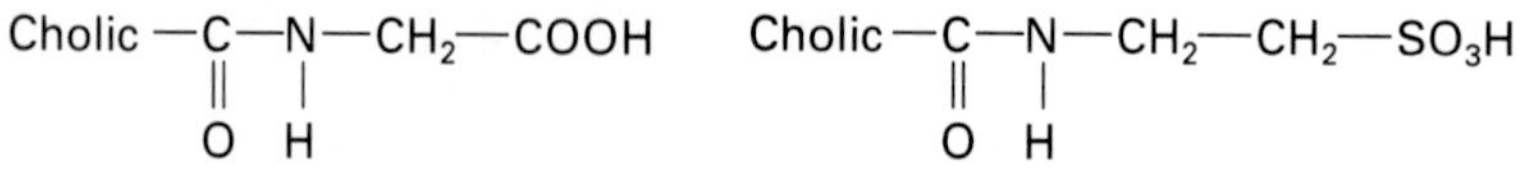

Cholic $-\overset{\overset{\textstyle O}{\|}}{C}-\overset{\overset{\textstyle H}{|}}{N}-CH_2-COOH$ Cholic $-\overset{\overset{\textstyle O}{\|}}{C}-\overset{\overset{\textstyle H}{|}}{N}-CH_2-CH_2-SO_3H$

Glycocholic acid
(conjugated with glycine)

Taurocholic acid
(conjugated with taurine)

Figure 13-6. Conjugated bile acids.

dietary cholesterol; they are used pharmaceutically for that purpose. Campesterol, with the smaller methyl group instead of the ethyl group in the side chain, is much better absorbed.

Bile salts are by far the most abundant metabolite of dietary and endogenously synthesized cholesterol. The structure of cholic acid is shown in Figure 13-3. The four polar groups that surround the hydrophobic part of the molecule are all oriented on one side of the molecular plane. This makes for an apolar side of bile salts where lipids can interact, and a polar side that interacts with water. Thus, bile salts act as the body's detergents. Different animal species have different proportions of various bile acids and their conjugates in the bile. Cholic acid has three hydroxyl groups, chenodeoxycholic acid and deoxycholic acid have two, and lithocholic acid has one. Furthermore, the carboxyl group can be present as either the free acid or conjugated to either glycine or taurine (Figure 13-6). Conjugation imparts a greater water solubility to these molecules, making them less likely to precipitate in a watery medium (e.g., bile).

Other important metabolites of cholesterol include the sex hormones, such as estradiol and progesterone (female), and testosterone (male). Adrenal cortical hormones, derived from cholesterol, include those that regulate mineral metabolism (aldosterone) and those that affect glucose metabolism in particular (e.g., cortisol and corticosterone).

The D vitamins are steroids, formed from cholesterol via 7-dehydrocholesterol, under the influence of the sun's ultraviolet light. Earlier, in the context of calcium metabolism, the text discussed the hydroxylation reactions by which the hormonal substance, 1,25-dihydroxycholecalciferol, is formed from vitamin D_3.

Esterification and saponification

The reaction between an alcohol, such as glycerol or cholesterol, and an organic acid, such as fatty acid, is called **esterification,** because an ester bond is formed under the exclusion of water:

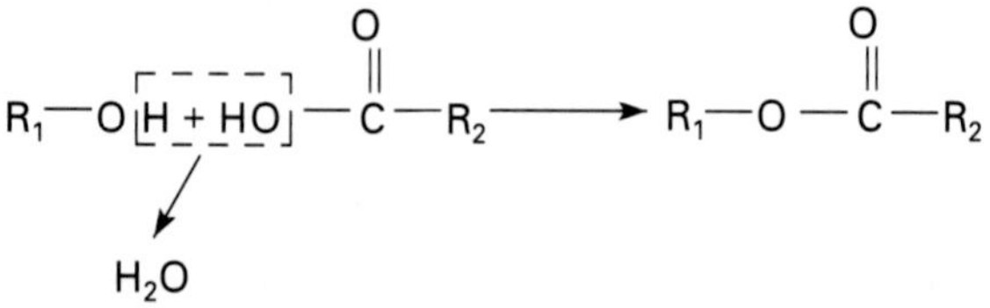

$$R_1-O\underset{\underset{\textstyle H_2O}{\swarrow}}{\lceil H + HO \rceil}-\overset{\overset{\textstyle O}{\|}}{C}-R_2 \longrightarrow R_1-O-\overset{\overset{\textstyle O}{\|}}{C}-R_2$$

Cholesterol is typically esterified with essential (unsaturated) fatty acids in circulating lipoproteins. Esterification thus creates a free-cholesterol and free-essential fatty acid gradient for transfer of these compounds from one tissue to another via circulating plasma lipoproteins.

The reverse reaction, whereby an ester bond is hydrolytically cleaved and free acid and alcohol are generated, is called **saponification,** which literally means soap formation, soaps being free fatty acids:

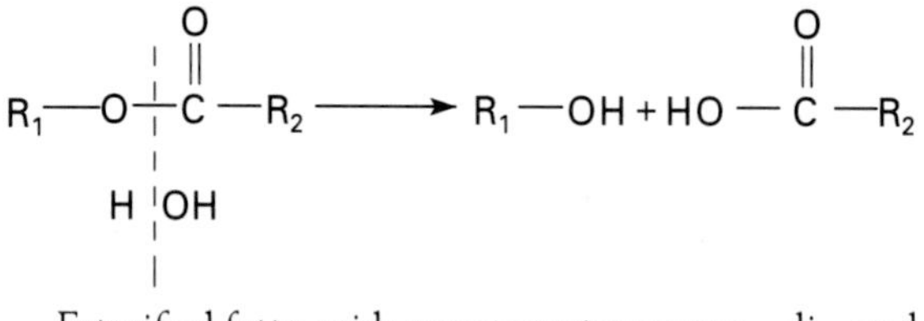

$$R_1-O\underset{\underset{\textstyle H \ OH}{|}}{\overset{\overset{\textstyle O}{\|}}{\underset{|}{C}}}-R_2 \longrightarrow R_1-OH + HO-\overset{\overset{\textstyle O}{\|}}{C}-R_2$$

Esterified fatty acids are present as mono-, di-, and triglycerides, phospholipids, sterol esters, and waxes. In lipid analysis of biological material, the isolated lipid mixture is usually boiled with alkali to hydrolyze the ester bonds and to produce water-soluble salts of the organic acids. Lipids that are not water-solubilized by the alkali treatment are called **nonsaponifiable.** Examples of saponifiable lipids are triglycerides and phospholipids; nonsaponifiable are cholesterol and steroid hormones.

Phospholipids

Lecithin is an example of a phospholipid. Because of numerous future references to lecithin, in which the structural details of the molecule are important, it is

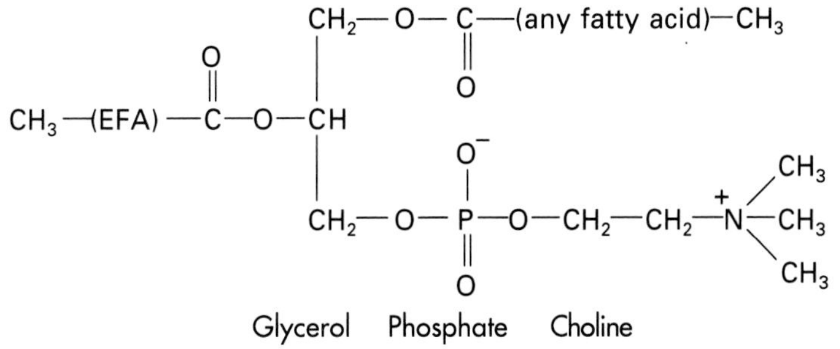

$$CH_2-O-C-(any\ fatty\ acid)-CH_3$$

Figure 13-7 structure showing:

$$CH_3-(EFA)-\overset{O}{\underset{\|}{C}}-O-CH$$

with glycerol, phosphate, and choline groups:

$$CH_2-O-\overset{O^-}{\underset{O}{\overset{|}{\underset{\|}{P}}}}-O-CH_2-CH_2-\overset{+}{N}\overset{CH_3}{\underset{CH_3}{-CH_3}}$$

Glycerol   Phosphate   Choline

Figure 13-7. Phosphatidyl choline, a lecithin. *EFA,* Essential fatty acid.

important to now consider its structure (Figure 13-7).

The centrally located three-carbon glycerol moiety contains two α-carbons separated by a β-carbon. With all three alcoholic OH— groups esterified to fatty acids, glycerol forms a triglyceride. In the case of a lecithin, one α-OH group can be esterified by any long-chain fatty acid. The β-position is more specific: it has a strong preference for a crescent-shaped polyunsaturated fatty acid, especially arachidonate. On the other α-position, phosphoric acid forms a double ester: on one side, it is esterified to glycerol, and on the other to the —OH group of choline.

Choline is a quaternary amine; it can be biosynthesized from ethanolamine by three subsequent methylation reactions in which methyl groups are provided by the essential amino acid methionine. In addition, choline is taken in with the diet, and the intestinal flora produces some. But there are circumstances, to be discussed later, that lead to choline deficiency, so that lecithins cannot be produced in adequate amounts. Lacking lecithins, the liver could not form lipoproteins, hence it could not package fats for export, so fats would accumulate, causing fatty liver degeneration. Because of this, choline is often included in vitamin mixtures. Phospholipids, in which choline's place is occupied by ethanolamine are called **cephalins.** By successive methylations a cephalin can be converted into a lecithin. Another important choline-containing phospholipid is **sphingomyelin.**

It is important to note that lecithin is a zwitterion: it has a negative charge (phosphate) and a positive charge (choline). These charges make for greater interaction with water, and, thus, for greater solubility. In fact, lecithin has lipid and water solubility. Hence, one function of lecithin is to stabilize lipoproteins

and emulsions in aqueous surroundings; for instance, stabilizing fat emulsion droplets in the gut by attaching lecithin molecules to the outside of those droplets in preparation of the fats being absorbed into mucosal cells.

Glycolipids

Cerebrosides and sulfatides occur in myelin; their structures contain galactose. Glycolipids also occur in lipoproteins. A reason why various glycolipids and phospholipids are found in the same biological structures (myelin, lipoproteins, cell membranes) is that, because of great similarities in their three-dimensional structures, they substitute for each other in the interdigitation of a continuous lipid matrix. Earlier, when reviewing cell membranes, the structures of glycolipids and lecithins were compared. (See Figure 6-3.)

Lipoproteins

Lipoproteins contain protein and lipid, and usually a small amount of carbohydrate. Lipoproteins are characterized in various ways: (i) by the identities of proteins and classes of lipids they contain; (ii) by their density; differences in densities among lipoproteins are caused by the fact that certain lipoproteins are protein-rich and therefore dense, while others are lipid-rich, making them less dense; classes of lipoproteins with different densities can be separated by ultracentrifugation; (iii) by their electrophoretic behavior, which separates them in classes similar to those obtained by ultracentrifugation. On the basis of their electrophoretic mobility and their ultracentrifugational pattern, lipoproteins are split into two main classes, namely α- and β-lipoproteins, each of which are divided into many subclasses. The main function of lipoproteins is to transport lipids in the bloodstream in a water-miscible form.

Micelles, emulsions, liposomes

Lipoproteins are one form in which lipids can be transported in aqueous surroundings; but not the only form. There are at least two situations in which proteins are not available for lipid transport; one is lipid absorption from the intestine, since proteins are digested there; the other is lipid elimination via bile. In these situations, amphoteric molecules, such as bile salts and lecithins, provide lipid transport. To this end, lipids are first saponified, so that their exposed polar —OH and —COOH groups can interact with water and with the amphoteric substances.

Most bile salts can form micelles (Figure 13-8) under proper conditions. In dilute solution they are present as individual molecules, but when the concentration of bile salts in the solution reaches a critical micellar concentration (CMC about 2mM), the molecules align themselves to form an organized structure, called a **liquid crystal,** or **micelle** (or **micel**). By lipid-lipid interaction between the apolar regions on the particle, internal coherence is established, while stability in the aqueous medium derives from water interaction with the outwardly directed polar groupings on the particle. Thus a stable, structured fat droplet in water is formed. In an oily surrounding, the micelle turns inside-out, exposing the lipid tails for interaction with the oil, and including a water droplet inside the polar region of the particle.

Molecules of different lipid classes can be incorporated in the bile salt micelle, thereby generating a "mixed micelle." Typically, one mixed micellar particle from the intestinal lumen might contain 47 long-chain fatty acids or monoglycerides, 2 lysolecithins, 2 cholesterols, some glycerol, and usually 1 fat-soluble vitamin (A, D, E, or K). Thus, they are normally small particles.

By the churning action of the stomach and gut motility, emulsion droplets (Figure 13-9) are formed from fats in the gastrointestinal tract. These emulsion particles contain largely apolar lipids (triglycereides). They are stabilized by having lecithin in their outer core to interact with the internal fat and with the water environment. Emulsion droplets have no internal structure and are quite large compared to micelles.

Liposomes are particles formed when a mixture of the appropriate lipids in the right proportions is sonicated in an aqueous medium. This way, lipid bilayers form around an aqueous core (Figure 13-10). The aqueous core may contain any water-soluble compound, such as proteins or drugs. Liposomes have

proven to be a fruitful research tool. Recently, they have become prominent as a means of administering foreign proteins to animals in a manner impervious to the immune system of the recipient. Also, by way of liposomes furnished with specific ligands, toxic drugs can be targeted to the exact cells of choice when those cells have the proper receptors for the ligands on their surface.

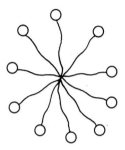

Figure 13-8. A micelle.

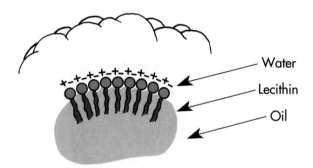

Water

Lecithin

Oil

Figure 13-9. Segment of an emulsion droplet.

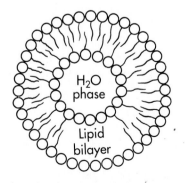

H_2O phase

Lipid bilayer

Figure 13-10. A liposome.

METABOLIC PATHWAYS: PHYSIOLOGICAL FUNCTIONS AND RATE CONTROL
Dynamic equilibrium

Adipose stores are in a constant state of flux. As shown by turnover studies of ^{14}C-labeled fatty acids, triglycerides stores are constantly degraded, their fatty acids either burned by some tissue or else transported to the liver, repackaged into lipoproteins, and redeposited in adipose tissue. In this section, the text considers the various metabolic pathways of lipid metabolism that allow the dynamic equilibria to exist.

Oxidation of fats

Neutral fats are stored as triglycerides. Oxidation of fats, thus, starts with hydrolysis of triglycerides—either by a lipase present in tissue cells or by lipoprotein lipase action on circulating lipoproteins. The free glycerol generated in tissues that lack glycerokinase (adipose tissue, muscle) is excreted into the bloodstream from where the liver removes it for the purpose of either triglyceride formation or gluconeogenesis. The free fatty acid liberated may be catabolized within the same tissue for energy purposes, or else excreted into the bloodstream where it is bound to albumin, offered as nutrient to other tissues and for the remainder taken up by the liver. A fatty acid is activated with CoA on the outside of mitochondria, then shuttled by a carnitine-carrier system across the mitochondriaal membranes, where it is next oxidized via the pathway of β-oxidation within mitochondria (Chart VIII).

Transport of activated fatty acids into mitochondria via the carnitine shuttle

Located on the outer mitochondrial membrane is the enzyme thiokinase, which activates fatty acids with CoA at the expense of either ATP or GTP. Fatty acyl-CoA, being too large a molecule to permeate the mitochondrial membranes, is converted with retention of the high-energy bond to fatty acyl-carnitine under the influence of the enzyme carnitine acyltransferase (CAT). After transport across the inner mitochondrial membrane by a translocase, fatty acyl-carnitine is reconverted by CAT to fatty acyl-CoA by combining with CoA from the mitochondrial pool (Figure 13-11). This liberates carnitine, which returns to shuttle another fatty acid molecule.

CAT has an important function in controlling fatty acid metabolism because of the fact that CAT is powerfully inhibited (allosterically) by malonyl-

CoA. The latter compound is formed as an intermediate in fatty acid biosynthesis. Therefore, when intracellular conditions prevail that stimulate fatty acid biosynthesis, and, thus, the level of malonyl-CoA rises, CAT is inhibited, so that fatty acids are not transported into mitochondria to their β-oxidative demise. On the other hand, fasting or hyperthyroidism increases CAT activity and, thus, powerfully increases β-oxidation.

The chemical structure of carnitine includes a quaternary amino group:

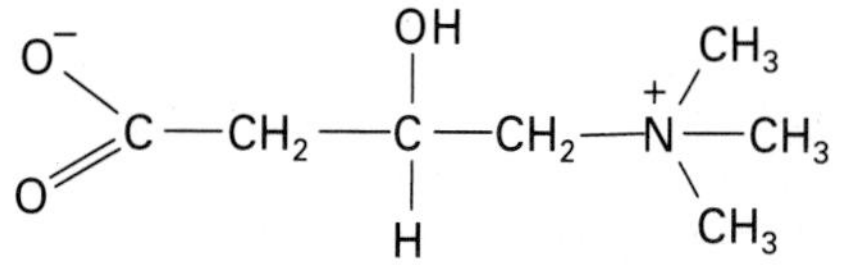

The compound can be synthesized in the body, particularly the liver, from the corresponding primary amine by successive methylations. Carnitine is also plentiful in milk. These methyl groups are derived from the essential amino acid methionine. It is known that diets deficient in methionine produce an accumulation of triglycerides in the liver (fatty liver). One explanation is that without methionine the formation of carnitine is impaired; fatty acids can then no longer be oxidized or converted to ketone bodies in mitochondria, so that the liver can do no better than storing them as triglycerides in the cytoplasm. Another explanation, discussed earlier, is that the formation of lecithin (containing the quaternary amine choline), and, thus, lipoproteins, is impaired.

β-Oxidation of fatty acids linked to the TCA cycle and oxidative phosphorylation

β-Oxidation of fatty acids occurs in mitochondria and in peroxisomes. In mitochondria, fatty acyl-CoA cycles through the pathway of β-oxidation (see Chart VIII) as if going through a meat slicer: with each successive "crank" of the cycle, one molecule of AcCoA is sliced off, ready for further metabolism, while one NADH and one reduced flavoprotein (FpH$_2$) are formed.

Peroxisomal β-oxidation was discussed earlier. In sum, it differs from its mitochondrial counterpart in these respects:

- Entry of fatty acyl-CoA does not require the carnitine shuttle.
- Oxidation is catalyzed by different enzymes, such as oxidases; it requires high oxygen tension, so

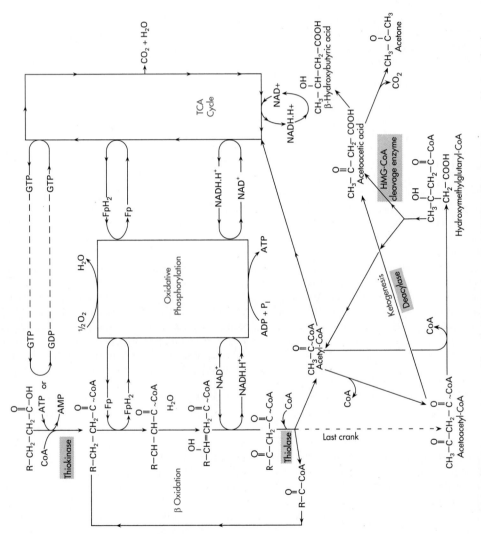

Chart VIII. Beta oxydation of fatty acids (relations to oxidative phosphorylation and ketone body formation in liver).

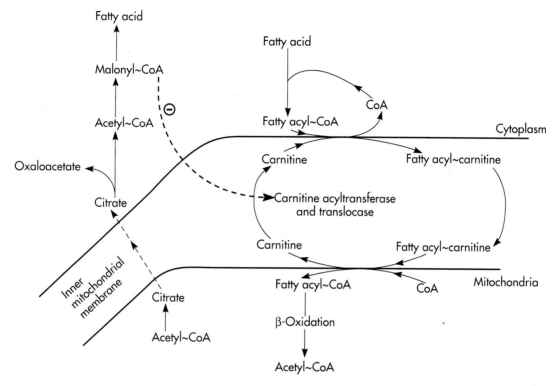

Figure 13-11. Carnityl acyltransferase activity in the inner mitochondrial membrane is allosterically inhibited by malonyl-CoA. Therefore conditions that stimulate synthesis of fatty acids *(left)* cause inhibition of fatty acid demise via β-oxidation *(right).*

it occurs predominantly in the liver and kidneys; it produces H_2O_2.

- It will not completely oxidize a fatty acid; rather, after removing some AcCoA, medium-chained fatty acids (e.g., octanoic acid) are exported via a carnitine shuttle; both AcCoA and the octanoate may then be further oxidized in mitochondria.
- Though any fatty acid larger than C8 can be oxidized, peroxisomes have a preference for very long-chained fatty acids, C20 and longer, that are poorly handled by mitochondria.
- Peroxisomal β-oxidation is not linked to energy production and, thus, can destroy fatty acids under conditions when mitochondrial β-oxidation is inhibited; thus, peroxisomal β-oxidation is inducible when needed; for instance, during fasting and high-fat feeding, by lipid-lowering drugs, and for thermoregulation.

In mitochondria, generation of AcCoA by β-oxidation of fatty acids is directly linked with, and metabolically regulated by, the TCA cycle and oxidative phosphorylation. (See Chart VIII.)

- GTP, the energy source for priming fatty acids with CoA, is generated in the TCA cycle at the substrate level.
- In the processes of β-oxidation of fatty acids and AcCoA combustion in the TCA cycle, flavoproteins (Fp) and NAD^+ accept electrons. FpH_2 and NADH thusly formed must be reoxidized via oxidative phosphorylation, otherwise, by lack of electron-acceptors, oxidation of fatty acids and AcCoA would stop. Oxidative phosphorylation, in turn, is controlled by the cell's need for energy (ATP/ADP and NADH/NAD ratios). Only when the cell needs energy is the ratio of ATP/ADP low, so that oxidative phosphorylation and TCA cycle activity increase; this produces GTP and oxidized redox cofactors with which fatty acid oxidation can take place to provide the cell

with the necessary energy. But when the ATP/ ADP ratio is up, oxidative phosphorylation diminishes, less NAD^+ and Fp are regenerated, TCA activity decreases, and fatty acids are not oxidized.

Energetics of fatty acid oxidation can be summarized as follows: 1 AcCoA oxidized in the TCA cycle yields 12 ATP. One crank of the β-oxidative cycle produces an NADH and a FpH_2, together worth 5 ATP. Considering that the β-oxidation of palmitate (C16) requires 7 passages through the oxidative path (35 ATP) and produces 8 AcCoA (96 ATP), while the equivalent of only 2 ATP are invested, the equivalent of 129 ATP worth of free energy is released. Since this is about 1000 Kcal, and the caloric value of palmitate is 2340 Kcal/mol when combusted in a bomb-calorimeter, better than 40% of the available energy is obtained in the form of useful free energy (ATP, NADH) by fatty acid oxidation. Carbohydrate combustion via the E-M path plus the TCA cycle also yields chemical energy with over 40% efficiency.

Tryglyceride is the most concentrated form in which the potential energy of the body can be stored. Its caloric value per unit mass is more than twice that of carbohydrate or protein, and it is associated with less water in storage. Fatty acids also provide more metabolic water upon oxidation than do carbohydrates or proteins, a characteristic that certainly makes fatty acid oxidation advantageous to mammals occupying dry environments and to birds migrating long distances.

Hepatic formation and extrahepatic utilization of ketone bodies

The reason for bringing up the topic of ketone body formation and utilization at this point, whereas bovine ketosis is discussed much later, is that metabolism of ketone bodies is another mitochondrial process that is intimately linked with fatty acid oxidation (see Chart VIII) and can thus be best understood in that context.

Ketone body formation

The compounds acetoacetate and hydroxybutyrate are the only freely soluble circulating lipids. Known as ketone bodies, they arise (from the partial oxidation of fatty acids) from the liver and can be used by most if not all aerobic tissues (e.g., muscle, brain, fetal liver, kidney, mammary gland, small intestine) except the adult liver. They are known to be important lipid-fuel in starvation and other conditions. The ketone bodies are misnamed, for they are not bodies, and hydroxybutyrate is not a ketone. The appellation ketone was given towards the end of the last century by German physicians who found that the urine of diabetic patients gave a positive reaction with reagents used to detect ketones. In these circumstances, not only acetoacetate but also acetone (propanone) would contribute to the reaction. Acetone, formed by the spontaneous decarboxylation of acetoacetate, is detectable only when the concentration of the latter is abnormally high. Acetone is not further metabolized but excreted through the kidneys and lungs (where it accounts for the characteristic sweet smell on the breath of severely diabetic patients).

Under physiological conditions, only the liver is able to synthesize ketone bodies (although the rumen wall will also contribute some ketone bodies to the circulation). It is probable that the flux-generating step for ketone-body formation is lipolysis of triglyceride in adipose tissue, so that the physiological pathway spans more than one tissue and includes adipose tissue, blood, and liver. Usually the pathway is considered to start at the level of long-chain fatty acids in the liver. Thus the first sequence of reactions in ketone body formation involves the activation of fatty acids, the transport of acyl-CoA from the cytosol into mitochondria, and the oxidative cleaveage of long-chain acyl-CoA to acetyl-CoA in the process of β-oxidation. The conversion of acetyl-CoA to ketone bodies requires three more stages: condensation of two molecules of acetyl-CoA to form acetoacetyl-CoA, deacylation of acetoacetyl-CoA, and reduction of some of the resulting acetoacetate to hydroxybutyrate. These processes all take place in mitochondria of the liver.

On the way down from the last crank in the β-oxidation of a fatty acid, "R" (see Chart VIII) has been diminished in size to just a CH_3-group, part of the compound acetoacetyl-CoA. At this point, when acetoacetyl-CoA has been formed, the pathway in the liver differs from that in extrahepatic tissues.

In extrahepatic tissues, acetoacetyl-CoA is thiolytically cleaved into two molecules of AcCoA and then oxidized in the TCA cycle. In the liver, deacylase activity prevails over thiolase, so that CoA is hydrolytically removed from acetoacetyl-CoA, and the ketone body acetoacetate is formed. (See Chart VIII.) This ketone can be reduced to hydroxybutyrate (the most abundant ketone body in the blood and urine), or it can be decarboxylated to acetone. But whatever their form, the adult liver cannot metabolize ketone bodies, and, thus, secretes them into the bloodstream. From there, extrahepatic tissues pick them up and use them as their preferred fuel.

Two hepatic pathways for ketone body production

Under normal dietary conditions, the liver constantly produces ketone bodies as a by-product of β-oxidation of fatty acids, since deacylase activity removes CoA from acetoacetyl-CoA. (See Chart VIII.) But under conditions of carbohydrate shortage leading to ketosis (discussed below) the liver copes with an enormous influx of fatty acids from the bloodstream by converting them to ketone bodies. It is helpful to consider that from one large fatty acid molecule, say stearate, only one acetoacetyl-CoA is formed that may be converted to acetoacetate by deacylase activity. At the same time, however, seven AcCoA molecules are generated. The pathway whereby that AcCoA is converted to ketone bodies is, thus, quantitatively the more important. This pathway (see Chart VIII), named after the Nobel laureate Lynen who discovered it, starts out by condensing two molecules of AcCoA, forming acetoacetyl-CoA; then a third AcCoA is added and another CoA is removed, leaving hydroxymethylglutaryl-CoA (HMG-CoA); finally, HMG-CoA is cleaved into one molecule of AcCoA plus one molecule of acetoacetate. Thus, the net of this pathway is:

$$2 \text{ Acetoacetyl-CoA} \rightarrow \text{Acetoacetate} + 2 \text{ CoA.}$$

Extrahepatic utilization of ketone bodies

Under conditions of normal health and proper nutrition, the liver does not form more AcCoA than it needs for metabolic functions and for energy production via combustion in the TCA cycle. The liver's limited rate of ketone-body production from acetoacetyl-CoA by deacylase activity is then offset by enzyme activities of extrahepatic tissues that activate ketone bodies with CoA to prime them for subsequent catabolism. The activated ketone body is thiolytically (using CoA) split into two molecules of AcCoA, which are then combusted in the TCA cycle.

Under normal conditions, muscles remove ketone bodies from the bloodstream as fast as the liver produces them, so that no ketone bodies accumulate. Actually, ketone bodies are preferred fuel for muscles; when muscle cells are incubated in a medium that contains a mixture of glucose, fatty acids, and ketone bodies, the muscle will take up the ketones first.

Conditions for ketosis

When carbohydrates are in short supply (fasting; lactation or pregnancy without dietary supplementation), shifts in the hormonal balance, allowing the body to cope with dwindling glucose reserves, cause degradation of triglycerides in adipose tissue at a rate that outweighs redeposition of fats. Excessive amounts of fatty acids are dumped into the bloodstream. Since tissues do not increase their intake of nutrients above their needs, the excess fatty acids have to be handled by the liver. The liver's capacity to repackage and export the incoming fatty acids in the form of lipoproteins is compromised under these conditions. Part of these fatty acids are esterified and accumulate, giving rise to fatty liver, but the liver's limited storage capacity for fat and the use of glycerol phosphate for gluconeogenesis limits the rate of triglyceride formation from excess fatty acids. At this point there is only one viable option: storing the fatty acids as such would be detrimental to the liver cells, so it is not done. Hence, the alternative is to destroy the excess fatty acids so that their metabolites become water-soluble. Massive amounts of fatty acids are β-oxidized in peroxisomes and mitochondria of the liver, and that leads to excessive mitochondrial ketone body formation for two reasons: (i) the large amounts of AcCoA produced by fatty acid oxidation saturate energy demands, raising the ATP/ADP and NADH/NAD$^+$ ratios, slowing down TCA cycle activity, and leaving AcCoA for ketone body production via the HMG-CoA (Lynen) pathway; and (ii) the activity of HMG-CoA cleavage enzyme increases greatly during fasting. As a result, the liver's ketone body production exceeds the energy demands of the muscles and, thus, ketone bodies accumulate in the blood (ketonemia) and spill over in urine (ketonuria). A reason for conversion of acetoacetate to hydroxybutyrate, the main ketone body in the blood, is to reoxidize NADH for continued β-oxidation in times when oxidative phosphorylation is down. (See Chart VIII.)

Since the mitochondrial NAD$^+$/NADH concentration ratio is normally maintained approximately constant at about 8.0, this sets the ratio of hydroxybutyrate/acetoacetate concentration in the liver, and hence that released into the blood, to within the range of 3 to 6. Thus, a considerably greater amount of hydroxybutyrate than acetoacetate is produced by the liver. Why two, rather than one, ketone bodies are produced is not entirely clear. Comparative studies indicate that acetoacetate is the more "primitive" ketone body, as it occurs in the absence of hydroxybutyrate in invertebrates and in some fish. However, hydroxybutyrate is the better fuel since it is more reduced, so why has acetoacetate persisted? The answer may be that to produce solely one or the other ketone body in large amounts could render ketone-body synthesis dependent on the redox state of the liver. However, if an equilibrium mixture of the two is produced, changes in the redox state of liver mitochondria simply alter the ratio of ketone bodies released.

Of some clinical importance is the fact that, in diabetic coma, the concentration ratio of hydroxybutyrate/acetoacetate can rise to as high as 15, probably due to disturbances in the hepatic NAD^+/NADH concentration ratio and the intracellular pH. Since a frequently used rapid test for ketonuria (using Clinistix or a similar material) detects only acetoacetate (and acetone), this can result in a serious underestimate of the extent of ketonuria.

Biosynthesis of fatty acids

There are two systems for fatty acid biosynthesis. Most important, quantitatively, is fatty acid synthesis from AcCoA, which takes place in the cytoplasm of the cell and mainly yields palmitate (C16) as an end product. But fatty acids other than palmitate abound in animal tissues; for example, in several animal species, including humans, oleic acid (C18, one double bond) is the most abundant fatty acid in the body's triglyceride stores.

Elongation of palmitate to stearate (C18) and desaturation to oleate takes place in the smooth endoplasmic reticulum. Most diets are much richer in carbohydrates than in fats, and, since carbohydrate storage capacity is limited, those carbohydrates are converted to fats that are characteristic for the species.

Another source of fat, of course, is the ready-made mixture of fatty acids absorbed from the diet; that is, the route by which the body has to obtain essential fatty acids. But also a large proportion of other fatty acids in human tissue are of dietary origin. The type of fat an animal deposits, hard or soft, can be influenced by diet. Also, the composition of milk fats reflects the diet.

Cytoplasmic fatty acid synthesis from acetyl-CoA

Like glycogenesis and glycogenolysis, lipogenesis (fatty acid biosynthesis) was previousley thought to be merely the reversal of oxidation. However, it now seems clear that unlike β-oxidation of fatty acids, fatty

acid biosynthesis is characterized by the following:

- It occurs in the cytoplasm.
- It is a reductive process, the reductant being NADPH.
- It requires a separate pathway from the reversal of oxidative reactions.
- Intermediates are covalently linked to acyl carrier protein, while those in β-oxidation are linked to coenzyme A.
- Many of the enzymes associated with fatty acid biosynthesis are organized into a multienzyme complex (called fatty acid synthetase).
- Fatty acid elongation takes place by sequential addition of 2-carbon units until palmitate (C16) is formed. Further elongation and/or desaturation are carried out by other enzyme systems.

This extramitochondrial system has been found in the cytoplasm of many organs and tissues including liver, kidney, brain, lung, mammary, and adipose tissue. Cofactor (or coenzyme) requirements for fatty acid biosynthesis are as follows:

ATP

Manganese

NADPH

Bicarbonate (a source of CO_2)

Biotin

The pathway of cytoplasmic fatty acid synthesis from AcCoA is illustrated in Chart IX. In the cytoplasm, the multi-enzyme complex is present, which combines with an activated acetyl group forming a high-energy acetyl-enzyme bond. Elsewhere in the cytoplasm, malonyl-CoA is produced from AcCoA plus CO_2 at the site of AcCoA carboxylase, the key enzyme. The multi-enzyme complex, already associated with acetate, establishes a high-energy bond with the malonyl group (releasing free CoA), and then reacts the acetyl's carboxy-end with the reactive middle-carbon of malonic acid; in this reaction, the same CO_2, attached to an AcCoA by AcCoA carboxylase, is removed, and an acetoacetyl group bound to the enzyme complex is left. In the following reactions at the site of the multi-enzyme complex, the —CO group of acetoacetyl-enzyme complex is reduced to a —CH_2 group; the reduction involves two NADPH-reducing equivalents, and forms butyryl-enzyme complex. The latter compound accepts another malonyl-CoA, which after loss of CO_2 and β-reduction reactions, yields the fatty acid that is two carbon atoms longer. After seven malonyl-CoA have been successively tagged onto the original AcCoA, and the last β-reduction reactions have been completed, palmi-

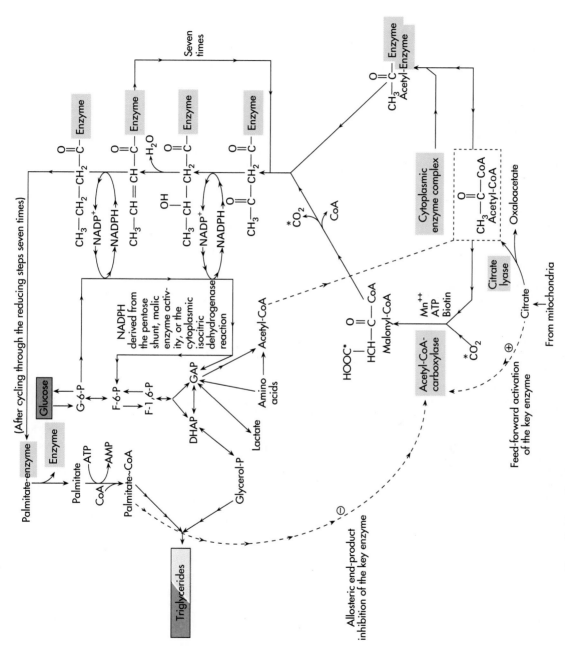

Chart IX. Cytoplasmic fatty acid synthesis (relation to glucose metabolism and NADPH generation).

tate-enzyme complex ensues. Free palmitate is then released by hydrolysis and activated to palmityl-CoA, in which form it reacts with glycerol phosphate for storage as triglyceride or for biosynthesis of phospholipids.

Rate-limiting in cytoplasmic fatty acid synthesis is the AcCoA carboxylase reaction in which AcCoA combines with CO_2 from bicarbonate ions to form malonyl-CoA. The enzyme activity requires manganese ions, ATP, and the B vitamin biotin to shuttle CO_2. The factors that modify this enzyme activity regulate the entire pathway of cytoplasmic fatty acid synthesis. Citrate, which shuttles AcCoA out of mitochondria for cytoplasmic fat synthesis, is an essential activator of AcCoA carboxylase via an allosteric feed-forward effect. Insulin activates AcCoA carboxylase for the purpose of storing dietary intake as fat. Unesterified fatty acids are allosteric inhibitors of AcCoA carboxylase. Therefore, when the free fatty acid level is high, no cytoplasmic fatty acid synthesis can occur. In fasting, for instance, free fatty acid levels in the blood are high, because glucose and energy demands establish a neuroendocrine environment that stimulates saponification of triglycerides by lipase activity and impairs reesterification of free fatty acids. The liver then forms ketone bodies from AcCoA since AcCoA carboxylase (and, thus, cytoplasmic fatty acid synthesis) is inhibited.

As free fatty acids inhibit fatty acid synthesis, palmitate must be immediately removed for its synthesis to continue. Palmitate forms triglycerides by esterification with glycerol phosphate. Adipose tissue, which lacks glycerokinase activity, obtains the necessary glycerol phosphate, either from imported glucose or from glucogenic precursors, such as lactate or amino acids. Therefore, under conditions of carbohydrate shortage or insulin deficiency, fatty acid synthesis in adipose tissue is depressed. The same is true in muscle. Liver cells do contain glycerokinase; yet, insulin is needed for hepatic fatty acid synthesis, because low insulin causes elevated fatty acid levels, which inhibit AcCoA carboxylase. Hence, fatty acid synthesis in all tissues requires insulin and the availability of glucose.

Biotin is required as a CO_2 shuttler, not only for AcCoA carboxylase, but also for the conversion of pyruvate to oxaloacetate via the pyruvate carboxylase step of the DCA shuttle, for conversion of propionate to succinyl-CoA in ruminants by propionyl-CoA carboxylase, and for purine biosynthesis. Biotin is also a cofactor in deaminase reactions of amino acids.

The availability of NADPH profoundly influences the rate of fatty acid biosynthesis. (See Chart IX.) Since each two-carbon addition requires two reducing steps, both specific for NADPH, no less than 14 NADPH molecules are required for the synthesis of 1 mol of palmitate. Different sources of NADPH have been considered in animals, but the pentose shunt may be the most important relative to the reactions catalyzed by malic enzyme and cytoplasmic isocitrate dehydrogenase. The pentose shunt is particularly active in tissues where fatty acid synthesis or sterol synthesis (which also requires NADPH) occurs at rapid rates; for example, in adrenal cortex, liver, adipose tissue, and lactating mammary glands.

Relations between glucose metabolism and fatty acid synthesis are indicated in Chart IX: (i) glucose can serve as a source for NADPH regeneration via the pentose shunt; (ii) glucose can deliver glycerol phosphate, without which esterification of palmitate would not be possible and fatty acid biosynthesis would stop; and (iii) glucose can be degraded to AcCoA, the building stone for fatty acid synthesis. Finally, glucose activates AcCoA carboxylase activity via the insulin response. Thus, glucose contains all the ingredients needed for its efficient conversion into fats.

Citrate is an effective precursor for fatty acid synthesis (Figure 13-12). (i) Citrate transports mitochondrial AcCoA to the cytoplasm with the help of citrate lyase; (ii) citrate can generate NADPH in the cytoplasm via isocitrate dehydrogenase or via malic enzyme after converting oxaloacetate (generated by citrate lyase) to malate; and (iii) citrate activates AcCoA carboxylase allosterically. The central position of citrate, linking carbohydrate catabolism and the mitochondrial formation of AcCoA with the extramitochondrial (smooth ER) syntheses of sterols and triglycerides, is indicated. It is important to note that citrate's feed-forward activation of AcCoA carboxylase allows stimulation of triglyceride synthesis without increased cholesterol formation.

Extramitochondrial isocitrate dehydrogenase is a substantial, if not main source of NADPH in ruminant animals. Since acetate (derived from the rumen) is the primary source of extramitochondrial acetyl-CoA, there is no necessity for it to enter mitochondria and form citrate prior to incorporation into long-chain fatty acids. Ruminants, therefore, are less dependent on malic enzyme and citrate lyase since they

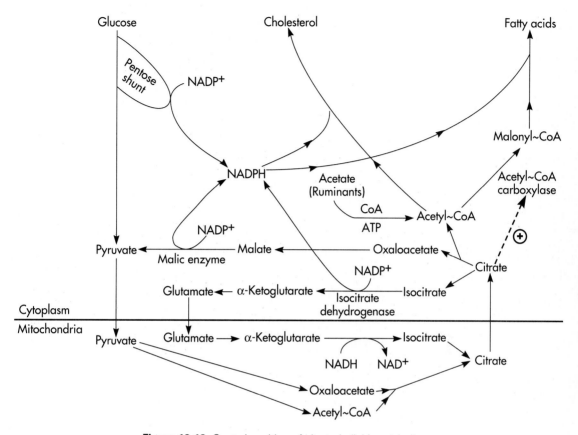

Figure 13-12. Central position of citrate in lipid metabolism.

have increased levels of readily available acetate and are less dependent upon glucose catabolism as a source of mitochondrial acetyl-CoA.

Another insight into control over pathways of lipid metabolism is the finding that three key enzymes—which catalyze the rate-controlling steps in fatty acid synthesis (AcCoA carboxylase), cholesterol biosynthesis (HMG-CoA reductase), and hydrolysis of triglycerides and cholesterol esters (hormone-sensitive lipase)—are regulated by a common, AMP-activated protein kinase. Elevated levels of fatty acyl-CoA activate a kinase enzyme that phosphorylates and thereby activates the AMP-activated protein kinase. The result is phosphorylation, and thereby inactivation of the key enzymes of both fatty acid and cholesterol syntheses. This mechanism offers a sensitive feedback control over fat synthesis. Moreover, simultaneous inhibition of cholesterol synthesis, at

times when fat synthesis is blocked, prevents increasingly available AcCoA from rushing toward cholesterol synthesis. Finally, phosphorylation of hormone-sensitive triglyceride lipase by AMP-activated protein kinase (which does not activate the lipase) prevents the lipase from being activated by cAMP-dependent protein kinase; hence, the lipase remains inactive and further fatty acid release from fat stores is inhibited.

Thus far, the discussion has been restricted to even-chained fatty acids, such as palmitate, stearate, oleate, and the polyunsaturated EFA's. In most animals and in humans odd-chained fatty acids are present only in minute amounts. But in ruminants, because of the abundance of propionate formed by ruminal bacteria, odd-chained fatty acids are produced in slightly larger, albeit still very small, amounts and, thus, occur in meat and dairy products. Their biosynthesis entails the use of propionate instead of acetate as the primer molecule, and for the rest, it goes along the same pathway.

Elongation and desaturation of fatty acids

The main product of cytoplasmic fatty acid biosynthesis from AcCoA is palmitate, the saturated C16 fatty acid. To convert palmitate, and dietary fatty acids with chain lengths of C10 or greater, to the specific fatty acids needed for certain functions and structures or for storage as triglycerides, the chain is elongated by successive C2 increments, to C18, C20, C22, etc. In addition, a double bond may be introduced to produce palmitoleic acid (C16:1) or oleic acid (C18:1), the most abundant fatty acid present in human triglyceride stores. Fat stores vary in their degree of unsaturation in response to diet; as discussed earlier, the microflora of the rumen saturate plant oils, so ruminant fat is highly saturated regardless of diet.

Elongation and synthesis of monounsaturated fatty acids take place in the smooth ER of the cell. Malonyl-CoA is used as a source of acetyl units, and for each C2 addition two reductions occur at the expense of NADPH.

INTESTINAL DIGESTION AND ABSORPTION OF LIPIDS

General features of gastrointestinal physiological chemistry were considered earlier. Presently, the text shall establish the forms in which various dietary lipids enter the circulation and become available for intermediary metabolism.

Gastrointestinal digestion of lipids; involvement of various organs

By chewing and mixing with saliva and stomach fluid, food is homogenized to some extent, forming a pasty chyme. Digestion of lipids occurs mainly in the duodenum after bile and pancreatic fluids have been admixed. These fluids, whose release is under the control of duodenal hormones (secretin, cholecystokinin), are concentrated in bicarbonate with which stomach acids are neutralized and the proper pH is generated for hydrolysis of esterified fatty acids by pancreatic and intestinal enzymes. Thus, pancreatic lipase saponifies neutral fats (triglycerides), and the pancreas and intestines both contribute cholesterol esterase and phospholipase enzyme activities.

Most lipids are either sparingly soluble in water or not at all, and this constitutes a problem, since the human body is an aqueous medium. In end stations of lipid metabolism, lipids may be sequestered in cells as non–water-miscible entities. Examples are the fat droplets in adipose tissue cells; cell membranes in which a lipid bi-layer may be present; droplets of cholesterol esters in adrenal cortical cells, ready for the production of corticosteroid hormones when needed. During intermediate phases of metabolism, however, lipids must be transported as complexes that are stable and miscible with water. The forms in which lipids are complexed for their transport are (i) lipoproteins; (ii) lipids bound to transport proteins in plasma (albumin) or intracellularly; (iii) fine emulsion droplets; and (iv) micelles.

Bile salts are important endogenous compounds for emulsification of lipids and for formation of mixed micelles. The main functions of the liver in lipid metabolism deal with transport: (i) formation of lipoproteins for lipid transport in blood; (ii) removal of tissue cholesterol from the body by reverse transport via high-density lipoproteins and excretion of cholesterol in bile; and (iii) elaboration of bile, needed for transport of lipids from the lumen of the gut to the outer surface of mucosal cells.

Intestinal absorption of lipids

For lipids to be absorbed they must first be converted to more polar compounds by processes that take place primarily in the lumen of the small intestine. By the churning action of the intestine plus the detergent action of bile salts, lipids are finely emulsified in the proximal gut (Figure 13-13). Triglycerides are then converted to the more polar 2-monoglycerides and free fatty acids under the influence of pancreatic lipase, which hydrolyzes the ester bonds in the 1 and 3 positions in two fast steps. A transferase reaction attempts to shuttle the remaining fatty acid from the 2 to a 1 position to prepare it for lipase cleavage. This reaction, however, is slow and, consequently, monoglycerides and free fatty acids are the main metabolites absorbed by the gut mucosa other than free glycerol, formed to a small extent by complete hydrolysis of triglycerides.

Pancreatic lipase, in conjunction with colipase, a pancreatic peptide, acts at the aqueous-lipid interface of the emulsion particles in the presence of bile salt micelles. (See Figure 13-13.) Free long-chain fatty acids and monoglycerides diffuse from the lipid phase of the emulsion particle into bile salt/lecithin/cholesterol micelles secreted by the liver and delivered

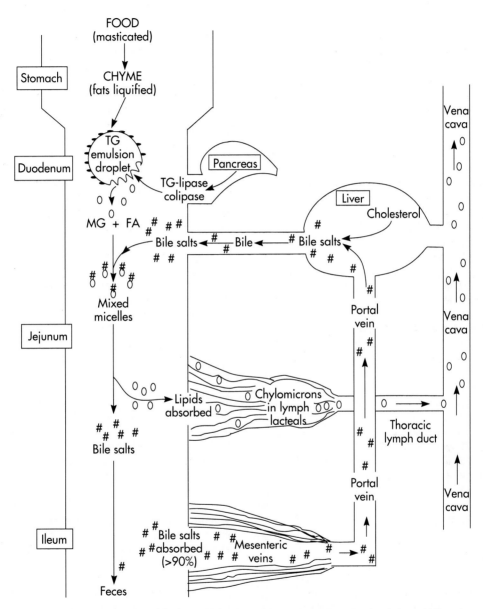

Figure 13-13. Intestinal digestion and absorption of fats; enterohepatic circulation of bile salts. Bile salt (mixed) micelles *(#)* circulate enterohepatically from liver via bile to gut and back to the liver via mesenteric and portal blood circulation. Dietary lipids, broken down to monoglycerides *(MG)* and free fatty acids *(FA)* are absorbed *(O)*, reconstituted in the form of triglycerides, incorporated into chylomicrons, and transported via the lymphatic system to the vena cava.

to the intestinal lumen via the bile. Since very non-polar compounds (triglycerides) cannot enter micelles, the digestive enzymes, yielding products with increased polarity, promote micelle formation.

The luminal surface of the intestine is coated by an unstirred water layer approximately 0.1 mm thick. To reach the brush border of mucosal cells, substances must first diffuse through that water layer. In the case of lipids, this diffusion may be the rate-limiting step in their absorption; emulsion particles are too large to diffuse at appreciable rates through the water layer, but the particle size of the micelles is small enough to do so. Therefore, micelles are the major vehicles for lipids to the brush border of the mucosal cells. Lipids are absorbed from the micelles in the proximal gut, bile salts much more distally in the ileum.

Inside the intestinal mucosa

The major pathway to triglyceride resynthesis within mucosal cells is the **monoglyceride acylation pathway.** Here, a 2-monoglyceride is joined with two fatty acyl-CoA derivatives to form triglyceride plus 2 CoA. The second, less utilized "scavenger pathway" (which is the major pathway in liver and adipocytes) is the **phosphatidic acid pathway.** Here, glycerol phosphate is joined with two fatty acyl-CoA derivatives to form phosphatidic acid. By removal of the phosphate group and addition of another fatty acyl-CoA, triglyceride is formed.

The small intestine does contain glycerokinase activity and, hence, for triglyceride resynthesis via the phosphatidic pathway, it can utilize free glycerol as long as it has not passed through the mucosal cell into the portal vein. However, for maximal efficiency of fat absorption in the gut, the diet should contain carbohydrates that yield glucose during digestion. This is another important link between carbohydrate and lipid metabolism.

Dietary phospholipids are partially degraded by pancreatic and intestinal phospholipases and for the rest, absorbed intact. The constituents of phospholipids, including choline, inositol, EFA, fatty acids, and galactose, are absorbed from the diet and used by many cells, but mainly in the liver for the biosynthesis of phospholipids, cerebrosides, sulfatides, and related compounds.

Cholesterol esters are hydrolyzed in the lumen of the gut by cholesterol esterase enzymes originating from pancreas and gut mucosa. Free sterol is then absorbed and reesterified in mucosal cells. Plant sterols, though structurally closely related to cholesterol, are virtually unabsorbed. In fact, plant sterols hamper the intestinal absorption of cholesterol and are for that purpose used as a cholesterol-lowering drug in human medicine.

Enterohepatic circulation

This term denotes an excretion/reabsorption cycle, from the liver, to the bile duct, intestines, mesenteric/portal bloodstream, and back to the liver. (See Figure 13-13.) Essentially, two classes of compounds can be distinguished in bile: (i) waste products of metabolism; that is products that the liver either generates or removes from the bloodstream, detoxifies, and then excretes into bile; and (ii) valuable components, such as bile salts and phospholipids, that serve important functions. The enterohepatic circulation, while allowing the biliary waste products to be excreted in feces, causes the valuable compounds, for the most part, to be reabsorbed and circulated back to the liver to perform their functions over and over. The reabsorption of bile salts, for instance, is about 90 to 95% effective and occurs mainly in the ileum. Administering drugs, such as cholestyramine, that bind bile salts and, thus, prevent their absorption, causes fecal elimination of bile salts; this necessitates increased rates of bile salt biosynthesis from cholesterol in the liver, so that cholesterol levels in the blood decline.

LIPID TRANSPORT IN THE BODY; ROLE OF LIPOPROTEINS
Transport of dietary lipid (metabolites) from gut mucosa into the lymph and blood

The transport of lipids that are to some extent water-soluble poses no special problem: a portion of the dietary phospholipids, short- and medium-chainfatty acids (C2-C12), bile salts, and some of the lipid-type vitamins (A, D, E, and K) all have hydrophylic properties that allow them to be transported, bound to albumin, via the portal vein to the liver. Then, the liver can either metabolize them further (cf., hepatic disposal of dietary carbohydrate and protein), or package them in the form of very low-density lipoproteins (VLDL) and secrete them into the bloodstream, so that other tissues can obtain them.

The problem of transporting poorly water-soluble dietary lipids is solved by the formation of chylomicrons in the gut mucosa. (Chyle is lymph; and micron is the upper particle size.) Chylomicrons (often called **chylos**) consist of a central core of triglycerides, comprising over 85% of the chylo weight, and cholesterol, mostly esterified (ca. 5%); on the periphery, phospholipids (ca. 7%) and a thin coat of proteins (1 to 2%) provide stability for the particle in aqueous surroundings. Chylos are the most lipid-rich and protein-poor of all lipoproteins, and, therefore, have the lowest buoyant density: they can be skimmed from the top of serum or lymph after centrifugation. Size and composition of chylos depend on relative rates of lipid and apoprotein synthesis and upon composition of dietary fat. Larger chylos are produced after consumption of high fat loads at the peak of intestinal absorption, and also when protein synthesis is inhibited. Chylos arise solely from the intestinal mucosa and contain triglyceride of dietary origin only.

Chylomicrons contain apoprotein (apo) A and apoprotein B_{48}, so named because its molecular weight is 48% of the liver's B_{100} apoprotein found in the VLDL, IDL, LDL (very low-, intermediate-, and low-density lipoprotein) family. Interestingly, intestinal B_{48} and hepatic B_{100} are coded in the same gene and the 2152 amino acid structure of B_{48} is identical to the amino-terminal half of apo B_{100}. In the intestines, though, during or after transcription, a $C \rightarrow U$ change in mRNA alters codon #2153 into a stop codon. In the liver, this change does not occur, so that a preapo B_{100} of 4563 amino acids is produced from which a 27 residue signal peptide is cleaved. It shall be shown that the distinction between apo B_{48} and B_{100} is meaningful, because cell surface receptors for LDL recognize apo B_{100}, but not apo B_{48}. Therefore, the chylomicron family of lipoproteins is distinct from the VLDL/IDL/LDL family.

The apoproteins are synthesized in mucosal cells, then combined with the dietary lipids, packaged into secretory vacuoles in the Golgi apparatus, and released as chylomicrons into intercellular spaces that are canalized as lacteals of the intestinal lymphatics. The lacteals join into larger mesenteric lymph channels that merge into the thoracic lymph duct; from there chylos finally enter the bloodstream in the left subclavian vein.

It is important to note well: most dietary lipids enter the circulation by way of the lymph and are presented to all tissues; this differs principally from the route taken by water-soluble nutrients. The latter are first directed to the liver via the portal vein. Chickens lack the lymphatic route of lipid transport.

Another lipoprotein present in intestinal lymph is VLDL. The origin of VLDL in the blood is mostly hepatic, but intestines do contribute. In the bloodstream, VLDL carry endogenously synthesized lipids, mainly triglycerides synthesized in the liver from dietary carbohydrates, toward deposition in fat cells. In the intestinal lymph, VLDL carries primarily intestinally produced (not dietary) triglycerides (i.e., triglyceride produced by the phosphatidic acid pathway). Hence, while the extent of chylomicron formation is related to dietary fat intake, and, thus, is variable, the secretion of VLDL into intestinal lymph is relatively constant. Chylomicrons and VLDL share a common catabolic fate at the "hands" of lipoprotein lipase.

Metabolism of chylomicrons

After a fatty meal, serum becomes turbid, milky-looking, because of a large number of chylomicrons. This phenomenon is called **postprandial lactescence.** Chylomicrons are rapidly removed from the bloodstream (they have a half-life of just minutes), which results in clearance of the lactescence (Figure 13-14).

In lymphatics and upon entering the bloodstream, nascent chylomicrons (and VLDL) acquire apoproteins of the C and E classes from circulating HDL. The presence of both phospholipids and apo C_{II} is required for recognition and enzymic degradation by lipoprotein lipase (LPL).

The enzyme LPL (formerly called **clearing factor**) is located on the endothelial surface of blood capillaries, mainly those associated with adipose tissue, skeletal muscle, heart, lung, and other tissues, but not with the liver. The enzyme is synthesized within the tissues and then transported to the endothelial surfaces of capillaries. There it recognizes circulating chylomicrons (and VLDL) by their apo C_{II}, which binds to and activates LPL. The enzyme then hydrolyzes the triglyceride core of the chylos (or VLDL) and the fatty acids so liberated are taken up by the tissues, where they are reesterified and stored as triglycerides.

Since the occurrence of chylos is a postprandial event, and therefore coincides with high glucose and insulin levels, it is helpful that LPL in adipose tissue is activated by insulin; at the same time, insulin stimulates glucose entry into the cells. This way, fatty acids and glucose (for glycerol-P production) enter the cell simultaneously to yield triglycerides for storage. Uptake of fatty acids from chylos and storage in adipose tissue are inversely related to muscular activity, which causes LPL activation in the muscle.

Evidence for the extracellular location of LPL is provided by the ability of heparin, injected intravenously, to release LPL into the circulation. Although

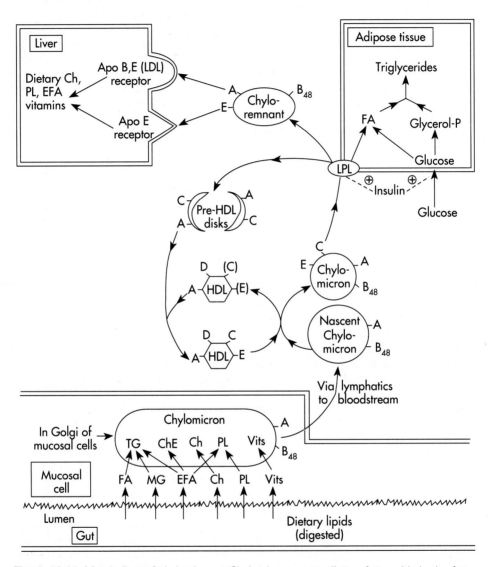

Figure 13-14. Metabolism of chylomicrons. Chylomicrons carry dietary fatty acids in the form of triglycerides to adipose tissue where lipoprotein lipase *(LPL)* deposits them in the fat stores. Chylomicron remnants transport other dietary lipids and lipids formed in the gut mucosa (e.g., cholesterol esters, *ChE*) to the liver. Specific apoproteins (capital letters on periphery of lipoproteins) direct lipoproteins to receptors on target cells. *HDL,* High-density lipoproteins; *LDL,* low-density lipoproteins; *FA,* fatty acids; *MG,* monoglycerides; *Ch,* cholesterol; *PL,* phospholipids; *EFA,* essential fatty acids; *A,D,E,K,* fat-soluble vitamins.

this effect may not be of physiological significance, it is useful in diagnosis. The activity of LPL is often measured in samples taken from patients following heparin injection.

Hydrolysis of the triglyceride core by LPL reduces (mature) chylomicrons to approximately half of their size. This renders a portion of their surface lipids and proteins redundant; part of the chylomicron's phospholipids and some cholesterol, together with apoproteins A and apo C_{II}, are shed from the surface of the particle as bilayer discs, which are thought to be precursors of plasma HDL. The loss of apo C_{II} decreases the affinity for LPL, hence, the particle is released.

The resulting particles, called **chylomicron remnants,** contain dietary sterols and sterol esters, fat-soluble vitamins (A, D, E, and K), phospholipids, some triglycerides, and apoproteins. Apo E is of special importance, for it is the apoprotein that directs the chylomicron remnant to the liver. As long as apo C is present on the chylo surface, it shields the chylo from binding to apo E receptors on the surface of liver cells. This way, dietary triglycerides can be directed to fat cells and not the liver for storage. But, after losing the apo C to HDL, the remnant is recognized and removed from the blood by binding to receptors on liver cells that recognize apo E.

There are two kinds of apo E receptors: one recognizes both apo B_{100} and apo E and is called the apo B, E (LDL) receptor, since it binds LDL; the other is specific for apo E only. One may ask, what may be the functionality of having two apo E receptors on the surface of liver cells? The LDL receptor is down-regulated when the cell's cholesterol needs have been met. If this were the only apo E receptor available, uptake of dietary sterols would be impeded; but the specific apo E receptor is not down-regulated, and, thus, dietary sterol intake can be handled by the liver under all conditions. Virtually all cholesterol in chyloremnants is brought from its intestinal origin to the liver, where it is either used in membrane or lipoprotein biosynthesis or excreted into bile as free cholesterol or bile salts.

Although the liver does not contain lipoprotein lipase (LPL), and, hence, extrahepatic tissues get a first crack at incoming dietary lipids, it does contain a heparin-releasable hepatic lipase that may participate in the clearance of chylomicron and VLDL remnants from the circulation. This enzyme has properties different from those of LPL. The lactating mammary gland has high LPL activity, and dietary lipids readily find their way into milk. In adipose tissue, LPL activity is high in the fed state and low during fasting, whereas in heart muscle LPL activity increases between meals and during fasting, causing a shift in those tissues toward fat utilization. The K_m value of LPL for triglycerides is ten times higher in adipose tissue than in heart tissue; since the triglyceride concentration goes down in fasting, LPL in heart tissues is still saturated, while that in adipose tissue is not, so that fat traffic is directed to the heart.

Transport of endogenously synthesized lipids; metabolism of VLDL, IDL, and LDL

The bulk of VLDL is produced in the liver for the purpose of transporting lipids, mostly triglycerides, that are biosynthesized from dietary carbohydrates and amino acids postprandially or from recirculating fatty acids in periods between regular meals. VLDL contain about 60% triglycerides, 14% phospholipids, 20% cholesterol and 6% protein. Required for the production of VLDL are lipotropic factors. Major proteins of hepatic nascent VLDL include apoproteins B_{100} and E; other apoproteins are present in smaller amounts. In similar fashion as described for chylos, VLDL acquire apo C from HDL in the bloodstream; VLDL originating in the gut are devoid of apo E and must acquire apo E and apo C from HDL. Lipoprotein lipase (LPL) recognizes and binds VLDL by the attached apo C_{II}, whiich also activates LPL. The triglyceride core of VLDL is saponified and fatty acids are taken up by the adjacent fat and muscle cells (Figure 13-15).

While delivering their dietary lipid bounty for storage, VLDL lose most of their triglycerides and become cholesterol-enriched. By concomitant shedding of surface lipids and apoproteins (giving rise to nascent HDL), VLDL become VLDL remnants, also called **IDL** (intermediate-density lipoproteins); together, chylomicron remnants and VLDL remnants are called **beta-VLDL.** IDL have a fast rate of turnover: being rich in apo B_{100} and apo E, approximately half of the IDL are removed from the circulation by hepatic receptors, primarily mediated by apo E. The other half converts to LDL (low-density lipoproteins) by losing more triglycerides and all apoproteins other than B_{100}. The composition of LDL is about 21% protein, as much as 50% cholesterol, 22% phospholipids, and only 7% triglycerides. While each class of lipoprotein contains a characteristic mixture of apoproteins, LDL contains exclusively apo B_{100}.

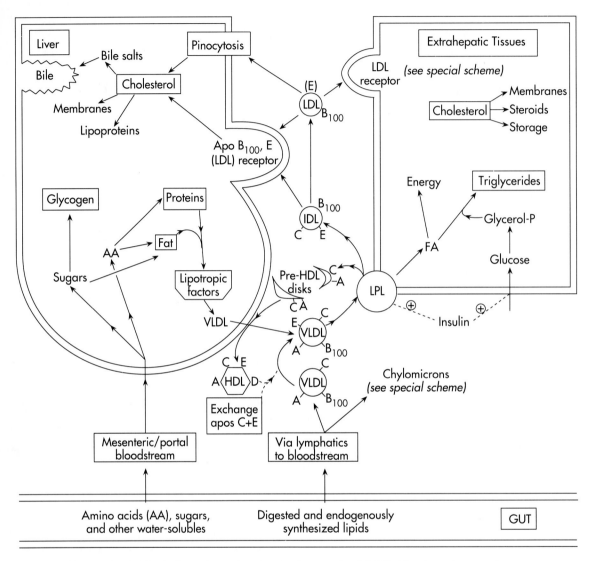

Figure 13-15. Metabolism of very-low-density lipoproteins (VLDL). Mostly endogenously synthesized triglycerides are transported from liver and gut in the form of VLDL towards fat depots in tissues. *IDL,* Intermediate-density lipoproteins. Other abbreviations as in Figure 13-14.

The bulk of LDL is taken up and metabolized after binding to LDL receptors on liver and extrahepatic cells (Figure 13-16). The rest is cleared by various tissues via receptor-independent mechanisms. Depending on animal species, more than half of the LDL receptors may be located in the liver. After endocytosis, released cholesterol elicits three regulatory responses with respect to cholesterol homeostasis: (a) it suppresses HMG-CoA reductase, the rate-limiting enzyme activity of cholesterol synthesis; (b) it activates cholesterol ester formation by cholesterol acyltransferase; and (c) it down-regulates LDL receptors on the cell surface.

In extrahepatic tissues, cholesterol delivered via LDL receptors can be used for membrane construction or steroid biosynthesis. Up- or down-regulation of LDL receptors controls cholesterol intake into those cells according to need. In the liver, cholesterol can

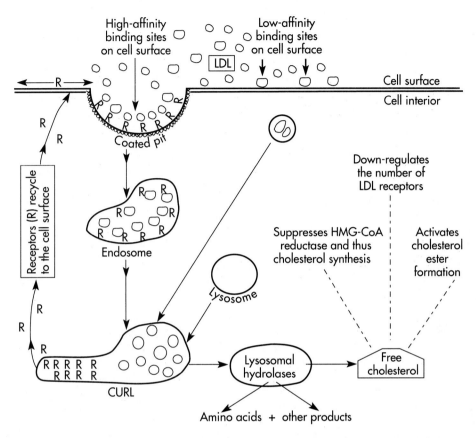

Figure 13-16. Metabolism of low-density lipoproteins *(LDL)*. Note down-regulation of LDL-receptors by free cholesterol released from lysosomally digested LDL. *CURL,* Compartment of uncoupling receptor from ligand.

be resecreted in newly formed VLDL or HDL, or secreted in bile after conversion to bile salts or as free or esterified cholesterol.

A major factor controlling steady-state concentrations of LDL is the generation of LDL from sources other than VLDL catabolism; that is, direct secretion of LDL. Direct synthesis yields LDL_2 with identical apoprotein, but a slightly higher density than the LDL_1 derived from VLDL catabolism. The direct pathway has been described for patients with familial hypercholesterolemia and other hyperlipidemias, and for normal subjects. The pathway can be regulated by treatment with cholesterol-lowering agents, such as cholestyramine and lovastatin, an HMG-CoA reductase inhibitor.

In patients with familial hypercholesterolemia, there may be a marked reduction (heterozygotes) or total absence (homozygotes) of functional LDL receptors, giving rise to chronically elevated LDL levels in the blood. In type III hyperlipoproteinemia (associated with premature atherosclerosis) the metabolic defect is caused by a variant form of apo E that binds poorly to lipoprotein receptors.

In rats, cholesterol feeding or hypothyroidism leads to a decreased number of hepatic LDL receptors and increased plasma LDL levels. Increased numbers of hepatic LDL receptors and decreased plasma LDL result from hyperthyroidism, administration of estrogens, and hypocholesterolemic drugs, such as the combination of colestipol or cholestyramine (binding bile salts in the gut) with mevinolin or compactin (inhibiting HMG-CoA reductase). Insulin, estrogen and triiodothyronine increase the specific binding of LDL to cultured hepatocytes. These observations may explain the hypercholesterolemia and increased risk of atherosclerosis associated with poorly controlled diabetes, post-menopause, and hypothyroidism.

Watanabe heritable hyperlipidemic (WHHL) rabbit

Considerable animal research has been focused on improving our understanding of the pathogenesis of hypercholesterolemia, particularly familial hypercholesterolemia (FH). An animal model of FH, the WHHL rabbit, was described in 1973 by Yoshio Watanabe, a veterinarian at Kobe University in Japan. Through selective inbreeding, Dr. Watanabe developed and began studying a colony of these hyperlipidemic rabbits. Initially the similarity between the WHHL rabbit and human FH was not appreciated, in part because the WHHL rabbit also exhibited hypertriglyceridemia. It is now known that the hypertriglyceridemia relates in part to the fact that normal rabbit LDL contains a relatively high content of triglyceride in contrast to human LDL. Thus, high LDL in the WHHL rabbit produces not only hypercholesterolemia, but also significant hypertriglyceridemia.

The WHHL rabbits proved invaluable in explaining a previously puzzling feature of homozygous FH. Kinetic studies using radiolabeled LDL indicated that these animals not only degraded LDL more slowly, but also appeared to overproduce LDL. How, then, does a genetic defect in the LDL receptor lead simultaneously to overproduction and reduced degradation of LDL? The answer to this question lies in the complex biosynthetic pathway for LDL.

As indicated above, the liver not only removes LDL from the circulation, but also IDL. IDL typically has a fast rate of turnover, being rich in apo B_{100} and apo E. However, the apparent overproduction of LDL in WHHL rabbits is due to the failure of IDL to be removed from plasma by the liver, therefore it remains in the circulation and is converted in increased amounts to LDL. Although experiments of similar detail as those conducted in rabbits cannot be carried out in humans, observations are consistent with the hypothesis that enhanced conversion of IDL to LDL occurs in human FH homozygotes, thus accounting for much of the apparent overproduction of LDL.

Reverse cholesterol transport; metabolism of HDL

HDL, also called **alpha-lipoproteins** based on their electrophoretic behavior, are small particles with high protein (ca. 50%) and high phospholipid (ca. 27%) content that carry cholesterol (ca. 20%, mainly esterified) in vascular and extravascular systems. The principal function of HDL is cholesterol and EFA distribution and redistribution among tissues and to ensure that tissue cholesterol returns to the liver.

HDL are the most heterogeneous class of lipoproteins, arising from various sources and containing several subclasses. In sequence of decreasing density (increasing cholesterol ester content), there are HDL_3, HDL_2 (which can be subdivided in a major fraction that lacks apo E and a minor fraction that contains apo E), and HDL_c (so-called in animals), or HDL_1 (in humans), or HDL-with-apo E; the latter are formed from HDL_2 after cholesterol feeding, and contain additional cholesterol esters and apo E.

It is difficult to characterize newly formed (nascent) HDL, because of their continuous modification while in circulation, commencing immediately upon secretion. Unlike lipoproteins containing integral apo B as a nonexchangeable marker, HDL are comprised of only exchangeable, peripheral apoproteins. Although only the liver and gut contribute apo A_I, apo A_{II}, and apo C to mammalian HDL, apo E (and cholesterol) may be derived from many cell types. Phospholipid disks containing apo E are HDL precursors secreted mainly from the liver, but, in smaller amounts, from almost any cell. The gut, which produces no apo E, secretes apo A_I-phospholipid disks as HDL precursors.

The origin of the nascent HDL disks is quite diverse: they are secreted from liver, gut, and various other cells, and, in addition, they arise intravascularly, on the vascular endothelial surface from apoproteins and lipids that split away from VLDL and chylomicrons as a result of surface area reduction, during lipoprotein lipase digestion (Figure 13-17). Three enzymes play an essential role in the transformation of nascent pre-HDL disks into mature spherical subclasses of HDL: (i) the circulating plasma emzyme, lecithin cholesterol acyltransferase (LCAT), which esterifies cholesterol with an EFA derived from the β-position of lecithin; lysolecithin, thus formed, returns to the liver; (ii) lipoprotein lipase (LPL); and (iii) hepatic triglyceride lipase (HTGL).

- LCAT, activated by apo A_I, esterifies free cholesterol at the HDL periphery. Since cholesterol esters are hydrophobic, they move into the center core of HDL, making the particle expand from a flat disk to a sphere. This initial sphere is HDL_3. As the particle continues to accept apolipoproteins and lipids from chylo and VLDL degradation by LPL and from peripheral tissues,

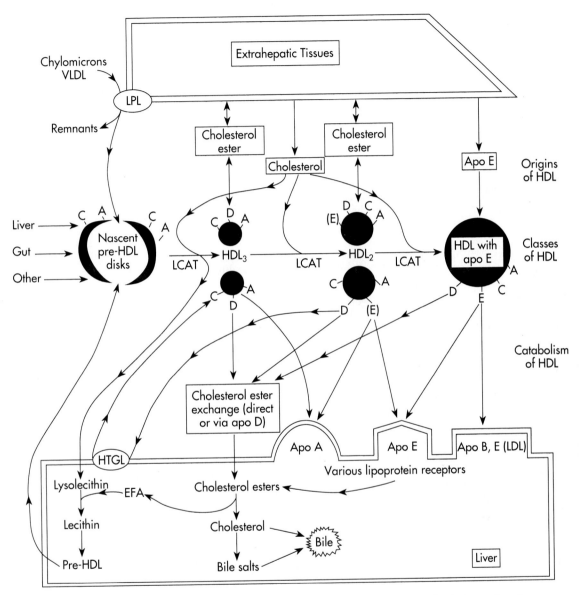

Figure 13-17. Metabolism of high-density lipoproteins (HDL). *LCAT,* Lecithin-cholesterol acyl-transferase; *HTGL,* hepatic triglyceride lipase. Other abbreviatons as in previous figures.

it is transformed into HDL_2. The main difference between these HDL is the presence of an extra apo A_I molecule and an approximately doubled cholesterol ester content. By depleting the HDL surface of free cholesterol, LCAT activity creates a free-cholesterol gradient for transfer of cholesterol from tissues or from other lipoproteins to HDL.

- LPL, situated on endothelial cells of blood vessels, principally in adipose and skeletal muscle tissues, is activated by apo C_{II} and then hydrolyses triglycerides from chylos and VLDL. In the course of this lipolysis, HDL_3 acquires cholesterol, phospholipids, and apo A_I, and progressively, with the help of LCAT, turns into HDL_2. Therefore, the level of HDL_2 reflects the efficiency of LPL lipolysis; this explains the elevation of the HDL_2 level under certain circumstances, such as during physical exercise.

- HTGL is involved in the transformation of HDL_2 back to HDL_3 in the liver.

Just as there are several different mechanisms and sites of origin of HDL, so do various modes of HDL catabolism exist, related to the various functions of HDL. In general, HDL carries cholesterol from sites of excess to sites of need. For example, HDL partakes in reverse cholesterol transport; that is, cholesterol transport from tissues to liver, where cholesterol is eliminated via bile. As such, HDL act antiatherogenically.

HDL catabolism and functioning is outlined in Figure 13-17.

HDL itself is taken up by the liver. In the case of HDL-with-apo E, the hepatic apo E receptors are involved. Cholesterol-loaded cells release their cholesterol to acceptors in interstitial fluid, especially the phospholipid-rich, nonapo E containing HDL. As HDL become cholesterol-enriched they acquire apo E and, in turn, the presence of apo E facilitates the acquisition of additional cholesterol by HDL. Because of LCAT, the HDL-with-apo E double in size due to cholesterol ester uptake, in concentric rings in the core of the particle. Such cholesterol-ester–enriched, swollen, HDL-with-apo E bind avidly to LDL receptors by virtue of apo E. (HDL without apo E do not bind to LDL receptors.) This way, cholesterol is transported from peripheral tissues to the liver by HDL-with-apo E, which is present in the plasma and interstitial fluid of most animal species.

It is not clear whether other specific receptors that are devoid of apo E exist for HDL. Apo A_{IV} is a ligand responsible for HDL binding to primary rat hepatocytes, and that apoprotein binds to a receptor site distinct from apo-E–dependent receptors.

The addition of apo E and cholesterol to HDL_2, especially after cholesterol feeding, produces HDL_c, which binds to the liver's apo E receptors.

Cholesterol esters of HDL are taken up at a fractional rate that is several-fold greater than is apo A_I by liver and steroidogenic tissues, which suggests an independent catabolic fate of these constituents: selective uptake. By this process, HDL can deliver cholesterol to most body cells without complete degradation through a lysosomal process.

The liver accounts for the large majority of cholesterol esters taken up in excess over apo A_I. To the extent that these HDL cholesterol esters arise from free cholesterol that leaves extrahepatic cells and is then esterified by LCAT, the pathway contributes greatly to reverse cholesterol transport.

Selective uptake is quantitatively very important. One mechanism for selective uptake, and reverse cholesterol transport, is the cholesterol ester transfer-protein (apo D)–mediated transfer of cholesterol esters from HDL to lower-density lipoproteins followed by LDL-receptor–mediated endocytosis (or nonspecific removal) of the lower-density lipoprotein. In addition, there may be a direct exchange of cholesterol esters from HDL to tissues.

In extrahepatic tissues, selective uptake is regulated according to the cholesterol needs of cells via up- or down-regulation of LDL receptors on the cell surfaces. Cholesterol feeding suppresses it; hypocholesterolemia enhances it in tissues that normally do not exhibit selective uptake (muscle, adipose tissue, skin), and in adrenals and ovaries, which take up cholesterol for the purpose of steroid biosynthesis. Thus, at very low levels of plasma cholesterol, HDL cholesterol esters move from the liver to other sites and, therefore, selective uptake of cholesterol esters in extrahepatic tissues delivers cholesterol to steroidogenic tissues (adrenals, ovaries). The selective uptake and retention of HDL cholesterol esters by isolated fat cells reflects a dynamic cholesterol storage pool in adipose tissue. Therefore, selective uptake in extrahepatic tissues is an important process in maintaining cholesterol homeostasis. In contrast, regulation of selective uptake in the liver has not been demonstrated: the liver acts as a cholesterol ester "sink." In normal cells, there appears to be enough cholesterol available to keep the selective uptake pathway down-regulated in all tissues except the liver and steroidogenic tissues.

The relative extents of the various catabolic routes for HDL vary with animal species and conditions. In humans and rabbits, HDL-with-apo E are in relatively low concentration under normal conditions (more so after cholesterol feeding) and cholesterol elimination is largely mediated by cholesterol ester transfer protein (apo D). In this way, cholesterol esters are transferred from HDL to VLDL, IDL, and LDL and then taken up by the liver for subsequent biliary elimination.

HDL participates in the redistribution of cholesterol among cells. When the sciatic nerve is damaged, as part of the inflammatory reaction, monocytes rapidly enter the site of injury and become macrophages. Macrophages now produce a lot of apo E in phospholipid-containing disks that can bind and thus scavenge cholesterol from cellular and myelin debris.

HDL-with-apo E delivers that cholesterol to the macrophages, where it is stored. Upon axon regeneration, high levels of LDL receptors, expressed on the tips of neurites, take up HDL-cholesterol for biogenesis of membranes. Later on, Schwann cells, expressing LDL receptors, take up HDL-cholesterol for remyelinization of the axon.

HDL, and notably HDL_2, are factors that protect against cardiovascular disease. HDL_2 is subject to the influence of numerous dietary, genetic, and hormonal factors, while HDL_3 seems to be more independent. Some factors that regulate HDL include:

- Genetic control: plasma HDL is especially elevated in Greenland Eskimos and black Americans; especially low in Asians.
- Gender: normal HDL cholesterol in females is 0.55 g/L; in males, 0.45 g/L.
- Excessive weight correlates negatively with plasma HDL levels, and so do plasma triglyceride levels.
- Dietary: alcohol in moderation, not enough to damage the liver, raises plasma HDL_3 levels. Tobacco lowers plasma HDL. Diets rich in carbohydrates lower HDL, especially HDL_2, with a corresponding lowering of apo A_I compared to apo A_{II}. Dietary cholesterol induces formation of HDL_1 (or HDL_c in animals), which is rich in cholesterol ester and apo E. This particle, recognized by the liver's apo B,E (LDL) and apo E (remnant) receptors, competes with LDL for hepatic uptake and catabolism. As HDL_1 precipitates together with LDL in a heparin-manganese solution, the two lipoproteins are measured together, which may account in part for the elevation in LDL cholesterol level reported after intake of a high-cholesterol diet.
- Exercise, especially endurance sports, increases lipolytic activities of muscle and adipose tissue. It raises HDL, especially HDL_2, and lowers triglycerides.
- Endocrine: estrogens and thyroxine increase HDL cholesterol, and testosterone lowers HDL cholesterol, especially HDL_2. Insulin increases HDL cholesterol by activating LPL and LCAT, and by increasing apo A_I synthesis.

Symptomatic treatment of hypercholesterolemia is based on the above. Cholestyramine or cholestipol, given orally, binds bile salts in the intestines and removes them in the feces, thus preventing their recirculation to the liver. Consequently, the liver must synthesize more bile salts for which purpose it takes up cholesterol from the bloodstream, and that lowers plasma cholesterol levels. Normally, the liver responds to lowered plasma cholesterol levels by increasing its rate of cholesterol synthesis, but that compensation could also be prevented by simultaneously administering agents that inhibit HMG-CoA reductase (the rate-controlling step in hepatic cholesterogenesis), such as mevinolin, compactin, or lovastatin. A third measure in the treatment of hypercholesterolemia is to lower the dietary intake of cholesterol. But remember, the dietary intake of excess calories in any form (carbohydrates, lipids, or proteins) ultimately leads to conversion to fat in the liver, resulting in the production of excessive amounts of lipoproteins and, thus, elevation of LDL cholesterol in serum.

LIPIDS IN PLASMA
Meaning of a plasma sample

Lipid metabolism is in a state of dynamic equilibrium among various processes and functions located at distant sites within an organism, and the levels of different lipid classes in plasma reflect that equilibrium. Lipoproteins are secreted, often in nascent forms, from many different cells, and in the circulation their composition is continuously changing because of cellular uptake, two-way interactions on the surfaces of tissue cells, and exchange of lipids and apoproteins among various lipoproteins. Added to this is the variability caused postprandially by dietary composition or, during fasting, by increased fat mobilization from stores and shortage of lipotropic factors and glucose. Neuroendocrine control mediates lipid homeostasis. Therefore, one must realize that the lipid composition of a plasma sample reflects a stop-motion picture of a very dynamic complex.

Relation to diet and time after a meal

After a meal, when storage of the dietary bounty is the order of business, dietary lipids enter the bloodstream, orchestrated by insulin, in the form of chylomicrons, causing postprandial lactescence. Dietary carbohydrates and proteins, ingested in excess over the body's storage capacities for glycogen and proteins, are converted mainly in the liver (in most animal species) to triglycerides and exported in the form of VLDL. Lipoprotein lipase activity, activated by insulin and apo C_{II}, clears the blood of chylos and VLDL, allows delivery of triglycerides' fatty acids to fat cells and muscles, and generates remnants of chylomicrons and VLDL. Chylo-remnants are quickly removed from the circulation by the liver's apo E receptors. The VLDL-remnant, IDL, is in part rapidly removed by the liver, and the rest is converted to LDL_1. LDL_1 turns over more slowly while being removed by all cells needing cholesterol (including liver; LDL receptor up-regulation). The liver exports a small amount of the incoming dietary cholesterol from chylo-remnants into the circulation in the form of LDL_2. When cholesterol-rich diets are fed, elevated levels of HDL-with-apo E are observed. Below-average levels of "free fatty acids" are found in plasma postprandially, since insulin inhibits lipolysis of triglycerides in fat cells (Figure 13-18). The term free fatty acids is confusing: it means, nonesterified fatty acids; in the blood, they are albumin-bound to solubilize them.

In periods between regular meals, metabolism shifts to a state of economy since insulin-antagonistic hormones take control. In adipose tissue, triglycerides are broken down at a rate in excess of their resynthesis, so there is a net release of free fatty acids (bound to albumin) in the bloodstream. These fatty acids are offered to tissue cells for nutrition and, if unused, removed from circulation by the liver. The liver uses them in part to provide energy for its numerous functions, and the rest are reesterified to triglyceride and released in the form of VLDL into the bloodstream from where LPL removes them either for energy supply to tissues or for redeposition in fat stores. As the rate of fatty acid release from stores is balanced by their utilization in cells and reesterification in the liver, their levels in the circulation remain constant. (See Figure 13-18.)

Upon prolonged fasting, when critical shortages develop in carbohydrates (needed to supply glycerol

phosphate in fat cells for redeposition of fatty acids in the form of triglycerides in fat stores) and lipotropic factors (needed for hepatic VLDL synthesis), metabolic economy is sacrificed for the purpose of survival. The imbalance beteween increased fatty acid release from adipose tissue (caused by neuroendocrine stimulation of triglyceride lipase) and diminished fat redeposition (caused by lack of glycerol phosphate) is reflected in elevated levels of free fatty acids in plasma. (See Figure 13-18.) The liver, running out of lipotropic factors, cannot match the increased influx of fatty acids with increased VLDL export. To some extent, fatty acids are esterified in the liver and accumulate there (causing "fatty liver"), but the bulk of incoming fatty acid is degraded to ketone bodies (acetoacetate and β-hydroxybutyrate) and secreted into the bloodstream, giving rise to ketonemia, ketoacidosis, and ketonuria.

Diagnostics

The relative proportions in which the various lipoprotein classes occur in plasma, allowing for the influences by diet and the time of day relative to meal intake, fall within narrow limits for each animal species. Since the presence of various lipoproteins in blood reflects all of lipid metabolism, and metabolism in general, the lipoprotein profile of plasma has profound diagnostic meaning in distinguishing various disorders (e.g., the HDL/LDL ratio in atherosclerosis).

Measurement and classification

Various methods are used for measurement and classification of lipoproteins in plasma (Table 13-1).

- Differences among lipoproteins in their relative proportions of lipids and proteins are exploited in ultracentrifugation methods. After adjusting the density of the medium to a known value (e.g., by adding salts), lipoproteins of specified densities can be either floated up or spun down ultracentrifugally. This method gives rise to classifications of high, intermediate, low, and very low density lipoproteins.
- Electrophoresis is the method of choice in clinical laboratoria, since it is faster and less expensive than ultracentrifugation. Because the velocity of running of lipoproteins in an electrical field depends on the number of electrical charges on proteins, and is impeded by the drag of inert lipids, it is clear that the small, protein-rich HDL run fastest (hence, called α-lipoproteins); they are followed by LDL (β-lipoproteins); chylomi-

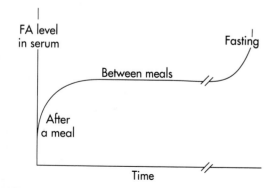

Figure 13-18. Free fatty acid *(FA)* levels in serum in relation to the time of meal intake.

Table 13-1	Classification and composition of major lipoprotein classes in human plasma			
Density, ultra-centrifugation	Chylomicrons d < 1.006	VLDL d < 1.006	LDL 1.019 < d < 1.063	HDL 1.063 < d < 1.210
Electrophoretic mobility	Origin	Pre-β	β	α
Composition*				
Total proteins	1-2	6-10	18-25	44-55
Total lipids	98-99	90-94	75-82	45-56
Apoproteins				
Major	B_{48}, C_I, C_{II}, C_{III}	B_{100}, C_{III}, E	B_{100}	A_I, A_{II}
Minor	A_I, A_{II}, A_{IV}, E	A_I, A_{II}, C_{II}, D	C_I, C_{II}	B_{100}, C_I, C_{II}, C_{III}, D, E
Major lipid	Dietary triglycerides	Endogenous triglycerides	Cholesterol	Phospholipids + cholesterol
Lipid analysis*				
Triglycerides	75-90	50-65	4-9	1-7
Phospholipids	3-9	10-20	15-24	25-32
Cholesterol†	3-14	20-31	50-58	15-26

*Expressed as percent (w/w) of particle weight.
†Extreme variations have been reported for the ratio of esterified to free cholesterol: 0.67-2.0 in chylomicrons; 0.25-4.0 in VLDL; 0.19-7.5 in LDL; and 0.23-4.0 in HDL.

crons remain near the origin. After the electrical run has been completed, the lipoproteins can be fixed, stained for either protein or individual lipids, and densitometrically scanned, so that a permanent record of scans can be kept.
• More or less specific precipitation and ultrafiltration procedures are also used.

ADIPOSE TISSUE AND LIPID METABOLISM
Functions

Storage and release of fats for energy purposes is the prime function of adipose tissue. Large adipose stores are found in (i) the subcutaneous connective tissues; (ii) the abdominal cavity; (iii) the perirenal, pericardial, and epididymal fat pads; and (iv) interspersed in most tissues. Each animal species, and each organ within an animal, tends to store its particular fatty acids in the triglyceride compartment. However, the fat composition of the diet does have an influence on the composition of a tissue's fat store; for example, feeding mostly oils does lead to deposition of softer fats in most animal species. In ruminants, dietary unsaturated fatty acids are hydrogenated and, thus, hardened in the rumen.

Dynamic triglyceride equilibrium

Direction and rate of adipose tissue metabolism are regulated by availability of adequate levels of glucose (and insulin) in the blood. Triglyceride metabolism is in a state of dynamic equilibrium (Figure 13-19).

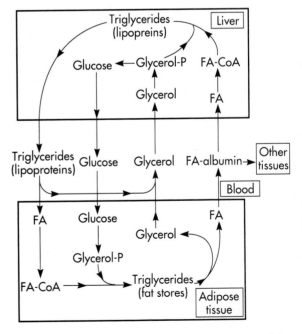

Figure 13-19. The glucose-glycerol cycle in support of the dynamic equilibrium of triglyceride stores, *FA,* Fatty acid.

Under the influence of adipolytic triglyceride lipase, (TG-lipase), also called hormones-sensitive lipase, triglycerides are hydrolyzed, yielding free fatty acids and free glycerol, while triglycerides are concurrently synthesized from fatty acyl-CoA and glycerol phosphate.

The fat cell has a problem in that it cannot reuse the glycerol liberated by hydrolysis of its triglyceride stores, because the cell lacks glycerokinase activity. Therefore, free glycerol is excreted into the bloodstream, from where the liver and kidneys remove it for gluconeogenesis. The consequence of this glycerol drain from adipose tissue is that fat cells need a constant supply of glucose from blood to reensemble triglycerides. The glucose-glycerol cycle (see Figure 13-19) performs this function. It is instructive to trace this cycle in the global picture of animal metabolism. (See Chart I, Chapter 10.)

Glucose uptake by adipose tissue requires insulin; adipose tissue is very sensitive to insulin (Figure 13-20):

- Insulin enables glucose uptake by the fat cell and stimulates glucose metabolism inside the cell.
- Insulin inhibits TG-lipase activity powerfully, which has a fat-sparing effect.
- Insulin activates lipoprotein lipase activity on the vascular endothelial cells in adipose tissue.

It is necessary to recall how these three facts add up: at the time lipoprotein lipase releases free fatty acids from chylomicrons and VLDL, sufficient glucose is available within the fat cell to produce glycerol phosphate and deposit these fatty acids in fat stores.

Because lipogenesis from glucose yields ATP, a futile cycle (see Figure 13-20) is needed to spend ATP, since ATP buildup impairs lipogenesis (cf., phosphofructokinase and pyruvate dehydrogenase).

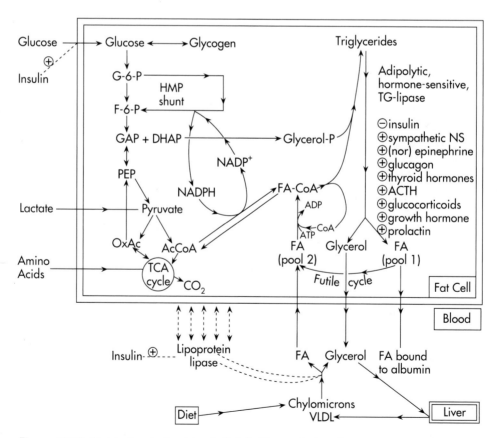

Figure 13-20. Metabolism in the fat cell. *G-6-P,* Glucose-6-phosphate; *F-6-P,* fructose-6-phosphate; *GAP,* glyceraldehyde phosphate; *DHAP,* dihydroxyacetone phosphate; *PEP,* phosphoenolpyruvate; *OxAc,* oxaloacetate; *FA,* fatty acid.

Relation to mealtime

After a meal, under the direction of insulin, metabolism is geared toward storage of the dietary bounty. Glucose, insofar as it is not utilized for refilling glycogen stores and for energy, is converted to fatty acyl-CoA and glycerol phosphate and stored as fat. The relative extents to which liver and adipose tissue participate in postprandial fat synthesis vary among animal species and with age. The level of free fatty acids (albumin-bound) in serum drops, since fat release from adipose tissue is slow because of the inhibition of TG-lipase by insulin. The dynamic triglyceride equilibrium temporarily shifts toward net fat synthesis.

Between regular meals, blood glucose levels plateau, and metabolism is directed by insulin antagonists toward a state of economy: glucose is spent on high-priority items only, and fat for indiscriminate energy. The forementioned anabolic situation gradually shifts toward a state of net triglyceride degradation and higher, but stable, levels of albumin-bound fatty acids in blood. Metabolically this is what happens: fatty acid synthesis from glucose ceases and adipolytic TG-lipase becomes more active as insulin titers in the blood drop and neuroendocrine influences stimulate TG-lipase. Thus, increasingly more fatty acids become available to fuel metabolism in various tissues and the serum free fatty acid level rises—up to a point; then the level of fatty acids in serum levels off, signifying that a new equilibrium has been reached. Then, gluconeogenesis in the liver provides enough glucose for upkeep of a constant blood sugar level, and this, plus increased PEP-carboxykinase activity in fat cells (allowing more glycerol phosphate production from lactate and amino acids from blood), provides the fat cell with ample capacity for triglyceride redeposition. The liver, using circulating glycerol liberated from adipose tissue during lipolysis, reesterifies plasma fatty acids and repackages them into VLDL. Hepatic export of VLDL and redeposition of their fats in adipose tissue keeps pace with the lipolytic production of free fatty acids in excess over that which tissues consume for energy; consequently, the plasma free fatty acid level is stable. (See Figure 13-18 and Chart I, Chapter 10).

Prolonged fasting (or a disease condition, such as diabetes) can upset the glucose balance to a life-threatening extent. At such a point, metabolism sacrifices its characteristically economic use of body stores and shifts to a mode of survival. In plasma, the glucose level is low, fatty acid levels rise significantly above their norm, and ketonemia is observed. The neuroendocrine milieu causes a lopsided shift in the body's dynamic triglyceride equilibrium toward degradation. The sympathetic branch of the autonomic nervous system and norepinephrine are the most powerful and fast-acting of the influences on TG-lipase. Also, upon prolonged fasting, two different pituitary factors are elaborated; these factors are slower-acting, since they cause TG-lipase synthesis. The liver cannot cope with the rapid influx of fatty acids from plasma as (i) it runs out of certain lipotropic factors (e.g., choline, methionine, inositol) needed to package triglycerides into VLDL for export, which leads to pathologic storage of triglyceride (fatty liver); and (ii) it has no viable alternative but to convert the excess fatty acids to ketones, having to use glycerol for gluconeogenesis (survival).

Neuroendocrine control

Adaptive modification of TG-lipase activity resembles, in every respect, that of liver phosphorylase discussed earlier. Three principally different kinds of TG-lipase stimulation exist:

- Promoting TG-lipase synthesis (glucocorticoids);
- Activating TG-lipase via the adenylate cyclase and Ca^{++}/calmodulin systems mediated by receptors for various hormones and the autonomic nervous system; TG-lipase is active in the phosphorylated form;
- Inhibiting phosphodiesterase activity, so that the level of cAMP remains high (e.g., caffeine).

Insulin inhibits TG-lipase by lowering the level of cAMP and increasing the level of phosphodiesterase.

Outspoken differences exist in the lipolytic responses to various hormones in different animal species. Human adipose tissue is unresponsive to most lipolytic hormones apart from thyroxine and the catecholamines. However, in the rabbit, guinea pig, pig, and chicken there is a lack of a significant lipolytic response to catecholamines. In birds, lipogenesis is confined to the liver, where it is particularly important in providing lipids for egg formation. There is also a pronounced lipolytic effect of glucagon in birds. It appears that in the various species studied a variety of mechanisms have evolved for fine control of lipid metabolism.

It seems probable that TG-lipase activity in adipose tissue is mainly controlled by liberation of norepinephrine in most animal species through activity of the sympathetic nervous system. Evidence for this statement is that a ganglionic blockade with hexamethonium or a depletion of norepinephrine with reserpine leads to severely impaired triglyceride mobilization from adipose tissue. Also, differences between α-and β-adrenergic innervation greatly influences the degree of fat mobility at various sites in the body, as does absence or presence of the potentiating influences of thyroid hormones.

Brown adipose tissue

Brown adipose tissue (BAT) consists of small cells with many mitochondria (hence, its color) and lipid droplets. In contrast, white fat cells contain few mitochondria and a single lipid droplet. BAT is amply perfused with blood.

BAT mitochondria possess a unique uncoupling protein in the inner membrane that transfers protons from outside to inside the inner mitochondrial membrane without concomitant ATP formation. This feature allows BAT to combust large amounts of fuel (glucose or fatty acids, depending on the time after a meal) for the purpose of heat production. The uncoupling protein is induced for the purpose of nonshivering thermogenesis; for instance, immediately after birth, during exposure of an animal to cold, or during arousal from hibernation. Hibernating animals have more BAT than nonhibernators. When cold-adapted rats are infused with norepinephrine (the hormone which switches on nonshivering thermogenesis), there is a threefold increase in their respiration, and at least 60% of that increased oxygen uptake can be attributed to brown fat, which accounts for less than 2% of their body weight. Uncoupling protein is depressed during pregnancy and lactation, conditions when the animal needs to conserve metabolic energy.

Lipogenesis from glucose results in net ATP production that can become rate-limiting at the level of phosphofructokinase, pyruvate dehydrogenase, or oxidative phosphorylation. Therefore, different mechanisms for lowering the ATP/ADP ratio exist in tissues with high rates of lipogenesis. In white adipose tissue, where the rate of lipogenesis is much lower than in BAT, sufficient ATP utilization occurs via the triglyceride/fatty acid futile cycle. ATP generation by lipogenesis in other tissues can be offset by other futile cycles (e.g., phosphofructokinase/fructose-1,6-bisphosphatase in the liver). In BAT, the unique uncoupling system for oxidative phosphorylation allows for the enormously high rates of lipogenesis after a meal, which leads to the next topic.

A major metabolic and functional characteristic of BAT is its high capacity to postprandially convert glucose to triglyceride and store it as fat. During cold acclimation, BAT possesses the highest hexokinase activity of any major glucose-utilizing tissues in the body; also pyruvate dehydrogenase activity is high. Hence, BAT can play a significant part in the removal of glucose after a meal.

Understandably, as oxidative phosphorylation is uncoupled, lipogenesis in BAT is accompanied by thermogenesis. Hence, increased BAT activity after dinner accounts for a large part of the postprandial heat development (specific dynamic action).

BAT has a weight-regulating function shown in many animal species. Young animals resist obesity by responding to overfeeding with a compensatory increase in postprandial heat production, which, of course, decreases feeding efficiency. Although BAT amounts to less than 2% of body weight in rats, its thermogenic capacity is sufficient to double the metabolic rate (energy consumption rate).

BAT thermogenesis (induction of the uncoupling protein) is controlled by the sympathetic nervous system. BAT activity declines with age, this is commonly due to reduced sympathetic drive, and the resulting fall in thermogenic capacity may be responsible for the poor cold tolerance and greater propensity to obesity seen in many older animals.

LIVER AND LIPID METABOLISM

The liver is the hub of lipid metabolism, and is responsible for lipid homeostasis. It communicates with peripheral cells by means of lipoprotein secretion and reabsorption, mediated by specific receptors. It synthesizes lipids (e.g., fats from dietary carbohydrates and amino acids; phospholipids for lipoprotein synthesis; and cholesterol for bile salt formation), stores vitamins A, D, E, and K, and, uniquely, it eliminates lipids in bile (e.g., cholesterol, bilirubin, and steroid derivatives).

The liver does not store much fat under normal conditions. Rather, the role of the liver in lipid metabolism is concerned mainly with transport. The text has already related, in passing, to the importance of lipoprotein and bile formation as means of lipid transport, and the consequences of disturbances of hepatic liver transport (fatty liver and ketosis). Here, the discussion shall briefly focus on those topics.

Lipoprotein formation

Lipids are synthesized in smooth ER, combined with protein and carbohydrates in Golgi, packaged there in vesicles, and exported out of the cell by exocytosis.

In this manner, the liver secretes very low-density lipoproteins (VLDL) in which it packages triglycerides, formed from fatty acids that were either synthesized in the liver postprandially or taken up from the bloodstream between regular meals.

Ingredients that go into the synthesis of VLDL (Figure 13-21) include: various proteins, cholesterol, cholesterol esters, phospholipids, triglycerides, and carbohydrates. It is important to recall that lipoproteins have a characteristic composition. Hence, if only one of the ingredients for VLDL is not available in the liver at the time the lipoprotein must be formed, the entire synthesis cannot occur, hence, the liver retains stranded fats (fatty liver). A substance that prevents abnormal accumulation of fats in the liver is called a **lipotropic factor;** for example, choline, methionine, and inositol. Vitamin E is a lipotropic factor, because it protects EFA, a constituent of phospholipids and cholesterol esters. The mineral selenium is listed as a lipotropic factor, because it is a component of an enzyme (glutathione peroxidase) that degrades peroxides and, thus, protects EFA-containing structures. Pantothenic acid is a lipotropic factor, being part of the structure of CoA.

Fatty liver

The extensive accumulation of lipids (mainly triglycerides) in liver is abnormal for an organ unaccustomed to storing lipids. Fatty liver infiltration (i.e., steatosis)

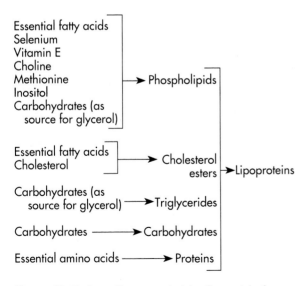

Figure 13-21. Ingredients needed for lipoprotein formation in liver.

may be generally referred to as either the milder fatty liver syndrome, the more severe fatty liver condition, or fatty liver disease. In severe cases, the liver becomes enlarged, soft, edematous, brownish-looking, and may contain over 50% of its wet weight in the form of fat. When this situation becomes chronic, cirrhosis and impaired liver function develop.

Factors that may lead to the accumulation of triglycerides in the liver include the following.

- When the level of fatty acids in plasma becomes elevated to such an extent that the liver's rate of lipoprotein synthesis from those fatty acids cannot keep up with the rate at which they are absorbed, the liver esterifies them to triglycerides, which it is then forced to store. This situation may arise during starvation or as a result of feeding diets that are rich in certain fats.
- Lack of carbohydrates or of the ability to utilize carbohydrates (e.g., starvation, diabetes, pregnancy, or lactation) causes plasma fatty acid levels to rise, which may produce fatty liver and ketosis (discussed below).
- Any condition that restricts availability of even one of the components that make up a lipoprotein may cause fatty liver; for example, feeding diets deficient in EFA or choline. Lack of essential amino acids in the diet limits synthesis of the protein moiety of lipoproteins. Moreover, when essential amino acids are lacking, methionine shortage limits production of the choline moiety of phospholipids; also, methionine deficiency causes a lack of carnitine (and, thus, a lack of fatty acid oxidation), leading to triglyceride accumulation. Too much cholesterol in the diet may tie up so much EFA for esterification that not enough EFA are available for phospholipid production.
- Antibiotics, such as puromycin, inhibit protein (e.g., apo-protein) synthesis and are conducive to fatty liver.
- Hepatotoxins, such as Pb, As, and CCl_4, all interfere at one point or another with lipoprotein synthesis or with the release of lipoproteins from the liver to the blood.

Any one of these pathophysiologic conditions, or a combination of them, could lead to inhibited transport of fat from the liver and to steatosis, provided lipid is available to the liver in normal or in increased amounts. As a general rule, most agents that lead to steatosis, however, appear to do so mainly by interference with egress of lipid (i.e., VLDL) from the liver.

Ketosis

Under normal conditions, the liver produces ketone bodies during β-oxidation of fatty acids, but the rate of ketone-body production is normally matched by the rate at which tissues remove them from the circulation, since ketone bodies are preferred fuel for energy production. Hence, ketone bodies do not normally accumulate in blood, and therefore only traces are lost in urine.

Under abnormal conditions of ketosis, the levels of ketone bodies are elevated in both blood (ketonemia) and urine (ketonuria). Both acetoacetic acid and β-hydroxybutyric acid are strong acids, and their accumulation in the blood constitutes a form of acidosis, called **ketoacidosis.** Increasingly, plasma H^+ is exchanged for intracellular K^+, so that transmembrane potential (Donnan) differences are lowered to the point where neurologic control over heart muscle contraction may be lost, which is fatal. The loss of ketoacids in urine and elimination of acetone via the breath (detectible on the breath of a heavily ketotic cow) constitutes a tremendous energy drain from the body: a ketotic animal loses weight rapidly.

The common denominator of all causes of ketosis (with the exception of spontaneous bovine ketosis) is a lack of carbohydrates or a deficiency in carbohydrate utilization; for instance, fasting, diabetes mellitus, or pancreatic lesions. The condition can be aggravated by putting an extra burden on carbohydrate metabolism, such as pregnancy and lactation. Ruminants are more prone to ketosis than monogastrics, because they do not obtain glucose from the diet; instead, they have to synthesize all their glucose by gluconeogenesis from small end products of microbial metabolism.

When the body's carbohydrate stores become depleted, neuroendocrine factors that control gluconeogenesis (and, thus, survival) stimulate TG-lipase in adipose tissue, so that increased amounts of fatty acids are released and the level of free fatty acids in plasma rises. The liver removes from the circulation excess fatty acids not taken up by extrahepatic tissues, but cannot repackage them fast enough as VLDL, because of a lack of lipotropic factors. Hence, fatty liver develops. The need to maintain blood glucose will eventually divert most glycerol in the direction of gluconeogenesis, so it is unavailable for the esterification of incoming fatty acids. The latter are then β-oxidized (in mitochondria and peroxisomes) to AcCoA, which, in turn, is converted (via the Lynen pathway) to ketone bodies that are secreted in large quantities into the bloodstream.

Muscles, using ketone bodies as their preferred fuel, will increase their ketone combustion, but they cannot burn up more than the equivalent of their energy need, which means that ketone combustion leaves more fatty acids in the bloodstream for the liver to be converted to ketones: a sum-zero proposition. Also, the brain, the body's largest glucose consumer, adapts its metabolism by gradually increasing its use of ketones for energy. Another contribution to survival is made by the combined effect of low pH on the liver and kidneys. In the liver, glutamine production is stimulated, while in the kidneys, the low pH stimulates glutaminase, producing NH_4^+ ions to electrically neutralize the acids to be excreted and, thus, to keep the losses of K^+ ions in the urine down. But this, too, is a stop-gap measure, since it augments the negative nitrogen balance. Both for glutaminase and for gluconeogenesis, amino acids are spent and the ultimate result may be decreased plasma albumin concentrations and edema.

Fetal ketone-body utlization

Ketone bodies originate in the mother from fatty acids derived from maternal fat stores that accumulated largely during the first two trimesters of pregnancy. During the third trimester, the greatest amount of fetal development occurs, a time that coincides with an ever-increasing glucose drain by the conceptus; utilization of maternal fat stores; and, therefore, a maternal liver poised toward ketone-body production. Ketone bodies produced from incoming fatty acids are not only utilized by the mother but also cross the placenta by passive diffusion where they are utilized in several ways by the fetus:

- As fuel in lieu of glucose.
- As an inhibitor of glucose and lactate oxidation with sparing of glucose for biosynthetic disposition.
- For inhibition of branched-chain ketoacid oxidation, thereby maximizing formation of their parent amino acids (valine, leucine, and isoleucine).

Enzymes capable of oxidizing ketone bodies in the fetus are found in a variety of tissues including the kidney, liver, brain, and musculoskeletal system. Unlike fetal liver, the postnatal liver loses its ability to oxidize ketone bodies, thus becoming a ketone-body exporter only. However, ketone bodies can be used as oxidative fuels by adult skeletal muscle and by the pregnant uterus and adult brain.

In addition to salvaging branched-chain amino acids from oxidation, ketone bodies from the mother are utilized for lipid synthesis in fetal brain and in other tissues, including adipose tissue, pancreas, liver, and lung. The type of lipids include not only neutral lipids but phospholipids and sterols, which indicates that ketone bodies can be used for both structural component synthesis and energy storage in the fetus. Finally, it has been shown that ketone bodies inhibit de novo biosynthesis of pyrimidines in fetal rat brain slices. Thus, during maternal starvation ketone bodies may maximize chances for survival by restraining cell replication and sustaining protein and lipid stores in fetal tissues.

Neonatal ketone body production and utilization

It has been established that neonates of a number of mammalian species exhibit increased concentrations of ketone bodies in the circulation throughout the suckling period. This raises two questions:

- What is the physiological advantage of hyperketonemia to the neonate?
- How is the availability of ketone bodies regulated?

The milk of most mammals has a high fat content relative to that of carbohydrate. Therefore, during the suckling period the neonate must both conserve its limited supply of glucose for cells that depend exclusively on this substrate and provide sufficient alternative substrates (fatty acids and ketone bodies) for the energy requirements of developing tissues. Ketone bodies have advantages over free fatty acids in that they are nontoxic in the physiological range of concentrations (0.1 to 5 mM), and they are water soluble; however, they are carboxylic acids and therefore at high concentrations will affect acid-base balance.

When one compares factors influencing ketogenesis in the suckling animal to those in the starved animal, it becomes readily apparent that the physiological situation occurring in each situation (i.e., suckling vs. starvation) is similar: (i) plasma-free fatty acids are increased; (ii) the plasma insulin/glucagon ration is decreased; (iii) hepatic carnitine levels are increased; and (iv) hepatic lipogenesis is decreased.

It appears that during the early postnatal period ketone bodies are preferred over glucose as substrates for synthesis of phospholipids and sphingolipids in accord with requirements for brain growth and myelination. Thus, during the first 2 weeks of postnatal development, when the accumulation of cholesterol and phospholipids accelerates, the proportion of ketone bodies incorporated into these lipids increases.

An increased proportion of ketone bodies is also utilized for cerebroside synthesis during the period of active myelination.

In the lung, acetoacetic acid serves better than glucose as a precursor for the synthesis of lung phospholipids. The synthesized lipids, particularly dipalmityl-phosphotidylcholine, are incorporated into pulmonary surfactant, and thus have a potential role in supplying adequate surfactant lipids to maintain lung function during the early days of life. Studies demonstrate that ketone bodies and glucose could play complementary roles in the synthesis of lung lipids by providing fatty acid and glycerol moieties of phospholipids, respectively. The preferential selection of acetoacetic acid for lipid synthesis in brain, as well as lung, stems in part from the active cytoplasmic pathway for generation of AcCoA and acetoacetyl-CoA from acetoacetic acid via the actions of cytoplasmic acetoacetyl-CoA synthetase and thiolase. Enhanced fetal catecholamine and glucocorticoid levels during parturition (i.e., stress hormones) stimulate surfactant production by type II alveolar epithelial cells of the lung.

STUDY QUESTIONS

1. Name the saturated C16 fatty acid; name a glucogenic VFA; name the lipid composed of glycerol plus three fatty acids; name a ketone body; list four vitamins that are lipids.

2. *a.* Name one of the essential fatty acids (EFA).
   b. Name an EFA-derived class of hormones.
   c. Name an EFA-derived class of compounds released from mast cells during allergic reactions.

3. *a.* Name the general lipid category to which lecithin belongs.
   b. List two dietarily essential constituents of lecithin.

4. Name the histological structure, covering nerve axons, in which sulfatides and cerebrosides are found.

5. List the vitamin, hormone, and detergent all derived from cholesterol.

6. List the vitamin whose function in lipid systems is comparable to that of vitamin C in aqueous systems.

7. List the intestinal hormone that stimulates lipase release from the pancreas.

8. Name the aggregate structures in which lipids are transported: (i) from duodenum to jejunum; (ii) from lumen of the gut into mucosal cells; (iii) from the gut mucosa into the circulation; and (iv) in bile.

9. List the compound that stabilizes fat emulsion droplets in the gut.

10. Why are monoglycerides a main product of triglyceride digestion in the intestinal lumen?

11. Identify two pathways for triglyceride synthesis within mucosal cells of the small intestine.

12. What is the fundamental difference in the immediate postabsorptive destination of dietary ingredients that are water-soluble as opposed to those that are lipidlike?

13. Give the name and function of the route whereby bile salts are passed via the bile duct into the gut and then returned to the liver via the portal circulation.

14. *a.* By what action in the gut does cholestyramine lower plasma cholesterol?
    b. For what purpose would one administer compactin or mevinolin during cholestyramine treatment?
    c. Is cholestyramine a drug?

15. *a.* List a lipoprotein of intestinal origin that transports dietary lipids.
    b. List a lipoprotein of intestinal or hepatic origin that transports endogenously synthesized lipids.

16. *a.* List two classes of essential dietary ingredients carried by chylomicron remnants.
    b. What directs a chylomicron remnant to its final destination?

17. *a.* Name the enzyme activity that clears postprandial lactescence.
    b. Where is this enzyme located and what activates it in adipose tissue after a meal?

18. Explain the postprandial drop in the free fatty acid level in a dog's serum.

19. *a.* In what form does the liver export triglycerides it synthesized from excess dietary carbohydrates?
    b. What targets these fats toward adipose tissue for storage?
    c. List a lipoprotein class that accumulates after excessive caloric intake, causing hypercholesterolemia.

20. In times between meals and fasting, what allows VLDL to serve the energy needs of heart cells in preference to fat deposition in fat cells?

21. How are β-lipoproteins formed? How does their density compare with that of α-lipoproteins? Which lipid class is chiefly transported in β-lipoproteins?

22. *a.* What causes down-regulation of LDL-receptors on cell membranes?
    b. Why is it that liver cells can still remove cholesterol from the blood under conditions when extrahepatic cells cannot?

23. *a.* List six classes of compounds that make up a VLDL.
    b. Why is choline needed for hepatic lipoprotein production?
    c. What adjective describes the dietary factors involved in hepatic VLDL production and release?

24. What do HDL contribute to chylomicrons, so that incoming dietary cholesterol is targeted toward the liver?

25. List the plasma enzyme that allows the cholesterol-scavenger function of HDL. What essential compound does this enzyme transfer?

26. *a.* Define "reverse cholesterol transport."
    b. List a function of apoprotein D on HDL.

27. Will down-regulation of insulin receptors on adipose tissue cells: (i) Increase fat synthesis from glucose? (ii) Decrease the length of postprandial lactescence? (iii) Increase concentration of free fatty acids in plasma?

28. *a.* List a functional reason why fasting stimulates carnitine acyltransferase activity.
    b. List the allosteric negative control over this enzyme complex in times of fatty acid synthesis.

29. List the cofactor linking rates of β-oxidation and oxidative phosphorylation and explain why, under ischemic conditions, β-oxidation of fatty acids cannot continue. _____

30. *a.* Which compound links methionine availability to β-oxidation of fatty acids?
    b. Which compound links increased Ac-CoA carboxylase with decreased carnitine acyltransferase activity?

31. During fasting, when fatty acid in the blood is high, how can the liver β-oxidize more fatty acids than mitochondrial control mechanisms allow?

32. Where in the liver cell are ketone bodies synthesized? Can the adult liver catabolize ketone bodies?

33. How can the liver produce ketones between regular meals and why don't those ketones build up in the bloodstream?

34. Why is the Lynen pathway of hepatic ketogenesis needed for survival during fasting?

35. Name the ketone body obtained by reduction of acetoacetate. Give a functional reason for that reduction.

36. *a.* List the common denominator in various instances of ketosis.
    b. List a condition in sheep under which ketosis often develops.
    c. For what purpose does the liver use incoming glycerol during ketosis?
    d. List an odiferous compound in the breath of a ketotic patient.

e. List a critical mineral distribution upset during ketoacidosis.

37. What benefit has an animal from the fact that renal glutaminase activity is stimulated by ketoacidosis?

38. About the rate-controlling step of fatty acid synthesis in the cytoplasm:
   a. Name the enzyme catalyzing this step.
   b. List the feed-forward activator of this enzyme, whose level increases after a meal.
   c. List the feedback inhibitor of this enzyme, whose level increases during fasting.
   d. List an essential organic cofactor and a trace mineral involved.
   e. List an endocrine stimulator of this step.

39. Which redox cofactor is required for cytoplasmic fatty acid synthesis, and which processes regenerate the proper redox state of that cofactor?

40. Why must fatty acid synthesized in cytoplasm be immediately esterified for fatty acid synthesis to continue?

41. Why does cow fat contain more odd-chained fatty acids than does dog fat? How do ruminants obtain essential fatty acids?

42. Which two processes are needed to convert palmitate to oleate?

43. Explain how the action of insulin on citrate lyase is consistent with that hormone's mission to lower blood glucose.

44. How does an AMP-dependent protein kinase prevent runaway cholesterol synthesis from Ac-CoA when fatty acid synthesis is blocked?

45. What is the functionality behind negative feedback by bile acids on hepatic cholesterol synthesis?

46. What is the purpose of the glucose-glycerol cycle between liver and adipose tissue?

47. If you knew that a compound (e.g., caffeine) had a negative effect on phosphodiesterase activity, what then would be the effect on the level of free fatty acids in plasma?

48. List two concomitant insulin effects at the plasma membrane of fat cells that allow triglyceride deposition after a meal.

49. List the purpose for which G-6-P dehydrogenase is activated in fat cells after dinner.

50. Interpret: blocking β-adrenergic receptors of fat cells inhibits the release of fatty acids.

51. List the futile cycle in adipose tissue and give the putative need for it.

52. List two reasons why, in times of starvation, there can only be little fat synthesis in adipose tissue.

53. *a.* List the function of brown adipose tissue immediately after birth.
   b. List one putative function of brown adipose tissue associated with the occurrence of a conspicuously high level of hexokinase.

54. *a.* Explain thermogenesis in brown adipose tissue after a meal.
   b. What mechanism underlies thermogenesis in brown adipose tissue during cold stress?

55. The main liver functions in lipid metabolism deal with transport: list (i) the liver's involvement in intestinal lipid absorption; (ii) the liver's role in lipid transport in the bloodstream; (iii) the liver's role in reverse cholesterol transport; and (iv) the role of hepatic lipid metabolism during ketosis.

56. *a.* Why do certain antibiotics cause fatty liver? Why do some cause selenium deficiency?
   b. To explain why methionine deficiency leads to fatty liver, list two important quaternary amines formed by methylation reactions and, in addition, one protein-synthesis related factor.

57. *a.* For what purpose does the fetus use ketone bodies?
   b. How might ketone-body utilization by the fetus enhance chances for survival during maternal food deprivation?

58. What is the physiological advantage of hyperketonemia to the neonate?

14 Nitrogen metabolism

This chapter deals with the main classes of compounds that contain nitrogen: proteins, amino acids, purines, pyrimidines, nucleosides, nucleotides, nucleic acids, and porphyrins. (See left-hand side of Chart II.) The text shall look into the functions of these N-compounds in metabolism more elaborately than it has in previous chapters.

As part of homeostasis in the adult organism, nitrogen balance must be maintained; that is, the total uptake of dietary nitrogen must equal nitrogen excreted in urine plus feces and exudates. Dietary nitrogen compounds and their digestion, metabolism, and excretion products will be considered in the context of nitrogen balance under normal and some pathologic conditions.

AMINO ACID METABOLISM
General functions and main metabolic reactions of amino acids

Several of the numerous functions of amino acids have already been discussed; for example, the function and synthesis of proteins and peptides; transamination and glutamate dehydrogenase reactions involved in the conversion of amino acids into gluconeogenic and ketogenic intermediates; replenishment of TCA cycle intermediates; lipotropic functions of methionine; and conjugation of bile acids with glycine or cysteine-derived taurine (Figure 14-1).

Essential amino acids

Though most amino acids can be endogenously synthesized from their corresponding α-ketoacids, some cannot, and must be included in the diet; these are the essential amino acids.

Different animal species have different amino acids that they cannot synthesize in adequate amounts, and, thus, have different dietary requirements for es-

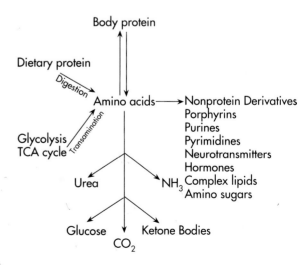

Figure 14-1. Sources and utilization of amino acids.

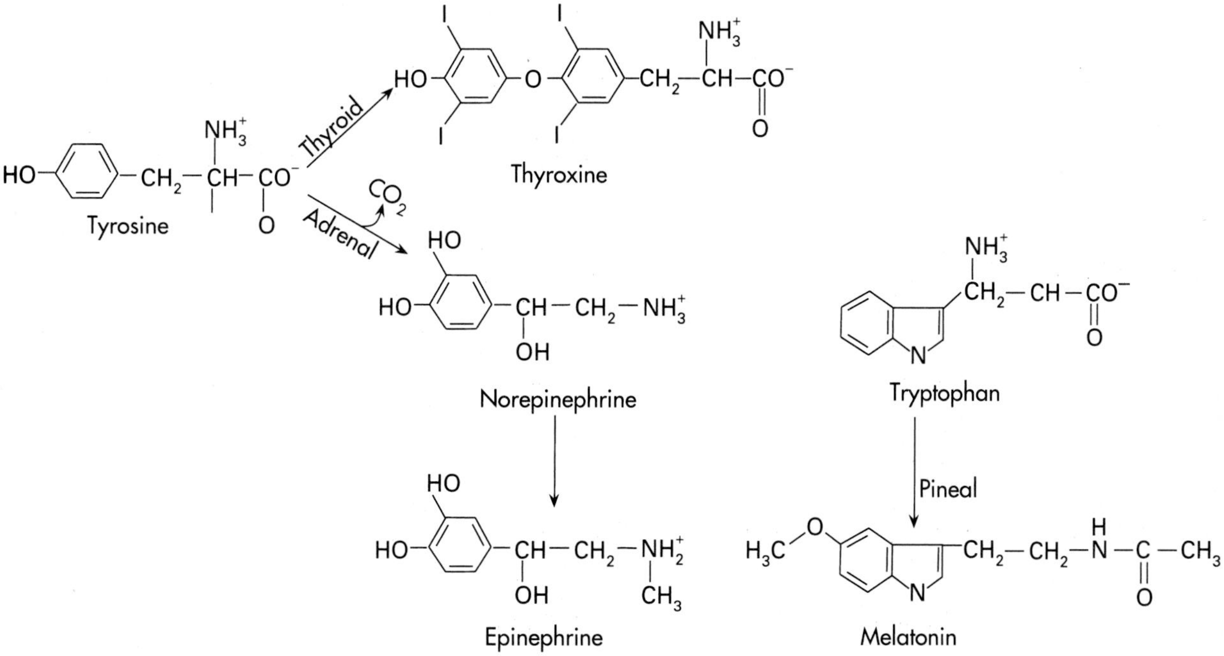

Figure 14-2. Hormones derived from single amino acids.

sential amino acids. For humans and most animals, histidine, leucine, isoleucine, lysine, threonine, tryptophan, valine, and methionine are essential. Arginine is essential for growing animals in general, and glycine for young chickens.

Protein synthesis is the most important function for which essential amino acids are truly essential. Their biological half-lives are longer than are those of the nonessential amino acids, since the latter are spent preferentially on various amino acid functions.

Synthesis of nonproteinaceous hormones

Amino acids are precursors not only for hormones that are proteins, but also for small-molecular, non-

proteinaceous hormones such as melatonin, thyroxine, epinephrine, and norepinephrine (Figure 14-2).

It is important to realize that hormones are, chemically speaking, a very diverse group of compounds, ranging from lipids (steroids, prostaglandins) through proteins (prolactin), and small peptides (ADH), to simple compounds derived from single amino acids (thyroxine, melatonin, epinephrine, and norepinephrine).

Taurine

Taurine (2-aminoethane-sulphonic acid), discovered in ox bile in 1827, is formed by oxidation of the $-SH$ group of cysteine to $-SO_3H$, and decarboxylation:

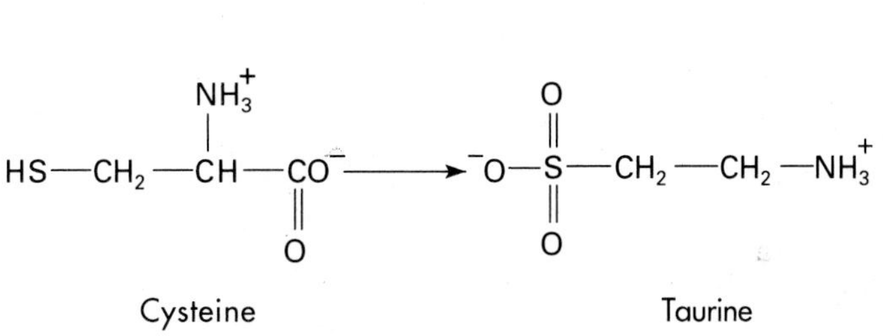

It has been known for nearly 150 years that taurine and glycine occur in conjugation to bile acids (e.g., taurocholate, glycochenodeoxycholate), yet only within the past 15 years has it been shown that cats have only a limited capacity to synthesize and store taurine, and consequently must obtain it routinely from the diet. Taurine deficiency in cats leads to several pathophysiological symptoms including central retinal degeneration and blindness, reproductive failure, retardation of body growth and skeletal deformations in kittens, and dilated cardiomyopathy. Although the mechanisms of taurine action have yet to be elucidated, it is nonetheless clear that taurine is a subtle modulator of important processes in cells such as energy metabolism, cell division, osmotic balance, prostaglandin metabolism, antioxidation, muscle contraction, and the conjugation of xenobiotics. It is thought that the greater part of its activity reflects either the influence it has over ionic fluxes in cells, particularly that of calcium, or that through its control of glutamate synthesis it indirectly regulates the excitation threshold of cellular membranes.

Removal of ammonia from the blood

Ammonia formation, resulting from amino acid catabolism, occurs in all tissues, but is especially prevalent in the liver and kidneys during gluconeogenesis. Also, NH_3 is produced in the gut by bacteria, resulting in high ammonia levels in portal blood. In systemic blood, by contrast, the ammonia level is normally low at all times; this has to be so, because ammonia is strongly toxic to the nervous system.

There are four active processes in tissues that keep blood ammonia levels low:
- Keto acids plus NH_3 produce amino acids, mostly alanine (from pyruvate), aspartic acid (from oxaloacetate), and glutamic acid (from α-keto-glutarate).
- Amidation of glutamic acid produces glutamine; amidation of aspartic acid produces asparagine.
- Renal formation of ammonium salts; excreted in urine.
- Formation of urea in the liver by the urea cycle (Figure 14-3).

By urea formation, the liver detoxifies two ammonium ions at the expense of four high-energy phosphate equivalents:

$$2 \, NH_3 + CO_2 + 4 \sim P \rightarrow Urea + 4 \, P_i$$

In humans and other ureotelic mammals, urea accounts for over 90% of all nitrogenous wastes. Since ammonia is toxic, this is one of the most important

liver functions in metabolism. The enzyme arginase is present only in the liver; therefore, occurrence of arginase in the bloodstream is diagnostic for hepatocellular damage.

METABOLISM OF PURINES AND PYRIMIDINES

Two classes of nitrogen-containing compounds, the purines and pyrimidines, are vitally important to all tissues: they are building blocks of DNA, RNA, and high-energy phosphate compounds, such as ATP, GTP, and UTP. In combination with several vitamins, these compounds make up the active form of vitamins (e.g., with riboflavin as FAD, with niacin as NAD^+ and $NADP^+$, and with pantothenic acid in coenzyme A).

Cells that divide rapidly or that have high rates of protein biosynthesis, such as skin, intestinal mucosa, liver, pancreatic cells, or the champion hen oviduct cells, have high requirements for purines and pyrimidines. Even the stable cell populations of adult muscle and nervous tissue have internal turnover of RNA and protein, although at slower rates, and, hence, need these compounds.

Nucleic acids are synthesized from scratch whenever needed. This is very thoughful of nature, since the body does not have to derive anything from the diet in order to synthesize vital nucleic acids, provided that the body keeps up with its B vitamin requirements, which, other than the bacterial flora, the diet has to provide.

Biosynthesis of purines

Purines are synthesized from nonessential amino acids with the aid of B vitamins (Figure 14-4).

Adenine and guanine are the most important purines:

Adenine
(6-aminopurine)

Guanine
(2-amino-6-oxypurine)

Guanine is readily biosynthesized from adenine. In the structures of nucleosides and nucleotides, the pentose sugar ribose is attached to nitrogen-9.

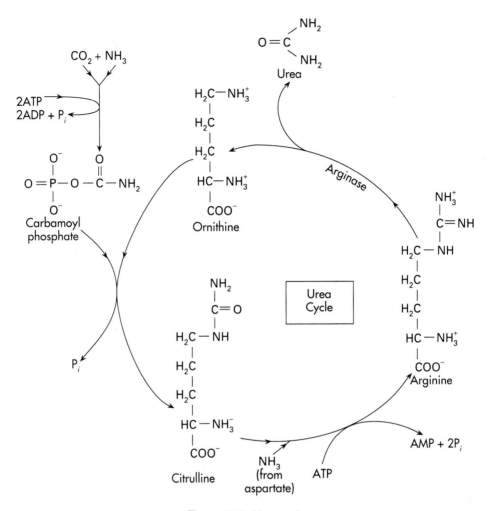

Figure 14-3. Urea cycle.

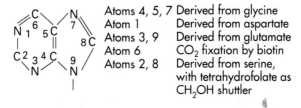

Atoms 4, 5, 7 Derived from glycine
Atom 1   Derived from aspartate
Atoms 3, 9   Derived from glutamate
Atom 6 CO_2 fixation by biotin
Atoms 2, 8   Derived from serine, with tetrahydrofolate as CH_2OH shuttler

Figure 14-4. Ingredients of purine biosynthesis.

Purine nucleotide biosynthesis starts with the conversion of ribose-5-phosphate to 5-phosphoribosyl-1-pyrophosphate (PRPP) and linking PRPP to an ammonia that is to be nitrogen-9 in the end. The synthesis is regulated by demand for the product; as long as the product is needed, it is incorporated into nucleic acids or into NAD or FAD. As soon as demands are met, the free product inhibits further production by allosteric inhibition of PRPP synthesis.

Biosynthesis of pyrimidines

Like purines, the biosynthesis of pyrimidines requires no essential compounds, except B vitamins (Figure 14-5). Control over the rate of pyrimidine nucleotide synthesis is through feedback inhibition and repression/derepression control over enzyme activities.

Because the diet is no significant source, purines and pyrimidines that are used by the body are, by and

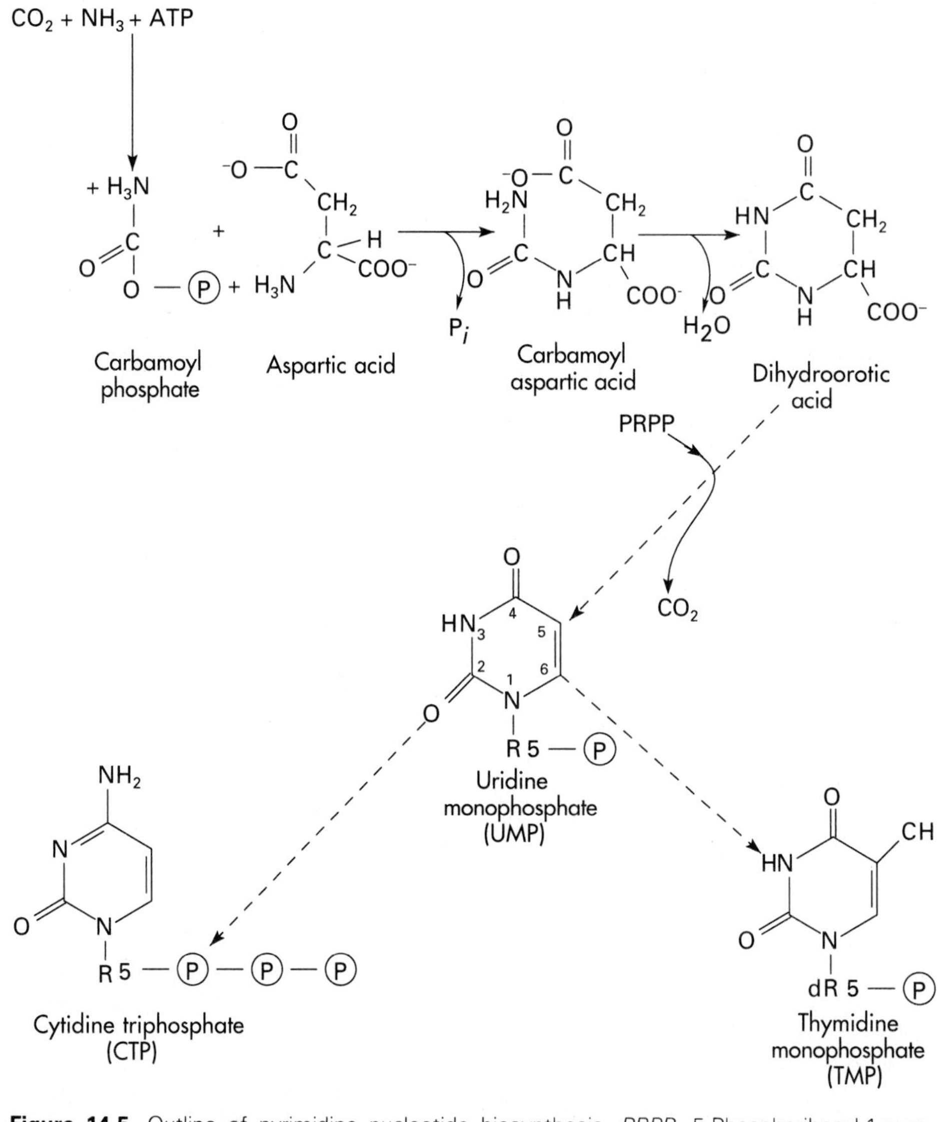

Figure 14-5. Outline of pyrimidine nucleotide biosynthesis, *PRPP,* 5-Phosphoribosyl-1-pyrophosphate.

large, synthesized from endogenous materials. Synthesis of purine and pyrimidine bases requires B vitamins and nonessential amino acids (glycine, serine, aspartate, and glutamine). Hence, the need for purine and pyrimidine biosynthesis does constitute a constant leak in the TCA cycle.

The pentose sugars ribose and deoxyribose, needed for nucleotide and nucleic acid synthesis, are synthe-sized from glucose, either via the oxidative pentose shunt (liver) or via the nonoxidative portion of the pentose shunt (muscles), or via the uronic acid pathway (liver, kidneys). A small amount is passively absorbed from the diet.

Degradation of purines

Purines are broken down to uric acid, which may be further degraded to allantoin:

Uric acid   Allantoin

Most purine oxidation takes place in the liver and gut; the end products are excreted in urine. Catabolism of both dietary and endogenous purines leads to the formation of uric acid. In humans and other primates, uric acid is normally excreted in urine. In other mammals, uric acid is reabsorbed by the kidneys and transported to the liver, where the enzyme uricase converts it to allantoin, which is then excreted via the urine. The Dalmatian dog has a kidney tubular defect that does not allow this breed to reabsorb filtered uric acid. Dalmatians have a normal content of uricase in the liver, but, because much of the uric acid is filtered from the blood and lost as such in the urine, both allantoin and uric acid appear in the urine of this breed.

Uric acid is sparingly soluble in the blood and urine; even less so at acidic pH. When exceeding its solubility, uric acid precipitates out in the urinary tract and joints. This may cause urinary tract obstruction (urolithiasis) and a painful arthritic-type swelling of the joints (tophi). Primary gout is an inborn lack of control over purine biosynthesis; chronic overproduction of purines leads to excess uric acid and to the formation of kidney stones and tophi. The drug allopurinol, a competitive inhibitor of xanthine oxidase, prevents oxidation of purines to uric acid, and thereby relieves symptoms of primary gout. Secondary gout may occur when there is an abnormally elevated turnover of endogenous purines, such as in starvation, certain blood diseases (leukemias), and other wasting

conditions. Gout is normally a disease of primates. The Dalmatian dog is also susceptible to urinary tract problems from uric acid.

Degradation of pyrimidines

Pyrimidines are broken down mainly in the liver and yield β-alanine and β-aminoisobutyrate (BAIB):

$$\overset{+}{H_3N} - CH_2 - CH_2 - COO^-$$

β-Alanine

$$\overset{+}{H_3N} - CH_2 - \underset{\underset{H}{|}}{\overset{\overset{CH_3}{|}}{C}} - COO^-$$

β-Aminoisobutyrate

Those pyrimidine degradation products are excreted in urine. β-Alanine is formed from cytosine and uracil, BAIB from thymine, and, thus, from DNA. BAIB secretion in urine is monitored to estimate irradiation damage to DNA.

Inhibitors of purine and pyrimidine biosynthesis

Inhibiting biosynthesis of purines and pyrimidines is used as a form of chemotherapy in the treatment of various kinds of cancer. Malignant cells characteristically divide much more rapidly than normal cells and, hence, have a higher requirement for purines and pyrimidines, which makes them more vulnerable to the metabolic inhibitors. Of course, the inhibitors also impair purine and pyrimidine synthesis in normal cells; they are toxic to all body cells. Asazerine, a potent inhibitor of purine and pyrimidine biosynthesis, does so by blocking nitrogen transfers, but it has proved to be too toxic to normal cells and is, therefore, not routinely used as a chemotherapeutic agent. Aminopterin inhibits the one-carbon transfers in purine and pyrimidine biosyntheses, and is, therefore, of value in the chemotherapy of acute leukemias.

Ureotelic and uricotelic animals

Proteins are by far the most abundant nitrogen store for animals. Because amino acids yield urea as their main nitrogen excretion product in urine, mammals are termed **ureotelic.** In mammals, uric acid and allantoin are the urinary excretion products of purine catabolism. However, purines constitute only a small proportion of total nitrogen metabolism.

Birds and certain reptiles, on the other hand, excrete not only their purine waste, but also their amino acid nitrogen in the form of uric acid; this makes them **uricotelic** animals. The uric acid pathway of excretion of amino acid nitrogen has this advantage: uric acid is highly concentrated and is excreted in urine as a uric acid paste with minimal osmotic loss of water.

Teleost fish, like most aquatic animals, excrete amino acid nitrogen as ammonia; they are termed **ammonotelic.**

INTESTINAL DIGESTION OF NITROGEN COMPOUNDS FROM THE DIET
Protein digestion

Mainly single amino acids and short peptides are absorbed in adult animals, as is evidenced by the finding that protein balance is maintained when only free amino acids are fed, provided that all essential amino acids are administered. Evidence for absorption of small peptides as a major route of amino acid uptake is the observation that patients with Hartnup disease, who cannot transport free tryptophan across the mucosa, nevertheless grow almost normally. Caused by the presence of peptide hydrolases in the brush border and cytosol of mucosal cells, most of these peptides undergo hydrolysis to free amino acids as soon as they enter the mucosal cells. Insofar as they are not utilized for intestinal protein synthesis, free amino acids (and some small peptides) are routed via the portal vein to the liver.

Proteolytic enzyme activities

Protein-digesting enzymes in the gut lumen are classified as endopeptidases and exopeptidases. The former attack a peptide chain from within at the site of peptide bonds, between amino acids for which the endopeptidase is specific. Since these bonds between just the right amino acids are rare, endopeptidase activity leaves large peptide fragments. The endopeptidases are pepsin in the stomach and trypsin, chymotrypsin, and elastin coming from the pancreas. Neuroendocrine stimuli leading to secretion of these enzymes, and activation of the zymogen forms in which they are secreted, have been discussed earlier.

Among the exopeptidases are pancreatic carboxypeptidase and intestinal aminopeptidase, which digest the leftovers of endopeptidase digestion from their terminals. Aminopeptidases lop off one amino acid at a time, starting from the amino terminal of the peptide chain, and carboxypeptidases remove one amino acid at a time from the carboxyl ends of the peptide chains. The gut mucosa facing the lumen has enough peptidase activities, in the brush border and intracellularly to complete the last phase of digestion, so that single amino acids (and a few small peptides) remain.

Active absorption of L-amino acids

Since only L-amino acids are incorporated in proteins, the diet does not contain many D-amino acids. The L-amino acids are actively absorbed for which ATP and vitamin B_6 are required. When ATP formation is impaired (e.g., by dinitrophenol's uncoupling of oxidative phosphorylation), amino acid absorption is inhibited. Different routes exist in the gut mucosa for the active absorption of various amino acids and small peptides.

Absorbed amino acids are used in part for intestinal protein synthesis. The remainder are transported via portal blood to the liver, where numerous anabolic routes exist for incorporating them into larger macromolecules. The subsequent metabolic fates of absorbed amino acids are discussed below.

Degradation by intestinal flora

A proportion of the dietary amino acid is lost because of putrefaction and fermentation by intestinal flora. By decarboxylation of the α-carboxyl group, amines are formed, some of which are rather odoriferous, such as cadaverine (formed from lysine) or putrescine (formed from ornithine). Some are vasopressors, such as histamine (formed from histidine). More complete fermentation of amino acids yields gases (H_2S, methane), ammonium ions (which enter the bloodstream to be detoxified by urea formation in the liver), and various other small-molecular compounds.

Nucleoproteins

Pancreatic enzyme activities split nucleoproteins into proteins and nucleic acids, and then convert RNA and DNA by specific RNA-ase and DNA-ase activities to nucleotides. Intestinal mononucleotidases then produce nucleosides and continue to split the pentose moiety from the free bases.

REGULATION OF BODY PROTEIN METABOLISM

After the liver, gut, and kidneys have removed amino acids from the blood, the amino acids are not stored as such: their electrical charges and their low molecular weights make storage of free amino acids osmotically impossible. Hence, they are rapidly metabolized. Either they are incorporated into proteins and stored in the reservoir of structural cell components, or they are immediately used for one of their numerous functions or stored as fat. Free amino acids are every bit as dynamic as glucose and free fatty acids.

Metabolic properties of skeletal muscle

In this section, the text considers the metabolic requirements needed for maintenance of muscle structure and function. Later, the metabolic functions of muscle protein stores in support of whole body metabolism are reviewed.

Differentiation of muscle fibers

Muscle fibers may be differentiated on the basis of appearance and contraction characteristics.

- Type I fibers are red and exhibit slow-twitch contraction. They serve for prolonged contraction in sustained exercise (e.g., longissimus muscles for posture control). These muscle cells owe their dark color to myoglobin and mitochondrial cytochromes used for aerobic catabolism of fatty acids and ketone bodies. Given the abundance of these nutrients and the fact that these cells derive the necessary ATP for contraction from oxidative phosphorylation, red muscles do not fatigue easily. Type I fibers have a rich blood supply, numerous mitochondria whose number increases with training, small cell diameters, less of a sarcotubular system than type II fibers, and the Ca^{++} uptake and release from the sarcoplasmic reticulum is slow.
- Type II fibers are white and exhibit fast-twitch contraction. They serve for rapid bursts of activity of short duration. These cells contain few mitochondria (hence, their pale color) and derive their needed ATP mainly anaerobically from glycogenolysis, anaerobic glycolysis, and from phosphocreatine. These cells are rich in glycogenolytic and glycolytic enzymes, lactate dehydrogenase, phosphocreatine, and creatine phosphokinase (CPK), the enzyme involved in forming phosphocreatine from creatine at the expense of ATP. Lactate is used to store metabolic electrons, since oxygen is scarce. Type II fibers do not have a rich blood supply, but their cell diameters are typically large, and the uptake and release of Ca^{++} from their extensive sarcotubular system is rapid. Myosin ATPase activity is also high, giving these fibers a rapid and powerful contractile response.
- Type III fibers, called **intermediate fibers** because of their color, are fast-twitch fibers with high rates of aerobic metabolism and glycogenolytic activity.

The ratios of these muscle fiber types are mainly determined genetically and are not affected by training. For example, the Quarter Horse (7% Type I, 93% Type II) is good for high speed over short distances, The Thoroughbred (12% Type I, 88% Type II) has an intermediate ratio, while the Heavy Hunter (31% Type I, 69% Type II) can sustain a higher level of aerobic exercise for a longer period of time. Greyhound dogs (3% Type I, 97% Type II) are excellent athletes over short distances, but mongrel dogs (31% Type I, 69% Type II) may be better prepared for long-distance exercise. Elite human distance runners (79% Type I, 21% Type II), on the other hand, have a ratio that is almost the reverse of elite human sprinters (24% Type I, 76% Type II). Different muscles contain characteristic ratios of the three muscle types; for instance, gastrocnemius has a majority of white muscle fibers (to serve sprinters and jumpers) while soleus contains more of the red, slow-twitch fibers that are used by marathon runners and swimmers.

Energy sources for muscle contraction

The involvement of myosin ATP-ase in muscle contraction requires a supply of ATP. The different types of muscle fibers all have a full complement of glycogenolytic, glycolytic, and TCA enzymes; however, as red fibers contain more mitochondria than do the white fibers, Type I fibers rely more on oxidation of free fatty acids and ketone bodies, whereas Type II fibers obtain their ATP mostly from glycogen, glucose uptake, and hydrolysis of phosphocreatine.

Energy sources in muscles, then, can be categorized thusly:

- Fatty acids and ketones are an abundant source of ATP in fibers with adequate blood supply (oxygen) and numbers of mitochondria (i.e., red fibers).
- Glycogen stores are rather limited, but these, together with glucose uptake from the blood, must supply the bulk of ATP in the white fibers, since they must operate to a large extent anaerobically. Compared to ATP formation by oxidative phosphorylation in red fibers, ATP formation at the substrate level in white muscle is about 2.5 times faster. Stored glycogen can provide about 1.5 minutes worth of fuel for maximal muscle contraction. The glycogen stores can be built up by nutritional means (carbohydrate loading before an athletic event); but after exhaustion, it requires several days (depending on diet)

to replenish. It is important to note the critical role of Ca^{++}: not only is it needed for contraction, but also as part of the second-messenger system that activates the protein kinase that phosphorylates inactive muscle phosphorylase *b* to active phosphophosphorylase *a*. This enzyme is lacking, for example, in McArdle's glycogen storage disease.

- ATP and phosphocreatine are present in muscles in small amounts. These compounds, called the **phosphagen energy system,** could sustain muscle contraction for less than 10 seconds before being exhausted, and, thus, serve for short, vigorous bursts of power. A slow myokinase activity converting 2 ADP into 1 ATP plus 1 AMP is of little practical importance. Phosphocreatine, also called **creatine phosphate,** is especially important in white muscle, since it produces ATP at about four times the speed of oxidative phosphorylation.

Creatine — Phosphocreatine — Creatinine

- The combined anaerobic effect of glycoenolysis and phosphocreatine degradation in Type II white muscle fibers accounts for the fact that a good sprinter can run the 100-yard dash without taking a breath.

The enzyme activity of creatine phosphokinase (CPK) in plasma is often measured clinically as a measure of muscle damage. The catabolite of phosphocreatine, creatinine, is excreted from muscle into the circulation at the same rate at which the kidneys remove it; its constant level in blood is an internal reference in plasma clearance measurements, as discussed earlier.

Oxygen debt

During heavy exercise, all oxygen physically dissolved or bound to hemoglobin and myoglobin in

body fluids and tissues is soon used up. At this point, aerobic metabolism can continue only in red fibers, whereas white fibers must fuel their activity anaerobically; that is, from stored glycogen and, in the longer run, from glucose taken up from the bloodstream. The end product of anaerobic metabolism, lactate, is then reconverted to glucose in the liver (Cori cycle) for another round of muscle activity. Thus, to sustain its anaerobic activity, the muscle relies on the aerobic (fat burning) capacity of the liver. After cessation of exercise, the oxygen balance must be reestablished; continued hyperventilation then brings in enough oxygen to repay the oxygen debt that was incurred; that is, the stores of dissolved and bound oxygen in fluids and tissues are replenished, and, by aerobic metabolism, the phosphagen and glycogen stores are restocked.

Skeletal muscle metabolism in relation to meals

Muscle metabolism is postprandially fueled by glucose. High insulin levels stimulate glucose uptake and its oxidative metabolism in mitochondria. Oxidative pentose shunt (G-6-P dehydrogenase) activity is practically nonexistent in muscle. Glycogen is synthesized, mainly from lactate. Amino acids, especially the branched-chain ones (leucine, isoleucine, and valine), are taken up and deposited in the form of muscle protein, aided by insulin's inhibitory effect on protein breakdown.

Between meals, glucose and insulin levels decline and fatty acids liberated from adipose tissue are the muscle's main nutrient. Oxidation of fatty acids and ketone bodies, produced by the liver in increased amounts during fasting, inhibits pyruvate dehydrogenase activity and, thus, spares glucose for vital purposes. Skeletal muscle is the major protein reserve of the body. Branched-chain amino acids are degraded in skeletal and heart muscle (not in the liver) to TCA cycle intermediates at a rate which increases during fasting; their carbon skeletons are used to fuel muscle contraction, and their amino groups are shuttled in the form of alanine to the liver for elimination via the urea cycle. Other muscle proteins are, to a large extent, converted to alanine and shipped to the liver where they serve as substrate for gluconeogenesis.

Cardiac muscle metabolism resembles that of red muscle fibers. Since the heart muscle is loaded with mitochondria, fatty acids, ketone bodies, and lactate (during exercise) are its main nutrients, except after dinner, when fatty acid levels are low and glucose is abundantly available.

Role of the intestines and liver after a meal

In humans, the average dietary intake of protein is about 100 g per day. Add to that some 50 g protein of sloughed mucosal cells plus approximately 17 g of protein in gastrointestinal secretions to arrive at an intestinal load of circa 170 g per day. From that, only about 10 g ends up in the feces, while 160 g is absorbed.

Absorbed amino acids pass to the liver via the portal vein. The liver is the primary site for catabolism of the essential amino acids, with the exception of the branched-chain ones — valine and isoleucine (both glucogenic) and leucine (ketogenic) —which bypass the liver to be metabolized and/or stored primarily in muscle and kidneys. After dogs are fed a large meat meal, more than half of the incoming amino acids are degraded in the liver, yielding urea, fat, and carbohydrates, a small proportion are retained as liver protein, some are secreted as plasma proteins, and only 25% of the incoming load passes into the general circulation as free amino acids, predominantly the branched-chain ones.

By a sensitive and discriminating mechanism, the liver modulates the degradation of many of the essential amino acids in relation to the needs of the body. When dietary intake of an essential amino acid is increased beyond requirements, induction of the enzymes of the corresponding degradative pathway often occurs (e.g., tryptophan oxygenase).

The postprandial plasma levels of amino acids are also affected by dietary carbohydrate through an insulin-dependent mechanism: the plasma amino acid levels go down, especially the branched-chain amino acids, because of deposition in muscle through insulin-mediated transport.

Role of skeletal muscle in whole-body protein metabolism
Protein stores and nitrogen economy

Since 60% of the total body protein is present in muscle, it constitutes a large potential reservoir of amino acid precursors to support the liver's syntheses of plasma proteins and glucose between meals. However, muscle stores of glycogen and protein both subserve vital contractile functions, which would be compromised if these stores became unduly depleted. The glycogen store serves as a vital energy source to fuel rapid contraction and, therefore, needs to be maintained at a level that allows this function to be preserved even in situations of total carbohydrate deprivation. In fact, in the rat, diaphragm muscle glycogen falls to 40% of the fed level in the first 24 hours of starvation, but thereafter remains constant. So, any contribution of muscle glycogen to body glucose formation, via production of glycolytically derived gluconeogenic precursors (lactate, pyruvate, and alanine), is confined to the early period of starvation. In contrast, the protein content of the diaphragm muscle falls throughout the first 5 days of starvation in the rat, eventually stabilizing at about 60% of the fed level. Thus, muscle protein can provide a continuous supply of amino acid precursors for glucose formation over a longer period of starvation compared with muscle glycogen.

It is of considerable help for withstanding prolonged starvation that the body establishes a tighter nitrogen economy, so that a drastic slowdown in muscle protein turnover is observed; down to 20% of the original turnover rate. Important in this nitrogen economy is adaptation by the brain, the largest glucose consumer. By shifting to ketone body utilization, the brain takes up less glucose, so that hepatic gluconeogenesis is diminished and muscle protein is spared.

Hepatic gluconeogenesis from muscle proteins

The total of glucogenic amino acids released from muscle adds up to about 80% of all amino acids released; ketogenic amino acids constitute the remainder. Identities and relative amounts of glucogenic amino acids from muscle that are made available to liver and other tissues is depicted (Figure 14-6).

Alanine is by far the most important amino acid taken up by the liver. Alanine accounts for approximately 38% of all glucogenic amino acids released from muscle, and, in addition, some alanine is formed from glutamine in the gut and kidneys. Three different transport systems for amino acids have been discovered in the liver. One of them is the A system; A stands for alanine transport. The A system is induced by fasting and glucogenic hormones, such as glucagon, glucocorticoids, and catecholamines. This induction is abolished in the presence of antibiotics that cripple protein synthesis. Induction of the A system is, thus, an important gluconeogenic adaptation of the liver in times of need. Another gluconeogenic rate determinant is the level of alanine in the blood. Gluconeogenesis from alanine in the liver has such a high capacity that it is not saturated even at nine times the physiological alanine concentration. Therefore, the alanine concentration in blood, in addition to A system induction, regulates the rate of hepatic gluconeogenesis.

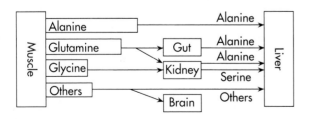

Figure 14-6. Relative amounts of glucogenic amino acids released from muscle. *Modified and reproduced with permission from Snell K: Alanine as a gluconeogenic carrier, Trends Biochem Sci 4:124-128, 1979.*

Export of alanine from muscle; glucose-alanine cycle

It is important to note that muscle releases alanine and glutamine far in excess of the proportion in which these amino acids occur in muscle proteins. Part of the alanine and glutamine released by muscle must be generated by converting carbohydrate and other amino acids to alanine and glutamine.

Production of alanine. For amino acids in muscle to serve as a source of alanine, they must first transaminate with α-ketoglutarate (Figure 14-7). This transamination in muscle is practically restricted to aspartate and the branched-chain amino acids valine, leucine, and isoleucine. Hence, these amino acids, derived from muscle proteins and from the bloodstream, serve as alanine precursors. It is clear from the figure, that there must be an adequate supply of pyruvate, so that alanine export can be sustained. In fact, pyruvate supply may be rate-limiting.

There are two sources from which pyruvate for alanine export is derived: (i) from muscle protein, via the ketoacids formed by transamination of amino acids (route #1 in Figure 14-7); and (ii) from extraneous glucose provided by the liver via the glucose-alanine cycle (route #2 in Figure 14-7). These two routes are discussed below.

Muscle protein. Pyruvate is derived from muscle protein (route #1). The keto acids formed from amino acids in muscle, insofar as they are glucogenic, all form pyruvate for alanine transport, either directly or indirectly via oxaloacetate and the phosphoenolpyruvate-carboxykinase (PEP-CK) reaction (Figure 14-8). Under conditions requiring a net alanine export (fasting, between meals) various gluconeogenic hormones stimulate PEP-CK, and simultaneously inhibit pyruvate dehydrogenase (PDH), so that effective production of pyruvate occurs and, thus, alanine is exported.

Glucose-alanine cycle. Pyruvate is derived from the glucose-alanine cycle (route #2). Amino groups must be transported from muscle and other extrahepatic tissues to the liver, where they are detoxified by means of the urea cycle (Figure 14-9). To this end, the liver converts alanine back to glucose, and muscles utilize the glucose to form pyruvate. Thus, the function of the glucose-alanine cycle is to recycle hydrocarbons and shuttle NH_3. To state this more precisely, it is essential to realize that glucogenic amino acids generate their own pyruvate for amino transport in the form of alanine. But, at the same time, ketogenic amino acids leave ammonia stranded without pyruvate. Therefore, only for transport of the amino group

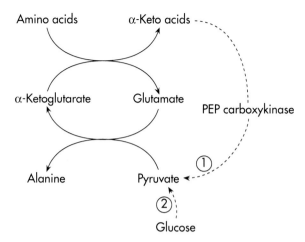

Figure 14-7. Conversion of amino acids to alanine in muscle. *PEP,* Phosphoenolpyruvate.

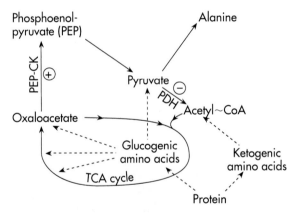

Figure 14-8. Pyruvate is derived from muscle protein. *PEP-CK,* Phosphoenolpyruvate carboxykinase; *PDH,* pyruvate dehydrogenase.

from ketogenic amino acids is the glucose-alanine cycle required. Thus, this cycle is not a means of net glucose synthesis in the liver, because, as behooves a cycle, all glucose formed in it is also used in it.

Three glucose cycles between the liver and other tissues. In addition to the glucose-alanine cycle, the text has discussed two other glucose cycles in which the liver comes to the rescue of a cell that lacks a certain pathway: the glucose-lactate (Cori) cycle between the liver and exercising muscle (lacking oxidative metabolism), and the glucose-glycerol cycle between the liver and adipose tissue (lacking glycerokinase). Alanine, glycerol, and lactate involved in glucose cycles yield glucose that cannot be used for extracycle purposes. However, alanine and glycerol are also the mainstays of net gluconeogenesis in the liver. This is understandable, since expenditure of tissue proteins yields extracycle alanine (and other glucogenic amino acids), and, likewise, expenditure of the fat stores (via fatty acid uptake by tissues) yields extracycle glycerol. These extracycle precursors give rise to the net production of glucose in the liver.

Protein balance

Balance experiments on a 70-kg man show that nitrogen homeostasis can be maintained on a daily intake of 32 g of high-quality dietary protein. This value equals the total of daily nitrogen losses in feces (10 g), urine (20 g), and from the skin (2 g). The customary protein intake in western countries is safely estimated at 100 g per day. Despite daily dietary intake of only 32 to 100 g of protein, 300 g of proteins are synthesized per day. This means that incoming amino acids are used and reused many times over in a dynamic equilibrium of protein synthesis and degradation.

The intensity of protein metabolism varies with

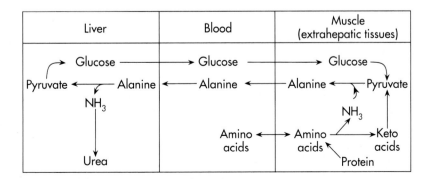

Figure 14-9. Pyruvate is derived from the glucose-alanine cycle.

the body size of the mammal. Some examples of this are as follows:

- Requirements for the essential amino acids, threonine and methionine, per kilogram of body weight of the mature rat are about four times that of humans.
- Slower turnover of serum albumin with increasing body size is found (Table 14-1).
- There is a parallel decrease in RNA content per liver cell, measured as RNA/DNA ratio, indicating a reduced rate of hepatic plasma protein synthesis in the larger species. (See Table 14-1.)

The conclusion from these data is that a quantitative description of amino acid homeostasis must take body size into account. Indeed, a similar argument has been raised against linearly extrapolating a rat's vitamin C requirement as an argument to recommend megadoses of that vitamin for human usage. Also, total energy requirements of the body are not linearly related to size.

Hormones and protein metabolism

Growth hormone, acting through somatomedins produced by the liver, is protein anabolic. It promotes the transport of amino acids into cells, thereby decreasing amino acid concentration in plasma. During starvation, growth hormone spares protein degradation in muscle tissue and decreases carbohydrate utilization, yet it simulates lipolysis and hepatic gluconeogenesis.

Insulin and the insulin-like growth factor (somatomedin) mobilized by growth hormone, promote transport of amino acids into cells and works protein anabolically. Furthermore, insulin stimulates the uptake of carbohydrate and thereby the energy generation needed for protein synthesis. Glucagon, the pancreatic antagonist of insulin, is protein catabolic.

Testosterone and synthetic derivatives of testosterone have both anabolic and androgenic (i.e., masculinizing) activities. Although clinical applications of anabolic steroids may be indicated in some of the following conditions, recreational abuse is condemned by most medical authorities:

- Wasting diseases of old age (Negative nitrogen and Ca^{++} balance)
- Reverse tissue-depleting processes
  Malnutrition
  Heavy parasitism
  Febrile conditions of nephritis
- Convalescence after surgery
- Delayed union of fractures
- Recovery of prolapsed disc or repair of damaged tendons
- Stimulate erythropoiesis
  Aplastic anemia and lymphomas

Epinephrine and TSH work protein catabolically and also lower amino acid concentration in the plasma. These hormones direct amino acids, among other nutrients, toward energy production.

Adrenal corticoids (glucocorticoids) are protein catabolic and, by stimulating phosphoenolpyruvate-carboxykinase and fructose-1,6-bisphosphatase activity, direct amino acids toward gluconeogenesis.

Glucorticoids decrease carbohydrate and amino acid uptake by muscle tissue.

NITROGEN BALANCE AND EXCRETION PRODUCTS

Normal adults are in nitrogen balance: Nitrogen intake in the diet equals nitrogen losses in urine and feces. When nitrogen intake is changed, a new balance is reached within a few days. The organism can change rapidly toward nitrogen economy when needed.

When more nitrogen is taken up than is excreted as wastes, one speaks of a positive nitrogen balance. Such is found during growth, tissue repair, pregnancy, and lactation. Negative nitrogen balance is encountered in starvation, malnutrition, trauma (blood and tissue losses), and diabetes (excessive demands upon gluconeogenesis and loss of NH_4^+ by the kidneys during acidosis).

Nitrogen in the diet

Protein is by far the major source of metabolizable nitrogen. It is important to consider the quality of dietary protein; that is, the essential amino acid content. Purines, pyrimidines, and porphyrins in the diet are minor nitrogen sources.

Table 14-1	Effect of body size on protein metabolism	
Species arranged in ascending body weight	Half-life (in days) of plasma albumin	RNA/DNA ratio
Mouse	1.2	4.45
Rat	2.5	3.05
Rabbit	5.7	2.44
Dog	8.2	1.69
Cow	20.7	1.29

Approximately 60% of digestible protein in the small intestine of ruminant animals is microbial protein (derived from the rumen). Much of this protein is synthesized from carbohydrate (cellulose) and nonprotein nitrogen (salivary urea).

Nitrogen in feces (the minor route for nitrogen excretion)

Primary amines (fermentation, putrefaction), taurine and glycine (as conjugates), bilirubin, and many other minor nitrogen products are found in feces. Dead bacteria are not to be considered a factor in nitrogen balance, because there is equilibrium between elimination of dead bacteria and the growth of new ones at the expense of dietary nitrogen.

Nitrogen in urine (the major route for nitrogen excretion)

- Urea is the main nitrogen compound in urine of ureotelic animals. It arises from detoxification of NH_3 generated by amino acid catabolism.
- Uric acid, from purine catabolism, is excreted by humans and the Dalmation dog, whereas subprimates convert their purines to allantoin. Birds do not excrete urea, but convert all nitrogen wastes into uric acid (uricotelic).
- NH_4^+ is found in urine, depending on acid-base and mineral balance.
- Beta-aminoisobutyrate and beta-alanine, from pyrimidines, are found in urine.
- Hippuric acid is found in relatively high concentration in equine urine (hence, its name), but it is present in the urine of all plant eaters. Hippuric acid is formed by conjugation of benzoic acid and glycine (Figure 14-10). This serves as the detoxifying mechanism for plant-derived phenolic compounds.
- The presence of methylhistidine in urine is a measure whereby muscle protein turnover is estimated. Methylation of histidine in the muscle proteins actin and myosin occurs after those proteins are synthesized. Upon breakdown of the myofibrillar proteins, methylhistidine cannot be reused for protein synthesis, since there is no codon for it. It is released into the circulation and its excretion in the urine, thus, offers an index of muscle protein turnover.
- D-Amino acids, porphyrin oxidation products (from heme and cytochrome catabolism), and other minor constituents are normally present in urine, and under abnormal conditions, so are amino acids and proteins.

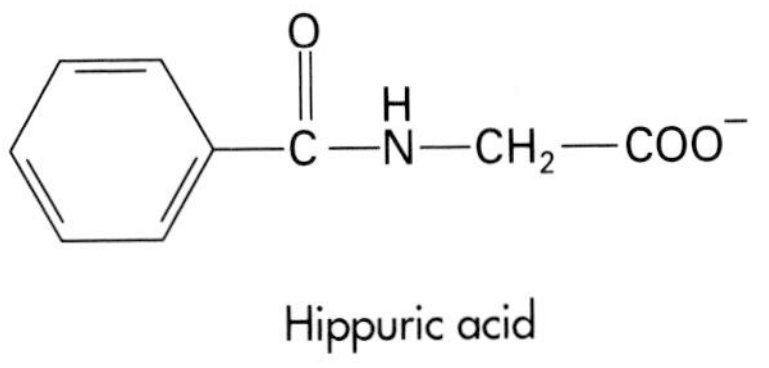

STUDY QUESTIONS

1. *a.* List two functions other than protein synthesis in which amino acids serve as building blocks for the biosynthesis of nitrogenous compounds.
   b. List three hormones synthesized from tyrosine.
   c. List an amino acid that has lipotropic properties.

2. *a.* What are amino acids not yielding glucogenic precursors called?
   b. Name one branched-chain, one aromatic, and one essential amino acid.

3. *a.* List the main process used by mammals to detoxify ammonia.
   b. Name a key enzyme involved in this process, and indicate what to conclude when the enzyme is found in the blood.
   c. List other processes for ammonia detoxification especially important in the brain.

4. List the compound formed in the liver during acidosis for detoxification of ammonia, so that ammonium ions are excreted in urine.

5. What is the main process by which amino acids are converted to their corresponding ketoacids for gluconeogenesis? List the vitamin involved.

6. What purpose is served by the glutamate dehydrogenase reaction, and what purpose by the glutaminase reaction?

7. About the biosyntheses of purines and pyrimidines:
   a. What control mechanism regulates biosynthesis of the bases that make up the structures of nucleic acids?
   b. Name two purine bases and list a nucleotide derived from one.
   c. Give an example of a dinucleotide.
   d. Which TCA intermediate leaks away for the synthesis of pyrimidines?
   e. List two B vitamins involved.
   f. Is there also an essential amino acid involved?

8. *a.* What is the metabolic end product of guanine degradation in humans?

Hippuric acid

Figure 14-10. Hippuric acid.

   b. List the metabolic end product of adenine degradation in most ureotelic species.
   c. Ureotelic animals convert cytosine and thymine to allantoin.

9. *a.* Translate "urolithiasis" and list one cause of it.
   b. List the origin and potential diagnostic value of methylhistidine in urine.

10. *a.* What is the main water source of birds at times when the ponds are frozen?
    b. List the adaptation in elimination of nitrogenous waste that the bird has made with respect to obligatory water losses.

11. *a.* Why are intestinal mucosal cells not digested by the human body's proteolytic enzyme activities?
    b. Why are pancreatic acinar cells not trypsin-digested?

12. *a.* List the gastric enzyme activity affecting milk-protein metabolism in young sucklings.
    b. Why can there not be pepsin and rennin activity in the stomach at the same time?
    c. List a factor, present in colostrum, that allows immune proteins to escape intestinal degradation.

13. *a.* Name a protein-anabolic hormone from the pituitary.
    b. List the cholecystokinin effect on the pancreas that affects protein metabolism.
    c. How do growth hormone and insulin establish their protein-anabolic effects?

14. List the risks associated with taking protein-anabolic steroids.

15. Is the human body's constant sloughing of intestinal mucosal cells a drain on the body's nitrogen stores? Explain.

16. *a.* Name two important quaternary ammonium compounds and indicate one function of each of them.
    b. Which essential amino acid must be available to produce adequate amounts of these compounds.
    c. What pathological condition may be observed when these compounds are lacking.
    d. For what purpose is creatine phosphokinase activity in plasma measured clinically?

17. What is the advantage for white muscle fibers of storing larger amounts of glycogen than red fibers, and why would a red muscle fiber obtain more mileage per mole out of its glycogen stores than would a white fiber?

18. List the reason and functional consequence of the fact that the ratio of Type II over Type I muscle fibers in Quarter Horses exceeds that in Heavy Hunters.

19. List the predominant site of deposition of leucine after absorption from the gut.

20. *a.* For what purpose is the A system for amino acid transport from the blood into the liver activated between meals?
    b. List the hormone responsible for this activation.

21. Describe the function of the glucose-alanine cycle between muscle and the liver. (Distinguish glucogenic and ketogenic amino acids.)

22. *a.* Give an argument for dynamic amino acid equilibrium based on a 70-g dietary intake and a 300-g endogenous biosynthesis in humans per day.
    b. Why could this argument not be used in the case of carbohydrate balance?

23. *a.* In humans, roughly what percentage of muscle protein can be spared for gluconeogenesis in times of fasting?
    b. What features, during fasting, prolong the time one can survive before having spent that critical (maximal) amount of muscle protein?

24. *a.* If the human body loses only about 32 g of protein-equivalent in urine, feces, and skin, why then must it ingest as much as 100 g of protein per day to remain in nitrogen balance?
    b. What metabolic fate awaits the protein eaten in excess of what is replaced in the body stores?
    c. Derive an expected difference in the efficiency of dietary nitrogen utilization in meal eaters versus nibblers.

25. *a.* List the form in which phenols are detoxified and excreted in urine.
    b. What can be learned from measuring urinary excretion of β-aminoisobutyrate (BAIB)? From methylhistidine?

15 Whole body metabolism

NORMAL CONDITIONS IN RELATION TO MEALS

Energy stores

Energy stores are primarily comprised of glycogen (limited), triglycerides (unlimited, best for indiscriminate energy production), and protein (expensive to use for energy, because its use involves detoxification of NH_3 in the form of urea for which much ATP is needed). Then there are the smaller elements: energy "currency" ATP and phosphocreatine (in muscles).

The following tallies are meant to bring out the relative sizes of energy stores:

- The average adult human has a total fuel reserve of 166,000 Kcal, consisting of about 85% lipids, 15% proteins, and 0.5% carbohydrates.
- Energy stores in a 70-kg lean human athlete (< 10% fat) can be expressed in walking distance equivalents:

ATP:	40 yards
Phosphocreatine:	120 yards
Glycogen:	1400 yards (anaerobic)
	10 miles (aerobic)
Fat:	630 miles

After taking in a large number of calories with a meal, those calories are not retained in the form of ATP currency, since the amount of ATP available is not nearly as high as the number of calories to be stored after a meal. Hence, the dietary calories are deposited in large reservoirs. First, the limited glycogen stores are restocked; the excess glucose is converted to fats and, together with dietary fats, stored as triglycerides. After a meal, amino acids are mostly stored as proteins in tissues and, for the remainder, converted to fat. The amount of energy currency (ATP) on hand is small and is constantly monitored and regulated via oxidative phosphorylation and production of ATP at the substrate level. For both of the latter processes, a store has to be tapped; determination of which store (glycogen, fat, or protein) depends on the tissue requiring it and on the time of day. For indiscriminate energy in most tissues, fat is spent predominantly. The glycogen stores being small, glucose is spared for vital purposes, such as for nutrition of the brain and erythrocytes. Proteins, too, are reserved for specific, essential purposes. When glucose runs low, protein stores via gluconeogenesis are tapped.

Defining postprandial, between regular meals, and fasting conditions

The following criteria are used to define metabolic conditions relative to meal intake:

- Postprandially, the parasympathetic branch of the autonomic nervous system prevails; influences of the sympathetic branch gain between regular meals, and especially during fasting.
- Carbohydrate availability is a bottleneck in overall metabolism. The postprandial state is characterized by a dietary glut that must be stored. Under the direction of insulin, carbohydrates are stored as glycogen, used for energy by various cells, or converted to fat. The between-meal state is defined as the time for glucose economy; stores of glucose and glucogenic precursors must be made to last until the next meal. Insulin antagonists (glucagon, glucocorticoids) prevail.

The fasting state denotes that glucose availability is inadequate. Emergency survival measures are taken at the expense of economy (e.g., ketonuria).

- The concentration of free fatty acids in serum is low postprandially, maintained constant between regular meals, and is elevated during fasting.
- Lactescence is present in postprandial serum.

Whole-body metabolism of carbohydrates, lipids, and nitrogen compounds at times immediately after a meal (postprandial), between regular meals, and during fasting is depicted for each of those three situations on an appropriate set of diagrams consisting of a global chart (Charts Xa to XIIa; cf., Chart I) and its pertinent metabolic scheme (Charts Xb to XIIb; cf., Chart II). In reviewing and comparing each of the dietary situations, it is best to use the relevant set of charts in tandem and retrace carbohydrate pathways, lipid metabolism, and the dynamics of nitrogenous compounds each in a different color, as has been done on the charts (Charts Xa′ to XIIa′ and Xb′ to XIIb′). One should start with the organismic approach (global chart, labeled a) and then, using the appropriate metabolic scheme (labeled b), consider control mechanisms over directions and rates of metabolic pathways (endocrine, feedback, feed-forward, etc.).

Postprandial situation: storage

In the time right after a meal, glucose and insulin levels are high. This is the time for storage of incoming nutrients and dietary essentials (Chart Xa and Chart Xb). Carbohydrates are stored as glycogen and used by various tissues for energy; amino acids are stored as proteins in muscles. From those, both can be retrieved in periods between meals. But, after filling the limited glycogen and protein stores, excess sugars and amino acids are converted to fat and stored, together with dietary fatty acids in the triglyceride stores. From that store, only the glycerol moiety can later be recalled for gluconeogenesis; the fatty acid moiety of the triglyceride stores is used for energy.

Liver

- Water-soluble compounds enter via the portal vein; vitamins and minerals are stored.
- Protein and glycogen stores are filled.
- Branched-chain, essential amino acids are allowed to pass through.
- Excess sugar and amino acids are converted to tri-

glycerides and exported as VLDL in the bloodstream.
- Chylomicron remnants enter the liver; they contain valuable phospholipids, proteins, and fat-soluble vitamins; vitamins A, D, and K are stored in the liver; vitamin E is stored everywhere.
- It is important to note insulin action: to lower blood glucose, it stimulates glycogenesis and lipogenesis from glucose.
- There is a net influx of glucose into the liver at this time.
- Following in the appropriate metabolic scheme are the insulin effects on key enzymes that direct postprandial metabolism toward storage of the dietary glut.

Extrahepatic tissues

- Chylomicrons' triglycerides are saponified by insulin-stimulated lipoprotein lipase activity, and their fatty acids are deposited in adipose tissue.
- Uptake of dietary glucose is insulin-stimulated in most extrahepatic tissues (e.g., muscle and adipose tissue). This glucose is used for filling glycogen stores, for energy, and for conversion to fat.
- Dietary amino acids are taken up and stored as tissue proteins; this, too, is under insulin control.

Bloodstream

- Glucose level is elevated.
- Amino acid levels, enriched in branched-chain amino acids, are elevated, but rapidly lowered under the influence of insulin.
- Lactescence, caused by chylomicrons and VLDL, is observed; it is cleared by lipoprotein lipase activities in extrahepatic tissues that produce chylomicron remnants and VLDL remnants, which are taken up by the liver.
- Plasma concentration of free fatty acids is lowered.

Between regular meals: economy

The situation between regular meals is characterized by the economic usage of the various body stores (Chart XIa and Chart XIb). The limited glycogen stores serve to provide glucose to tissues that require it for energy (e.g., brain tissues, erythrocytes) and to other tissues (muscle, adipose tissue) for typical carbohydrate functions, such as replenishing TCA cycle intermediates, providing glycerol phosphate for triglyceride deposition, and synthesis of glycoproteins and glycolipids. The protein stores are most economically parceled out over processes for which amino acids are indispensable; for example, resynthesis of proteins, nitrogenous compounds (such as nucleic acids, glutathione, and hemoglobin), and gluconeogenesis. The fat stores provide the energy necessary for maintaining the body's homeostasis. Constant levels of glucose, free fatty acids, amino acids, and ketones are maintained in plasma under the influence of the autonomic nervous system, which also finely tunes the balance between insulin and insulin-antagonistic hormones, glucagon acting chiefly on the liver, glucocorticoids, and epinephrine.

Liver

- To maintain a constant blood glucose level, the liver changes over to net glucose outflow.
- Glycogenolysis prevails over glycogenesis.
- Gluconeogenesis prevails over glycolysis. The most important precursors for gluconeogenesis in the liver are amino acids, imported mostly as alanine (from glucogenic amino acids in muscle) and via the glucose-alanine cycle (from muscle's ketogenic amino acids). The A system for amino acid transport into the liver is activated. Increased urea cycle activity detoxifies the amino wastes. In addition, a nitrogen-saving, net gluconeogenesis occurs from glycerol derived from adipose tissue's triglyceride degradation. Gluconeogenesis from lactate completes the glucose-lactate cycle (Cori), whereby anaerobic tissues are provided with energy.
- Fat, imported in part from the bloodstream, is used for energy. Fatty acid catabolism spares glucose; moreover, fatty acid oxidation promotes gluconeogenesis by providing NADH and ATP and by stimulating the formation of oxaloacetate and alanine via pyruvate carboxylase activation and inhibition of pyruvate dehydrogenase.
- Small amounts of ketones are produced (deacylase) and exported into the circulation from where they are removed by muscle cells. Since the rates of hepatic production and muscles' utilization of ketones are equal, the level of ketones in the blood remains low and constant.
- Enough lipotropic factors are present for VLDL production to close the lipid cycle between adipose tissue and the liver without the need for triglyceride accumulation in the liver.
- It is beneficial to review the sympathetic nervous effects and associated glucagon-glucocorticoid-epinephrine effects coming to the fore with falling insulin titers, then to follow in the metabolic chart for the between-meal situation and determine how

these hormones fulfill their mission of maintaining blood glucose by stimulating all glucose-producing and glucose-sparing processes (glycogenolysis, gluconeogenesis, proteolysis, and glycolysis).

Extrahepatic tissues

- Fat is used for energy; triglyceride lipase activity is stimulated by the sympathetic nervous system and by insulin-antagonistic hormones, resulting in increased release of fatty acids from fat cells to meet energy demands of extrahepatic tissues. Fatty acids released in excess over energy needs are repackaged by the liver in the form of VLDL, exported, and redeposited in fat stores.
- Glucose (and amino acids) are used for glycerol phosphate production in adipose tissue to redeposit triglycerides formed from fatty acids derived from VLDL.
- Ketone bodies are used by muscle as preferred fuel. Hence, ketone bodies do not accumulate in blood.
- In heart muscles, lipoprotein lipase activities increase, so that mostly fatty acids can fuel their metabolism.
- Glucose is spared for high-priority uses, such as nutrition of nervous tissue and erythrocytes.
- Tissue protein stores are broken down to amino acids, transaminated with α-ketoglutarate (producing glutamate and glutamine) and with pyruvate (forming alanine), and transported to the liver for gluconeogenesis.

Bloodstream

- Levels of glucose, amino acids, free fatty acids, and ketone bodies are "normal" and steady.
- Lactescence is cleared.
- In the appropriate set of charts, it is helpful to trace the following cycles: (i) lactate-glucose; (ii) glycerol-glucose; and (iii) alanine-glucose, and to review the functions of these cycles.

During fasting: survival

Upon prolonged abstention from food, the body runs out of essential factors, such as vitamins, minerals, essential amino and fatty acids, lipotropic factors, and glycogen (Chart XIIa and Chart XIIb). This is a life-threatening situation which is aggravated by the fact that the remaining body reserves cannot even be utilized to their best avail because the lack of those essential factors precludes economic use of body stores. Emergency measures (e.g., ketonuria) are now

Text continued on p. 364.

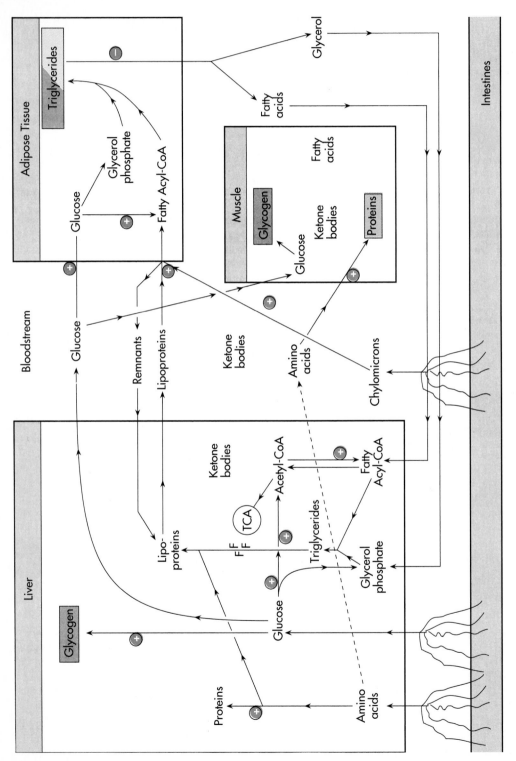

Chart Xa. Postprandial situation: storage. Insulin and feed-forward effects are marked. *F*, Lipotropic factors.

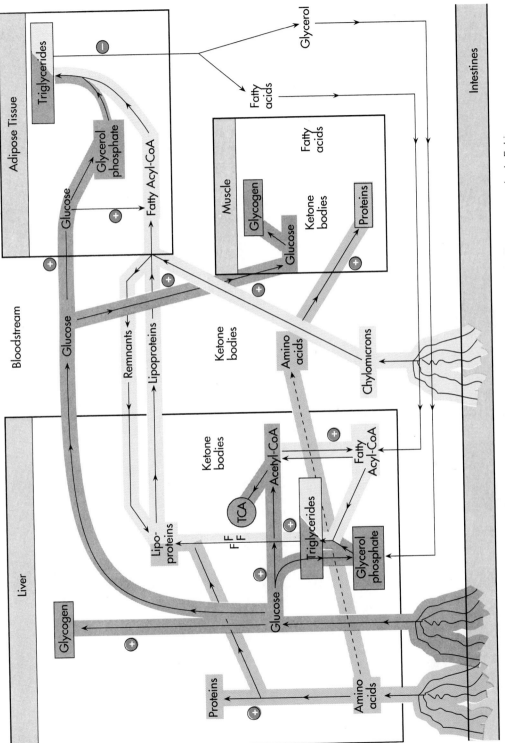

Chart Xa'. Postprandial situation: storage. Insulin and feed-forward effects are marked. *F*, Lipotropic factors. Carbohydrate, lipid, and protein pathways are identified by color.

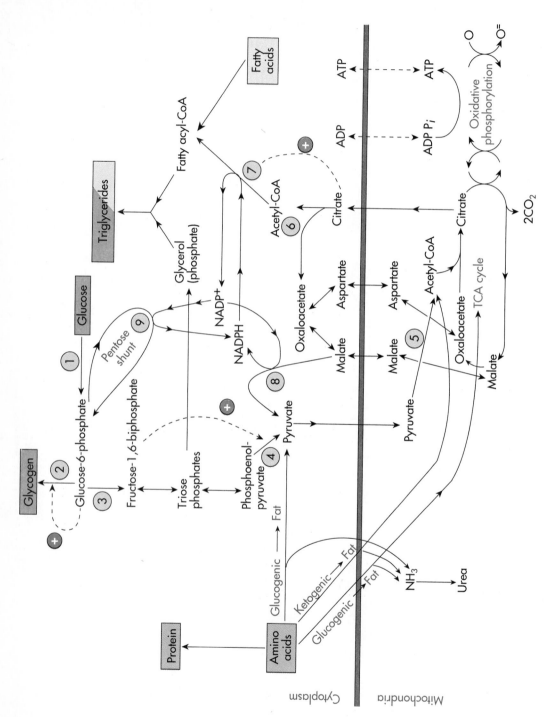

Chart Xb. Postprandial situation: storage. Insulin and feed-forward controls of inducible enzymes are marked. Place the key enzymes, indicated by number, and their functional control of pathways within the global picture of Chart Xa: *1*, glucokinase; *2*, glycogen synthase; *3*, phosphofructokinase; *4*, pyruvate kinase; *5*, pyruvate dehydrogenase; *6*, citrate lyase; *7*, acetyl-CoA carboxylase; *8*, malic enzyme; *9*, glucose-6-phosphate dehydrogenase.

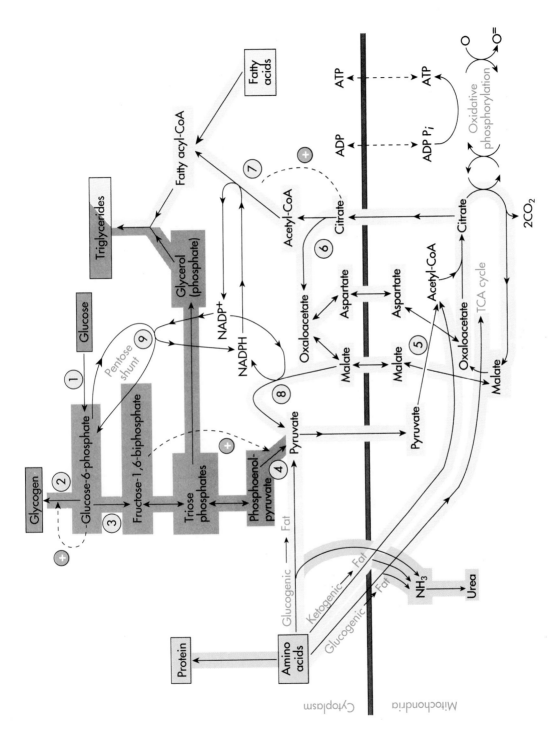

Chart Xb'. Postprandial situation: storage. Insulin and feed-forward controls of inducible enzymes are marked. Carbohydrate, lipid, and protein pathways are identified by color. Place the key enzymes, indicated by number, and their functional control of pathways within the global picture of Chart Xa': *1,* glucokinase; *2,* glycogen synthase; *3,* phosphofructokinase; *4,* pyruvate kinase; *5,* pyruvate dehydrogenase; *6,* citrate lyase; *7,* acetyl-CoA carboxylase; *8,* malic enzyme; *9,* glucose-6-phosphate dehydrogenase.

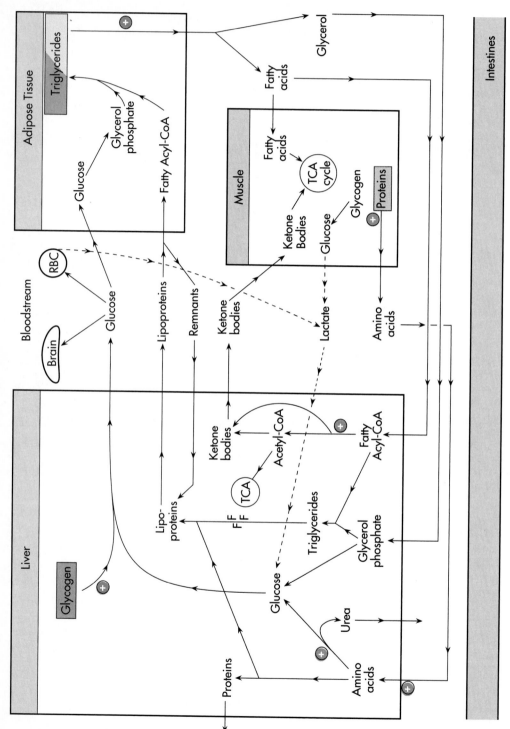

Chart XIa. Between regular meals: economy. Glucagon effects are marked. *F,* Lipotropic factors.

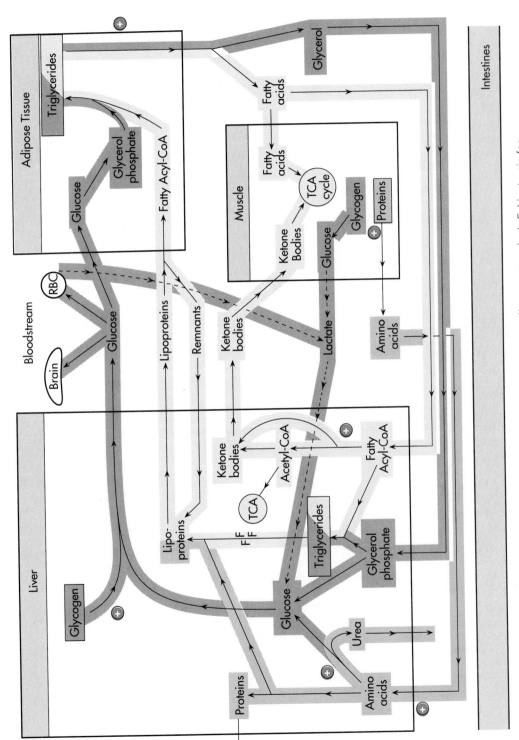

Chart XIa'. Between regular meals: economy. Glucagon effects are marked. *F,* Lipotropic factors. Carbohydrate, lipid, and protein pathways are identified by color.

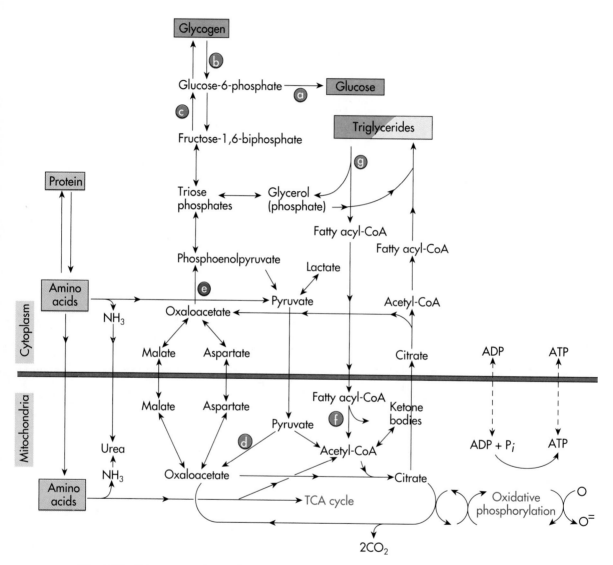

Chart XIb. Between regular meals: economy. Note the glucagon/glucocorticoid effects on key enzyme activities. Place the key enzymes, indicated by letters, and their functional control over pathways within the global picture Chart XIa: *a*, glucose-6-phosphatase; *b*, phosphorylase; *c*, fructose-1,6-bisphosphatase; *d*, pyruvate carboxylase; *e*, PEP carboxykinase; *f*, deacylase; *g*, triglyceride lipase.

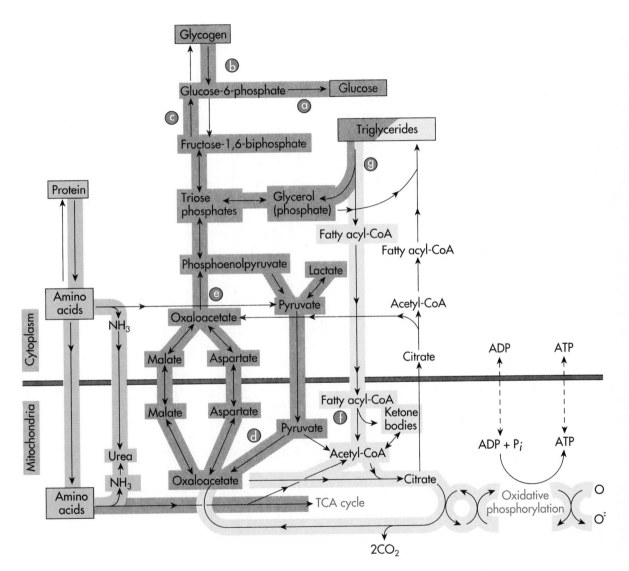

Chart XIb'. Between regular meals: economy. Note the glucagon/glucocorticoid effects on key enzyme activities. Place the key enzymes, indicated by letters, and their functional control over pathways within the global picture of Chart XIa': *a,* glucose-6-phosphatase; *b,* phosphorylase; *c,* fructose-1,6-bisphosphatase; *d,* pyruvate carboxylase; *e,* PEP carboxykinase; *f,* deacylase; *g,* triglyceride lipase.

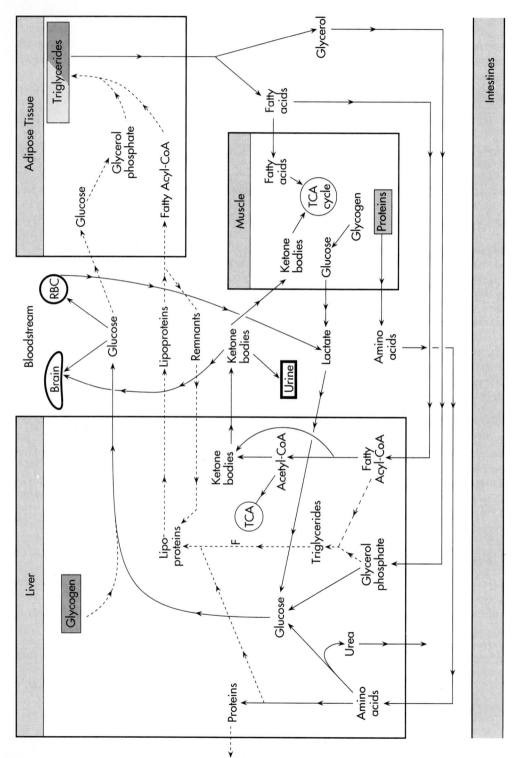

Chart XIIa. Fasting situation: survival. Solid lines represent the major pathways. *F*, Lipotropic factors.

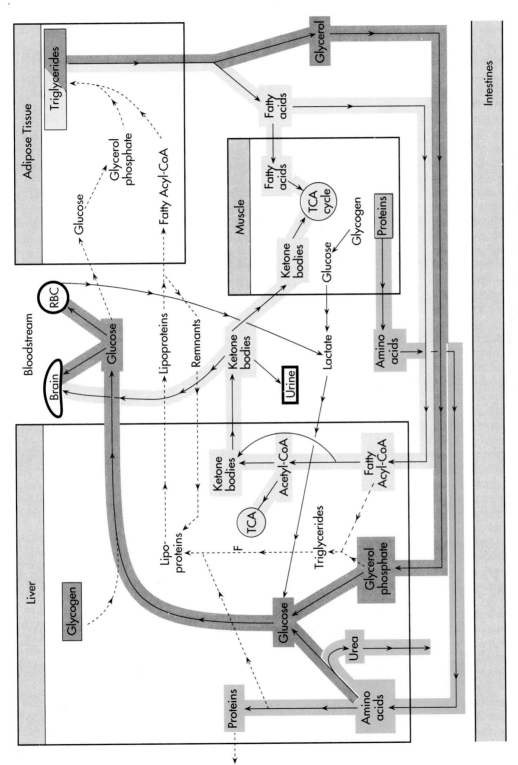

Chart XIIa'. Fasting situation: survival. *Solid lines* represent the major pathways. *F,* Lipotropic factors. Carbohydrate, lipid, and protein pathways are identified by color.

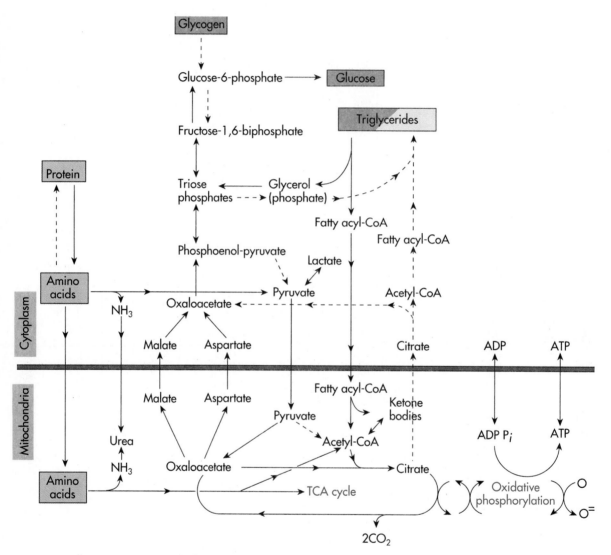

Chart XIIb. Fasting situation: survival. *Solid lines* represent the major pathways. Place the key pathways within the global picture of Chart XIIa.

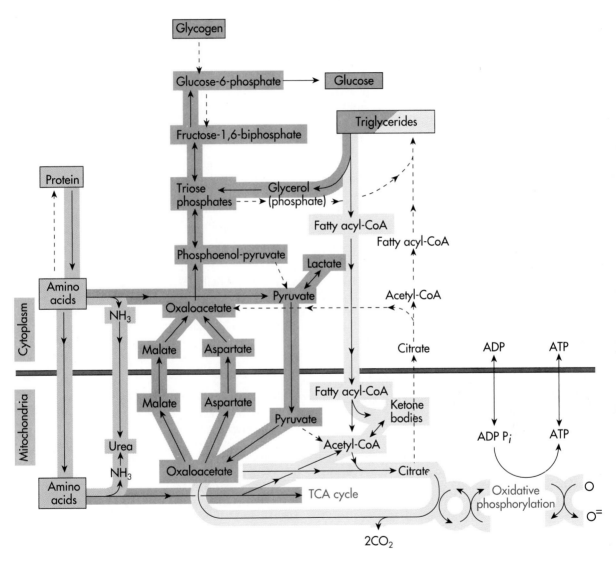

Chart XIIb'. Fasting situation: survival. *Solid lines* represent the major pathways. Carbohydrate, lipid, and protein pathways are identified by color. Place the key pathways within the global picture of Chart XIIa'.

taken, which may not be economic, but at least prolong survival.

Under the direction of the sympathetic nervous system and its associated release of insulin-antagonistic hormones (glucagon, glucocorticoids, epinephrine, and norepinephrine) proteolysis in tissues provides amino acids for hepatic gluconeogenesis, while increased lipolysis releases large amounts of fatty acids from fat stores. The supply of free fatty acids far exceeds the demands for energy and the liver's capacity to recycle them as VLDL, especially now that lipotropic factors are lacking. Triglycerides accumulate in the liver giving rise to fatty liver, and, for the most part, the liver converts incoming fatty acids to ketone bodies. The ensuing fasting ketosis with its associated acidosis, K^+ loss, and loss of huge amounts of energy in the form of ketonuria is life-threatening if not brought under control. However, ketone-body formation does have several advantages for survival: (i) ketone bodies are a means whereby fatty acids can be disposed of in a water-soluble form, voided in the urine; (ii) converting fatty acids to ketone bodies leaves glycerol for gluconeogenesis, since it is not used for triglyceride formation; (iii) the brain, the largest glucose consumer in the body, responds to the lack of glucose by shifting its metabolism toward utilization of ketone bodies; consequently, the liver is relieved of a major portion of its glucose production, and, thus, muscle protein is spared; and (iv) ketone bodies have an additional regulatory effect in that they stimulate the elaboration of insulin, which, in turn, protects the animal from a runaway breakdown of all of its body stores.

Extrahepatic tissues

- Triglyceride redeposition is strongly depressed, because of low insulin titers and the lack of precursors for glycerol phosphate.
- Triglyceride degradation is stimulated by the neuroendocrine controls that respond to the critical need for glucose. The result is an outpouring of free fatty acids (much in excess of tissues' nutritional needs), raising the level of free fatty acids in serum and the fatty acid load that enters the liver.
- Tissue protein stores are raided for gluconeogenesis.

Liver

- During fasting, various lipotropic factors run out, resulting in the accumulation of triglycerides (fatty liver).
- Excessive amounts of fatty acids enter from the bloodstream.

- Glycerol, used for gluconeogenesis, is in short supply, so fatty acids cannot be reesterified to triglycerides at their rate of entry.
- Nonesterified fatty acids easily enter mitochondria (carnitine acyltransferase is active, since the concentration of malonyl-CoA is low), where they are β-oxidized to AcCoA, then converted to ketone bodies via the Lynen pathway.
- Ketone bodies are exported from the liver into the bloodstream in increasingly large amounts, and when their production rate exceeds their rate of consumption, ketoacidosis develops.

Bloodstream

- Ketoacidosis
- Elevated K^+ level
- Elevated free fatty acid level
- Low plasma glucose level
- Decreased plasma protein level; decreased oncotic pressure; edema in tissues

Summary of metabolic liver functions

To appreciate the liver as the center of metabolism, this section briefly reviews metabolic liver functions and relates them to the regulation of the blood glucose level (in which the liver figures prominently) and to the apparent paradox of having opposing pathways going on concurrently in the liver, a quandary that appears to be linked to inhomogeneity (zonation) within the hepatic parenchyma.

Blood glucose homeostasis

The blood sugar level is fairly constant in a given animal when variations, due to circadian rhythm, different breeds, sex, nutrition, and stress of handling, are taken into account. But large differences exist between animal species. Whereas in humans and other monogastrics, glucose levels at around 100 mg/dl are common (rising after a meal to 120 to 130 mg/dl, and falling between meals to 80 mg/dl), and in ruminants, blood glucose levels of approximately 40 to 60 mg/dl are found.

Regulating the blood glucose level is a complex organismic function, under general direction of the neuroendocrine system, in which the liver plays a key role (Figure 15-1).

Monitoring and adjusting the blood sugar level is controlled via the autonomic nervous system and its associated endocrine releases that affect key enzyme activities. In addition to their autonomic nervous release, hormones are secreted in response to the presence of either secretagogues (e.g., glucose, amino

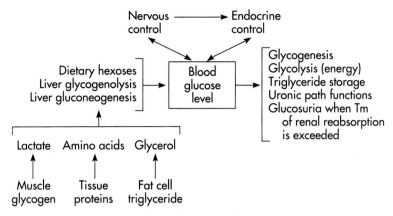

Figure 15-1. Regulation of the blood glucose level.

acids, ketones) or different hormones in blood.

Under neuroendocrine direction, various tissues (e.g., muscles) aid in blood glucose control by shifting toward glucose utilization postprandially and toward glucose economy (fat and ketone body combustion) thereafter. Between meals, muscles' protein stores support hepatic gluconeogenesis. The brain uses ketone bodies during fasting. The kidney, to a limited extent, shares in gluconeogenesis and has the additional function of spilling glucose into urine at times of severe hyperglycemia. A danger of severe hyperglycemia is osmotic dehydration of tissues (e.g., brain). Adipose tissue postprandially converts glucose to fat and deposits the fat in its triglyceride stores. Between meals, triglyceride stores contribute glycerol for hepatic gluconeogenesis; for three fatty acid molecules combusted in tissues, one glycerol becomes available for hepatic gluconeogenesis. The liver postprandially takes up glucose for glycogenesis, energy, and lipogenesis. Between regular meals, the liver is unique: whereas extrahepatic tissues only take glucose from the bloodstream (or utilize their own glycogen), the liver donates glucose to the circulation, which is referred to as "metabolism upside-down." The bulk of that glucose is derived by glycogenolysis and the remainder by gluconeogenesis from amino acids, glycerol, and lactate. (See Figure 15-1.)

Lipid transport

The liver has a pivotal role in maintaining the body's lipid balance by providing means of lipid transport in media that are either devoid of proteins (bile; gut) or that contain them (bloodstream).

The liver produces bile salts, cholesterol, and phospholipids that form mixed micelles for the transport of water-insoluble wastes and lipids in bile and intestines. The enterohepatic circulation recycles bile salts for multiple rounds of duty.

For lipid transport in plasma, the liver produces very low-density lipoproteins (VLDL) that postprandially carry dietary energy and cycle and recycle fatty acids between fat cells and liver between meals. In addition, the liver provides adipose cells with glucose from which to generate glycerol phosphate needed for triglyceride formation. High-density lipoproteins (HDL) are formed in the liver and elsewhere; their cholesterol-scavenging function entails lecithin cholesterol acyltransferase (LCAT) activity, which esterifies cholesterol at the expense of an essential fatty acid removed from HDL-lecithin. Lysolecithin, thus formed, is converted back to lecithin in the liver. Cholesterol esters contained in HDL are finally excreted in bile. These cholesterol-excretory functions, added to uptake of dietary cholesterol from chylomicron remnants and formation of VLDL and LDL, and cholesterol neogenesis for the purpose of bile and lipoprotein formation, establish the liver as the center of cholesterol metabolism as well. Another hepatic contribution to the transport of lipids and other water-insolubles in the blood is the production of albumin. Ketone body formation is a normal byproduct of fatty acid oxidation in the liver, which provide energy in times between meals; these ketones are metabolized by muscles. During fasting, increased ketogenesis solubilizes excess fatty acids and helps in survival.

Protein metabolism

Postprandially, the liver destines amino acids either for storage extrahepatically or for conversion to liver and plasma proteins or to fat. Between meals, activation of amino acid uptake in the liver via the A system and the glucose-alanine cycle allows mobilization of tissue protein stores for the purpose of hepatic gluconeogenesis. Furthermore, the liver is the source of most plasma proteins that function to provide oncotic pressure and to transport minerals, vitamins, lipids, hormones, and waste products. Many of these proteins contain sugar chains derived, in part, via the uronic acid pathway.

Storage functions

The liver stores minerals (e.g., iron) and vitamins (e.g., A and D) and dispenses them by means of special mineral-carrying proteins (e.g., ceruloplasmin; transferrin) and vitamin-carrying proteins (e.g., transcobalamine). The liver also stores blood and glycogen.

Waste removal from the bloodstream

Clearing the blood of waste is an important function for which the liver has various mechanisms. Ammonia is removed mostly via the urea cycle, but under acidotic conditions, wherein the bicarbonate availability is lowered, glutamine production takes over, followed in the kidney by ammonium ion elimination under the influence of enhanced glutaminase activity. Bilirubin and other waste materials, cleared from the blood, are conjugated in the liver with glucuronic acid, glutathione, or other compounds, and either excreted in bile or refluxed back into the bloodstream for urinary elimination. Hormones (e.g., steroids) are also inactivated that way. Another mode of drug and waste disposal and hormone inactivation is by chemical modifications, such as oxidation by cytoplasmic cytochromes P450 and B_5, decarboxylation, oxygenation, methylation, etc.

Hormonal balance

The liver occupies a central position in regulating the hormonal control system by various means. Hormones are inactivated by conjugation (e.g., steroids, catecholamines), chemical modification (e.g., thyroxine to reverse-triiodothyronine), or enzymic degradation (e.g., insulinase and glucagon breakdown) or activated (e.g., conversion of tetra- to triiodothyronine). The liver synthesizes specific hormone-binding proteins (e.g., transcortin) and somatomedins (insulin-like activity).

Metabolic zonation of liver parenchyma

The large number of liver functions are distributed over the various cell types present in the liver. For metabolic functions, it is meaningful to distinguish reticuloendothelial (Kupffer) cells from parenchymal cells. The former remove particulate matter from the bloodstream by phagocytosis; they also possess receptors for glycoproteins and lipoproteins (used for the removal of these proteins). Digestion products from the Kupffer cells are metabolized further in liver parenchyma. Minor metabolic activities of endothelial cells in the liver have been reported. Most of the typical liver functions occur in parenchymal cells.

The liver parenchyma (Figure 15-2) is richly perfused with blood; about 30% of the cardiac output normally flows through the liver, with hepatic blood flow matintained by both hepatic arterial and portal venous circulations. There appears to be considerable species variation in the proportional input of these two circulations to total hepatic blood flow. Hepatic arterial blood flow has been measured as being 2% of total hepatic blood flow in guinea pigs, 20% in dogs, and as much as 35% to 40% in humans. The far greater proportion of hepatic blood flow being portal venous in guinea pigs (and perhaps ruminants and other animals dependent upon cecal fermentation), suggests that the liver would receive mainly oxygen-poor blood. This does not appear to be the case, for in guinea pigs the portal venous blood reaching hepatocytes is still 80 + % saturated with oxygen.

Portal venous blood is under a low pressure of about 9 mmHg. Various conditions (postprandial absorption, exercise) affect that venous pressure and, thus, have a major impact on the extent of liver perfusion. Hepatic arterial blood enters the liver at a higher pressure, is under control of the autonomic nervous system, and is thought to maintain nutrition of connective tissue (and particularly the walls of bile ducts). It also brings vitally needed oxygen to the liver which is needed to drive the numerous metabolic reactions that maintain viability of the organism. Loss of oxygen to the liver (from either hepatic arterial or, in the case of guinea pigs, portal venous blood) can be lethal because it often causes necrosis of basic liver structures. Incoming arterial blood, after it supplies structural elements of the liver, merges with portal venous blood at the origin of sinusoids (the **periportal zone**; also termed zone #1) where the oxygen tension is thus relatively high in comparison with the drainage areas around hepatic venules (the **perivenous zone**; also termed zone #3). Between zones #1 and #3 a less well-defined zone #2 is located. The endothelial lining of blood vessels perfusing the liver parenchyma is extremely porous and, thus, allows passage of even large protein molecules (but not

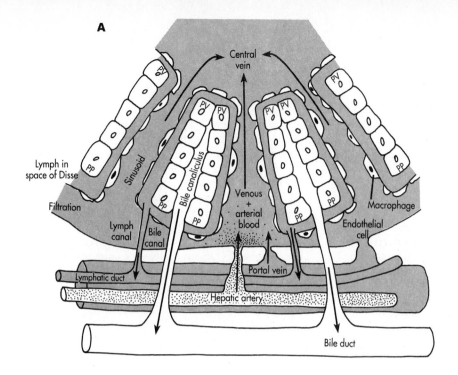

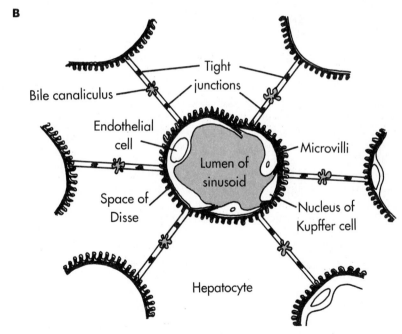

Figure 15-2. Basic structure of a liver lobule. **A,** Hepatic arterial and portal venous blood mixing in sinusoids lined with endothelial cells and macrophages (Kupffer cells). Pores in that lining allow protein-rich lymph to filter into the space of Disse that is connected via lymph canals with lymphatic ducts. Plates of hepatocytes, their microvilli protruding into the space of Disse, take up protein-bound and other materials and transport wastes into the bile canaliculi. Note that the flow of both bile and lymph is countercurrent to the bloodstream. (PP = periportal hepatocytes, Zone 1, and PV = perivenous hepatocytes, Zone 3.) **B,** A cross-section through a lobule in a plane, perpendicular to that of **A,** in which six hepatocytes surround a sinusoid. Note the rich vascularization; tight junctions between liver cells preclude paracellular transport of compounds from blood to bile canaliculi.

erythrocytes) from plasma into the Disse's space. Reaching into the Disse's space are the numerous microvilli belonging to the parenchymal cells that aid in the various transport and exchange processes at the cell surface in contact with plasma protein-bound compounds. The lymphatic system, among other features, returns escaped proteins to the bloodstream. Countercurrent to the direction of bloodflow runs the biliary system; it consists of bile canaliculi located between plates of hepatocytes; canaliculi merge into larger vessels and ultimately into a common bile duct. (See Figure 15-2.) Both afferent and efferent nerves of sympathetic and parasympathetic branches of the autonomic nervous system run parallel, and are attached to, incoming blood vessels; they can be severed or stimulated in an isolated, perfused liver to study direct nervous effects (not hormone-mediated) on key enzyme activities.

Periportal cells can be distinguished from perivenous cells in several ways. Having adapted to exposure to higher oxygen tension, periportal cells have a greater mitochondrial volume, more peroxisomes, and more key enzyme activities belonging to oxidative pathways (fatty acid oxidation, TCA cycle, oxidative phosphorylation) and the pathways that utilize energy so generated (gluconeogenesis). Perivenous cells are higher in downhill processes, which do not require oxygen for energy production, such as glucose uptake and conversion to glycogen and fat. Table 15-1 provides a more complete listing of functional differences inherent on metabolic zonation of liver parenchyma. These listings are based on zonal distribution of subcellular structures and key enzyme activities. All liver functions, such as formations of urea, bile, and ketone bodies, are polarized in one of the zones.

The zonal distribution of all key enzyme activities illustrates once more how certain parts of metabolism belong together. For example, in periportal cells, PEP-carboxykinase (gluconeogenesis) and succinate dehydrogenase (TCA cycle for energy) are active; in perivenous cells, glucokinase, citrate lyase, and all NADPH producing enzymes, all needed for conversion of glucose to fat, are concentrated. In addition, rates of hormone degradation vary zonally, so that the ratio of insulin to insulin-antagonists is higher in perivenous cells. (One can observe how this agrees with the zonation of pathways.) Also, innervation and gene expression for key enzyme synthesis are zonally distributed. The sum of these zonations adds up to a clear-cut zonation of metabolic liver functions.

Urea formation and metabolic paradoxes discussed earlier will now be reviewed in the context of metabolic zonation of liver parenchyma.

Ammonia removal. Ammonia is taken up by periportal cells and converted to urea; urea cycle enzyme activities are highest periportally. Though the capacity of the urea cycle is high, its affinity for ammonia is low. Hence, to lower the ammonia concentration under its toxic level, there is a high-affinity system located exclusively in the perivenous cells, where ammonia combines with glutamate to form glutamine. Glutamine circulates via the bloodstream back to periportal cells where it delivers ammonia for urea production. During metabolic acidosis, urea cycle is down (paucity of bicarbonate), glutamine synthase is

Table 15-1	Metabolic zonation of liver parenchyma
Periportal zone	**Perivenous zone**
Oxidative energy metabolism	
Fatty acid oxidation	
Citrate cycle	
Respiratory chain	
Glucose release	Glucose uptake
Gluconeogenesis	Glycolysis
Glycogen synthesis from pyruvate	Glycogen synthesis from glucose
Glycogen degradation to glucose	Glycogen degradation to pyruvate
Amino acid utilization	Liponeogenesis
Amino acid conversion to glucose	
Amino acid degradation	
Ureagenesis from amino acid nitrogen	
Ammonia-detoxification	
Urea formation	Glutamine formation
Glutamine utilization	
Cholesterol synthesis	Ketogenesis
Protective metabolism	Xenobiotic metabolism
Glutathione peroxidation	Monooxygenation
Glutathione conjugation	Glucuronidation
	Mercapturic acid formation
Bile formation	
Cholic acid excretion	
Bilirubin excretion	

From Jungermann K: Metabolic zonation of liver parenchyma, Seminars in liver disease 8:329-341, 1988

activated, and glutamine is broken down in the kidneys by elevated glutaminase activity to deliver ammonium ions to urine.

Glucose paradoxes. During postprandial glycogenesis in the liver (in contrast to muscle), a large proportion of dietary glucose is first glycolysed to lactate/pyruvate and then converted to glycogen via gluconeogenesis. This leads to the following quandaries: (i) how can glycolysis and gluconeogenesis be activated concurrently; (ii) since pyruvate kinase activity is high (for conversion of glucose to fat), how then can phosphoenolpyruvate (PEP), formed via the DCA shuttle from lactate/pyruvate, escape from being converted to pyruvate and still be available for gluconeogenesis; and (iii) why wouldn't the postprandially prevailing high ratio of insulin over its antagonists inhibit gluconeogenesis?

Metabolic zonation provides the following answers (Figure 15-3): postprandially, glucose is taken up perivenously and converted there to glycogen and lactate. Via the bloodstream, lactate returns to the liver where periportal cells convert it to glycogen via gluconeogenesis. Between meals, in perivenous cells glycogen breakdown yields lactate. Periportal cells use lactate and alanine for gluconeogenesis and also provide blood glucose by glycogenolysis. The perivenous zone always takes up glucose; the periportal zone always releases it. The above three quandaries, thus, find their solutions in different zonations of various pathways and hormonal ratios.

The following summarizes the discussion of metabolic zonation: Periportal hepatocytes catalyze predominantly oxidative energy metabolism of triglycerides and amino acids, urea formation, gluconeogenesis (both for postprandial glycogen stores and for glucose release between meals), cholesterol synthesis and bile formation, and glutathione conjugation. Perivenous hepatocytes preferentially mediate glucose uptake for glycogen and fat synthesis, ketogenesis, glutamine formation, and most detoxification reactions.

DISEASE CONDITIONS: BOTTLENECKS OF METABOLISM

Metabolism as a whole is well equipped to maintain homeostasis in the face of adversities. However, there are some critical conditions that must be met before the organism can function properly; they are "bottlenecks of metabolism."

Bottlenecks of metabolism

1. Carbohydrate stores are limited and yet carbohydrates have vitally important functions. Therefore a sustained carbohydrate supply is critical.
2. Fats are insoluble and yet must be transported in aqueous media, such as bile, intestines, and the bloodstream.
3. Nutritionally essential compounds (the ones the body needs but cannot synthesize adequately) must be supplied; for example, vitamins, minerals, essential fatty acids and amino acids.
4. Pacemaker enzymes are affected by genetic influences and by environmental conditions, such as cofactor availability, allosteric effects, and hormonal and nervous signals.

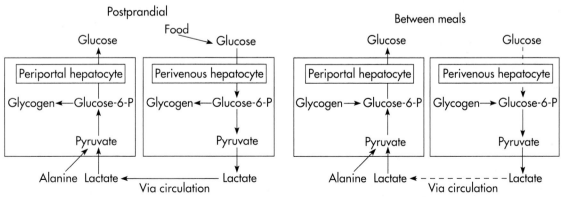

Figure 15-3. Hepatic glucose metabolism with metabolic zonation. *Reproduced with permission from Jungermann K: Metabolic zonation of liver parenchyma, Seminars in Liver Disease 8:329-341, 1988.*

Lacking control over bottlenecks; metabolic disorders

Abnormalities (disorders) of metabolism become apparent predominantly at the sites of the four bottlenecks detailed above. The following metabolic disorders, discussed earlier in more detail, exemplify the lack of control over bottlenecks. For therapeutic purposes, it may be helpful to distinguish conditioned (dietary, surgical, iatrogenic, environmental) and genetic (inborn) disorders.

Carbohydrate related disorders

The most prevalent disorder stemming from carbohydrate deficiency is ketosis caused by fasting, malnutrition, diabetes mellitus, multiple pregnancy, and overproduction of milk. Inborn enzyme deficiencies may lead to glycogen storage disease or galactosemia.

Fat related disorders

Lack of lipotropic substances in the diet leads to fatty liver, followed by loss of liver function. Dietary liver poisons have similar effects. Cholelithiasis and atherosclerosis list among their possible causes a deranged control over lipid (cholesterol) solubility.

Disorders related to a lack of nutritional essentials

- Lack of calories leads to fasting edema, fatty liver, and ketosis.
- Lack of lipotropic factors, such as selenium, methionine, and lecithin, causes fatty liver.
- Lack of minerals is responsible for various metabolic disorders, such as osteoporosis, anemia, hypothyroidism, and diminished activities of key enzyme reactions that involve trace minerals, such as Se, Mb, Mn, Zn, Cu, Fe, etc.
- Lack of essential fatty acids may cause cell aging, atherosclerosis, sterility, and other disorders.
- Lack of essential amino acids leads to protein deficiency and derailment of both carbohydrate and lipid metabolism.
- Lack of vitamins leads to various avitaminoses with symptoms ranging from anemia to scorbus, rickets, impotence, etc.

Disorders stemming from genetic and conditioned effects on key enzyme activities

- Disorders stemming from lack of cofactor availability include avitaminoses. Pernicious anemia is a vitamin B_{12} deficiency caused by the lack of intrinsic factor, which may be due to deficienct diet, gastrectomy, or genetics.
- Deficient allosteroic control over rate-controlling enzymes is among the causes for gout (uncontrolled purine synthesis and conversion to uric acid) and various kinds of hyperlipidemia.
- Lack of proper hormonal control over key metabolic activities may result from insufficient hormone production (e.g., diabetes, hypothyroidism) or surgical removal of an endocrine organ without proper hormonal compensation; it may also be a consequence of having genetically or conditioned abnormal hormone receptors (e.g., atherosclerosis).
- A patient may have a molecular disease, that is, an inborn deficiency in a key enzyme activity (e.g., phenolketonuria, galactosemia) or in the structure of hemoglobin with associated loss of oxygen-carrying capacity (e.g., sickle cell anemia).

STUDY QUESTIONS

1. Fill in the blanks and answer all questions: right after dinner, metabolic activities peak, so as to assimilate the incoming dietary digestion products. The liver is the clearing house for all water-soluble products entering via the portal vein, together with the pancreatic endocrine substance, (a) _____.
Since storage capacities for carbohydrates and nitrogen compounds are very limited, and the liver cannot let these small, osmotically active, compounds pass right through into the bloodstream, it has no alternative but to convert most of these compounds to (b) _____. Liver does not store much (b) and therefore must package (b) into large aggregates, called (c) _____, that are exported so that (b) can be stored elsewhere. The various factors that contribute to the formation of (c) are collectively called (d) _____, and a trace element among these factors is (e) _____. When one of these factors is lacking, the resultant pathologic condition of the liver is called (f) _____. Give one reason (g) why eating low-quality protein could lead to (f).

Now back to the situation of the liver cell postprandially, and consider the following three key enzymes: for what purpose (h) would G-6-P dehydrogenase be stimulated? For what purpose (i) would citrate lyase be stimulated? Which biotin-dependent key enzyme (j) would be stimulated?

2. *a.* List the vehicle that transports dietary vitamin A to the liver.
  b. List the compound transported via the enterohepatic circulation.

3. *a.* List the particulate form in which dietary lipids are transported from the intestines.
  b. List the technical term for the appearance of postprandial plasma.

4. List the three insulin-related effects on adipose tissue that stimulate postprandial fat deposition.

5. What links the postprandial increase in hepatic glucokinase with activation of glycogen deposition?

6. List a redox-related advantage when a TCA/malate/pyruvate/AcCoA route is followed to convert an amino acid to fat.

7. List three feed-forward effects working in tandem postprandially to metabolize glucose.

8. *a.* In periods between regular meals, the liver maintains blood glucose levels by two main mechanisms (pathways): name them.
  b. List the two body stores that serve to maintain blood glucose.

9. List the effects of glucagon on the hepatocyte plasma membrane in support of gluconeogenesis:
  a. Specifically to allow import of amino acids derived from muscle protein.
  b. Applying to gluconeogenesis in general.

10. List the important extrahepatic sources of gluconeogenic precursors.

11. The following cycles, involving the liver and one tissue, each have the liver perform a function that the extrahepatic tissue lacks but needs.
  a. In the glucose-lactate cycle, liver makes up for erythrocytes' lack of _____.
  b. In the glucose-glycerol cycle, liver makes up for adipose tissue's lack of _____.
  c. In the glucose-alanine cycle, liver makes up for muscles' need for _____.
  d. Evaluate these cycles with regard to their contribution of net gluconeogenesis.

12. *a.* List the branch of autonomic nervous system and the associated hormone release that control postprandial metabolism.
  b. How does the sympathetic nervous system translate hyopglycemia into glucose release from the liver?

13. Fill in the blanks: in response to hypoglycemia, a hypothalamic releasing hormone orders the pituitary gland to elaborate the hormone (a) _____, and this hormone, in turn, orders the adrenal cortex to produce hormones called (b) _____; in addition, the pancreas releases the hormone (c) _____. Under the influence of these hormones, the liver corrects the hypoglycemia in two ways: by activating the key enzyme (d) _____ that raids the carbohydrate stores; and by stimulating gluconeogenesis as a result of activation of its key enzymes, named (e) _____. At the same time, glucose utilization is spared as much as possible by the hormonal stimulation of adipose tissue's key enzyme, namely (f) _____, that guards fat stores. In the liver, the utilization of fat for energy purposes leads to formation of a by-product that is muscles' preferred fuel, namely (g) _____, and this spares even more glucose. The effect of these hormones on nitrogen metabolism is that in the blood, the level of a certain amino acid, namely (h) _____, increases, signifying that muscle proteins are being used for the process of (i) _____.

14. About the meager carbohydrate stores in the body:
  a. Approximately how much sugar is stored in the human liver?
  b. Why can't muscle contribute directly to the blood sugar level?
  c. What limits the liver's utilization of glycerol (from fat cell triglycerides) for gluconeogenesis?

15. List three mechanisms whereby the liver establishes half-lives of hormones. For which one of these is the uronic acid pathway needed?

16. Contrasting activities of antagonists allows the body to cope with adversities in either direction:
  a. Name the antagonist of the sympathetic nervous system.
  b. Name the antagonist of calcitonin.
  c. Name the antagonist of glucokinase.

17. *a.* List the key enzyme that directs pyruvate toward combustion.
  b. List the key enzyme that directs pyruvate toward gluconeogenesis.
  c. In periods between meals, which compound inhibits enzyme *a* and at the same time activates enzyme *b*?
  d. List the pathway (source) from which this compound is derived?

18. About the roles of the liver in lipid metabolism:
  a. List the hepatic lipid transport functions in the blood, gut, and bile.
  b. Under which conditions and for what reasons does the liver produce excessive amounts of keto acids from fatty acids?

19. What abnormality in plasma composition would result from chronic down-regulation of LDL receptors?

20. List the liver functions that (i) enable HDL to continue gobbling up cholesterol; and (ii) get rid of HDL cholesterol.

21. *a.* Which special high-energy compound (in addition to glycogen) is present in muscle?
    b. What is the muscle's preferred food taken up from the bloodstream between regular meals under resting conditions?
    c. Why doesn't the muscle use this same food during heavy exercise?

22. What is the economical significance for the muscle of the fact that β-oxidation of fatty acids raises the citrate level, which then inhibits phosphofructokinase?

23. About the fasting situation in an animal:
    a. List the key word that describes metabolism.
    b. In the blood there is a life-threatening shortage of what?
    c. List the purpose for which the uronic pathway in the liver continues to operate.
    d. Fasting edema is the result of the loss of what?
    e. Fatty liver is the result of the lack of what?
    f. What causes low plasma pH (list the metabolic product)?

24. *a.* List the adaptation of nonruminant-brain metabolism sparing muscle protein during fasting.
    b. List a reason why erythrocytes cannot possibly adapt in the same manner as the brain does.

25. Name the enzyme whose increased activity during fasting allows fat cells to utilize nonglucose compounds for the production of glycerol-phosphate.

26. *a.* List how, in the liver between regular meals, the rates of fat catabolism and gluconeogenesis are linked?

    b. Would these two processes have to be located in the perivenous or periportal zone? Explain.

27. *a.* List the process in the liver that takes care of the toxic nitrogenous waste products from amino acids between regular meals.
    b. Under which condition, and in which zone, does the liver produce more glutamine than urea?
    c. What is the metabolic fate of hepatic glutamine (i) under normal conditions; and (ii) during acidosis?

28. About plasma proteins formed in the liver:
    a. List the most abundant plasma protein and give two functions of that protein.
    b. List functions of: angiotensinogen; transferrin; transcobalamine; and transcortin.

29. List two mechanisms whereby the liver transforms xenobiotics into excretable products.

30. List the names and functions of nonparenchymal liver cells.

31. List a glucose paradox relating to glycogenesis for which the concept of metabolic zonation of liver parenchyma has to be invoked.

32. Regarding bottlenecks of metabolism in humans and disorders that derive from them:
    a. What results from a lack of cobalt?
    b. What results from a lack of selenium?
    c. What are clinical signs of an inborn lack of G-6-P activity?
    d. After a gastrectomy, what must be chronically administered to patients to avoid anemia?

METABOLIC RATE, RESPIRATORY QUOTIENT, AND CALORIMETRY

A simple and yet fundamental approach to the metabolic economy of an organism is to assess its energy exchange with the environment. Transformation of energy necessarily accompanies the variety of chemical reactions that make life possible, such as growth, mental activity, reproduction, movement, and respiration. Total metabolism, which is manifest as the energy released by all chemical transformations in the body, must ultimately derive from oxidation of foodstuffs. Dietary energy, whether used for maintenance of body structure and functions or for temperature regulation, appears in two forms in an adult, nonlactating, non–weight-gaining animal. Those two forms are heat, which under all conditions is the major form, and external mechanical work. It is important to realize that, if external work is not done, all energy contained in the diet will appear as heat. Actually, pyramids do not last forever, and energy spent on them, too, will ultimately appear as heat.

Metabolic rate

The rate of heat production in an animal at rest is a measure of the rate at which the animal is metabolizing (i.e., oxidizing) its metabolic substrates. This rate of heat production by an animal has therefore been defined as the animal's metabolic rate:

$$\text{Metabolic rate} = \text{Rate of heat production}$$

The metabolic rate of an adult animal consists of energy needed for upkeep of the body's vital processes, additional energy required to cope with changing internal and external environments, and energy spent on physical activity, growth and tissue repair, pregnancy, and milk production (see below).

Different forms of dietary energy

Not all of the chemical energy entering the body will appear as heat. Energy taken in as food is called the **gross energy**. Its value is determined by total chemical combustion in the bomb calorimeter. Bomb calorimeter values are identical to the gross energy content of food to an animal, because energy release is independent of reaction mechanism:

Bomb calorimeter:

$$C_6H_{12}O_6 + 6O_2 \longrightarrow 6CO_2 + 6\ H_2O + \text{Heat}$$

Animal:

$$C_6H_{12}O_6 \xrightarrow{\text{Glycolysis}} 2\ \text{Pyruvate} \xrightarrow{\text{TCA cycle}} \begin{array}{l} 6H_2O \\ 4CO_2 \\ \text{Heat} \\ \text{ATP} \end{array}$$

$$2CO_2 \qquad \text{Heat}$$

To be subtracted from the gross energy of the diet is energy contained within feces, including both digestible and nondigestible dietary components. One of the most important nondigestible compounds in monogastric animals is cellulose. Fecal energy also includes sloughed intestinal cells, bile salts, bacterial products and cell bodies, etc. Gross dietary energy enters the gastrointestinal tract and fecal energy is

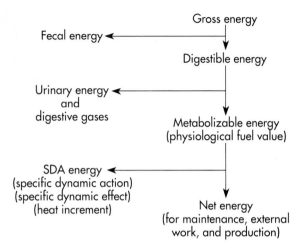

Figure 16-1. Energy losses from foodstuffs.

lost at the end; what remains is called **digestible energy** (Figure 16-1).

Digestible energy is not a fair estimate of the energy available to an animal, for it includes energy contained in gaseous digestion products and urinary energy, which will be lost. Gaseous digestion products, such as methane, are of quantitative importance in herbivores, especially ruminants. Methane is eructated in rumen gas, a part of which enters respiratory passages to be reabsorbed in the lungs. Urinary energy loss is the main reason why bomb calorimetry of the caloric intake of animals does not match metabolic heat production when protein is fed; for in the bomb calorimeter, even the nitrogen of protein is oxidized and contributes heat, whereas in metabolism, nitrogen is excreted as urea at the expense of energy. In contrast, good agreement between calorimetric and metabolic heat productions are found for carbohydrates and fats.

Subtracting urinary energy and the energy contained in gaseous products of digestion from digestible energy yields **metabolizable energy,** also termed **physiological fuel value.** Part of that is available as net energy for the body's maintenance, extenal work, and milk and egg production. Another part of the metabolizable energy is unavoidably lost as heat because of specific dynamic action.

Values reported for caloric equivalents of foodstuffs are the equivalents of the metabolizable energy, and amount to the following:

> 4 kcal/g for carbohydrates;
> 4 kcal/g for proteins; and
> 9 kcal/g for fats.

Practical example of the use of physiological fuel values

Suppose one is faced with a dog of 20 lb weight, and the owner wants to know how much of diet brand X he should feed the animal per day. Analysis of the contents of the can of dog food lists:

Crude protein	25%	(@ 4 kcal/g = 100 kcal/100 g of diet)
Crude fiber	4%	
Fat	8%	(@ 9 kcal/g = 72 kcal/100 g of diet)
Moisture	10%	(water)
Ashes	4%	(minerals)

The sum of the noncarbohydrate ingredients listed on the can is 51% of the contents. This leaves 49% of the diet for carbohydrates (@ 4 kcal/g = 196 kcal/100 g diet). Adding up the caloric contents in the forms of protein, fat, and carbohydrates yields 100 + 72 + 196 (= 368) kcal/100 g diet.

Given that a pound equals 454 g, then the dog's diet contains 1,671 kcal/lb. As a dog needs about 30 kcal/lb per day, the 20-lb dog would need 600 kcal per day; that is, 600/1671 or 0.356 lb of diet per day.

Measuring metabolic rate by direct calorimetry

In direct calorimetry, an animal is placed in a calorimeter, for example, an insulated container directly surrounded by ice. Knowing that it takes 80 kcal/kg to melt ice, then a guinea pig melting 0.37 kg of ice in a 10-hour period had a 10-hour heat production of 0.37 × 80 kcal = 29.6 kcal.

Different types of calorimeters measure transfer of heat to water insulation or to sensitive thermocouples in insulation materials. The best ones also measure heat loss by water vaporization from the animal, for which measurement of vapor pressure, temperature, and air velocity must be monitored.

Direct calorimetry, thus, is a difficult tool to use. The equipment is expensive to build and maintain, and too cumbersome for routine use. These objections, and advances in biochemistry, nutrition, and metabolism, have led to the development of indirect calorimetry.

Respiratory quotient; indirect calorimetry

Indirect calorimetry is based on the fact that, because the animal body ultimately derives its energy from oxidation of ingested foodstuffs, the magnitude of energy exchange (heat production) can be computed from observed values of oxygen consumption, CO_2 production, and urinary urea-nitrogen loss. To this end, the respiratory quotient (RQ) is applied, which is defined as the ratio of volume of CO_2 produced over volume of O_2 consumed. As derived below, the RQ value is highest for carbohydrate and lowest for fat combustion. Given this, RQ has meaning in vitro as well as in vivo. For example, in the fasted animal the in vitro RQ of the brain is lowered, because ketone bodies, in part, substitute for glucose as fuel (one can verify for him or herself that acetoacetate has the same RQ as does glucose, but β-hydroxybutyrate has a lower RQ); postprandially the RQ of the whole body increases because of sugar combustion, whereas later on fats are the main fuel, and so the RQ drops.

The following stepwise example demonstrates the procedure of indirect calorimetry. (The short cut listed below can be taken.)

Carbohydrate combusted

It is important to recall that a gram-molecule of a solid equals the molecular weight in grams, and that of a gas equals 22.4 L at atmospheric pressure.

$$C_6(H_2O)_6 + 6\ O_2 \rightarrow 6\ CO_2 + 6\ H_2O + heat$$
$$180\ g\ glucose + 134.4\ L\ O_2 \rightarrow 134.4\ L\ CO_2 + H_2O + 4 \times 180\ kcal$$

For carbohydrates: RQ = 6/6 or 1.0
134.4 L O_2 produce 720 kcal, or
1 L O_2 produces 5.36 kcal.

Fat combusted

If one takes, for example, the combustion of tripalmitin (TP):

$$C_{51}H_{98}O_6 + 72.5\ O_2 \rightarrow 51\ CO_2 + 49\ H_2O + heat$$
$$806\ g\ TP + 1624\ L\ O_2 \rightarrow 1142\ L\ CO_2 + water + 9 \times 806\ kcal$$

For lipids: RQ = 51/72.5 or 0.7
1624 L O_2 produce 7254 kcal, or
1 L O_2 produces 4.47 kcal.

Mixture of carbohydrate and fat combusted

If one supposes that a fraction (f) of the oxygen consumption was used for fat combustion, leaving $(1 - f)$ for carbohydrate oxidation, the observed RQ would then be $0.7 \times f + (1 - f) \times 1$, which equals $1 - 0.3 \times f$. For example: if the RQ was 0.8, then $1 - 0.3 \times f = 0.8$ and f = 0.67. One would conclude that 67% of the measured O_2 consumption was used for fat combustion (@ 4.47 kcal/L) and the remainder for carbohydrates (@ 5.36 kcal/L). The sum of these caloric releases would constitute the metabolic rate.

Protein combusted

An exact RQ prediction for protein combustion is precluded by proteins' variable structures. On the average, 16% of a protein's weight is nitrogen, excreted in urine as urea-N. Accurate protein feeding experiments have revealed that 1 g of urea nitrogen in urine corresponds with 6.25 g of proteins oxidized (approximately 25 kcal worth), 4.8 L of CO_2 produced, and 5.9 L of O_2 consumed. Thus, for proteins, 1 L O_2 produces approximately 4.23 kcal.

Mixture of carbohydrate, fat, and protein combusted

In computing the metabolic rate of a dog on regular chow, the following data were observed over a 24-hour period: 139 L of O_2 consumed; 120 L of CO_2 produced; and 10 g of urea-N excreted in urine. From these values, the metabolic rate follows:

- 10 g urea-N means that 62.5 g of proteins were oxidized (approximately 250 kcal worth), 48 L of CO_2 produced, and 59 L of O_2 consumed.
- This leaves 120 L − 48 L = 72 L of CO_2 and 139 L − 59 L = 80 L of O_2 for carbohydrate plus fat catabolism; that is, the nonprotein RQ equals 72 L / 80 L, or 0.9 L.
- Calculating the fraction (f) of oxygen consumption used for fat combustion, as above: $1 - 0.3 \times f = 0.9$ and, thus, f = 0.333. Therefore: 33.3% of the nonprotein oxygen consumption was used for fat combustion; that is, 26.67 L of O_2, each producing 4.47 kcal, for a total of 119 kcal worth of fat combustion.

The remainder of the nonprotein O_2 consumption was used for carbohydrate oxidation; i.e., 53.33 L of O_2 each producing 5.36 kcal, for a total of 286 kcal worth of carbohydrate combustion.

The metabolic rate thus equals 250 kcal + 119 kcal + 286 kcal = 655 kcal per 24 hours.

A short cut

The above procedure is somewhat laborious to use for routine work. Hence, often only the O_2 consumption is measured (no CO_2 and no urinary urea-N). Under fasting conditions, a liter of O_2 consumption represents a caloric equivalent of 4.825 kcal in rats on standard chow; slightly different values are obtained for other animals. These values are good enough for routine work and adequate to compare a given animal on a certain diet in one situation with another; for instance, to estimate what effect a certain treatment may have on the metabolic rate.

Standardizing values of metabolic rate

The interpretation of metabolic rate values is difficult, because many conditions in an animal affect the energy requirement and, thus, alter the metabolic rate.

- Weight and size of an animal relate to its energy requirement. Obviously, the larger animal requires more calories. Pound for pound, though, the larger animal is more efficient than the smaller one; for example, a 300-g rat requires approximately 100 kcal/kg per day, a 3-kg cat approximately 50, an 81-kg human approximately 23, and a 150-kg pig only 18. A useful equation to standardize metabolic rates per kg body weight for warm-blooded animals of widely different sizes and different species is:

Metabolic rate (kcal) = 70 × [Body weight (kg)]$^{3/4}$.

This formula predicts a linear relation between the logarithms of metabolic rate and body weight, and that indeed is found (Figure 16-2).

Of course, animals require different numbers of kcal/kg when their shapes deviate from the conventional four-legged model, or when they have different skin coverings (fur, scales, naked), or especially, when they are cold-blooded; in all of these cases, heat exchange with the environment is nonstandard.

- Exposure to hot or cold environments influences heat exchange, and, thus, alters the metabolic rate.

- Exercise requires calories, and, thus, increases metabolic rate; both duration and intensity of exercise must be considered.
- Shortly after a meal, large amounts of heat are produced by digestion in the intestines and by specific dynamic action.

Because of these influences, care must be taken to ensure that metabolic rates are measured and expressed in standardized fashions; that is, the patient should have had nothing to eat for a standard length of time before the measurement; the patient must be at rest during the measurement; metabolic rates must be measured at standard environmental temperature (also humidity must be controlled); and the metabolic rate should be expressed per unit of body weight. When these factors are carefully monitored, one can obtain a standard value for the metabolic rate of a given animal species, of a given sex (lower for female than for male), at a given age bracket (rising during periods of rapid growth), and under given climate conditions (for humans, the metabolic rate in the tropics is lower than in the arctic regions).

Basal metabolic rate

The term basal metabolic rate (BMR) denotes the minimal caloric requirement to maintain energy homeostasis. Thus, BMR is a theoretical concept. BMR comprises energy expenditures for essential processes, such as cardiac contraction, respiration, kidney func-

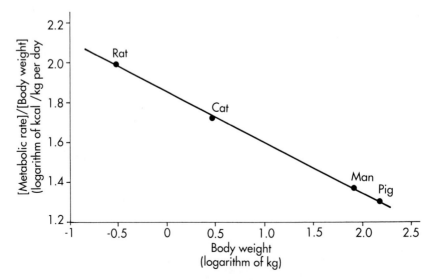

Figure 16-2. Linear relation between the logarithms of metabolic rate and body weight. Diameter of circles is ±10% deviation.

tion, sodium pump, brain activity, and body temperature maintenance.

It is not practical to measure BMR values, because the measurement itself will establish in the patient all sorts of conditions that raise his or her BMR; for example, apprehension (nervous and hormonal effects) and mental activities (work). Hence, for practical purposes, and as a reference, the resting metabolic rate (RMR) is measured under standardized and reproducible conditions of complete relaxation, after 12 hours of fasting, and at ambient temperatures. Resting metabolic rate values are about 3% above basal metabolic rate values.

Energy expenditure

Energy expenditure = RMR + work + maintenance increments

- RMR in the equation above reflects the energy cost of synthetic activities necessary to keep the body alive.
- Work is defined here as energy spent on physical activity, growth, tissue repair, pregnancy, and milk production.
- Maintenance increments include factors, other than physical activity, that raise energy expenditure above the BMR, such as psychological stress, exposure to cold, or thermic effects of food or drugs (e.g., caffeine).

Rates of energy requirements per unit of mass of various body tissues are grossly disproportionate (Table 16-1). Fat cells have a sluggish rate of metabolism compared to all other cells; hence, different body composition helps to explain the lower metabolic rate of females compared to males. It is striking that the size and metabolic rate of the human brain matches that of the liver.

Table 16-1	Weights and energy requirements of aerobic tissues in humans	
Tissue	**Weight (%)**	**Energy needs (%)**
Brain	2	20
Liver	2	20
Muscle	35-40	20
Adipose	20	2-5

Weights are expressed as % of body weight; energy needs as % of the body's metabolic rate. From: Owen OE: Resting metabolic requirements of men and women, Mayo Clin Proc 63:503-510, 1988. By permission.

Use of metabolic rate values in medicine

With the standardized value for the metabolic rate, several conditions in patients can be gauged.

Nutritional status

In times of starvation, the metabolic rate declines, since the body economizes on energy expenditure. Similar data were presented earlier for protein balance: (i) the intensity of protein metabolism varies in proportion to the body size of the animal; and (ii) when dietary protein is in short supply, the animal economizes on nitrogen expenditure. For people on weight-reducing diets, this energy-economizing feature is one of the reasons why pounds lost earlier come off more readily than later ones.

Disease conditions

Raising body temperature (fever) is calorically costly. In humans, the metabolic rate increases 12% per degree centigrade fever. Other conditions that also increase cellular activity raise the metabolic rate (e.g., cancer).

Hormonal balance

Hormonal balance profoundly affects the metabolic rate. Imbalance in the insulin/glucagon ratio, improper rates of production of corticosteroids, catecholamines, growth hormone, and other endocrine-related factors (e.g., receptors) all affect the efficiency with which the body is able to utilize dietary energy, and, thus, the metabolic rate. Especially, thyroid hormones must be considered in this respect.

Thyroid hormones

Thyroxine (T4) and triiodothyronine (T3), both secreted by the thyroid gland, increase oxygen consumption in most all tissues with the exception of brain and anterior pituitary, lymph nodes, lung, spleen, testes, uterus, and retina. In the normal state (euthyroid), the thyroid hormones maintain the rate of metabolism in tissues that is optimal for their normal functioning. Thyroid hormones are slow-acting, since they affect transcription of key enzyme mRNA in the nuclei of cells. Their elaboration from the thyroid is controlled via hypothalamic TRH that stimulates release of pituitary TSH.

In hypothyroidism, that is, when hormonal production by the thyroid is abnormally decreased or lacking, the metabolic rate is decreased, body temperature is below normal, mental and physical reflexes are slow, and carbohydrates and other foodstuffs are converted to fat. Other clinical signs of hypothyroidism include infertility, myxedema, thin haircoat, bradycardia, decreased blood pressure and volume, renal Na^+ loss, and constipation.

Excess thyroid secretion causes the body tissues to increase their rates of metabolism. As a result of increased metabolic rate in hyperthyroid animals, their rate of oxygen consumption is increased. For example, when rats were made hyperthyroid by including iodinated casein in their diet, a 23% increased metabolic rate was indicated by measurement of their oxygen consumption rate (Figure 16-3). The increased rates of metabolism that accompany severe hyperthyroidism cause depletion of the body's reserves of carbohydrate, protein, and fat. Thus, the hyperthyroid animal is usually underweight and may exhibit evidence of muscular wasting. Other metabolic effects of hyperthyroidism include hyperglycemia with an associated tendency to become diabetic because of exhaustion of the pancreatic insulin-producing cells, and an increased rate of intestinal absorption of glucose, resulting in abnormal glucose tolerance. An augmented rate of heat production, which accompanies the increased rate of metabolism, is enough to elevate the body temperature. Cardiac output is increased by the direct action of thyroxine on the heart, so that increased systolic blood pressure and heart rate are common clinical signs of hyperthyroidism. Excessive thyroid secretion also affects the central nervous system, causing irritability, restlessness, and often muscular tremors. Other clinical signs of hyperthyroidism include diarrhea, increased renal Ca^{++} excretion, exophthalmos, and decreased circulating levels of creatine phosphate, K^+, and cholesterol.

The actions of thyroid hormones and catecholamines are intimately related with many signs and symptoms of hyperthyroidism, reflecting increased sympathetic nervous system activity. Thyroid hormones act to increase the number of beta-adrenergic receptors in myocardial tissues, skeletal muscle, adipose tissue, and lymphocytes and to decrease myocardial alpha-adrenergic receptors. Therefore, hyperthyroidism enhances beta-adrenergic receptor activity in the body (e.g., heart rate and contractility, glycogenolysis, lipolysis, insulin and glucogen secretion, cutaneous vasodilation, renin secretion).

QUANTITATIVE ASPECTS OF NUTRITION
Nutrition

Earlier, the qualitative aspects of nutrition underlying the concept of a balanced diet were established: adequate intake of carbohydrates to ensure efficient metabolism of protein and lipids; amino acids to maintain nitrogen balance; essential amino acids in high-quality proteins; essential fatty acids of the n-6 and n-3 families; vitamins; minerals; and water.

Based on previous discussions of metabolic rates, the quantitative element of nutrition can now be

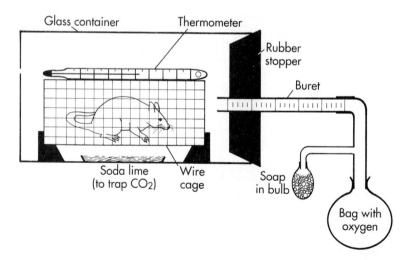

Figure 16-3. Measuring rate of oxygen consumption in a rat. Pinching the bulb with soap solution generates a bubble which is carried by the oxygen stream into a buret. The time it takes for the bubble to move over the length of the buret is measured. Oxygen consumption is corrected for temperature fluctuation.

added; that is, the total caloric requirement of the animal. Feeding fewer calories leads to weight loss, while excess calories increase body weight. Of course, dietary allowance must be made for special performance, such as growth, pregnancy, lactation, and external work.

In mixing the dietary ingredients that meet the total caloric requirement of an animal, one must usually adhere to the values of 4 kcal/g worth of metabolizable energy obtained from either carbohydrates or proteins, and 9 kcal/g from fat. These values, though, may not be a reasonable estimate of the expendable net energy of the diet for at least two reasons.

- The first reason for caution, already discussed, is that one assumes that all essential dietary factors are present in adequate amounts and that carbohydrates, proteins, and fats are mixed in proportions that allow their optimal utilization. If such a balanced diet is not given, then the above caloric values of nutrients may be in error. For instance, fats may contain 9 kcal/g of metabolizable energy when part of a balanced meal, but if they are eaten as sole nutrients, they cannot be absorbed or metabolized and, thus, have no caloric value.
- A second reason to be cautious in applying standard calorie values of nutrients deals with the variability of energy loss caused by specific dynamic action.

Specific dynamic action

Synonyms for specific dynamic action (SDA) are specific dynamic effect, heat increment, and thermogenic effect.

Specific dynamic action (SDA) is that fraction of metabolizable energy that is unavoidably lost as heat instead of becoming part of the net energy pool. Heat increments were demonstrated, for example, in fasted dogs. When 25 g of protein were metabolized, 130 kcal of heat were produced instead of the 100 kcal expected, that is, + 30%. When a 100-kcal portion of fat was metabolized, 113 kcal of heat were produced (+ 13%), and when 100 kcal worth of carbohydrates were metabolized, 105 kcal (+ 5%) of heat were produced. These values were obtained when pure foodstuffs were fed to fasted dogs. However, when the foodstuffs were mixed before feeding, the SDA was much lower. Also, when the pure foodstuffs were fed to well-nourished dogs, lower SDA values were observed. Hence, the SDA of a diet is not a constant factor; instead, it depends on the nutritional state of the animal and on the composition of the diet. For this reason, no standard deduction of SDA from the listed (metabolizable) caloric values of nutrients can be made.

SDA is not caused by the peristaltic actions of the intestines and the secretions of bile and pancreatic juices. This fact was discovered from injecting amino acids intravenously and finding that SDA was only slightly lower than when the amino acids were given orally. SDA reflects increased metabolic activity of tissues needed for storage of dietary components in the body (i.e., glucose to fat conversion); urea synthesis; protein synthesis; etc. Such activities may be considered as energy investments required to bring metabolizable energy into the net energy pool; the price of "doing business" with nature. Because of a high rate of metabolism, the temperature in the liver exceeds that in the gut. The thermogenic action of brown adipose tissue, especially after dinner, contributes greatly to SDA.

Meal eating versus nibbling

Affecting the magnitude of SDA are the profound metabolic consequences (both qualitative and quantitative) of feeding meals, as opposed to continuous feeding. Such is the case even though the total caloric intake over a given period may be equal. The reason for this is that dietary carbohydrates and proteins soon fill their limited stores and then, for the remainder, are converted to fat. This affects the body (carcass) composition. It also affects feeding economy: no matter how big the size of a meal, carbohydrates and proteins must be fed regularly anyway, since not enough of them can be stored to bridge prolonged withholding. By continous feeding (nibbling), on the other hand, resupply of carbohydrates and proteins keeps pace with their rates of utilization. Consequently there is less conversion to fat, and, thus, less metabolic heat loss and less nitrogen loss as urea, smaller SDA, and more efficient feeding. Of course, these arguments do not apply to ruminants.

STUDY QUESTIONS

1. Define metabolic rate (MR) and list the three components that constitute it.

2. What is dietary energy, discounted for urinary and fecal energy losses, called?

3. With the physiologic fuel value of carbohydrates being approximately (fill in the blank) _____ kcal/g, and that of fats approximately _____ kcal/g, explain why the kcal/g value of proteins is only roughly _____ kcal/g, despite the fact that amino acids chemically look at lot more like fats than like carbohydrates, and in the bomb calorimeter, amino acids yield much higher caloric values.

4. *a.* Is it accurate to say that, in an animal at rest, all metabolizable dietary energy ultimately appears as heat?
   b. Would your answer change if the qualifier "metabolizable" were deleted? Would your answer change if the animal were not at rest?

5. Caloric values on chow cans are (choose one): gross / net / digestible / metabolizable energy values. Give a synonym for metabolizable energy.

6. *a.* If a 25-lb dog needs roughly 30 kcal/lb body weight per day, how many grams per day must the dog be fed of a diet that contains 10% fat, 20% protein, 10% water, 5% fiber, 5% minerals, and, for the rest, carbohydrates?
   b. Would a dog twice as big need twice as many calories per day?

7. Leaving out the carbohydrates from a diet would have what effect on the metabolizable energy of fat?

8. Using the simplest method for indirect calorimetry, what volumetric measurement is done to determine the metabolic rate of an animal on a standard diet?

9. Two tricky questions:
   a. List the physiological fuel value of a meal consisting solely of 100 g of corn oil.
   b. Estimate the respiratory quotient (RQ) in muscle during heavy exercise.

10. *a.* The whole animal's RQ in the postprandial state exceeds that between meals. (True/False)
    b. As the brain adapts to fasting by shifting toward ketone body metabolism, its respiratory quotient remains unchanged. (True/False)

11. *a.* Per pound of weight, rats have a higher basal metabolic rate than elephants. (True/False)
    b. Based on different body composition, explain why males, on a per-kg basis, have a higher metabolic rate than females.

12. If a dog weighs 10 times more than a rat, is it fair to say that the dog's daily vitamin C requirement is 10 times more than the rat's?

13. *a.* List the hormonal condition that greatly increases an animal's MR.
    b. How does dinitrophenol raise the MR?
    c. Fasting decreases the MR. (True/False)

14. *a.* Is the MR increased during cold stress?
    b. Is the RQ increased during cold stress?

15. What is meant by resting MR and how does it differ from basal MR?

16. List two considerations that must be given to estimate available net energy from the metabolizable energy value listed on a container of food.

17. *a.* Give one explanation for specific dynamic action.
    b. Reason as to why metabolizable energies on food containers have not been corrected for SDA.
    c. Explain why the caloric loss caused by SDA is less in continuous feeders than in meal eaters.

18. Which small-scale tissue contributes greatly to heat increment?

19. *a.* Give four symptoms of hyperthyroidism.
    b. Why does hyperthyroidism predipose to diabetes?
    c. Give the train of endocrine events leading ultimately to elaboration of thyroxine from the thyroid gland.

17 Comparative ruminant metabolism

Characteristic of ruminants is the presence of the forestomachs (rumen, reticulum, and omasum) proximal to the true or glandular stomach (abomasum) in their digestive tracts. Many of the unique features of ruminant metabolism center around anaerobic fermentation of foodstuffs by ruminal bacteria and protozoa. Ruminant metabolism, though interesting and important in its own right, is reviewed in comparison with other animals to offer additional perspectives into metabolism in general.

GASTROINTESTINAL DIGESTION AND ABSORPTION
Digestion; ruminal flora

Ruminants differ greatly from many animals in that they can utilize cellulose, which is resistant to digestion by enzymes of mammalian origin. The utilization of cellulose and other crude fibers is largely dependent upon microbial metabolism in the ruminal-reticular complex. Cellulose is by far the most abundant organic compound in the world, and since plant material may contain up to 20% of cellulose or crude fiber, the ruminant is an important link in the food chain between the plant and animal world. Another unique feature of the ruminant is that significant quantities of nonprotein nitrogen can be incorporated microbiologically into high-quality bacterial and protozoal protein. The bacteria and protozoa, in turn, become available to the ruminant animal for digestion in the abomasum and small intestine. Indeed, the rumen is a site of major importance when considering assimilation of nonprotein nitrogen for metabolic pur-

poses. Protein endogenous to the diet is also broken down by microflora and becomes available to the ruminant animal as microbial protein, partially digested protein, amino acids, and fatty acids. Furthermore, ruminal microflora synthesize vitamin K and virtually all the B-complex vitamins, provided that adequate cobalt is present for vitamin B_{12} synthesis.

The relationship between ruminal flora and the host animal is a symbiotic one. The microflora benefit by being provided with a secure niche in which to live and the necessary ingredients (the ruminant's food and water intake) to thrive and multiply. In return, the ruminant benefits from microflora by utilizing their end products of metabolism and, in addition, by digesting microflora in the abomasum and small intestine.

The rumen is well equipped to handle the requirements of its microbial population. It is large, some 40 gallons in a medium-sized cow, and can therefore accommodate considerable quantities of bulky foods. Herbivores must eat a lot, since plants constitute a lean ration. The rumen has a fairly stable pH (approximately 6.8) depending on diet, and temperature (38 to 40° C), is well mixed, and richly vascularized for uptake of certain products of microbial metabolism. Devoid of its microbial population, the rumen would serve no digestive function since it lacks exocrine secretory glands.

Bacteria contained in the rumen are predominantly gram-negative cocci and short rods. They are numerous, rougly 5×10^{10} per gram of rumen material, and are composed of many genera and species. The protozoa in the rumen are predominantly ciliates and number approximately one million per gram of rumen material.

Microbial metabolism in the rumen is anaerobic in nature, because oxygen is not present. Hence, for electron balance, oxidative processes (electron removal) must be accompanied by reductive processes (electron acceptance); for instance, the production of CO_2, and oxidized products of carbohydrates and proteins, is accompanied by the generation of reduced products, such as CH_4 (methane), hydrogen gas, and volatile fatty acids (VFA). In this environment, polyunsaturated fatty acids (e.g., EFA) become saturated to a large extent.

Carbohydrates and proteins both serve as important substrates presented to the microbial population of the rumen. By microbial metabolism, these compounds can serve for synthesis of microbial protein and other microbial constituents, as well as take part in oxidative pathways leading to CO_2, and as reductive pathways leading to CH_4 and VFA. The volatile fatty acids—acetate, propionate, and butyrate (and, to a lesser extent, valerate and isovalerate)—are important microbial waste products. VFA are transported across the ruminal epithelium in unionized form to enter ruminal veins and subsequently provide roughly two-thirds of the ruminant's daily caloric needs.

Acetate and butyrate are ketogenic or lipogenic, and, thus, not capable of contributing to glucose synthesis. In the process of absorption, the ruminal wall converts almost half the butyrate to the ketone body β-hydroxybutyrate, the other half of the butyrate is converted in the liver. Propionate serves as a critically important precursor of glucose in the ruminant liver. The other compounds of major importance for gluconeogenesis are amino acids. Approximately 50% of the glucose synthesized arises from propionate and the other half from amino acids. The exact proportion of each utilized for gluconeogenesis depends upon the chemical composition of the diet and on the physical manner in which it is prepared (Table 17-1). For example, diets containing extensive roughage, primarily cellulose, favor production of acetate by microflora. Diets that contain relatively more concentrate (grain) favor production of propionate. If the concentrate source has been heated or cooked (flaked, expanded), propionate production by microflora is further enhanced. Under conditions of increased propionate production, more glucose arises from propionate. This frees amino acids for protein synthesis, since it lessens their use for gluconeogenesis.

Table 17-1	Effects of chemical composition and physical treatment of diets on digestibility
Substrate added	**3-Hr gas production**
None (control)	1 ml
Expanded milo	130 ml
Plain milo	47 ml
Casein	37 ml
Aspartic acid	32 ml
Cellulose	11 ml
Sucrose	113 ml

Digestibility of diets was demonstrated by incubating equal volumes of ruminal contents, obtained from a rumen-fistulated cow, for three hours with various nutrients in closed containers provided with gas-volume measuring equipment. Especially noteworthy is the effect of expansion on digestibility of milo and the relatively slow rate at which cellulose is digested.

Large glucose requirement of lactating cow

One disadvantage of ruminant microbial metabolism is that the microbes ferment essentially all the dietary carbohydrate to acetic, propionic, and butyric acids. Consequently, a ruminant receives little or no alimentary carbohydrate and is entirely dependent upon gluconeogenesis to supply its necessary glucose. Ruminants need glucose for the same functions as do monogastrics. Through selective breeding, however, science has made some of these glucose functions quantitatively more important. For example, cows have been bred to produce much larger quantities of milk than nature intended. The adaptive physiological changes that occur in the coordination of metabolism of body tissues that support lactation (so called homeorrhetic adaptations) are illustrated by the observation that the lactating udder of the goat utilizes 60 to 85% of the glucose (largely produced by hepatic gluconeogenesis), 14 to 41% of the acetate, and a significant proportion of the amino acids available to the animal as a whole. In the lactating dairy cow producing 80 lbs of milk per day, an amount of glucose equivalent to the blood glucose pool turns over every 5 minutes, with mammary gland uptake accounting for 50 to 85% of total glucose turnover. Although the majority of glucose is used for lactose synthesis in the mammary gland, glucose is also used for glycerol, fatty acid, and milk protein synthesis. In ewes, the glucose demand has also been extended beyond nature's intent, because the ewe has difficulty supporting 2 fetuses sumultaneously (twin lamb syndrome), particularly in the third trimester (i.e., the dead of winter), when food is scarce and fetal growth is maximal.

To accommodate these excessive demands for production, the laws of nature were violated. The cow's rumen, large as it is, cannot physically contain the vast amounts of the natural (lean) diet needed for high productivity; so, calorically concentrated, non-natural rations are fed. In doing so, the probability of metabolic problems for the ruminant are greatly increased. For example, feeding high-grain supplements may cause lactic acidosis; and adding urea as a nitrogen source to the diet may lead to ammonia toxicity.

INTERMEDIARY METABOLISM
Carbohydrates

Most of the dietary carbohydrate is converted through fermentation in the rumen, and can be accounted for by the amounts of VFA, methane, and CO_2 produced. Although some starch may escape fermentation when certain grains are fed, it is to little avail to the ruminant, since maltase activity in the small intestines may be insufficient to complete hydrolysis of maltose to glucose. Moreover, absorption of glucose from the small intestine can occur from fairly high glucose concentrations, since active transport of glucose in ruminants is rather rudimentary, as has been demonstrated in sheep. Thus, in nearly all circumstances, 90 to 100% of the circulating glucose in cats and ruminant animals is derived from gluconeogenesis occurring chiefly in the liver. This pathway is permanently "switched on." Indeed the rate of gluconeogenesis is greatest after a meal in cats and ruminants, when the supply of gluconeogenic precursors is greatest (i.e., amino acids and propionate, respectively). In addition, minor quantities of valerate, isovalerate and L-lactate, produced by rumen microflora, are available for gluconeogenesis. During fasting, glycerol from triglycerides increases its relative contribution to the pool of gluconeogenic ingredients.

Renal gluconeogenesis is important in ruminants: approximately 10% of glucose synthesized is derived from the kidneys (in sheep), of which 65% is from glutamine, lactate, and pyruvate and 12% from glycerol. Unlike the rat, glycine is a poor gluconeogenic source; the substantial hepatic uptake of glycine may reflect a requirement for hippuric acid synthesis and for bile acid conjugation.

Except for quantitative differences in gluconeogenic precursors, gluconeogenesis in nonruminants and ruminants is quite similar. In ruminants, however, the DCA shuttle, of prime importance in gluconeogenesis, has both mitochondrial and cytoplasmic pyruvate carboxylase activities, in addition to cytoplasmic PEP-carboxykinase. Therefore, in cattle, pyruvate does not have to enter mitochondria for carboxylation to oxaloacetate on its way to gluconeogenesis. The ruminant is, however, primarily geared to produce glucose from precursors provided by microflora. Fatty acid synthesis from acetate, like gluconeogenesis from pyruvate, does not involve mitochondria; acetate does not need to be produced inside mitochondria from pyruvate, since it abounds in the bloodstream among VFA generated from carbohydrates in the rumen.

Another noteworthy feature of ruminants is that gluconeogenesis is not very sensitive to insulin; one must administer insulin intraportally to see inhibition. Earlier the fact was discussed that in nonruminants, too, insulin does not affect hepatic metabolism nearly to the same extent as it does extrahepatic metabolism, its main function in the liver being that of a glucagon antagonist. It was noted that in periportal cells gluconogenesis takes place postprandially. Insulin's main functions are to stimulate glycogenesis in the liver and extrahepatic fat and protein deposition. Insulin release in ruminants is stimulated not only by glucose, but also by propionate, butyrate, isovalerate, and valerate, the postprandial signals of plenty.

Figure 17-1 features glucogenic and lipogenic ingredients derived from the diet in support of the ruminant's milk production.

Nitrogen metabolism

Proteins vary a great deal in the extent to which they are degraded in the rumen (Table 17-2). Feeding ruminants proteins that are relatively resistant to microbial degradation in the rumen (escape protein) can improve the animal's nitrogen economy: (i) by minimizing losses that are incurred when dietary protein is transformed to microbial protein; and (ii) by not allowing the production of adequate amounts of ammonia for maximal microbial growth. The latter increases the opportunity of feeding inexpensive nonprotein nitrogen (urea), because it lessens the risk of ammonia overproduction and toxicity.

Manipulating nitrogen transactions in the rumen to increase the pattern and outflow of amino-nitrogen has produced encouraging increases in wool growth, body growth, and milk protein yield. For optimal milk

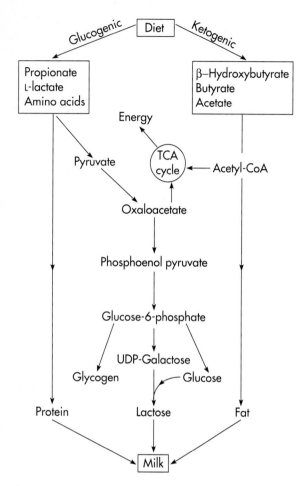

Figure 17-1. Dietary ingredients used for milk production by ruminants.

Table 17-2	Estimates of protein escaping destruction in the rumen

Feedstuff	% Protein escaping ruminal digestion
Casein	10
Grass silage (unwilted)	15
Oats	20
Barley	20
Whole soybeans (unprocessed)	20
Alfalfa silage (< 35% DM)	20
Peanut meal	25
Sunflower meal	25
Alfalfa hay	25
Alfalfa silage (> 55% DM)	30
Cottonseed meal (solvent)	30
Corn silage	30
Soybean meal	30
Cottonseed meal (expeller)	35
Extruded whole soybeans (300°F)	40
Corn	40
Sainfoin	50
Brewer's grains	50
Distiller's dried grains	55
Corn gluten meal	55
Fish meal	60

Reproduced, with permission, from Satter LD: Protected Protein and NPN, Anim Nutr & Health, 38(11):14-18, 1983.

production, escape proteins (also, though misleadingly, called *bypass proteins*) may be fed especially during early lactation when calorie availability, in the form of fat released from adipose tissue, exceeds protein intake. It is economically important that the milk production rate in early lactation be maximized, since this sets the pace for milk production in the later phases.

Two notes may be added to the above considerations on feeding escape proteins:

• The decision to feed escape proteins cannot be based simply on the ongoing rate of milk production in a cow. One must also take the phase of lactation into account. For it makes a great deal of difference whether 70 lb of milk are produced in early lactation, when negative energy and nitrogen balances prevail, or after peak lactation when the animal's food intake is in excess of expenditures.

• Not only the degree of escape determines the economic use of a given protein. It is of critical importance to also consider the quality of the protein, especially its content of the essential amino acids lysine and methionine. These amino acids, whose concentration is generally low in plant proteins, may be rate-limiting for growth and milk production. Therefore, depending on the ration fed, one may settle for a lesser escape in favor of higher lysine and methionine availability.

The major nitrogenous constituents of the ruminant's diet are proteins, nucleic acids, free amino acids, and nonprotein nitrogen sources (NPN; e.g., urea). In the rumen, these materials are degraded into NH_3 and carbon skeletons. Dietary NPN, free amino acids, and nucleic acids are extensively degraded, while preformed proteins are degraded to a variable degree, depending largely on their solubility in the rumen. The NH_3, in turn, is incorporated into microbial cells. Some ammonia is absorbed and converted in the liver to urea; then, urea is either voided in urine or, via saliva, recycled into the rumen, where urease regenerates ammonia from it. A function of urea recycling is to help the liver get rid of bicarbonate (for urea production) and, thus, regulate acid-base balance. Plants contain large amounts of organic acids whose metabolism yields a bicarbonate burden that must be coped with.

The microbial cells, undegraded dietary protein (escape protein), and some free amino acids pass with the digest from the rumen-reticulum through the omasum and abomasum to the small intestine (Figure 17-2). Thus, the lower gut's digestive and absorptive apparatus is presented with a mixture of nitrogen compounds, consisting of plant (dietary) and microbial proteins, nucleic acids, and some free amino acids and peptides. Roughly 60 to 80% of the amino acids

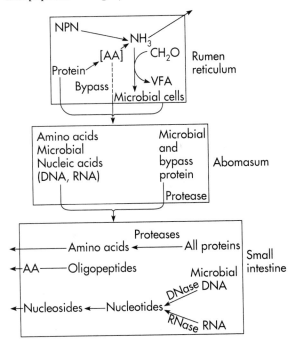

Figure 17-2. Overview of ruminal and postruminal nitrogen metabolism; *VFA,* Volatile fatty acids; *NPN,* nonprotein nitrogen; *AA,* amino acids; *DNase,* deoxyribonuclease; *RNase,* ribonuclease. *Reproduced with permission from Bergen WG: Postruminal digestion and absorption of nitrogenous compounds, Fed Proc 37:1223-1227, 1978.*

in the gut are derived from microbes; hence, about two thirds of milk proteins were once microbial proteins in the rumen.

A general accounting of dietary crude protein and nonprotein nitrogen (NPN) in the ruminant digestive tract is as follows:

- 85% of dietary nitrogen intake with typical ruminant rations is in true protein form and 15% in natural NPN form.
- The amount of nitrogen recycled into the reticulorumen (from salivary urea or urea which diffuses from systemic blood) is equal to 12% of the normal dietary nitrogen intake.
- 40% of true dietary protein escapes degradation by microbes in the rumen and goes to the intestine, while all the dietary NPN and recycled nitrogen pass through the ruminal ammonia pool.
- 90% of all ruminal ammonia produced is incorporated into microbial nitrogen.
- 80% of microbial nitrogen is in true protein form and 20% in nonutilizable NPN form.
- 80% of microbial true portein will be digested and absorbed in the small intestine (metabolizable protein).

The pancreas of ruminants has 100 to 200 times more ribonuclease activity than that of dogs or primates. Absorption mechanisms in ruminants, though similar to those of other animals, show the highest rate of amino acid uptake in the mid to lower ileum. This is caused by a slow rate of neutralization of abomasal digesta in ruminants, which then delays activation and peak activity of pancreatic proteases to the mid jejunum. Essential amino acids (methionine, threonine, isoleucine, leucine, phenylalanine, lysine, histidine, and arginine) are absorbed faster than nonessential ones. Postprandially, amino acid levels in plasma remain unchanged or decline in mature sheep, while in nursing lambs, and in nonruminants, this level increases (Figure 17-3).

For the purpose of gluconeogenesis in the liver, muscle proteins are catabolized. In muscle, the majority of glucogenic amino acids are converted to alanine, glutamine, and (specific for the ruminant) also to aspartate before release into the bloodstream. Leucine, being a ketogenic amino acid, cannot be converted to the above three nitrogen-transport forms, and, thus, leucine accumulates in muscle during protein breakdown. Increased leucine concentrations inhibit protein catabolism and, thus, help to regulate the release of amino acids from muscle. Ketone bodies

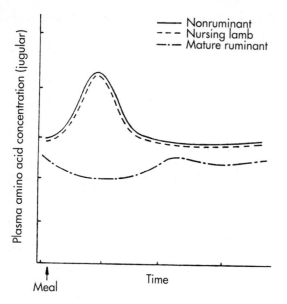

Figure 17-3. Postprandial changes in circulating amino acid levels. *Reproduced with permission from Bergen WG: Postruminal digestion and absorption of nitrogenous compounds, Fed Proc 37:1223-1227, 1978.*

in elevated concentrations also inhibit protein catabolism.

Proteins released from muscle are transported between organs (Figure 17-4). The liver removes amino acids from the bloodstream, with increased rate during fasting. The gut removes glutamine from the blood, but releases alanine. The kidneys (in sheep) postprandially add glutamine to the blood; roughly half of all the glutamine the liver receives comes from the kidneys. Renal gluconeogenesis, insofar as it is derived from amino acids, leaves ammonia that must be transported, in the form of glutamine, to the liver for urea production. But during fasting, glutamine is removed by the kidneys for increased gluconeogenesis and urinary ammonia excretion; renal glutaminase activity is induced by acidosis.

Glucagon increases hepatic removal of amino acids, especially alanine and glutamine, for use in gluconeogenesis. Insulin stimulates muscle to promote protein synthesis. Consequently, the amino acid concentration in the blood declines postprandially in a mature ruminant. (See Figure 17-3.) This amino

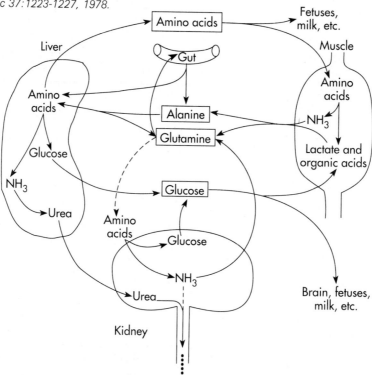

Figure 17-4. Nitrogen transport between organs in ruminants. *Dashed line indicates acidosis or starvation. Reproduced with permission from Bergman EN: Glucose metabolism in ruminants as related to hypoglycemia and ketosis, Cornell Vet 63:341-382, 1973.*

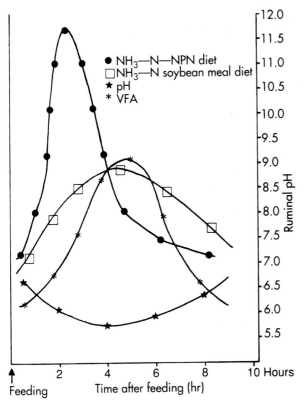

● NH₃—N—NPN diet
□ NH₃—N soybean meal diet
★ pH
* VFA

Figure 17-5. Defining the postprandial state in a ruminant. *Reproduced with permission from Bergen W and Owens F: Extent and limits of manipulation in nitrogen metabolism, Anim Health & Nutr 40(10):32-36, 1985.*

acid decline coincides with postprandially increased VFA levels in the blood because VFAs stimulate insulin secretion. The postprandial state in a ruminant is defined by a rise in the concentrations of dietary metabolites and a drop in pH in the rumen after a meal (Figure 17-5).

Over 92% of the N-compounds of a cow's milk consist of proteins synthesized de novo in the mammary gland from amino acids extracted from blood. Interestingly, the mammary gland takes up essential amino acids in excess of that secreted in milk, but takes up nonessential amino acids in short supply. The mammary gland thus converts essential amino acids to nonessential ones.

Lipid metabolism

Over 90% of de novo fatty acid synthesis in adult ruminants takes place in adipose tissue; for this purpose, predominantly acetate (the main ruminal VFA)

is used. Only small amounts of glucose are converted to fat in ruminants.

The liver is practically of no importance for fatty acid synthesis in adult ruminants. Of the VFA arriving in portal blood, propionate is used for gluconeogenesis, and acetate is not absorbed by the liver. Although butyrate is not used for gluconeogenesis, it nonetheless enhances hepatic glucose production by stimulating phosphorylase and pyruvate carboxylase activity and also by generating needed energy to drive gluconeogenesis. The liver is a net exporter of acetate for the purpose of fat synthesis in adipose tissue, especially in early lactation; it is important to note that this is a significant alternative to ketone body production. Endogenously produced mitochondrial AcCoA is not a precursor for lipogenesis since (i) citrate lyase activity is low, so that there can be no export of AcCoA out of mitochondria; and (ii) high PEP-carboxykinase activity in the liver of ruminants pulls oxaloacetate in the direction of gluconeogenesis, with lipogenesis losing out. Another important consequence of low oxaloacetate concentration in the liver is that AcCoA, formed during fatty acid oxidation, does not as readily engage in TCA cycle activity, and, thus, forms ketone bodies. In adipose tissue, malic enzyme activity is low, and, thus, NADPH needed for fatty acid synthesis must be generated by the pentose phosphate shunt and cytoplasmic isocitrate dehydrogenase, which may be rate-limiting.

Ruminant plasma contains few chylomicrons; endogenously synthesized and dietary lipids are primarily transported in the form of VLDL. VLDL levels drop during lactation, because of the low K_m of lipoprotein lipase in the udder; increased plamsa lipid levels are present for 80 to 90% in the form of cholesterol-rich LDL and phospholipid-rich HDL.

Homeorrhesis

The text previously defined homeostasis as follows: maintaining the steady state of nonequilibrium by controlling the dynamic processes of anabolism and catabolism of body stores. Homeorrhesis deals with a steady flow of metabolites; for example, partitioning of nutrients for muscle (protein) or adipose (fat) tissue growth; or flow of dietary and body constituents into milk production. Homeorrhetic control of growth and milk production is poorly understood, even though it is known that certain dietary and nutritional factors are involved and certain pharmacological agents can affect it. Besides the scientific importance of understanding growth control, there are huge economic interests involved here; for instance, livestock produces billions of pounds of adipose tissue in excess of that necessary for normal biological functioning of the animals. If homeorrhetic control of fat formation were better understood, it might be curtailed and dietary energy economized. Likewise, understanding of homeorrhetic control of milk production might lead to better feeding economy. To illustrate the effects of homeorrhetic control over partitioning body mass away from fat and toward muscle protein, the text shall look at repartitioning agents, including an endocrine factor (growth hormone) and beta-agonists (clenbuterol; ractopamine).

Insulin and growth hormone (somatotropin) are both protein-anabolic hormones, but this is where their similarity stops. Insulin is primarily involved with the synthesis and deposition of protein and fat stores after a meal, and, thus, is regarded as a homeostatic control agent. Similarities shared by growth hormone in this regard are in large part due to the effects of somatomedins (e.g., insulin-like growth factor I), which are produced by the liver in response to growth hormone. In contrast, growth hormone alone is one of the homeorrhetic agents that controls the partitioning of nutrients over protein and fat stores and their use for milk production. Under the influence of growth hormone, proteins accrue, while fat stores dwindle. These effects seem desirable for the production of leaner pig meat, since daily intramuscular injections of porcine somatotropin for an 8-week period decreased ham fat from a control value of 21% to 13.6% of carcass weight, while increasing ham protein from a control value of 18.2% to 19.7%. The effects of growth hormone on milk production are equally revealing (Figure 17-6). When growth hormone was administered to cows during early lactation (i.e., when the cow is in negative energy and nitrogen balance), increased milk yield was accompanied by increased fat and decreased protein content of the milk produced. However, later in lactation, when the cow is in positive energy balance, the administration of growth hormone resulted in vastly (41%) increased milk yield and no compositional changes in milk fat, protein, or lactose. Commercial amounts of growth hormone are produced by the recombinant-DNA method; the hormone thusly obtained differs from natural somatotropin by having one additional methionine. It is of interest to note that the recombinant somatotropin's effect on milk production exceeds that of the natural hormone.

On the downside, it should also be realized that

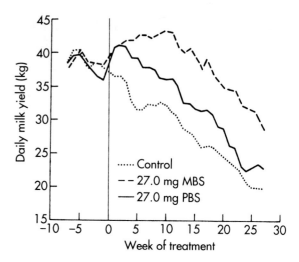

Figure 17-6. Administering bovine somatotropin increases milk yield. Treatment commenced at week zero, circa 84 days after parturition. Daily doses of pituitary *(PBS)* and engineered methionyl bovine somatotropin *(MBS)* are indicated. *Reproduced with permission from Bauman DE, Eppard PJ, DeGeeter MJ, and Lanza GM: Responses of high-producing dairy cows to long-term treatment with pituitary somatotropin and recombinant somatotropin, J Dairy Sci 68:1352-1362, 1985.*

growth hormone is potentially diabetogenic, meaning that it can create an altered state of chronic hyperglycemia. In this regard, growth hormone stimulates hepatic gluconeogenesis (and therefore more glucose for milk production) and decreases glucose utilization in muscle tissue by decreasing insulin receptor and hexokinase activty. Much of growth hormone's mammogenic and galactopoietic activy is accounted for by its structural similarity to prolactin.

Clenbuterol and ractopamine, both synthetic compounds, are beta-agonists; they stimulate beta-adrenergic receptors normally activated by epinephrine in response to sympathetic nervous system activity, and, hence, are classed under sympathomimetic agents. Beta-adrenergic receptor activation is typically associated with enhancing such activities as heart rate and contractility, glycogenolysis, gluconeogenesis, lipolysis, insulin and to a larger extent glucagon secretion, cutaneous vasodilation, and renin secretion. The striking effects of these repartitioning agents in steers, poultry, sheep, and pigs include decreased fat and increased protein contents of the carcass. For example, in Hereford steers weighing approximately

350 kg, clenbuterol administered at 10 mg per head per day reduced fat depth measured at the 12th rib by roughly 40% while increasing the longissimus muscle area at the 12th rib by 10%, compared to normal controls; carcass protein increased by 13%, while fat diminished by 20%. In finishing swine, ractopamine at a dose of approximately 60 mg per day increased the loin eye area by 14%, while reducing the fat depth at the 10th rib by 14%; in the carcass, dissected lean increased by 12%, while dissected fat decreased by 14%.

Ketone bodies

Since their discovery in the urine of diabetic patients in the latter part of the 19th century, ketone bodies have had a checkered history, being variously considered as indicators of disturbed metabolism and as important fuels. Their association with the diseased state (ketoacidosis) branded them initially as undesirable metabolic products. However, the demonstration in the 1930s that various tissues could oxidize ketone bodies led to the suggestion that they could be important as a lipid fuel. In 1956, evidence was presented that long-chain fatty acids provided the important lipid fuel in starvation, so that ketone bodies were again neglected as a fuel and were once more associated in the minds of biochemists, physiologists, and clinicians with pathological conditions. Even in 1968, doubts were present in at least some minds as expressed in a review by G.D. Greville and P.K. Tubbs (*Essays in Biochem* 4:155, 1968):

Clearly it is not obvious in what ways ketogenesis in fasting is a good thing for the whole animal; should the liver be regarded as providing manna for extrahepatic tissues, or does it simply leave them to eat up its garbage?

Research since that time has provided strong support for the view that ketone bodies have an important role to play in the transport of lipid fuels in blood. Furthermore, recent developments indicate that, as well as being a fuel, ketone bodies play an important role in integrating fuel mobilization and utilization in the whole animal.

Ketone bodies are produced predominantly in the liver but also in the forestomach (mostly rumen) epithelium. In liver tissue they are generated from partial oxidation of long-chain fatty acids arising from triglyceride stored in adipose tissue. Thus, the question arises, "why should one lipid fuel be converted into another in the liver?" To answer this question, it is necessary to look at the limitations of fatty acids

as fuel. The problem of transporting long-chain fatty acids in nontoxic form in the aqueous medium of blood has been solved by binding them to albumin. However, this has an important drawback; although the total concentration of fatty acids in blood can increase to approach 2 mM, the free (noncomplexed) concentration will be much lower (possibly as low as 10 μM) since a large proportion is complexed with albumin. The rate of diffusion into the cell will consequently be low. This may restrict fatty acids from fulfilling their role of providing fuel that will be utilized in preference to glucose. This restriction will be particularly important if fuels must diffuse over long distances within tissues in which there is a high rate of energy demand. If fatty acids are converted to ketone bodies, which are freely soluble and do not require albumin for their transport, the concentration of lipid fuel can be maintained at much higher levels in blood and interstitial fluid. The ketone-body concentration in blood may rise to 2-3 mM after a few days starvation and to 7-8 mM after prolonged starvation. At these levels, ketone bodies can compete effectively with glucose, which has a normal concentration of approximately 5 mM in blood. This ability of ketone bodies to provide a ready replacement for glucose plays two particularly important roles:

- As provision of readily diffusible fuel for essential muscles. There are a number of muscles in the body associated with vital physiological functions (e.g., heart for the circulation of blood, diaphragm for respiration, some smooth muscles for digestion and absorption of food, the myometrium during parturition, etc.). If hypoglycemia coincided with a reduction in the blood supply to these muscles (e.g., during hypotension or hypoperfusion), insufficient fuel (i.e., fatty acids and glucose) might reach these vital muscles resulting in their fatigue, and hence precipitate a life-threatening situation. In such circumstances, a high concentration of ketone bodies, which could diffuse rapidly into these vital tissues, could replace glucose as fuel. Such vital muscles do indeed possess high activities of enzymes in the ketone body utilization pathway.

- As provision of fuel to the brain during periods of starvation. Measurements of arterio-venous differences across the brain of several animal species (including humans) indicate that ketone bodies progressively displace glucose as a fuel for this organ during starvation. After about 3 weeks of starvation, the human brain gains most (60%)

of its energy from the oxidation of ketone bodies, with the remainder provided by the oxidation of glucose. Further starvation does not appear to alter this degree of dependence on ketone body oxidation. The increased rate of oxidation appears to depend solely on the increase in the blood concentration of ketone bodies. It has been suggested that fatty acids cannot provide a fuel for brain tissue because, unlike ketone bodies, they are bound to serum albumin and therefore have difficulty diffusing across the blood-brain barrier. In contrast to that of monogastric animals, the adult ruminant brain has apparently not adapted as well to ketone body utilization and is therefore more dependent upon glucose oxidation.

The ratio of β-hydroxybutyrate to acetoacetate is normally greater than 10:1 in ruminant animals. As is typical for ruminants, ketone levels in the blood are high after a meal; of course, they are also high in the fasting state.

Acetoacetate (AcAc) is formed from acetate in the mitochondria and can pass into the cytosol, where it can be enzymatically converted to β-hydroxybutyrate (BHB):

This conversion of AcAc to BHB in the cytosol of hepatocytes, rather than in mitochondria, is unique to ruminants. This characteristic appears to account for the different pattern of change in serum AcAc to BHB concentration ratios that occurs during intense fatty acid oxidation in ruminants, as compared to monogastric species:

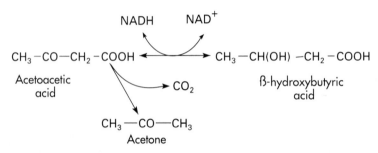

- In monogastrics, the ratio of AcAc to BHB in serum decreases with increased oxidation of fatty acids. This probably reflects the low ratio of NAD to NADH that occurs in the mitochondria caused by extensive oxidation of fatty acids; high concentrations of NADH favor the production of BHB.
- In ruminants, the ratio of AcAc to BHB appears to be proportional to the rate of ketogenesis, and does not appear to be influenced by the ratio of NAD to NADH in mitochondria. This stands to reason: under conditions of ketogenesis, gluconeogenesis is also active, and this process uses cytoplasmic NADH, so that less NADH is available for BHB formation.

Why two ketone bodies are produced rather than one is not entirely clear. Comparative studies indicate that AcAc is the more "primitive" ketone body since it occurs in the absence of BHB in invertebrates and some fish. However, BHB is the better fuel since it is more reduced, so why has AcAc persisted? The answer may be that to produce solely one or the other ketone body in large amounts could render ketone-body synthesis dependent on the redox state of the liver, particularly in nonruminant animals. However, if an equilibrium mixture of the two is produced, changes in the redox state of liver mitochondria simply alter the ratio of ketone bodies released.

Ketogenesis and gluconeogenesis are related directly; that is, as one increases so does the other. Several factors may be considered to explain this correlation: (i) When the demand for glucose is great, oxaloacetate is removed from mitochondria for the production of glucose. Not enough oxaloacetate may remain to combine with acetate in the TCA cycle, and, thus, ketone bodies are formed. (ii) Translocation of fatty acids from cytoplasm into mitochondria, needed for β-oxidation, is mediated by the carnitine acyltransferase (CAT) system, which, in turn, is controlled by glucose availability, both directly and indirectly (hormonally). Fatty acid transport is stimulated during periods of high glucose demand and rapid gluconeogenesis, and is depressed when cellular glucose supplies are ample. This explains the synchronization of gluconeogenesis and ketogenesis. The glucose affect on CAT may also help to explain why, in early lactation feeding, high-grain diets diminish ketogenesis: increased propionate production raises glucose levels and, thus, inhibits CAT activity. (In addition, increased insulin release inhibits triglyceride lipase activity in adipose tissue, and, thus, less fatty acid is available for ketogenesis.)

During prolonged fasting, the gastrointestinal tract of the ruminant does not contribute ketone bodies; all ketones are then formed in the liver from fatty acids taken up from the circulation. These fatty acids are less well packaged in VLDL form, since the ruminant's liver quite easily runs out of lipotropic factors during fasting: (i) essential fatty acids are a problem because of a shortage of digestible microbes from the rumen; (ii) cholesterol must be synthesized, since the ruminant does not consume any in its herbivorous diet, bacterial membranes do not contain it, and de novo cholesterol synthesis is depressed during fasting; (iii) choline becomes depleted; methionine administration brings relief; and (iv) the apoprotein availability is limited. Thus typically, fatty liver infiltration and ketone body overproduction are observed.

It is important to recall that under fasting conditions the brain of nonruminants shifts its metabolism toward utilization of ketone bodies; this relieves the gluconeogenic burden on the liver and, in doing so, spares muscle proteins. In contrast, neither the ovine nor the bovine brain has adapted well to ketone body utilization. Hence, even during fasting, the ruminant brain represents a constant, large glucose drain.

To alleviate the lack of polyunsaturated fatty acids (EFA), one may administer linoleic acid, one of the EFA, encapsulated in formaldehyde-treated proteins, so that they are protected from ruminal digestion and hydrogenation. A side effect of this treatment is that the fat in adipose tissue stores is softened. After feeding encapsulated EFA, one must increase vitamin E (and/or Se), particularly in young animals. Milk produced this way contains more EFA, but may be low in total fat content. (See below.)

Appetite control by VFA

An interesting role for VFA in ruminant metabolism and nutrition is their proposed involvement in appetite control. Acetate is particularly important in this respect. As food is consumed, the rate of fermentation in the rumen increases, the concentration of VFA (primarily acetate) in the blood subsequently increases (since acetate is not absorbed by the liver) and depresses appetite. A period of ruminating (cud chewing) follows. The effect of acetate in depressing appetite is thought to result from a direct action of

this VFA on the brain. As fermentation in the rumen subsides, the concentration of acetate in the blood declines, appetite is renewed, fresh food is provided to ruminal microflora, and the fermentation rate is stimulated.

METABOLIC DISORDERS AND MANAGEMENT

As a way of illustrating and applying intermediary metabolism in a comparative manner, the text briefly discusses a few ruminant disorders that are, in essence, consequences of (i) the peculiar features of ruminal digestion; (ii) controlled genetic selection for high milk production and multiple offspring (stretching the limits); and (iii) industry's greed to squeeze the last penny worth of profit out of livestock operations, which necessitates feeding artificial diets (high-concentrate; nonprotein nitrogen).

Ammonia toxicity

Economic considerations make the substitution of proteins in the diet by cheaper nonprotein nitrogen (NPN) sources desirable. Feeding escape proteins allows the inclusion of increased proportions of NPN as ruminal microflora assimilate that NPN into their proteins. When excess urea is added to a ration, microbial urease activity releases ammonia in excess of what the liver can handle. The neurotoxic effects of increased ammonia levels in the blood and the alkalosis caused by H^+ ion binding to ammonia lead to muscle twitching, uncoordinated movement, convulsions, coma, and death.

Lactic acidosis

To provide the necessary calories for the high production demands placed on ruminants, rations are supplemented with grain (concentrate). Much propionate is produced from grain, providing an adequate supply of gluconeogenic procursors. Feeding concentrate in excessive proportions leads to production of large amounts of lactic acid (both D- and L-acid) and a drop in rumen pH. This, in turn, depresses growth of several more desirable species in the ruminal microflora and enhances growth of lactate producers. The result is lactic acidosis with damage to the ruminal wall, allowing bacteremia (liver abcesses), and an osmotic effect on the ruminal lactic acid and satellite cations that pull large amounts of body water into the rumen. The latter may lead to death via hypovolemic shock.

Low milk-fat syndrome

Low milk-fat syndrome (LMS) is characterized by a marked depression in milk fat content; this constitutes an economic loss. It occurs after feeding a high ratio of concentrate over roughage to dairy cows; it is also noted when normal rations are fed, supplemented with protected (encapsulated) polyunsaturated fatty acids.

The etiology of this syndrome is somewhat multifaceted. Easiest to pinpoint is the LMS caused by polyunsaturated fatty acids; their presence in plasma lipoproteins inhibits the mammary gland's uptake and metabolism of triglyceride (from VLDL), and this lowers milk fat content. It is more of a problem to explain LMS caused by high concentrate/roughage ratios in the diet. It was formerly believed that LMS was the result of lowered acetate supply for the mammary gland's fat synthesis, but this proved to be incorrect, since the acetate supply was found to be unaltered. Three arguments point to the large production of propionate (glucogenic) from the high concentrate ration as the cause for LMS: (i) glucose injection intravenously also depresses milk fat yield; (ii) insulin secretion is stimulated by propionate or glucose, so that release of fatty acids from adipose tissue is suppressed, which causes lowered production of VLDL in the liver, and this limits the VLDL availability to the mammary gland for milk fat synthesis; and (iii) increased propionate production diminishes the production of vitamin B_{12} in the rumen; this causes impaired conversion of propionate to succinyl-CoA; instead, the intermediate, methylmalonate, increases in the blood, and this intermediate inhibits fatty acid synthesis in tissues (e.g., mammary gland).

Milk fever

Calcium, magnesium, and phosphates are normally present in extracellular fluids in relatively small amounts compared with sodium, bicarbonate, and chloride; but intracelluclar fluids contain large amounts of magnesium and phosphate ions as well as potassium. Should the "mineral" concentrations in blood (especially calcium and magnesium) fall below minimal levels, a condition known as **milk fever** is precipitated. In order to understand the pathophysiological symptoms observed with milk fever, one must be fully aware of the range of neuromuscular functions dependent upon the opposing actions of magnesium and calcium (see Chapter 8).

Milk fever, or **parturient hypocalcemia,** is one of the most serious and costly production diseases of cattle. It occurs close to parturition and is associated with the onset of lactation. More than 90% of cases occur between 24 hours before and 48 hours after parturition. Analysis of the incidence of milk fever reveals that it occurs in both dairy and beef cattle, but that in the former the disease is predominantly a calcium and phosphate imbalance, whereas in beef breeds the hypomagnesemic condition seems more frequent.

A typical case of hypocalcemic milk fever is accompanied by dullness, a dry nose and dilated pupil, a constricted anal sphincter, and a disinclination to eat. "Paddling" of the hind legs, with stiff extended joints and nervousness due to decreased muscle control, precedes collapse. A period of narcosis (CNS depression) may follow in which the neck may be typically kinked. Finally, coma supervenes, and the head may be turned onto the flank. Hyperglycemia is also frequently observed during the course of this disease.

Acute hypophosphatemia can accompany hypocalcemia in cases of milk fever. The lack of blood phosphate is then correlated with muscle weakness: a typical case shows acute lumbar pain, parturient edema of the brisket and udder, and an inability to rise. In many cases, calcium injections allay the more acute signs, but the apparently normal animal is still unable to rise. In other cases there is a temporary improvement but the animal relapses a few hours later and rarely responds to a second injection. These cases usually become chronic if treated first with calcium, and the animal may stay recumbent for several days, even if subsequently treated with phosphates.

The direct costs of treatment and prevention are only part of the economic losses incurred because of this disease. Some milk fever cases fail to respond to treatment and become "downer" cows, for which prognosis is much less favorable. Between 4 and 28% of cases relapse and may become downer cows, of which between 20 and 67% subsequently die or must be slaughtered. One of the most important consequences of milk fever is damage to nerves and muscles caused by the pressure of recumbency, such damage causing even more recumbency. Other, secondary causes of death are probably related either to the failure of neuromuscular transmission or to the paralysis of smooth muscle. The effects of such paralysis include the loss of the eructation reflex, which may result either directly in bloat or secondarily in pneumonia caused by inhalation of rumen contents.

Therapeutic use of vitamin D or its active metabolites may be of some value in the prevention of milk fever in dairy cattle. Fed cows receiving a high calcium prepartal diet become dependent upon intestinal calcium absorption and generally tend to reduce the output of PTH from parathyroid glands. Anorexia and gastrointestinal stasis that often occur near parturition interrupt the major inflow of calcium into the extracellular fluid pool. Outflow of calcium with the onset of lactation now exceeds the rate of inflow, and the cows develop a progressive hypocalcemia. On the other hand, calcium homeostasis may be maintained in cows fed a low-calcium prepartal diet. Bone resorption and intestinal absorption will both contribute to the inflow of calcium to the extracellular pool throughout pregnancy. The anorexia and gastrointestinal stasis that often occur near term may temporarily interrupt one inflow pathway. However, there is more likely to be an adequate pool of active bone resorbing cells capable of responding to (unsuppressed) PTH secretion under these dietary conditions in order to maintain and approximate balance between calcium inflow and outflow, thereby preventing the development of progressive hypocalcemia, and thus milk fever.

Ketosis
Description and etiology

Bovine ketosis, observed especially during the first two months of lactation, and ovine pregnancy toxemia, observed at the end of term with twin fetuses, are characterized by hyperketonemia, acidosis, ketonuria, hypoglycemia, fatty liver, loss of appetite, etc. The explanation for ketosis that occurs during early lactation is a negative energy balance caused by homeorrhetic hormones, such as prolactin and growth hormone, that establish a high rate of milk production in spite of the fact that dietary intake has not yet peaked (Figure 17-7). Fat stores are abundant at this time; their mobilization yields milk fat, but also a fatty acid burden, which is partly converted to ketone bodies in the liver. Proper management of the preparturient cow should keep her fat stores from becoming overabundant, so that ketone production early in lactation is limited. Also, she should be provided with grain in her diet for the ruminal microflora to generate enough propionate to support milk sugar production. Protein supply then may be rate-limiting for this early milk production; hence, the improved milk yield when protein is supplemented. Later in lactation, if enough energy, glucose, or protein are not available, then simply less milk is produced.

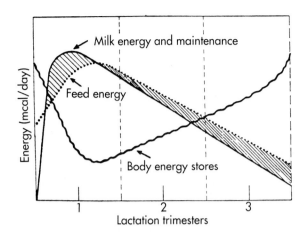

Figure 17-7. Relation between dietary, milk, and body energy during the lactation cycle. *Reproduced with permission from Kutches A: Feeding the dairy cow in the 80s, Anim Health & Nutrit 38(6):6-12, 1983.*

The etiology of bovine ketosis is multifactorial; four different types have been classified:
Underfeeding ketosis
- Primary underfeeding ketosis: the cow is not fed enough acceptable feed.
- Secondary underfeeding ketosis: the cow's feed intake is diminished because of illness.

Feeding ketosis
- Ketogenic ketosis: the cow ingests excessive amounts of ketogenic nutrients, such as butyric acid and medium-chained fatty acids present, for instant, in ground nuts.
- Spontaneous ketosis: the cow consumes a nutritionally adequate ration containing enough glucogenic precursors to provide glucose for milk production; the ensuing mobilization of fatty acids from triglyceride stores serves milk production, but also causes excessive ketone body generation in the liver. It is important to note that this is a case of ketosis in the presence of enough carbohydrates.

The primary underfeeding ketosis is similar to the kind of ketosis in nonproducing animals, already discussed. Because some 85% of total glucose production is used for milk sugar, a critical carbohydrate shortage develops, which leads to mobilization of fat from adipose tissue. The glycerol, thusly mobilized, contributes to hepatic gluconeogenesis. Fatty acids, in excess of tissue demands, enter the liver from where they cannot be exported as VLDL (lack of lipotropic factors). The extent of storage in the form of triglycerides is limited (fatty liver), and, thus, the liver must export these fatty acids in a water-soluble form; that is, after conversion to ketone bodies. Add to this the observation (in ewes) of decreased renal plasma flow, depressing glomerular filtration rate, thus diminising ketonuria and allowing accumulation of ketone bodies in the blood. Also, it has been observed in normal cows that the blood flow in the gastrointestinal tract region was cut in half after two days of fasting; the loss of appetite during ketosis may, thus, impair nutrient absorbability.

Secondary underfeeding ketosis usually accompanies any of the other types of ketosis, because a common characteristic of ketosis is loss of appetite.

Nutritional management to avoid ketosis

Care should be taken when adding a feed additive as a prophylaxis against bovine ketosis or ovine pregnancy toxemia. For example, sodium propionate is often suggested, because it is an excellent glucogenic precursor. However, propionate has several serious disadvantages as a feed additive: (i) exogenous propionate (e.g., dietary supplement) inhibits the metabolic activity of propionate-producing bacteria and favors the activities of acetate and butyrate-producing bacteria. This can lead to an unfavorable balance of microbial enzymes in the rumen, and, thus, to a severe shortage of glucogenic precursors when propionate-feeding is discontinued; (ii) above, it was noted that propionate elicits an insulin response and lowers vitamin B_{12} production, both leading to low milk fat syndrome; (iii) propionate feeding depresses appetite before an adequate quantity of food has been ingested; and (iv) ruminants seem to find feed containing propionate unpalatable; this dislike then depresses food intake and, thus, the availability of glucogenic precursors.

The ideal method for preventing ketosis has not yet been discovered. For cows, a dry period of 45 to 60 days is recommended to replenish body stores; this, in turn, increases milk yield. Restriction of total-calorie intake toward the end of pregnancy is recommended to avoid fat buildup in adipose tissue (fat-cow syndrome). This fat would be excessively released immediately after delivery, in early lactation, and, thus, contribute to the extent of ketosis. Toward the end of gestation, as part of the restricted calorie diet, the proportion of concentrate in the diet should be increased to culture propionate-producing bacteria in the rumen, which will help meet the glucose demands

during early lactation. The rumen pH-lowering effects of concentrate feeding may be buffered with a mixture of $NaHCO_3$ and MgO in the diet of the postparturient (lactacting) cow; however, the effect of these buffers in the rumen is too short-lasting.

To institute proper management procedures for dealing with bovine ketosis, it is of paramount importance that first criteria are established to differentiate between spontaneous feeding ketosis, the type not caused by carbohydrate shortage, and underfeeding ketosis; treatment of one form of ketosis may be totally ineffective for another.

An innovative method to combat spontaneous ketosis is to feed long-chained fatty acids in a form that protects them from ruminal catabolism; that is, bound to formaldehyde-treated or other escape proteins, or as calcium salts. To appreciate the advantage of providing the milk-fat components by fat feeding, instead of via mobilization from fat stores in adipose tissue, one should recall that a condition that leads to spontaneous ketosis is the feeding of high-concentrate rations. Large production of glucogenic precursors from this diet provides, via increased milk sugar formation, a stimulus for enhanced milk production. Fat mobilization from adipose tissue then becomes stimulated. This provides the necessary milk fat, but it also presents the liver with a large excess of fatty acids that are then converted to ketones (i.e., spontaneous ketosis). On the other hand, after feeding the necessary fatty acids in an escape form, these fatty acids enter the body's metabolism as chylomicrons. Hence, they are channeled to tissues with lipoprotein lipase (e.g., mammary gland) but not to the liver, and therefore these dietary fatty acids do not contribute to ketosis; in fact, they effectively combat it.

STUDY QUESTIONS

1. Compare symbiotic digestion of foodstuffs in the rumen to constitutive digestion of rumen microbes in the small intestine.

2. *a.* Does the ruminant derive more propionate from roughage (cellulose) than from concentrate (starches)?

   b. For what purpose would the concentrate source be flaked or expanded?

3. *a.* List two kinds of vitamins produced by ruminal microfloral.

   b. List the primary gluconeogenic precursor the ruminant absorbs from the gastrointestinal tract.

c. Why is it that in the rumen each oxidative process must be accompanied by the formation of a reduced compound? List two of these compounds.

d. Microbial fermentation products can be taken up directly from the rumen of a cow into the blood stream. (True/False)

e. List two examples of why the ruminant animal is an important link in the food chain between the plant and the animal world.

4. Why do "bypass" proteins bypass? Give a synonym for bypass proteins.

5. Give the metabolic fate for ruminally produced acetate and butyrate.

6. In cows, postprandial insulin release is inhibited to allow gluconeogenesis to take place. (True/False)

7. Compared to other animals:
a. Why does the adult ruminant's liver lack glucokinase?
b. Why does the cow not need citrate lyase activity in its liver cells?

8. Comparing ruminants to nonruminants:
a. Where do postprandial ketone bodies in the cow's plasma come from?
b. List the difference in postprandial lipoprotein composition of plasma.
c. Postprandially, in systemic blood, which VFA is the most elevated and for what purpose is that VFA used?

9. Even though in many animals and in humans, fatty acids are readily synthesized from glucose, in the cow this does not happen to any appreciable extent.
a. Explain why this finding in the cow is not surprising.
b. From which ruminally absorbed compound does the cow synthesize fat?
c. As a consequence of the lack of malic enzyme activity in ruminants' adipose tissue, what reaction, and from what ingredients, does the ruminant generate the necessary reduced cofactor for fatty acid synthesis?

10. Liver and adipose tissue share almost equally in fat production from VFA in the ruminant. (True/False)

11. *a.* What is meant by homeorrhesis?
b. List two desirable homeorrhetic effects of growth hormone administration to pigs.
c. Indicate the enzymic site of action where sympathetic nervous stimulation (e.g., by supplementing diets with the sympathomimetic agents clenbuterol or ractopamine) affects carcass composition of steers.

12. *a.* For what reason would one want to feed nonprotein nitrogen (NPN) to lactating cows?
b. Name and list some symptoms of the disorder

that may result from adding too much urea to a cow's ration.

c. Why does feeding escape proteins allow more NPN in the cow's ration?

d. The desirability of feeding a certain protein to cows depends on the extent of "escape" and, in addition, the "quality" of the protein judged by _____. (Fill in the blank.)

13. Name the compound in the bloodstream responsible for the ruminant's appetite control.

14. Would a high-calcium prepartive diet or a low-calcium one be more likely to be associated with parturient hypocalcemia?

15. About adding sodium propionate to the cow's diet as a prophylaxis against ketosis:
a. List one reason why one is tempted to do it.
b. List four strong objections against this practice.

16. *a.* Among lipotropic factors, what causes polyunsaturated fatty acids to be in short supply in ruminants?
b. What problem may be caused by feeding linoleic acid to a cow?

17. Give an insulin-related explanation for the occurrence of low milk-fat syndrome during mid-lactation when concentrate is fed.

18. Why would cobalt deficiency lead to bovine ketosis?

19. Explain what causes negative energy balance in a cow during early lactation.

20. Give an argument as to why feeding supplementary protein to the cow during early lactation is more advantageous than doing so after the first trimester of lactation.

21. Consider these observations in the cow during early lactation: (i) FFA in serum are high; (ii) liver clears the bloodstream of increasing amounts of FFA and returns them as lipoproteins into the bloodstream; and (iii) levels of VLDL in the blood are low compared to dry cows.
a. The lactating mammary gland of the cow has high lipoprotein lipase activity. (True/False)
b. Practically all milk fats are synthesized in the udder. (True/False)

22. *a.* List a rationale for adding concentrate to the cow's ration during mid-lactation.
b. Explain the effect this might have on milk fat content.
c. Explain how an abrupt change to a high-grain ration can cause a severe form of acidosis, and describe some symptoms of that syndrome.
d. To maximize the amount of concentrate in a diet while reducing the health hazard associated with it, what chemical supplement can one add to the diet?

23. *a.* Feeding ketosis is characterized by a high level of which VFA in the blood, as compared with underfeeding ketosis?

b. List another difference in serum composition to differentiate between spontaneous and fasting ketosis.

24. To explain ketosis during early lactation (choose):

a. (A) Lactation peaks early; (B) lactation gradually increases to a later maximum; (C) lactation is approximately level throughout.

b. Feed intake peaks: (A) before; (B) simultaneously with; or (C) later than lactation.

c. The cow is in a negative balance with respect to: (A) fat; (B) carbohydrate; (C) nitrogen.

25. *a.* Lipid mobilized from body stores is ketogenic, because it is transported in the blood in the form of _____. (Fill in the blank.)

b. Dietary bypass fat is not ketogenic, since it is offered to extrahepatic tissues in the form of _____ (name lipoprotein).

c. Explain how the feeding of calcium salts of long-chained fatty acids may help to combat spontaneous bovine ketosis.

26. List a clinical/behavioral symptom of any form of ketosis that often causes a secondary underfeeding ketosis to accompany (and, thus, confuse the picture of) feeding ketosis.

27. About management procedures for cows in dry periods:

a. Give a rationale for calorically limiting the cow's diet prior to the onset of lactation.

b. Give a reason for starting the cow on increased amounts of grain (relative to silage) at two to three weeks prior to calving.

c. List the reason for not feeding extra calcium prior to the onset of lactation.

28. How would one test whether the formation rate of a certain B vitamin by the intestinal flora in the lactating cow is sufficient for maximal milk production?

APPENDIX

Study questions on interpreting literature and clinical situations

STUDY QUESTIONS

1. Edema may be caused by (encircle true statements): (A) low blood pressure; (B) low hematocrit; (C) low plasma protein level; (D) low interstitial protein level; (E) low-protein diet.

2. "The hormone atrial natriuretic factor (ANF) promotes natriuresis and diuresis, blood pressure lowering, and inhibition of aldosterone biosynthesis, and possibly inhibition of renin secretion from the kidneys. Indeed, one could speculate that this system is the counterbalance to the renin-angiotensin system, which plays a fundamental role in cardiovascular regulation."
   a. List a condition that leads to increased ANF release.
   b. Before ANF was discovered, Na^+ concentration in serum was thought to be controlled via fluid balance by the kidneys' proper response to which hypothalamic/pituitary hormone?
   c. How do the kidneys react to low aldosterone output by the adrenals?
   d. What connects the kidneys' renin secretion (in response to lowered blood pressure) with increased thirst and aldosterone production?

3. What clinical symptom would be in evidence if:
   a. A pig ate the bark or leaves of an apple tree and the phlorizin contained therein lowered the transport maximum of renal tubular glucose reabsorption?
   b. An animal ingested dicumarol (an inactive look-alike of vitamin K) from sweet clover?

4. "Vitamin D must first be modified by 25-hydroxylation in the liver followed by 1-α-hydroxylation in the kidneys to produce the hormone 1,25-dihydroxyvitamin D_3 (DHC). This process is strongly regulated and is one of the major endocrine systems regulating plasma calcium and phosphorous concentrations. Furthermore, it is a major endocrine system regulating bone mass and state."
   a. What correlates renal 1-α-hydroxylation of 25-hydroxyvitamin D_3 with the serum calcium level?
   b. How is undue elevation of the serum phosphorous level prevented at the time of increased calcium and phosphorous mobilization from bone in response to hypocalcemia?

5. Autonomic neural and endocrine control of liver glycogenesis: "Intravenous injections of glucose or insulin have a minor effect on hepatic glucose uptake compared to the effect of oral doses of glucose in humans. These observations indicate that additional factors, other than insulin, can produce hepatic glucose uptake and glycogenesis."
   a. Which half of the autonomic nervous system would be stimulated by the monitoring of high glucose via oral, intestinal, and hepatic (portal) glucose receptors?
   b. List a hormonal and an enzymic way in which this nervous system influences glucose metabolism after oral glucose doses.
   c. List the effect of gastric inhibitory peptide after oral glucose doses.

6. A dog is afflicted with an adrenal cortical tumor secreting large amounts of glucocorticoids.
   a. Which other endocrine function may become overchallenged and finally exhausted?
   b. Explain osteoporosis in this patient.

7. It has been established that anaerobic metabolism provides little energy (if any) for the long-distance runner.
   a. How long does it take to deplete the liver glycogen reserves during sustained aerobic exercise?
   b. What are the three primary sources of fuel for the long-distance runner?

8. "In sheep, glycine is a poor gluconeogenic source; the substantial hepatic uptake may reflect a requirement for hippuric acid synthesis." List the purpose for which hippuric acid is produced.

9. Comparing lipogenesis in brown and white adipose tissue: "The biosynthesis of palmitate from glucose results in the formation of ATP. Lipogenesis generates NADH, which, when oxidized by the electron transfer chain, results in the conversion of ADP to ATP. Consequently, the high rates of lipogenesis in

brown adipose tissue (BAT) may be limited by the accumulation of ATP. If BAT is important in the removal of glucose from the bloodstream for conversion to and storage as triglyceride, the physiological uncoupling process, which is unique to BAT, is necessary to permit such high rates of lipogenesis.

"In white adipose tissue the rate of lipogenesis is much lower than that in BAT, so that sufficient ATP utilization may occur via substrate ("futile") cycling, especially the triglyceride/fatty acid cycle.

"The weight of interscapular brown fat in the rat and its rate of respiration increased in response to a single meal. These data suggest that brown adipose tissue plays a role in thermic effects of meals."

a. Define uncoupling, a reason as to why uncoupling is needed to allow more NADH oxidation via the electron transfer chain.

b. Show in which manner the "futile" cycle mentioned above disposes of ATP in white adipose tissue.

c. List the technical term for the heat development after a meal.

d. List the function of brown adipose tissue immediately after birth and during arousal from hibernation.

10. You are presented with a dog whose owner tells you the animal has fainting spells. Upon examining the dog, you notice that his sclera (eye white) is yellowish (jaundiced), and from the marks on his skin you suspect that the dog has been hit by a car. Palpation makes you wonder about the intactness of his abdominal organs. To confirm your suspicion, you take a blood sample and find high arginase activity.

a. Which organ is now surely incriminated?

b. Explain how that could also account for the jaundice.

c. Explain how the fainting spells could have been caused by the same organ's malfunction.

B Answers to study questions

(No answers are given for questions of which the word can be located in the index and then found in the text.)

Chapter 1

6. The K^+ level in blood is maintained homeostatically at the expense of tissue K^+.

7b. 80 mg/dl.

8. Nervous and endocrine controls.

9. Proteinaceous hormones include insulin, glucagon, prolactin; thyroxine and epinephrine exemplify hormones derived from a single amino acid; cortisol, estradiol, and aldosterone are examples of steroid hormones derived from cholesterol.

11. Hypothalamic ACTH-releasing hormone instructs the pituitary to release ACTH, which acts upon the adrenal cortex. Glucocorticoids are released, which direct the liver to make glucose available to the bloodstream.

14. Bile.

16a. Circadian rhythm is inborn; it may be entrained to the light-dark cycle, but does not depend on it.

17. The gut.

18. The pancreatic duct transports exocrine factors, such as bicarbonate solution and the digestive enzymes, whereas the endocrine pancreas influences the blood glucose level directly via insulin and glucagon releases, controlled by the autonomic nervous system and the paracrine factor somatostatin.

20. Insulin, being a protein, would be intestinally digested if given orally.

21. Bilirubin.

22b. Hemoglobin carries oxygen, which is needed to keep liver cells alive.

23. The fat cell combusts glucose to CO_2 and water. Labeling glucose with the radioactive isotope ^{14}C yields $^{14}CO_2$, which can be easily measured. Insulin must be present in the incubation medium to direct glucose transport across the fat cells' plasma membranes.

24. Myelin floats on top, because of its high lipid content. The smooth endoplasmic reticulum, ultracentrifugally obtained in the microsome fraction, contains lipid-synthesizing enzymes.

25. Adenylate cyclase.

26. The oviduct cell, because nucleoli manufacture ribosomal RNA, which is required for protein synthesis.

Chapter 2

1. Fatty acids consist of ($-CH_2-$) repetitions of molecular weight 14; thus, per 14 g, one mole of metabolic water is formed from the two hydrogens. Carbohydrates are repetitions of ($-CH_2O-$) and, thus, yield one mole of water per 30 g. Proteins are poor suppliers of metabolic water, because of obligatory water loss in urine accompanying the excretion of urea.

3. Apolar compounds are protein (albumin) bound for transport in the blood, and incorporated into bile salt micelles in bile.

4. Protein binding prevents glomerular filtration in the kidneys, but allows uptake by the liver and excretion in bile.

5b. Blood glucose is glomerularly filtered in the kidneys, but then actively reabsorbed in renal tubules to prevent urinary loss.

8. To lower the elevated HCO_3^-/CO_2 ratio, the kidneys allow bicarbonate loss in urine; the lungs conserve CO_2 by hypoventilation.

10b. Part of the added acid will associate with $-COO^-$ groups and neutralize the anionic charges, while not affecting cationic charges, thus bringing the protein closer to its isoelectric point.

11. Aspartic acid and lysine buffer in pH ranges beyond the mammalian body's limits of viability.

13. The net charge of albumin can be attributed to an excess of aspartic and glutamic acids over lysine, histidine, and arginine. Adding acid neutralizes anionic charges and, thus, lowers the net charge of the protein. In tissue cells, too, added H^+ associates with $-COO^-$ groups of proteins; this lowers net anionic charges on cellular proteins and frees part of the satellite K^+ to leave the cell.

Chapter 3

10. Ionogenic attraction between anionic phosphate and cationic histones.

15. A codon on mRNA for which there is no anticodon is a termination signal for translation.

17. The first translated amino acids may be part of a signal sequence that is edited out posttranslationally.

20. An agent that inhibits mRNase would prolong the lifespan of mRNA, and, thus, allow more protein copies to be translated; this might promote growth.

22. This could be termed induction or enhancement.

23. Phosphorylating IF-2 inactivates this initiation factor and, thus, stops protein synthesis. Diphtheria toxin and certain plant toxins stop protein synthesis by inactivating elongaton factor 2.

24. A risk is that additional nondesirable genes are excised and cloned.

25. Such an animal may exhibit an exaggerated fat breakdown.

27. Degeneracy of the genetic code; wobble.

28. DNA repair goes on in all phases of the cell cycle. Repair of radiation-damaged DNA is slow, because both strands of the DNA may have been broken.

30. These proteins may derepress an existing gene that codes for this prion protein.

31. Repression.

Chapter 4

1. ATP.

2. ATP conversion to ADP, P_i, and heat.

3b. Flavin (in FAD) and niacin (in NAD) shuttle electrons.

5. Vitamins and minerals.

6. Enzyme synthesis increases V_m. At a braching point, the enzyme with the greatest affinity (lowest K_m) for the substrate is favored to prevail; however, other controls may make the reaction with the higher K_m prevail.

9a. Lead combines with sulfides, and, thus, affects disulfide bridges, a chief determinant of tertiary protein structure.

10b. When enzyme activation is blocked by puromycin, the activation is due to synthesis of more enzyme protein.

11. Steroid hormones increase enzyme synthesis.

12a. Allosteric control requires one molecule of product per enzyme molecule; it works on the kinetics of the reaction. Product inhibition, working on the thermodynamics of the reaction, requires a large shift in concentration gradient.

15. The diagnostic value of serum enzymes is exemplified by arginase activity in case of liver disease, or a certain isozyme of lactate dehydrogenase for heart damage.

17. Bacteria acquire resistance to a penicillin.

20. Glucocorticoids stimulate gluconeogenesis from amino acids; to eliminate the ensuing ammonia, arginase, a key enzyme of the urea cycle, must be activated.

21. Phosphorylation or dephosphorylation.

23. Protein kinases phosphorylate enzymes; they are activated under the influence of second messengers produced at the plasma membrane, when certain hormones or nervous transmitter substances bind to their receptors.

Chapter 5

8. Main determinant of filtration pressure is blood pressure; that of absorption pressure is oncotic pressure of plasma.

11. A diet deficient in the essential amino acid lysine precludes adequate protein synthesis, so that the oncotic pressure of plasma may drop and edema ensue.

14. In fluid therapy, an albumin solution in a physiologic salt mixture is best for fluid retention. Infusion of K^+ salts at too rapid a pace can kill an animal.

17. The fact that the isoelectric point of most proteins is at an acidic pH, so that proteins carry a net anionic charge at physiologic pH.

18. As the electrical gradient would tend to move Cl^- out of the cell, the opposing chemical gradient must tend to move Cl^- back in; that is, the cholride concentration outside must be higher than inside the cell.

20a. When H^+ enters cells, it associates with proteins; this lowers the net anionic charge of the proteins and allows some of the satellite K^+ to leave the cells.

21. A drop in pH would lower the net anionic charge on a serum protein, which would hold fewer satellite cations in the serum.

Chapter 6

4. Insulin and a glucose transporter.

7. Special ion channels and ion pumps exist. Shielding polar groups on organic compounds facilitates their uptake into cells. On the other hand, phosphorylation of glucose prevents it from leaving the cell.

9. Low temperature causes loss of membrane fluidity.

10b. Calcium is needed for functioning of the cytoskeleton.

13. Tight junctions prevent paracellular transport; gap junctions promote lateral exchange of small molecules between cells.

20. Golgi assembles and targets new membrane proteins; also, aided by the presence of specific lectins on membrane surfaces, Golgi targets glycoproteins toward their final destinations (e.g., lysosomes).

22. Liposomes that contain an anticancer drug can specifically be targeted to certain hepatomas by incorporating an asialoglycoprotein into that liposome.

29a. Protein phosphatases undo the work of protein kinases.

30. The catecholamines affect phosphorylation of key enzymes by both the cAMP and the diglyceride/Ca^{++}/inositol trisphosphate systems of second messengers.

31. Oncogenes promote cell division by stimulating the production of phosphatidylinositol-4,5-bisphosphate, and thence diglycerides.

33. Hormonal activity is further determined by the presence of receptors on target cells, their degree of binding to plasma proteins, and their half-lives in the circulation.

35. Pathological consequences of the down-regulation of hormone receptors on cell surfaces include hypercholesterolemia and maturity-onset diabetes.

39. Inhibiting phosphodiesterase prolongs the life of cAMP in a cell and consequently stimulates the protein kinases responsible for activating the key enzymes involved in the breakdown of glycogen and triglycerides.

40a. The absence of ADH receptors in the kidneys results in nephrogenic diabetes insipidus, characterized by large-scale production of dilute urine.

Chapter 7

3. Platelet-derived growth factor.

10b. High altitude or blood loss stimulates the kidneys to produce erythropoietin for the purpose of hematopoiesis.

11. Since the red cell depends on glucose for nutrition, hexokinase activity is vital. A functional cytoskeleton, which requires calcium, lends plasticity to the erythrocyte, so that it can move through narrow capillaries.

12b. Because gastrectomy removes intrinsic factor, vitamin B_{12} must henceforth be taken by injection.

14. Hydrogen peroxide must be detoxified by glutathione-dependent enzymes that require selenium for their activity.

15. The pentose phosphate shunt generates NADPH.

18. Rapid breakdown of fetal hemoglobin provides the neonate with iron; at the same time, though, large amounts of bilirubin are produced, which the liver cannot handle, resulting in hyperbilirubinemia.

20. The chief mode of CO_2 transport in the blood is in the form of plasma HCO_3^-, produced inside the red cell by carbonic anhydrase, an enzyme that requires zinc for its activity.

22. Hydrophobicity of the heme pockets in hemoglobin retards the formation of methemoglobin; further offsetting the slow rate of formation of methemoglobin is reduction by an enzyme that derives reducing power (NADH) from glycolysis.

Chapter 8

8. Pancreatic fluid; large intestinal fluid.

10. These questions summarize control over oxygen delivery and CO_2 removal at sites of active metabolism, where pO_2 in the blood is lowered by oxygen uptake in cells and CO_2 is produced. Lowered pO_2 opens sphincters in the arterioles of the microcirculation, so that more blood is delivered; it also stimulates production of 2,3-diphosphoglycerate, which enhances oxygen dissociation from hemoglobin. Cooperativeness causes maximal oxygen unloading from oxyhemoglobin over a narrow range of declining pO_2. Increased pCO_2 also enhances oxygen unloading (Bohr effect). The lowering of hemoglobin's pK after the unloading of oxygen allows H^+ binding to hemoglobin and transport of HCO_3^- in plasma.

11. Lymphatics clear the interstitial space of proteins that have leaked out of the bloodstream; in doing so, they maintain the oncotic pressure gradient between bloodstream and interstitium needed for fluid reabsorption into the bloodstream.

16. Reduced volume and hyperosmolality of urine.

17. The psychogenic water drinker would continue elaborating excessive amounts of hyposmolar urine; the dog with diabetes insipidus of central origin would respond to administered ADH by concentrating the urine; however, when ADH receptors in the kidneys are defective (nephrogenic diabetes insipidus), ADH administration would be ineffective.

22. The water-retaining effect of high oncotic pressure in plasma and the water-losing effect of high blood pressure play a role in the glomerular filtration rate and in the rate of fluid absorption in peritubular capillaries.

26. Aldosterone counters hyperkalemia by releasing K^+ in exchange for Na^+ reabsorption and by promoting tubular K^+ secretion.

30. The Cl^- pump in the thick ascending Henle's loop curbs salt loss in urine and sets up the countercurrent multiplication mechanism, whereby the steep osmotic gradient in the deep medulla is maintained; ADH elaboration then causes water reabsorption, so that a small volume of hyperosmotic urine is excreted.

32. Diminished erythropoietin production may cause anemia; hyperventilation is a compensation to acidosis caused by increased bicarbonate loss; increased parathyroid hormone levels in the blood, in response to renal Ca^{++} loss, lead to increased release of Ca^{++} and phosphate from bone; hyperkalemia reflects poor Na^+ reabsorption, as so does hypovolemia; poor intestinal Ca^{++} absorption is caused from the renal failure to generate the necessary hormone 1,25-dihydroxycholecalciferol.

33. Total renal failure.

36b. Glutamine production in the liver, increased during acidosis, detoxifies ammonia for transport to the kidneys, where glutaminase releases the ammonia for excretion in urine as NH_4^+.

38. Bilirubin is albumin-bound, and, thus, not filtered.

39. (a) Injected 45 mg divided by recovered 8.35 mg/dl would indicate 5.39 dl plasma and, given a hematocrit of 45%, a blood volume of 9.80 dl in the 10-kg dog—a suspiciously high value. (b) C_0 = 10.00 mg/dl and hence there are 4.50 dl of plasma (4.5% of body weight, i.e., normal) or 8.18 dl of blood. (c) Dehydration reduced plasma volume and, thus, increased the dye concentration at time zero. (d) Extravasation of dye would have diminished the dye concentration in plasma at time zero.

40. 115.2 L of plasma cleared of creatinine per 24 hours.

41. (a) The level of K^+ in plasma is homeostatically controlled; (b) high dietary intake of K^+ will boost K^+ elimination; (c) in acidosis, H^+ for K^+ exchange in tissue cells elevates the plasma K^+ level resulting in increased urinary elimination of K^+.

43. (a) Aldosterone; (b) parathyroid hormone.

44. Acidemia leads to H^+ uptake by tissue cells, and, thus, to the lowering of the net negative charge of the intracellular proteins and a drop in transmembrane potential; cells become hyperexcitable.

45. (a) Ketone bodies are acids; (b) lactate is $C_3H_5O_3^-$; to produce 3 CO_2 plus 3 H_2O, lactate must first associate with a H^+, leaving a HCO_3^- stranded; also, for its conversion to glucose, lactate must associate with one proton.

46. The anion gap is 28 meq/L. This elevated anion gap points to the presence of organic acids in plasma; for example, lactic acidosis, or ketoacidosis. However, the anion gap is reduced in hypoproteinemic alkalosis (since both HCO_3^- and Cl^- will increase in order to fill the gap).

48b. The alkaline tide after a meal is not a permanent acid-base burden as the bicarbonate produced in the stomach is neutralized in the gut by bicarbonate.

49. (a) Voiding HCO_3^- leads to increased retention of Cl^-; (b) when not enough K^+ is available to exchange for Na^+ in the kidneys, H^+ is lost in the urine; (c) inhibition of carbonic anhydrase diminishes reabsorption of HCO_3^-; elimination of HCO_3^- plus satellite cations has a mild diuretic effect.

50. Increased production of ammonia in the gut prompts the liver to synthesize more urea, which gets rid of more HCO_3^-.

53. Glomerular filtration of increased amounts of Cl^- leads to reabsorption of increased Cl^- with a concomitant loss of HCO_3^-.

55. HCO_3^- is lost because of diarrhea, producing a metabolic acidosis and hyperventilation. The kidneys conserve HCO_3^-, eliminate NH_4^+ and titratable acid ($H_2PO_4^-$); hyperkalemia leads to increased urinary K^+ loss.

57. (a) pH = 6.1 + log[20/(20 × 0.03)] = 7.62; (b) an acidifying compound must be given, such as, ammonium hydrochloride; (c) too fast a ventilation rate has blown off too much CO_2.

58. Turnover amounts to less than one thousandth of the human body's calcium store per day.

66. Calcium mobilization from bone cannot keep pace with milk letdown.

69. The high phosphate content of an all-meat diet diminishes intestinal absorption of Ca^{++}. The ensuing hypocalcemia stimulates parathyroid hormone release, which will result in demineralization of bone.

70. (a) Plants contain minerals, but they also contain organic acids that produce insoluble calcium salts; (b) preparturient feeding of calcium will lower the parathyroid hormone level.

74. Secondary nutritional hyperparathyroidism; kidney disease resulting in lack of calcium reabsorption; inborn error in renal production of 1,25-dihydroxycholecalciferol.

Chapter 9

6. Horses can digest cellulose because of the microflora in their cecum. Another valuable contribution by intestinal microflora is the production of vitamins.

10. Intrinsic factor, produced in the stomach, is required for intestinal absorption of cobalamine (vitamin B_{12}).

11. Pancreatectomy removes amylase.

13. Renin is a circulating enzyme produced by JG cells of the afferent arteriole, that converts hepatically derived angiotensinogen to angiotensin I. Rennin is a milk-clotting enzme produced by the abomasum that converts casein to paracasein.

20. Elevated iron levels in plasma down-regulate transferrin, so that less iron is transported from the gut.

21. Parathyroid hormone, released in response to low calcium levels in plasma, stimulates the production of the hormone 1,25-dihydroxycholecalciferol, which aids in intestinal calcium absorption.

22. Orally administered antibiotics may kill the bacterial microflora.

23. Coprophagy provides the rabbit with the "waste products" of the cecal microflora (i.e., nutrients and vitamins).

Chapter 11

6. Vitamins C and E; Selenium.

11. Need for energy (i.e., ADP/ATP ratio).

13. Anaerobic glycolysis exemplifies ATP production at the substrate level.

14. Uncoupling may occur as a result of either blocking H^+ return to the mitochondrial matrix at the F_0-F_1 complex, or by not allowing the H^+ gradient to build up.

16. Uncoupling diminishes the efficiency of ATP production, and this necessitates the combustion of increased amounts of nutrients; hence, increased oxygen consumption.

18. In the liver, the rate of oxidative phosphorylation is determined by ADP/ATP ratio, that is, the need for energy; in an exercising muscle, oxygen availability becomes rate-limiting.

19. NAD^+/NADH.

21. Because the mammalian erythrocyte is devoid of mitochondria, it cannot convert pyruvate to AcCoA; converting pyruvate to lactate by lactate dehydrogenase regenerates NAD^+ from NADH, so that glycolysis (i.e., ATP formation at the substrate level) can continue.

22. Fat combustion requires mitochondria for β-oxidation and the TCA cycle.

23. Under ischemic conditions, oxygen supply is limited; this limits mitochondrial activity, so that anaerobic glycolysis must supply the tissue's energy; lactate is formed.

Chapter 12

3. Glucokinase, glycogen synthase, and phosphofructokinase are activated.

7. Glucagon can selectively mobilize glucose from hepatic glycogen stores without depleting muscle glycogen. Epinephrine effects glycogenolysis in muscle and in the liver.

9. Hypoglycemia evokes hormonal responses that stimulate gluconeogenesis; because of G-6-Pase deficiency, G-6-P thusly formed is not converted to glucose and activates glycogen synthase activity.

10. Phosphorylation activates phosphorylase and inhibits glycogen synthase activity.

13. Osmotic diarrhea; cataracts.

15. (a) Glucuronide conjugates are formed from, for instance, epinephrine; (b) production of ascorbic acid; (c) neonatal hyperbilirubinemia (jaundice); (d) no.

17. Blood glucose arises from glycogen and gluconeogenesis.

19. Inhibition of phosphofructokinase by ATP is overcome by $F-2,6-P^2$ for the purpose of converting glucose to fat.

30. Oxidative portion of the pentose shunt provides NADPH for fat synthesis; the nonoxidative portion provides pentoses for nucleic acid production needed for protein synthesis.

34. Parenchymal liver cell, postprandially.

35. Malate can shuttle NADH's reducing equivalent from cytoplasm to mitochondria; malic enzyme can produce NADPH.

38. Cobalt must be fed for the production of vitamin B_{12}.

40. Glycerol.

46. Production of glycerol phosphate.

47. Oxaloacetate; aspartate or malate.

50. Conditions that promote lipolysis antagonize lipogenesis.

52. Tissues produce no more lactate than the equivalent amount of glucose that they take up; hence, there is no net glucose production from lactate. From triglycerides, after combustion of fatty acids, glycerol remains for net gluconeogenesis.

53. Oxidation of fat and ketones requires mitochondria and oxygen. During exercise, the muscle may be short of oxygen.

55. Lactate brings in a reducing equivalent.

60. Some sympathetic neurons are thought to release peptide transmitters that in turn stimulate peptidergic receptors that would not have been blocked by anti-adrenergic drugs.

61. (a) Adrenaline (epinephrine), via cAMP, stimulates the release of material necessary to replenish TCA intermediates, so that fatty acids, simultaneously released, can be combusted efficiently. (b) Increase it by glycogenolysis and gluconeogenesis. (c) To cope with the ammonia production that accompanies conversion of amino acids to glucose.

65. To increase hepatic uptake of alanine, the most abundant amino acid released from the muscle's protein stores, for gluconeogenesis.

66. Glucocorticoids act via nuclear events that lead to increased enzyme protein synthesis; glucagon converts an inactive form of an already synthesized enzyme into the active form. Glucagon is synthesized and stored in vesicles, and therefore can be immediately mobilized into the circulation. Glucocorticoids, on the other hand, are synthesized upon demand.

69. (a) Down-regulation of insulin receptors. (b) When tubular glucose load exceeds transport maximum for tubular reabsorption of glucose, glucosuria ensues. Hyperglycemia may cause this to happen. On the other hand, glucosuria can also result from kidney defects or poisoning.

Chapter 13

7. Cholecystokinin effects the release of pancreatic enzymes.

11. The monoglyceride acylation pathway (primary), and the phosphatidic acid pathway (secondary "scavenger" pathway).

14. Inhibitors of the key enzyme of hepatic cholesterol synthesis are given to block a compensatory response to cholesterol lowering by cholestyramine administration. Since cholestyramine is not normally absorbed across the GI tract, some may have difficulty classifying it as a drug.

18. Free fatty acid levels in plasma decline postprandially because of insulin's inhibition of triglyceride lipase activity.

19. Hepatic VLDL are targeted to lipoprotein lipase on fat cells by apo C. Cholesterol-rich LDL accumulate in plasma.

20. Relative to fat cells, heart cells' lipoprotein lipase has the higher affinity (lower K_m) for VLDL.

22. In addition to the down-regulated LDL receptor, the liver has an additional apo E receptor.

28. Carnitine acyltransferase (CAT), when stimulated during fasting, allows β-oxidation of fatty acids, and when inhibited by malonyl-CoA, CAT will not counter fatty acid synthesis.

29. Reoxidation of NADH and ubiquinone. H_2 is required for continued β-oxidation of fatty acids in mitochondria.

30. Carnitine; malonyl-CoA.

31. Peroxisomal fatty acid oxidation.

34. During fasting, ketogenesis is the only available route for elimination of abundant fatty acids mobilized from fat stores; the glycerol that remains can serve to support the vitally important gluconeogenesis.

35. Formation of β-hydroxybutyrate from acetoacetate regenerates NAD^+ needed for continued β-oxidation of fatty acids.

37. During ketoacidosis, the urea cycle activity declines (because of decreased bicarbonate levels); ammonia formed from amino acids during gluconeogenesis must now be increasingly exported from the liver in the form of glutamine. Increased glutaminase activity in kidneys then serves to eliminate ammonia; also, elimination of NH_4^+ in urine curbs K^+ loss.

42. Elongation and desaturation.

43. Citrate lyase is a rate-limiting step in the conversion of glucose to fat.

44. The AMP-activated protein kinase, when activated, phosphorylates, and thereby inhibits, the key enzymes in both fatty acid and cholesterol synthesis.

45. Negative feedback of hepatic cholesterol synthesis by bile salts, the most important end product of cholesterol metabolism, prevents overproduction of cholesterol.

47. Inhibiting breakdown of cAMP would lead to continued stimulation of triglyceride lipase, and, thus, to elevated free fatty acid levels in plasma.

49. NADPH formation is needed for fatty acid synthesis.

50. An important stimulation of triglyceride lipase is by the sympathetic branch of the autonomic nervous system, via β-adrenergic receptors on fat cells.

52. Fasting stimulates CAT and thus β-oxidation of fatty acids. Low insulin levels fail to activate AcCoA carboxylase and to inhibit triglyceride lipase.

54. Fat synthesis from glucose releases heat. Brown adipose tissue has a special oxidative phosphorylation-uncoupling protein that is activated under cold stress.

55. (i) Bile; (ii) lipoproteins; (iii) uptake of cholesterol-loaded LDL and disposal of cholesterol in bile; (iv) ketone bodies provide a water-soluble way to eliminate fatty acids.

56. Not only is methionine an essential amino acid, needed for the protein moiety of lipoproteins, it is also a methylating factor needed for the formation of choline (part of lecithin) and of carnitine (needed for CAT activity).

Chapter 14

4. Glutamine.

5. Transamination and transdeamination; vitamin B_6 or pyridoxamine.

9. Causes of kidney stones include uric acid or insoluble calcium salts. Methylhistidine in urine indicates rate of turnover of muscle proteins.

10. In winter, birds rely on metabolic water and curb obligatory water losses by forming urates as nitrogen waste product.

12. Pepsin and rennin are active at different pH. Colostrum contains a trypsin inhibitor.

15. A small drain, since most of the protein of the sloughed cells is recovered following digestion and reabsorption of constituent amino acids.

16. Methionine is needed for production of carnitine and lecithin, a lack of which produces fatty liver.

17. Both questions relate to the fact that small numbers of mitochondria make white muscle fibers more dependent on anaerobic metabolism, in which glycogen can be used as fuel; white muscles catabolizing glycogen anaerobically to lactate obtain fewer calories per mole than red muscles, which can completely combust it to CO_2 and water.

18. Genetically, breeds of horses are endowed with different ratios of Type II over Type I fibers; the ones with a high ratio are fit for vigorous exercise for short duration.

20. Glucagon activates the A system to allow alanine uptake by liver for gluconeogenesis.

23. Some 40% of muscle protein can be spared for gluconeogenesis; the brain's ketone body utilization stretches this gluconeogenic reserve.

24. Nibblers are more nitrogen-economic, since they convert less of their dietary intake of amino acids into fat.

25. Urinary excretion of BAIB indicates thymidine (DNA) turnover; methylhistidine appearance rate in urine is a measure of muscle protein turnover.

Chapter 15

1. The liver must convert much of the dietary sugars and amino acids to fat. The trace element selenium is among the lipotropic factors that go into the production of VLDL. NADPH producing enzymes, the citrate shuttle for AcCoA (lyase), and AcCoA carboxylase are stimulated.

2. Lipid soluble vitamins are transported to the liver in chylomicron remnants. Bile salts recirculate enterohepatically.

5. Feed-forward activation of glycogen synthase by the product of the glucokinase reaction.

6. NADPH is produced.

9. Activation of the A system; activation of adenylate cyclase.

10. Muscle proteins and glycerol from fat stores contribute to net glucose synthesis. Lactate does not, since the glucose synthesized from it must be reused by lactate-producing tissues.

11. (a) Mitochondria; (b) glycerokinase; (c) ammonia detoxification, since muscles lack the urea cycle.

14. The liver uses glycerol to reesterify incoming free fatty acids for their incorporation in VLDL and return to the fat stores.

17. AcCoA, resulting from β-oxidation of fatty acids, inhibits pyruvate's destruction by dehydrogenase and activates pyruvate's use for gluconeogenesis via pyruvate carboxylase.

18. When carbohydrates are lacking, the liver produces ketone bodies to (i) make water-soluble products for elimination of abundant free fatty acids; (ii) be able to use glycerol for gluconeogenesis; (iii) provide the brain with ketone bodies, so that glucose (and, thus, tissue protein) will be spared.

20. Liver converts lysolecithin back to lecithin; also produces nascent HDL. HDL cholesterol is removed via the bile, mostly in the form of bile salts.

21. During exercise, muscle incurs an oxygen debt, hence, it cannot use its mitochondria and, thus, not combust ketone bodies for energy.

25. Phosphoenolpyruvate carboxykinase.

26. The higher oxygen tension, prevailing in periportal cells, is needed for fatty acid oxidation, so that NADH and AcCoA generated by this process can stimulate gluconeogenesis.

27. Glutamine, produced in perivenous hepatocytes, will normally be recirculated to periportal liver cells, where glutamine's ammonia is used for urea synthesis. During acidosis ammonia is increasingly eliminated as NH_4^+ ions in urine since: (i) urea cycle activity is down; (ii) hepatic glutamine synthase is activated; and (iii) renal glutaminase activity is stimulated.

29. The liver can chemically modify these compounds by oxidation, methylation, proteolytic activities, etc. In addition, it can leave the compound intact, but eliminate it in the form of a conjugate with glucuronic acid, glutathione, etc.

32. (a) Lack of cobalt blocks vitamin B_{12} formation by the intestinal flora, resulting in anemia. In ruminants, where cobalamine is involved in the conversion of propionate to succinate for gluconeogenesis, lack of cobalt leads to ketosis.
(b) Lack of selenium leads to fatty liver; also to white muscle disease, since selenium is involved in

the glutathione peroxidase reaction, which serves to protect cell membranes from the effects of hydrogen peroxide produced during metabolism.
(c) Glycogen storage disease; ketosis.
(d) Vitamin B_{12}.

Chapter 16

6. (a) A 100 G diet contains 10 g of fat (90 kcal), 20 g of protein (80 kcal), and 50 g of carbohydrates (200 kcal) for a total of 370 kcal. The dog needs 750 kcal/day (i.e., about 203 g of diet/day).
(b) Less than that; see Table 16-1.

7. Without carbohydrates in the diet, fats would be less absorbable.

9. (a) Approximately zero: not absorbable by itself.
(b) As oxygen consumption would be very low (particularly in white muscle), glucose would mainly serve as nutrient, but anaerobic glycolysis does not yield CO_2. So, the RQ in this muscle might be close to zero/zero (i.e., undetermined).

11. The female body contains more adipose tissue, which has a low metabolic rate. (See Table 16-2.)

13. Hyperthyroidism elevates MR; so do uncouplers of oxidative phosphorylation, such as dinitrophennol.

14. As cold stress increases the MR, it causes the animal to eat more; but since the animal does not switch diets, the ratio of CO_2 produced over O_2 consumed (or RQ) does not change.

16. Hormonal balance; composition of the diet; heat increment.

Chapter 17

5. Butyrate serves for energy production, mostly via ketone-body production; acetate is used for lipogenesis in fat cells.

7. Because practically no glucose is absorbed from the diet, hepatic glucokinase is not needed; acetate is derived from ruminal digestion, instead of mitochondrial pyruvate dehydrogenase; hence, the citrate lyase shuttle is unnecessary.

9. Glucose in a ruminant is a scarce commodity; there is no postprandial glucose glut that must be converted to fat.

11. Decreased carcass fat results from activation of triglyceride lipase by sympathomimetic agents.

12. Feeding escape proteins allows the microflora to digest more nonprotein nitrogen without production of toxic amounts of ammonia. Feeding NPN is economic, but the content of essential amino acids (methionine and lysine in particular) in the escape protein must be considered.

14. A high calcium prepartal diet.

16. Polyunsaturated fatty acids are in part hydrogenated in the rumen. Adding these fatty acids to the diet in an escape form leads to lowering of milk fat.

17. Propionate produced from concentrate elicits elaboration of insulin, which, in turn, inhibits triglyceride lipase.

19. Milk energy exceeds the caloric feed intake. (See Figure 17-7.)

20. Milk production rate early in lactation sets the pace for the entire period of lactation. Besides, after feed intake peaks, the intake of dietary protein may be adequate.

22. In midlactation the rate of milk production is determined by availability of milk sugar; adding concentrate, though, may lead to low–milk-fat syndrome. Lactic acidosis may, to some extent, be reduced by supplementing acid-base buffers (MgO and NaHCO₃); however, the buffers do not remain in the rumen long enough to be totally effective.

23. Feeding ketosis may be differentiated by a high serum level of acetate; also, the glucose level is not reduced.

25. Free fatty acids released from fat stores are ketogenic in the liver, but triglycerides entering from the diet in the form of chylomicrons and VLDL are not. Calcium salts of fatty acids escape ruminal digestion and enter the bloodstream as lipoproteins, so that lipoprotein lipase in the mammary gland can remove them; this spares the need for fat release from fat stores.

26. Anorexia.

27. Avoid fattening the cow; allow the growth of a propionate-producing microflora; do not inhibit parathyroid activity.

28. See if dietary vitamin supplementation increases milk yield.

Interpreting literature and clinical situations

1. Edema may be caused by low plasma protein levels, which, in turn, may stem from a protein-deficient diet.

2. ANF release responds to high blood pressure. Before ANF was discovered as a way to eliminate Na^+, the Na^+ level was thought to be maintained by ADH controlling water elimination and by aldosterone regulating the absorption of Na^+ with accompanying water. Hypertonicity of plasma leads to release of renin and activation of angiotensin, which evokes a thirst response and an increase in the level of aldosterone.

3. Phlorizin intake leads to glucosuria. Dicumarol competitively inhibits the synthesis of certain blood clot-

ting factors, thus prolonging the clotting time of blood.

4. The regulation of phosphate excretion to maintain phosphate balance is accomplished primarily by PTH, which inhibits phosphate reabsorption in the proximal tubule. Note that this effect of PTH is opposite to that of Ca^{++} (i.e., PTH enhances Ca^{++} reabsorption). To understand how PTH is regulated primarily by the concentration of ionized Ca^{++} in plasma, consider, for example, how phosphate balance is restored following an increase in plasma phosphate concentration. Some of the excess phosphate will complex with ionized Ca^{++}. The decrease in ionized Ca^{++}, in turn, stimulates secretion of PTH, which then inhibits proximal tubular reabsorption, enabling the kidneys to excrete the excess phosphate. PTH also stimulates Ca^{++} reabsorption in the thick ascending limb and distal nephron, and enhances 1-α-hydroxylation of vitamin D, thus enabling the plasma concentration of ionized Ca^{++} to return toward normal.

5. Glucose receptors stimulate the parasympathetic branch of the autonomic nervous system, which then elicits insulin release from the pancreas and activation of glycogen synthase in the liver. Gastric inhibitory peptide prompts insulin release (in an anticipatory fashion).

6. Large-scale gluconeogenesis necessitates increased insulin production; it also depletes the body's protein stores, including proteins of the bone matrix.

7. Any glucose taken by the muscles from blood must be replaced by degradation of liver glycogen or by gluconeogenesis. Experiments with both humans and other animals demonstrate that liver glycogen is depleted during sustained exercise in less than 30 minutes. As exercise continues, it is now apparent that glucose uptake by muscle can account for only 30% of the oxygen uptake; more than 60% being accounted for by the oxidation of fatty acids, particularly following 20 to 30 minutes of distance running. It can be calculated that the elite distance runner, if he (or she) relied solely on blood glucose for energy production, would utilize about 5 gm of glucose each minute (1 μmol/min/gm muscle). Although the maximum activity of hexokinase has not been measured in elite distance runners, it is about 1.0 μmol/min/gm in muscle of fit, normal subjects, which indicates that the long-distance runner could possibly support his or her mechanical activity using blood glucose generated from the liver. However, the total hepatic store of glucose is only 90 gm, which would provide the runner with fuel for only 20 min, so that muscle glycogen, glucose generated from lactate via the Cori cycle, and fatty acids from blood are required as essential fuels for the long-distance runner.

8. Hippuric acid serves to conjugate phenolic waste for urinary elimination.

9. Coupling of ATP formation (phosphorylation) to the electron transfer chain (oxidation) inhibits NADH oxidation under conditions when the ATP/ADP ratio is high. Therefore, to allow continued NADH oxidation when ATP/ADP is high, either oxidative phosphorylation must be uncoupled or else ATP must be hydrolyzed at the rate at which it is formed (futile cycle). These measures produce heat. Postprandially, this heat is a major component of the specific dynamic effect of foodstuffs. After birth and during arousal from hibernation, this heat serves for regulating the body temperature.

10. When arginase, an enzyme belonging to the urea cycle, is present in the blood, liver damage is indicated. Liver functioning may be compromised. Jaundice results from defective removal of bilirubin from the circulation, and fainting spells can be caused by hypoglycemia, caused by poor control over the blood sugar level.

Literature

RESPONSIBILITY TO KEEP CURRENT WITH THE LITERATURE

Having just been oriented in the area of physiological chemistry, the reader is responsible from here on for keeping up with new developments in the field. This is difficult, because the world literature in this area doubles almost every five years. The number-one objective of this text is to bring the reader's knowledge and vocabulary up to the level at which she or he can read contemporary literature and, thus, start the lifelong process of self-education. This section contains some practical suggestions toward that end.

HAVE A GAME PLAN

The most frustrating approach to keeping current with the literature is to enter a library without a game plan. Though one may come across some relevant articles, soon enough one finds oneself reading outside materials that are simply too tempting to brush aside. In addition, this haphazard approach in all probability will not cover the field. So what's next?

Valuable information on veterinary libraries in the United States, and on computer-assisted searching and retrieval of literature on veterinary sciences and animal culture is contained in the most current edition of the *AVMA Directory* in the section entitled "Directory of Information Sources," compiled and updated annually by Mr. E. Guy Coffee, Information and Documentation Service, Trotter Hall, College of Veterinary Medicine, Kansas State University, Manhattan, KS 66506. Another excellent and succinct guide to keeping current with the literature with the aid of the computer is an article entitled "Tapping Information Resources in Veterinary Medicine," J Vet Med Educ 17:30-32, 1990, written by Ms. Norma J. Bruce, a librarian in the Veterinary Medicine Library, Ohio State University, 229 Sisson Hall, 1900 Coffey Road, Columbus, OH 43210.

COMMUNICATION OF SCIENTIFIC INFORMATION

There are various ways in which current developments in a field are being communicated among scientists and practitioners, and which allow the individual to keep up with the current literature. Developing a habit of scheduling a small amount of time once a week to peruse the display of current journals in a library is strongly recommended. Attending an annual conference or workshop usually acquaints one with the developments that will appear in print during the following year. Also, printed abstracts of a conference or an annual review of a field of interest may be available. Generally, as a researcher or animal health professional, one belongs to a society that will hold an annual meeting and that publishes a monthly journal, such as the *AVMA Journal,* the *Journal of Animal Science,* or the *Journal of Dairy Science.* A personal subscription to a general science-oriented journal (e.g., *Science*) helps to broaden one's scope. To identify other highly relevant journals in an area of interest, one may consult the *Basic List of Veterinary Medical Serials 2nd Edition,* 1981, with revisions to April 1, 1986 (Boyd CT and others; The Serials Librarian 11(2):5-39, 1986).

Helpful and indispensable as all of these measures may be, they do not take the place of a systematic screening of some of the general indexes (e.g., *Index Veterinarius* or *Current Contents*) that cover the tens of thousands of scientific journals. The screening of indexed databases, and literature searching and retrieval, is facilitated by the use of a personal computer or one belonging to an abstracting service.

COMPUTER-ASSISTED LITERATURE SEARCHES AND UPDATING

There are five major online data bases in the English language that cover areas of interest to veterinarians and animal scientists. The most useful are the following:

- CAB ABSTRACTS, the online version of *Index Veterinarius, Veterinary Bulletin, Nutrition Abstracts,* and *Dairy Science Abstracts,* among others; and
- MEDLINE, produced by the National Library of Medicine and containing *Index Medicus* among a large number of other data bases.

For specific information, occasionally one will have to consult the following:

- AGRICOLA, produced by the National Agricultural Library, USDA, and pertaining to all aspects of agriculture, including animal culture and veterinary medicine;
- BIOSIS, the printed version of which are the *Biological Abstracts;* and
- SCISEARCH containing the popular *Current Contents.*

A comprehensive listing of over one hundred data banks that contain animal health related information is given in the *International Directory of Animal Health and Disease Data*

Banks, issued by the USDA National Agricultural Library.

To remain current with the literature, especially difficult if one lives in an isolated location, one can take advantage of a current awareness service provided by a librarian who will search one or more of the databases for specified search terms. Or one may subscribe to the Automatic SDI Service, which scans the current month file of MEDLINE and retrieves and mails the references that match a prestored list of specified search terms.

Alternatively, one may use a personal computer to communicate with other computers via the telephone, provided the PC is equipped with a modem and a telecommunications software program such as PROCOMM. You may then install on your personal computer GRATEFUL.MED, a software package that allows you to track down and retrieve information stored in the databases of the National Library of Medicine, or acquire the online retrieval of CAB ABSTRACTS from DIALOG Information Services or BRS (Bibliographic Research Service). Other programs can be purchased to assist the veterinarian with diagnostics and finding specialized literature.

In addition to online searches, most libraries provide CD-ROM (Compact Disk, Read Only Memory) services. Different CD-ROM disks are available for the various online databases (e.g., CAB or MEDLINE), and most libraries have an autotutorial manual for CD-ROM. Since the library pays for this service, it is offered free of charge to the client. A drawback is that the databases are copied on CD only intermittently, so that CD-ROM may not be current; it may trail the online CAB database by as much as one year.

For a quick orientation in a field, as may be needed when one must give a talk, write a paper, or attend a meeting, one can search CD-ROM databases, specifying recent years only, to identify the most recent review articles and current papers of interest. The very latest information (not contained in CD-ROM) can then be obtained by an online search of the most recent files of those databases most relevant to the topic. In addition, the latest issues of relevant journals on display in the library should be perused.

Index

Figures are indicated by *f*. Tables are indicated by *t*.

Reference Blood Chemistry Values in Domestic Animals*

The tabled values may be used only as a guideline. Each laboratory should establish its own set of reference values to eliminate variations due to methods, instruments, and personnel. The variability of a listed reference value within a given laboratory is in part inherent in the many factors that define a clinically 'normal' animal; e.g., breed, sex, age, diet and nutritional status, sampling time relative to meal intake, and stress. Excluded from this table are enzyme levels; variation in their reported values is so large as to render them meaningless for comparison unless identical assay methods are used.

Plasma Constituent/Units	DOG	CAT	HORSE	COW	PIG	SHEEP
Ammonia µg/dl	19-120	—	13-108	—	—	—
Bicarbonate meq/l	17-25	17-23	20-34	21-35	17-26	20-27
Bilirubin, total mg/dl	0.1-0.5	0.1-0.4	0-2.0	0-0.7	0-0.6	0.1-0.4
Calcium mg/dl	8.4-11.5	8.0-10.4	10.2-13.0	8.5-11.9	8.0-11.5	11.5-12.9
CO_2, total mmol/l	17-24	17-24	20-32	21-34	18-26	21-28
Chloride meq/l	105-120	115-125	98-110	97-111	95-105	96-113
Cholesterol, total mg/dl	130-260	90-170	75-140	75-125	40-120	35-70
Cortisol, resting µg/dl	0.5-6.8	0.3-3.3	1.3-6.5	0.4-0.8	2.8-3.2	1.5-3.0
Creatinine mg/dl	0.5-1.5	0.5-1.8	1.0-2.0	1.0-2.2	1.0-2.7	1.2-1.9
Glucose mg/dl	65-115	55-120	65-110	45-85	70-145	50-80
Iron µg/dl	30-180	68-215	73-140	57-162	91-199	166-222
Lactate mg/dl	2-13	—	10-16	5-20	—	9-12
Magnesium mg/dl	1.7-2.8	1.8-3.0	1.8-3.0	1.4-3.3	2.0-3.9	1.0-2.8
Osmolality mosm/kg	281-299	281-299	276-296	276-296	282-292	—
pH pH unit	7.31-7.42	7.24-7.40	7.32-7.44	7.35-7.50	—	7.40-7.46
Phosphate mg/dl	2.5-6.2	3.0-7.5	2.0-5.6	2.5-7.0	4.0-11	4.0-7.3
Potassium meq/l	3.6-5.7	3.3-5.5	2.3-4.7	3.5-5.8	4.4-7.1	3.9-6.0
Protein, total g/dl	5.4-7.8	5.4-7.8	5.2-7.9	6.0-8.5	6.0-8.8	6.0-7.9
Albumin g/dl	2.4-4.1	2.0-3.8	2.5-4.0	2.5-4.0	1.9-3.5	2.4-3.0
Albumin/Globulin	0.6-1.1	0.5-1.2	0.5-1.5	0.8-1.2	0.3-0.7	0.4-0.8
Fibrinogen g/dl	0.15-0.4	0.05-0.3	0.1-0.4	0.1-0.7	0.1-0.5	0.1-0.5
Sodium meq/l	140-155	143-159	132-150	132-156	135-155	136-154
Thyroxine ng/ml	6-40	10-50	9-30	40-86	—	—
Urea nitrogen (BUN) mg/dl	5-28	10-32	8-24	5-30	8-30	8-30
Urate mg/dl	0-2	0-1	0.9-1.1	0-2	—	0-1.9

Hematology Values/Units	DOG	CAT	HORSE	COW	PIG	SHEEP
Hematocrit (PCV) %	37-55	30-45	32-50	26-42	36-43	27-45
Hemoglobin g/dl	12-18	8-15	10-18	8-15	9-13	9-15
Red blood cell count $n \times 10^6/\mu l$	5.5-8.5	5-10	6-12	5-10	5-7	9-15
Platelet count $n \times 10^5/\mu l$	2-9	2-9	1-6	1-8	2-5	2.5-7.5
White blood cell count $n \times 10^3/\mu l$	6-17	5.5-19.5	6-14	4-12	11-22	4-12

Representative ranges were taken from those reported by Clinical Pathology laboratoria at Kansas State University and University of California, Davis; by Kaneko JJ: Clinical Biochemistry of Domestic Animals, 4th ed, 1989, Academic Press, San Diego; and by Duncan JR and Prasse KW: Veterinary Laboratory Medicine, 2nd ed, 1986, Iowa State University Press, Ames.